Biomechanics and Motor Control

Editor: Lael Dickson

AMERICAN
MEDICAL PUBLISHERS
www.americanmedicalpublishers.com

AMERICAN
MEDICAL PUBLISHERS
www.americanmedicalpublishers.com

Cataloging-in-Publication Data

Biomechanics and motor control / edited by Lael Dickson.
p. cm.
Includes bibliographical references and index.
ISBN 978-1-63927-931-9
1. Human mechanics. 2. Motor ability. 3. Biomechanics. 4. Human physiology.
5. Kinesiology. 6. Human physiology. I. Dickson, Lael.
QP303 .B56 2023
612.76--dc23

American Medical Publishers,
41 Flatbush Avenue,
1st Floor, New York,
NY 11217, USA

ISBN 978-1-63927-931-9 (Hardback)

Biomechanics and Motor Control

Biomechanics and Motor Control

Biomechanics and Motor Control

Editor: Lael Dickson

AMERICAN
MEDICAL PUBLISHERS
www.americanmedicalpublishers.com

AMERICAN
MEDICAL PUBLISHERS
www.americanmedicalpublishers.com

Cataloging-in-Publication Data

Biomechanics and motor control / edited by Lael Dickson.
p. cm.
Includes bibliographical references and index.
ISBN 978-1-63927-931-9
1. Human mechanics. 2. Motor ability. 3. Biomechanics. 4. Human physiology.
5. Kinesiology. 6. Human physiology. I. Dickson, Lael.
QP303 .B56 2023
612.76--dc23

American Medical Publishers,
41 Flatbush Avenue,
1st Floor, New York,
NY 11217, USA

ISBN 978-1-63927-931-9 (Hardback)

Contents

Preface

Biomechanics refers to the study of motion, structure and function of mechanical aspects of biological systems, at the cellular level or the level of organism as a whole. The movement in organisms is regulated by motor control, which comprises directed movement and reflexes. The integration of multimodal sensory information from proprioception and the external environment is needed to control the movement. The nervous system generates necessary signals for the muscles to carry out a specific task. Motor control is significant in organisms for interacting with external world, to carry out required activities, as well as for stability, posture and balance. In humans, all the movements require motor neurons to trigger action potentials, which cause the contractions of required muscles. The coordination of muscles is triggered by the impulses sent by motor cortex towards the motor units. This results in production of movements by a subset of muscles contracting in precise pattern temporarily for generating force at the right time. This book contains some path-breaking studies on biomechanics and motor control. It will serve as a valuable source of reference for graduate and post graduate students.

Significant researches are present in this book. Intensive efforts have been employed by authors to make this book an outstanding discourse. This book contains the enlightening chapters which have been written on the basis of significant researches done by the experts.

Finally, I would also like to thank all the members involved in this book for being a team and meeting all the deadlines for the submission of their respective works. I would also like to thank my friends and family for being supportive in my efforts.

Editor

1

The Spatial Distribution of Ankle Muscles Activity Discriminates Aged from Young Subjects during Standing

Fabio V. dos Anjos**, *Talita P. Pinto, Marco Gazzoni and Taian M. Vieira

Laboratorio di Ingegneria del Sistema Neuromuscolare, Dipartimento di Elettronica e Telecomunicazioni, Politecnico di Torino, Torino, Italy

****Correspondence:***
Fabio V. dos Anjos
fabio.vieira@polito.com

During standing, age-related differences in the activation of ankle muscles have been reported from surface electromyograms (EMGs) sampled locally. Given though activity seems to distribute unevenly within ankle muscles, the local sampling of surface EMGs may provide a biased view on how often and how much elderly and young individuals activate these muscles during standing. This study aimed therefore at sampling EMGs from multiple regions of individual ankle muscles to evaluate whether the distribution of muscle activity differs between aged and young subjects during standing. Thirteen young and eleven aged, healthy subjects were tested. Surface EMGs were sampled at multiple skin locations from tibialis anterior, soleus and medial and lateral gastrocnemius muscles while subjects stood at ease. The root mean square amplitude of EMGs was considered to estimate the duration, the degree of activity and the size of the region where muscle activity was detected. Our main findings revealed the medial gastrocnemius was active for longer periods in aged (interquartile interval; 74.1–98.2%) than young (44.9–81.9%) individuals ($P = 0.02$). Similarly, while tibialis anterior was rarely active in young (0.7–4.4%), in elderly subjects (2.6–82.5%) it was often recruited ($P = 0.01$). Moreover, EMGs with relatively higher amplitude were detected over a significantly wider proximo-distal region of medial gastrocnemius in aged (29.4–45.6%) than young (20.1–31.3%) subjects ($P = 0.04$). These results indicate the duration and the size of active muscle volume, as quantified from the spatial distribution of surface EMGs, may discriminate aged from young individuals during standing; elderlies seem to rely more heavily on the active loading of ankle muscles to control their standing posture than young individuals. Most importantly, current results suggest different conclusions on the active control of standing posture may be drawn depending on the skin location from where EMGs are collected, in particular for the medial gastrocnemius.

Keywords: postural control, standing, aging, electromyography, muscle activity

INTRODUCTION

Different mechanisms have been suggested to account for the control of human, standing posture. Of recent interest is the notion that bodily sways are arrested by timely, triggered bursts of calf muscles' activity (Loram et al., 2005; Vieira et al., 2012; Héroux et al., 2014). The physiological mechanism underpinning timed activation in standing is controversial; some suggest there is an internal clock triggering calf muscles' activation (Loram et al., 2009) while others believe activation is event-triggered (Bottaro et al., 2008). In spite of the potential sources accounting for such intermittent, postural activation, alternating periods of muscle activation with silencing seems advantageous. Periodically silencing postural muscles during standing may: (i) allow the nervous system to sense joint angles without interference from muscle contraction (Loram et al., 2011); (ii) compensate for intrinsic, feedback delays (Cabrera and Milton, 2002); (iii) reduce metabolic costs (Bottaro et al., 2008); (iv) not increase postural instability (Cabrera and Milton, 2002). In this view, the assessment of muscle activation may therefore reveal pivotal features of the control of standing posture, especially e.g., in persons with balance impairments.

Surface EMGs revealed, indeed, key differences in the activation of postural muscles with aging. From bipolar surface EMGs collected from the plantar flexor muscles, for example, previous studies reported that elderlies tend to stand with a more continuous and higher degree of activation than young individuals (Laughton et al., 2003; Nagai et al., 2011; Baudry et al., 2012). Moreover, while tibialis anterior is typically silent in young subjects during standing (Di Giulio et al., 2009; Masani et al., 2013), in aged individuals it is often recruited (Laughton et al., 2003). From the point of view of muscle activation, it seems therefore standing becomes progressively more demanding with aging. A crucial question arising from previous studies is whether the greater, prolonged activation observed locally (i.e., with bipolar EMGs) in plantar and dorsal flexors of aged subjects reflects the activation of the muscle as a whole.

The spatial distribution of surface EMGs over the whole muscle rather than the local sampling of surface EMGs with bipolar electrodes seems to more likely provide a genuine indication on the duration and degree of muscle activity. EMGs with different amplitudes have indeed been observed when sampled from different regions of a single muscle (Brown et al., 2007; Farina et al., 2008), suggesting activity does not distribute uniformly within the muscle volume. This uneven distribution of activity has been often observed for the calf muscles and for a number of circumstances, including standing (McLean and Goudy, 2004; Hodson-Tole et al., 2013; Reffad et al., 2014). Methodologically, these results suggest the local sampling of surface EMGs may not provide a representative view of the degree and duration of calf muscles' activation. Physiologically, the differential distribution of activity within the calf muscles may indicate a key mechanism contributing to the control of muscle force and thus of the standing posture. It is therefore possible that differences in the activation of postural muscles with aging are more expressive than previously appreciated.

This study questions, for the first time, whether the distribution of muscle activity differs between aged and young subjects during standing. Differently from previous studies, here we use arrays of surface electrodes to sample EMGs from different regions of individual, ankle muscles. More specifically, from surface EMGs collected serially from ankle plantar and dorsal flexors we ask: do young and aged subjects activate an equal proportion of their muscles for a similar duration during standing? If aging is associated with greater muscular effort for standing control (Nagai et al., 2011; Baudry et al., 2012), we therefore expect to observe EMGs with greater amplitude for a longer duration and in a larger muscle region in aged than young individuals.

MATERIALS AND METHODS

Participants

Thirteen young male volunteers provided written informed consent before participating in the study (mean ± SD; age: 26 ± 3 years; body mass: 72.4 ± 10.1 kg; height: 1.75 ± 0.06 m) and 11 aged (70 ± 6 years; 72.9 ± 12.5 kg; 1.72 ± 0.08 m). All participants were classified as minimally active according to the international physical activity questionnaire (IPAQ); short self-administered version (Tomioka et al., 2011). All community-dwelling older adults lived independently. We decided to include participants without a sedentary lifestyle because physical inactivity may further broaden the between-subjects variability often reported for stabilometric descriptors (Chiari et al., 2002). The experimental procedures considered in this study conformed with the *Declaration of Helsinki* and were approved by the Regional Ethics Committee (Commissione di Vigilanza, Servizio Sanitario Nazionale—Regione Piemonte—ASL 1—Torino, Italy). Volunteers did not report any balance impairments, neurological disorders, muscular injuries, or the intake of medications that could affect their standing balance at the occasion of experiments.

Experimental Protocol

Participants were instructed to stand upright barefoot on a force-plate, with eyes open and arms alongside the body. They positioned their feet at a comfortable orientation and distance, while keeping heels and toes at the same position along the force plate anterior-posterior axis (**Figure 1A**). Prior to starting experiments, the contour of both feet was marked on the force plate to ensure participants would keep the same feet position throughout the standing tests.

Two standing tasks were applied. In the first task, participants were provided with visual feedback of their CoP position in the anterior-posterior axis and were instructed to keep it at 65% of the longitudinal size of their support base for 60 s (**Figure 1B**). The size of the support base in the anterior-posterior axis was defined as the distance between the tip of the third metatarsal head and the tip of the calcaneus bone projected in the anterior-posterior direction (**Figure 1A**). The 65% figure corresponds roughly to 80% of the distance between the heels and the anterior limit of stability of healthy, young subjects (Duarte and Zatsiorsky, 2002); this figure was selected to ensure a somewhat high degree of calf muscles active loading while not threatening stability, in particular for the aged individuals. All elderly subjects tested could stand with their CoP at the target value without losing balance. This postural task was considered for the normalization of EMGs, as described below. In the second task, volunteers were asked to stand at ease for 60 s. Subjects were engaged in active conversation to ensure they would take their mind off the test and thus avoid any voluntary change in muscle activity (Loram and Lakie, 2002b). The trial started over in the

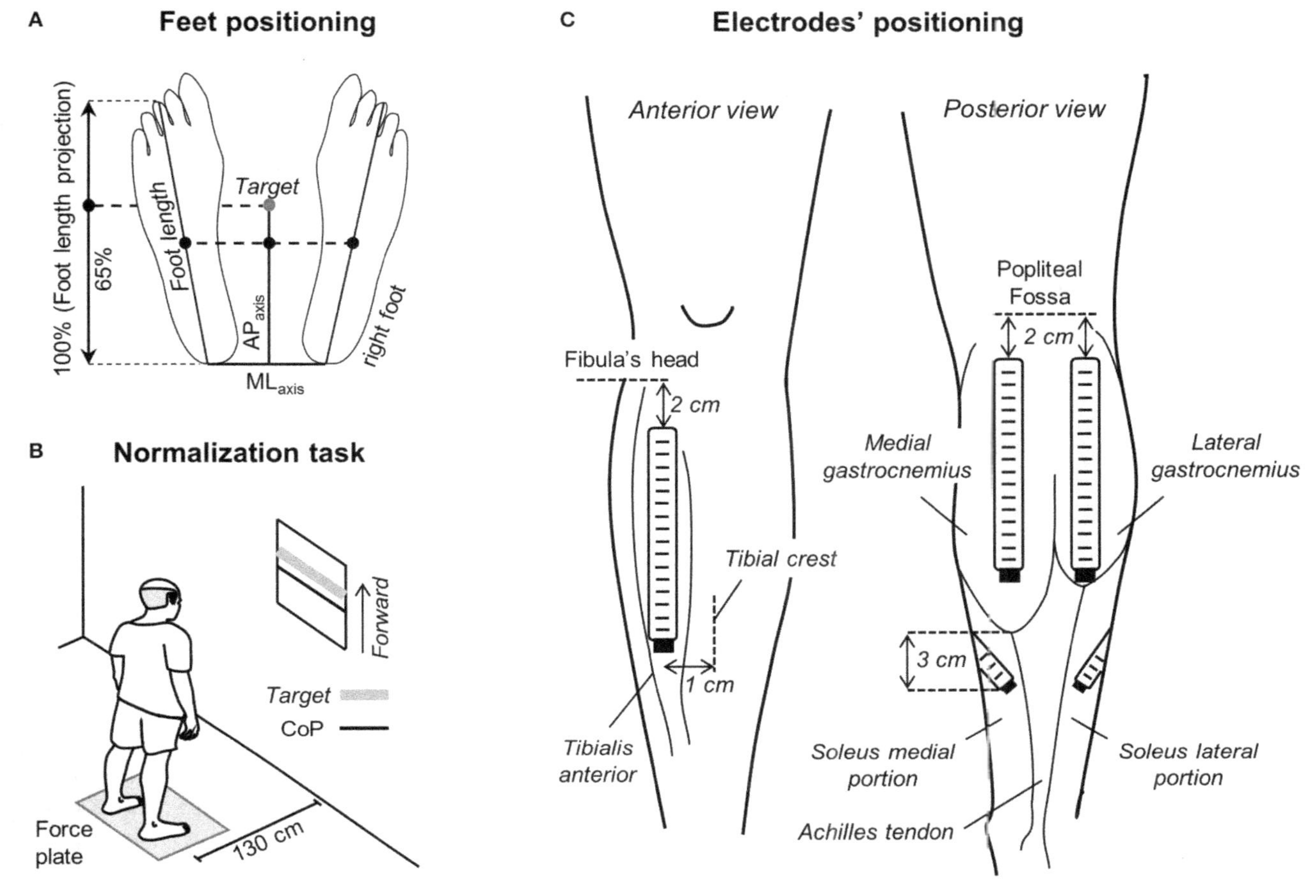

FIGURE 1 | Standing protocol and feet and electrode positioning. (A) Schematic illustration showing the procedure considered to measure feet length. The midpoint between the tip of left and right calcaneus bones was considered as the origin of the reference system for center of pressure (CoP) and foot length measurements. The target value, corresponding to 65% of the foot length projected on the anterior-posterior axis (AP_{axis}), was calculated and then considered for the normalization task shown in **(B)**. In such task, participants were asked to keep their CoP position in the AP_{axis} (black line) within 10% (±5%) of the target value (thick, gray line). **(C)** The positioning of electrode arrays is shown for the tibialis anterior muscle (left), for the medial and lateral gastrocnemius heads and for the soleus medial and lateral portions (right).

case gross body movements were noticed by the experimenter. The standing at ease task was applied three times, in accordance with previous evidence on excellent reliability of stabilometric descriptors (Pinsault and Vuillerme, 2009). Similarly, good-to-excellent reliability has been recently reported for EMGs detected from the calf muscles in aged individuals during standing (Gallina et al., 2016). Five minute intervals were applied between trials and their order was randomized.

Electrodes' Positioning

Linear arrays of surface electrodes were used to sample the distribution of ankle muscles' activity. Arrays were positioned over the plantar and dorsal flexors of both legs. Two arrays of 16 electrodes (10 mm inter-electrode distance) were used to detect surface EMGs from the medial and lateral gastrocnemius muscles. The most proximal electrode was located 2 cm distally to the popliteal fossa and arrays were aligned parallel to the longitudinal axis of each gastrocnemius' head (**Figure 1C**). Such positioning maximizes the representation of action potentials from muscle units residing in different, proximo-distal gastrocnemius' regions (Vieira et al., 2011). EMGs were sampled with one array of 16 electrodes (10 mm inter-electrode distance) from the tibialis anterior muscle, aligned 1 cm laterally and parallel to the tibial crest and with the most proximal electrode located 2 cm distally to the fibula's head (**Figure 1C**). Given the in-depth pennate architecture of tibialis anterior, as for gastrocnemius, such positioning is expected to provide EMGs representative of different, proximo-distal fibers. Two arrays with four electrodes each (10 mm inter-electrode distance) were used to sample EMGs from the soleus medial and lateral portions. For each soleus portion, arrays were aligned ~45 degree outward to the line connecting the junction between gastrocnemius' heads and the calcaneus tip. The lower border of both the medial and lateral arrays was positioned 3 cm distally to the medial gastrocnemius myotendinous junction (**Figure 1C**; Reffad et al., 2014). Gastrocnemii junction and their myotendinous junction were identified with ultrasound imaging (cf. Supplementary Material in Vieira et al., 2010b). Arrays were positioned after cleaning the skin with abrasive paste.

Electromyographic and Stabilometric Recordings

EMGs were recorded in single-differential derivation. All 51 single-differential EMGs were amplified by a between-individuals variable factor—from 5,000 to 10,000—to ensure the highest signal-to-noise ratio without saturation (10–750 Hz bandwidth amplifier; EMG-USB, OTBioelettronica and LISiN, Politecnico di Torino, Turin, Italy). CoP coordinates in the sagittal and frontal planes were computed from the ground reaction forces supplied by a piezoelectric force-plate (9286AA Kistler, Zurich, Switzerland). Reaction forces and surface EMGs were sampled synchronously at 2,048 Hz using a 12-bit A/D converter (±2.5 V input dynamic range).

Quantifying Muscle Activity during Standing

Raw surface EMGs were visually inspected. Whenever any channel in the array presented contact problems, likely due to high skin-electrode impedance, or massive power line interference, the corresponding channel was disregarded. Occurrences of low quality EMGs were infrequent (17 out of 1,224 EMGs detected in total) and were observed mainly in one channel per array. After controlling for signal quality, EMGs from tibialis anterior and gastrocnemius muscles were inspected for the identification of propagating potentials. Propagating potentials may be observed in the distal muscle region, where surface electrodes and muscle fibers may run in parallel direction. In such case, different electrodes sample from the same group of fibers rather than from different, proximo-distal fibers (cf. Figure 1 in Hodson-Tole et al., 2013). Channels providing propagating potentials were therefore excluded from analysis; from 0 to 8 channels per array were excluded for the 24 participants tested.

After visual inspection, EMGs were band-pass filtered with a fourth order Butterworth filter (15–350 Hz cutoff; zero lag, bidirectional filter). Then, the Root Mean Square (RMS) was computed over 40 ms epochs (Laughton et al., 2003), providing a total of 1,500 RMS values per channel. From these RMS values, three indices were considered to assess for how long, how diffusely and how much elderly and young activated their ankle muscles during standing.

Instants of activation were estimated by comparing the RMS values obtained during standing with the background activity. The background activity was defined from the RMS amplitude of EMGs collected with the ankle muscles at rest (Laughton et al., 2003). More specifically, for each channel in each array of electrodes we: (i) computed the RMS values over 40 ms epochs for EMGs detected during 3 s while participants were in supine position, providing a total of 75 RMS values; (ii) calculated the mean and the standard deviation for these RMS values; (iii) set the threshold defining the background noise level as the mean value plus three standard deviations; (iv) assigned Active or Inactive state to RMS samples respectively exceeding or not exceeding the background threshold. This procedure provided a series of Active-Inactive state values per channel. Given the EMGs detected by consecutive electrodes in the array sample from different fibers along the muscle proximo-distal axis, concurrent Active-Inactive events were often not observed between channels (**Figure 2A**). For this reason, to provide a global indication on the duration of muscle activity during standing, the muscle was deemed active whenever an Active state was observed across channels (cf. shaded areas in **Figures 2A,B**). The global series of Active-Inactive states indicates how long the ankle muscles were active throughout standing, regardless of where activity was observed in the muscle.

Based on the instants of activation, the spatial distribution and the intensity of muscle activity were computed. First, the number of channels detecting surface EMGs with RMS amplitude greater than 70% of the highest RMS amplitude in the array was identified. The 70% amplitude threshold was selected because it has been shown to provide a robust identification of channels located over active fibers within muscles pennate in the depth direction (Vieira et al., 2010a). The number of segmented channels multiplied by the inter-electrode distance was then normalized with respect to the muscle length (see below). Second, the degree of muscle activity was estimated by averaging the RMS values across all segmented channels for each muscle tested. This average RMS amplitude was then normalized with respect to the RMS amplitude averaged across channels identified during the normalization, standing task (**Figure 1B**), to compensate for the effect of anatomical differences between participants on the surface EMGs (Farina et al., 2002). It should be noted here the normalization of EMGs collected in a given condition with respect to that collected in a reference condition compensates for the effect of inter-individual differences on their amplitude though not on the spatial distribution of their amplitude. Finally, the size of the active region in the proximo-distal direction and the degree of activity were considered for analysis whenever any given muscle was active for at least 10% of the total, standing duration. Following previous evidence, occurrences of such sporadic activity was regarded as of marginal relevance for the control of standing posture (Héroux et al., 2014). Given we observed medial gastrocnemius was active for different durations (~20%) between legs in both aged and young subjects, the electromyographic indices and architectural muscle parameters (see below) computed from the subject's leg active for longer durations (left side for 10 young and 8 elderly subjects) were used for comparisons between groups.

Measurements of Ankle Muscles' Length and Subcutaneous Thickness

Parasagittal images from tibialis anterior and gastrocnemii were taken with a linear, ultrasound probe (10 MHz, 4 cm length; Echo Blaster 128, Telemed Ltd., Vilnius, Lithuania), with participants lying comfortably on a padded bed. Initially, the myotendinous junction was identified and marked on the skin. The length of tibialis anterior was then quantified as the distance between its myotendinous junction and the head of the fibula, whereas the

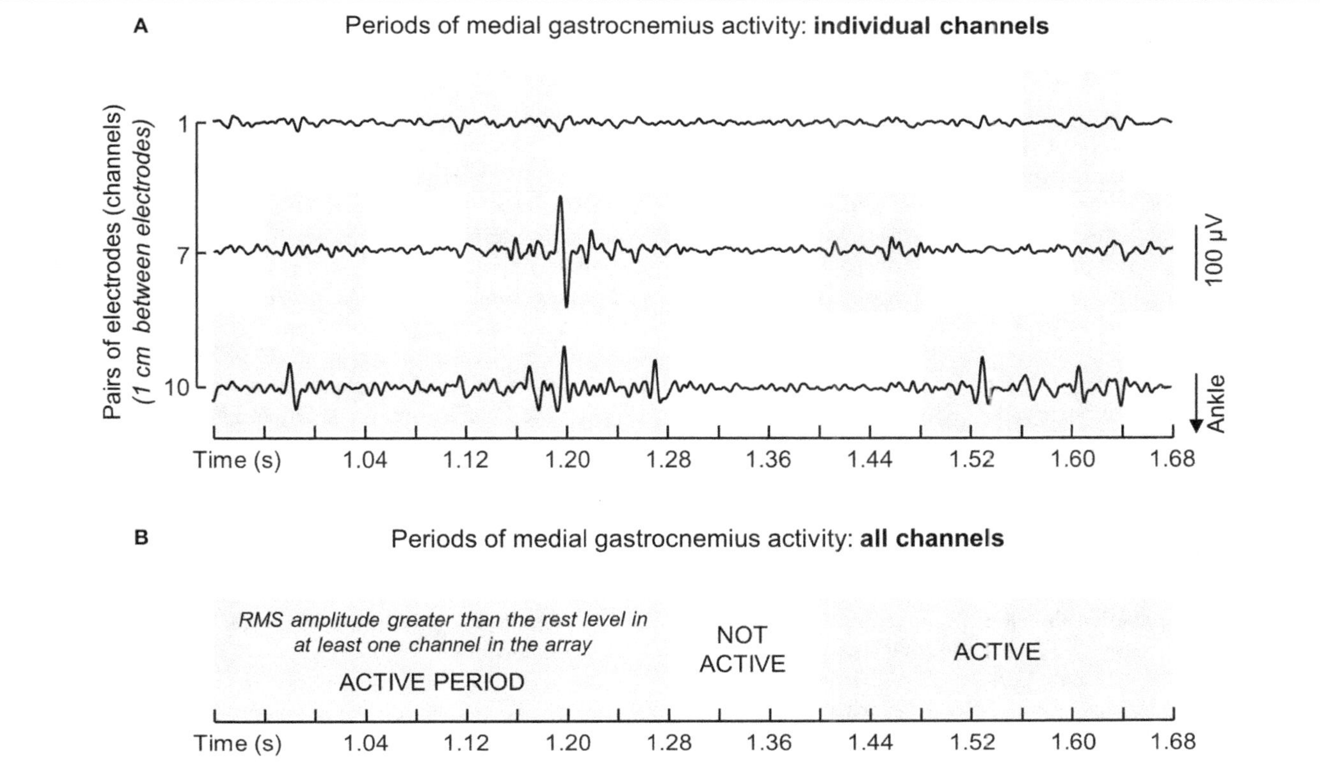

FIGURE 2 | Computation of instants of muscle activation. (A) Shows examples of single-differential EMGs detected by channels 1, 7, and 10 from the medial gastrocnemius muscle of a single participant. Note action potentials do not appear with equally high amplitude in the three channels. The muscle was considered active whenever for any given instants the RMS amplitude exceeded the background activity in at least one channel. Light gray rectangles in the grid denote periods within which the RMS amplitude of EMGs in each channel exceeded the background activity computed with the muscle at rest (see text). The resulting series of instants of muscle activity for this representative example is illustrated with a succession of white (Inactive state; muscle at rest) and gray (Active state; muscle active) rectangles **(B)**.

length of each gastrocnemius head was defined as the shortest distance between the myoetendinous junction and the popliteal fossa. Subcutaneous thickness and pennation angle were further quantified to assist in the interpretation of potential proximo-distal differences in the distribution of activity with aging. Subcutaneous thickness was computed as the distance between the skin/fat layer over the muscle and its superficial aponeurosis from parasagittal images obtained with the probe centered halfway the muscle length. Thickness measurements were taken from the central region of the proximal, central and distal thirds of the ultrasound images and then averaged, providing a representative indication on the general subcutaneous thickness per subject (Onambele et al., 2006). Finally, the pennation angle was estimated as the angle between a clearly visible fascicle in the image and the muscle deep aponeurosis (Avancini et al., 2015). Thickness and pennation angle values were obtained with the muscle at rest.

Quantifying the CoP Sway Area

The CoP sway area was considered to assess how largely young and elderly individuals swayed during the whole standing tests. The overall size of postural sways was estimated from the elliptic area conveying almost 85% of the total CoP samples during standing (Oliveira et al., 1996). The CoP elliptic area, as well as the EMG descriptors, were averaged across the three standing trials and considered for between-group comparisons. CoP data was 50 Hz low-pass filtered with a second order Butterworth filter to remove high-frequency noise.

Statistical Analysis

Non-parametric statistics were applied to compare the distribution of ankle muscles' activity between young and aged individuals, after ensuring the data distribution was not Gaussian (Shapiro-Wilk's W-test, $P < 0.03$ in all cases). The Mann-Whitney U-test was used to verify whether, during standing and for each muscle independently, the duration of the active period, the degree of activity, the relative size of the active region and the CoP elliptic area were different between groups. The same statistics was applied to assess regional differences in activity within soleus, by comparing the normalized RMS amplitude obtained for the muscle medial and lateral aspects. The level of statistical significance was set at 5% and data were reported using non-parametric, descriptive statistics.

RESULTS

Representative Examples of Variations in Ankle Muscles' Activity during Standing

Different ankle muscles were activated differently when young and aged individuals stood at ease. Descriptive considerations on these differences are summarized in this section based on the data shown in **Figure 3** for one young and one aged, representative participant. Lateral gastrocnemius was active for 6 and 17% of the whole standing trial for the young and aged subjects respectively. For the tibialis anterior muscle, the amplitude of EMGs remained below the background activity for the young subject during the whole standing duration while, for the elderly, bursts of activity were observed and provided an active duration of 36%. Conversely, EMGs with remarkably high amplitude in the soleus medial and lateral portions were observed consistently for both subjects (cf. shaded areas in **Figure 3**).

The medial gastrocnemius showed a somewhat different pattern of activity when compared with the other ankle muscles. Differently from lateral gastrocnemius, soleus and tibialis anterior, medial gastrocnemius was not completely silenced, was not activated almost continuously and did not show sporadic bursts of activity. For both participants whose data is shown in **Figure 3**, alternate periods of medial gastrocnemius activation and silencing were observed consistently during standing (**Figure 4A**). When considering the distribution of activity within medial gastrocnemius, EMGs with relatively high amplitude were detected by six channels in the young and by nine channels in the aged subject (cf. gray circles in **Figure 4B**).

Ankle Muscles' Activation in Elderly and Young Individuals during Standing

When considering group data, differences in the duration of ankle muscles' activity were observed between elderly and young subjects. The Mann-Whitney *U*-test revealed the medial gastrocnemius was activated for longer periods in aged (median, interquartile interval; 81.2, 74.1–98.2%) than young (58.8, 44.9–81.9%) individuals (**Figure 5A**; $P = 0.02$; $N = 24$; 13 young × 11 aged subjects). Similarly, notwithstanding the marked variability in the duration of active periods for the elderly, aged participants activated their tibialis anterior muscle during standing for a significantly longer duration than young subjects ($P = 0.01$; $N = 24$); tibialis anterior was rarely active in young (1.3, 0.7–4.4%) though not in the elderly (29.1, 2.6–82.5%). No group differences were observed in the duration of lateral gastrocnemius ($P = 0.07$) and soleus medial ($P = 0.90$) and lateral ($P = 0.26$) portions.

The degree and the distribution of activity within ankle plantar flexors varied differently between groups. The RMS amplitude of EMGs collected from the medial gastrocnemius

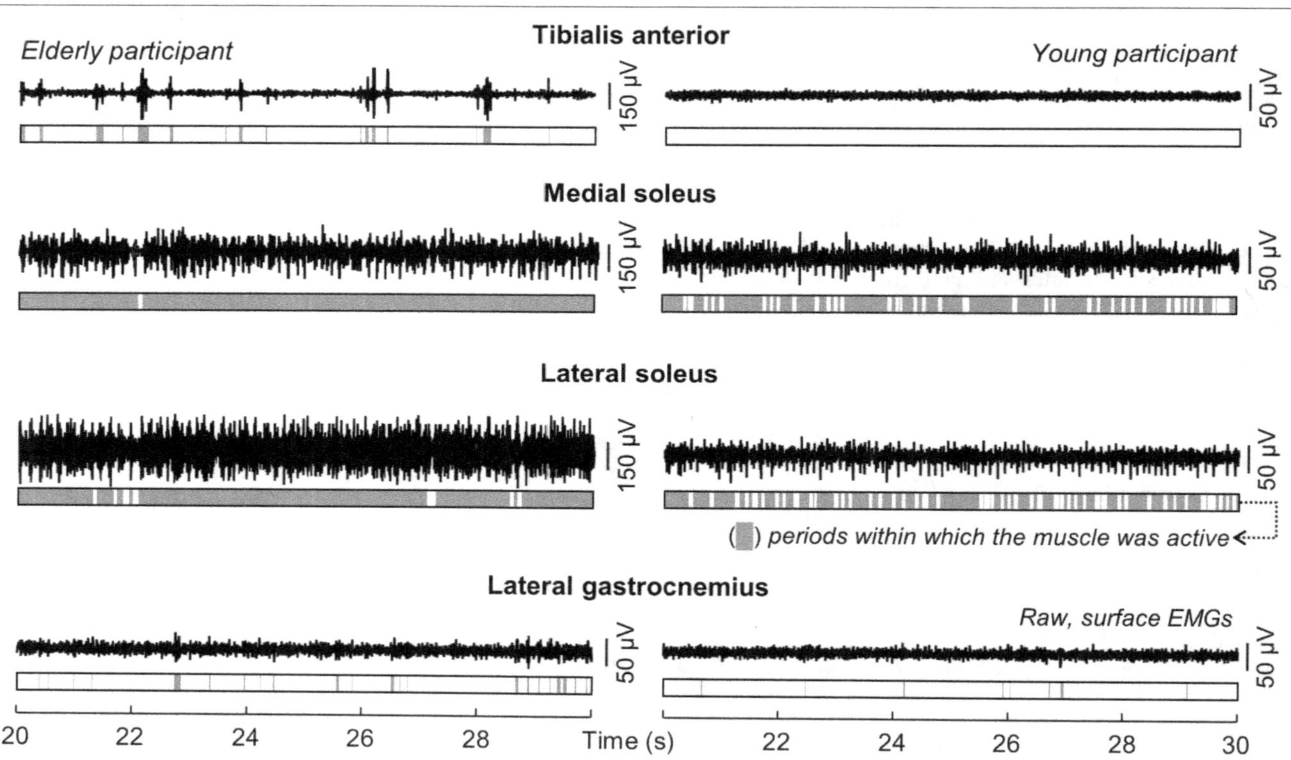

FIGURE 3 | Modulations in ankle muscles' activity during standing. Single-differential EMGs collected for a representative channel from the tibialis anterior, the soleus medial and lateral portions and from the lateral gastrocnemius of a representative young and elderly participant are shown for 10 s of standing at ease. Light gray areas in the bars indicate periods within which the RMS amplitude exceeded the background activity (i.e., Active state).

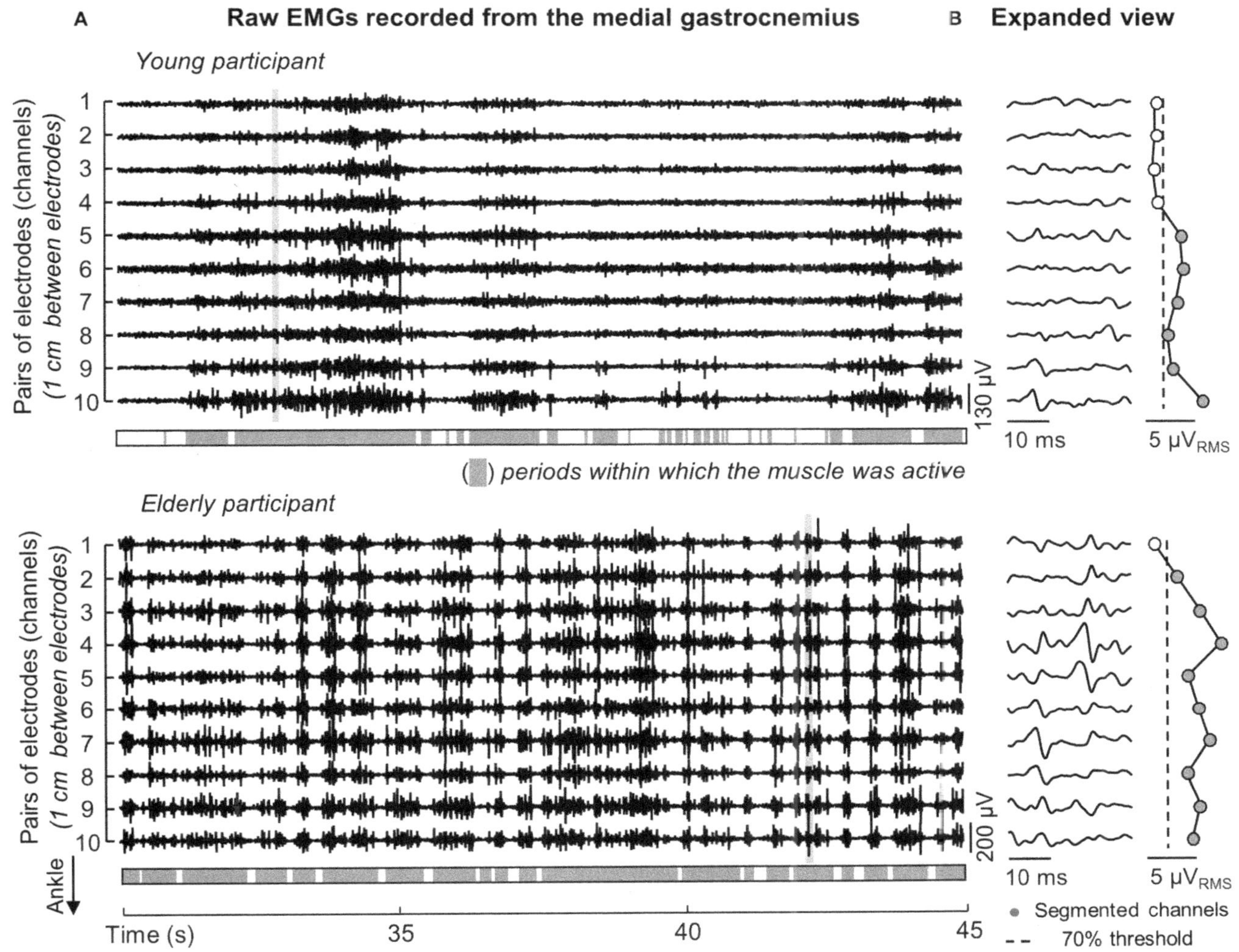

FIGURE 4 | Duration and distribution of medial gastrocnemius activity during standing. Raw EMGs detected by channels located over the gastrocnemius superficial aponeurosis, from channel 1 to 10, are shown in **(A)** for a young and elderly representative participant. Light gray areas indicate periods within which the RMS amplitude exceeded the background activity. **(B)** Shows an expanded view of all EMGs. Note different action potentials appear in different channels for each subject. Note also there is no delay between potentials detected by consecutive channels (e.g., channels 1–6 for the aged participant). The distribution of RMS amplitude across channels is represented from circles, with gray circles indicating the *segmented channels*; that is, channels detecting largest EMGs in the array (see text).

and from the medial and lateral soleus portions did not differ between elderly and young (**Figure 5B**; $P > 0.40$ in all cases; $N = 24$). No differences were observed between the RMS amplitude for EMGs collected medially and laterally from soleus muscle, both for young and elderly ($P > 0.70$ in both cases). In contrast, for medial gastrocnemius, EMGs with relatively higher amplitude were detected over a significantly wider proximo-distal region in aged (32.5, 29.4–45.6%) than young (29.8, 20.1–31.3%) subjects (**Figure 5C**; $P = 0.04$; $N = 24$). Given the lateral gastrocnemius and tibialis anterior of young individuals were active for a somewhat short period during the whole standing tests (less than 10% on average; **Figure 5A**), these muscles were disregarded from further consideration.

Medial Gastrocnemius' Subcutaneous Thickness and Pennation Angle

No differences in subcutaneous thickness were observed between groups ($P = 0.58$). Thickness values ranged from 1.6 to 2.7 mm for young and from 1.6 to 3.5 for aged participants. Similarly, the pennation angle did not differ significantly ($P = 0.37$) between young (range: 19.6–24.0 degrees) and aged subjects (17.2–25.0 degrees).

Differences in CoP Sway Area with Age

While aged participants stood at ease, their CoP occupied an area roughly twice (median, interquartile interval; 4.4, 3.8–9.6 cm^2) as large as that (2.3, 1.6–4.5 cm^2) confining the CoP of young participants ($P = 0.052$).

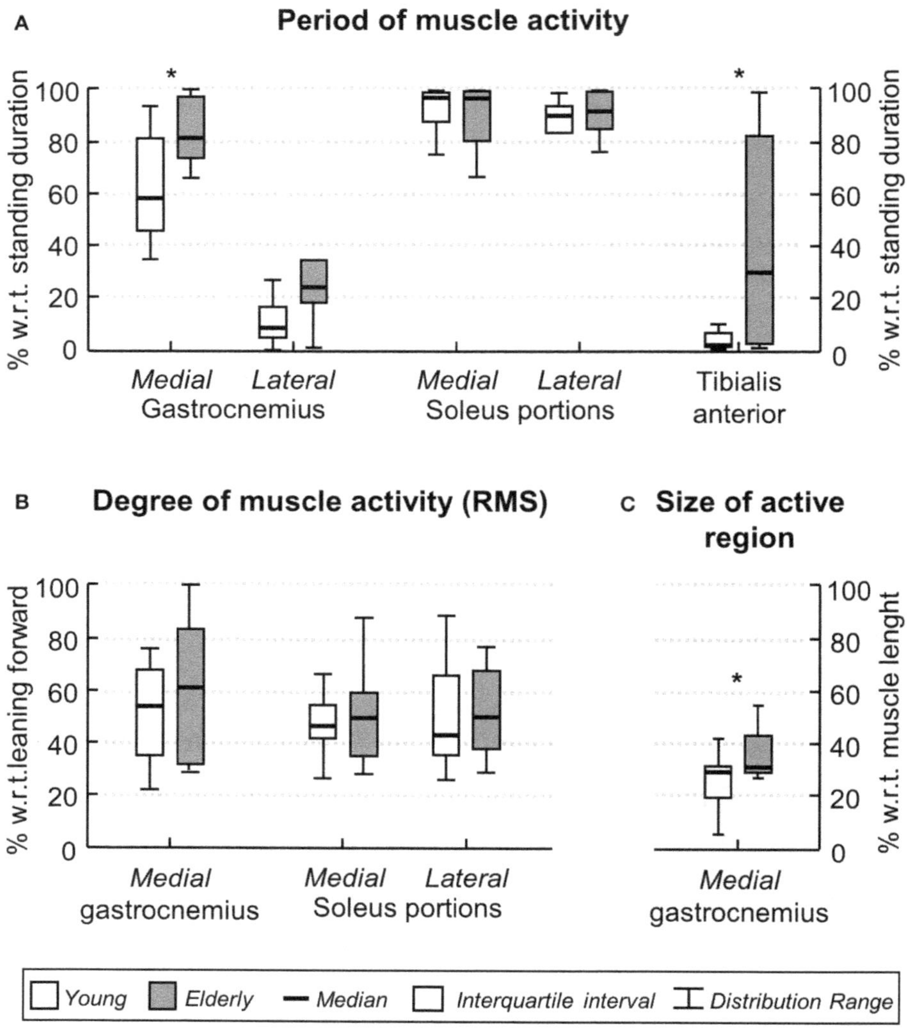

FIGURE 5 | Age-related differences in the ankle muscles' activity during standing. Boxplots in **(A)** show the relative period within which, during standing, young (white boxes) and elderly (gray boxes) individuals activated their ankle muscles. Group data in **(B)** corresponds to the normalized, RMS amplitude obtained for both groups from the medial gastrocnemius and from the medial and lateral soleus portions. The proximo-distal size of medial gastrocnemius region over which largest EMGs were detected in both groups is shown in **(C)**. Asterisks indicate significant differences between groups ($P < 0.05$).

DISCUSSION

In this study we used arrays of electrodes to investigate whether the temporal and spatial distributions of ankle muscles' activity differ between elderly and young individuals during standing. We hypothesized that elderlies would present greater EMGs, distributed over a larger muscle region and for a longer duration than young individuals. Surface EMGs from different regions of the ankle muscles were collected while subjects stood at ease to test this hypothesis. Our key results indicate that during standing: (i) tibialis anterior and medial gastrocnemius muscles were active for a longer duration in aged than young subjects; (ii) a greater proportion of medial gastrocnemius volume was active in elderlies. Collectively, these results indicate elderlies rely more heavily on the active loading of ankle muscles to control their standing posture than young individuals.

Preliminary, Methodological Considerations on Surface EMG Detection

Differently from previous studies, here we sampled surface EMGs with arrays of electrodes (**Figure 1C**). Our decision to sample activity from multiple locations of individual ankle muscles was motivated by recent evidence suggesting different muscle regions may be activated differently (Brown et al., 2007; Farina et al., 2008), in particular for pennate muscles (McLean and Goudy, 2004; Staudenmann et al., 2009; Vieira et al., 2011; Hodson-Tole et al., 2013); EMGs sampled locally (i.e., with a single pair of shortly spaced electrodes) may not provide a representative view of muscle activation. Indeed, as shown in **Figure 2**, EMGs in different locations may provide different estimations for the duration of gastrocnemius activity. Considering EMGs were represented with different amplitude in different muscle regions (**Figures 2, 4**), the duration of muscle activity would have been likely underestimated if we had not considered EMGs detected at different skin regions (cf. shaded areas for individual and all channels in **Figure 2**). Similarly, biased estimations on the degree of each calf muscles' activity would have been obtained if we had considered the RMS amplitude of EMGs detected locally. Depending on where EMGs were detected from, in particular for young individuals (**Figure 4**), their corresponding RMS values would provide either under- (white circles in **Figure 4B**) or over- (gray circles in **Figure 4B**) estimates of the degree of activity in the whole muscle. Through arrays of surface electrodes, we were able to obtain estimates of the duration and degree of activity presumably more representative of individual ankle muscles' volumes than previously appreciated. As discussed below, new insights have been gained into age-related differences in postural activation from such a high-density, surface EMG approach.

Are the Ankle Muscles Activated for a Similar Duration in Aged and Young Subjects?

The differences between aged and young individuals reported here were muscle dependent. When considering the duration of activity for lateral gastrocnemius and soleus muscles, statistic differences were not observed between groups. Both groups recruited lateral gastrocnemius for less than ~20% of the total, standing duration (**Figures 3, 5A**). The soleus muscle, on the other hand, was activated for periods roughly longer than 80% of standing. These results corroborate previous findings on the duration of calf muscles' activity, extensively reported for young subjects. Indeed, while the absence of activity in lateral gastrocnemius has been observed in some subjects (Masani et al., 2013; Héroux et al., 2014), it seems well-documented that soleus is recruited at almost all time during standing (Laughton et al., 2003; Héroux et al., 2014). Even though the temporal activation of postural muscles is not as commonly assessed for elderlies as it is for young individuals, Laughton et al. (2003) observed age similarities for the duration of soleus activity during standing. Extending the observation of Laughton et al. (2003), our current results suggest the duration of activity of the lateral gastrocnemius and soleus regions accessed by our surface electrodes is unlikely sensitive to aging.

Age differences emerged however in the duration of medial gastrocnemius and tibialis anterior activity during standing. Aged individuals activated their medial gastrocnemius muscle for a period ~20% longer, on average, than their young counterparts (**Figure 5A**). Similarly, tibialis anterior was active for a longer (~30%) period in aged than in young subjects (**Figure 5A**). The median duration of tibialis anterior activity observed here, both for young (~2%) and elderlies (~30%), is well in agreement with the duration of activity periods reported by Laughton et al. (2003) for this muscle. From a first inspection of results presented in **Figure 5A**, we feel inclined to consider the co-activation mechanism as responsible for the age differences in the timing of plantar and dorsal flexors' activation during standing. More specifically, while young subjects predominantly activated their plantar flexors, elderlies activated both plantar and dorsal flexor muscles during standing (**Figures 3, 4A, 5A**). In spite of controversies on whether co-activation may be detrimental or may compensate for poor control of posture, co-activation is often associated with increased postural sways (Nagai et al., 2011; Baudry et al., 2012; Warnica et al., 2014). Corroborating this common view, in the elderlies, we observed the CoP was confined within an elliptic area almost twice as large as that confining the CoP of young subjects. Regardless of the mechanisms underpinning age-differences in posture control, current results here suggest elderlies activate their ankle muscles for longer durations during standing than young subjects.

Do Elderly and Young Recruit Their Calf Muscles to a Similar Extent during Standing?

Two notes on our estimates of the degree of activity are necessary before interpreting results. Young subjects activated tibialis anterior and lateral gastrocnemius somewhat rarely (**Figures 3, 5A**). We therefore disregarded both muscles from age comparisons. A second observation concerns how we conceived muscle activity. While the amplitude of EMGs is traditionally considered to assess the degree of muscle activity, here we considered both the amplitude and the size of skin region where EMGs with relatively high amplitude were sampled (**Figures 2, 4**). As argued below, the extent to which elderly and young activate their calf muscles depends both on the amplitude and on the amplitude distribution of surface EMGs.

The proximo-distal distribution of the amplitude of medial gastrocnemius EMGs distinguished aged from young individuals during standing. While young subjects presented EMGs with relatively high amplitude in the gastrocnemius distal region, corroborating previous findings (Hodson-Tole et al., 2013), EMGs with similarly high amplitude were sampled from a larger, proximo-distal muscle region in aged individuals (c.f. gray circles in **Figures 4B, 5C**). Different sources could have accounted for a somewhat extensive distribution of EMG amplitude in the elderlies. A first issue to consider is the potential difference in muscle architecture between groups. Both subcutaneous thickness and pennation angle have shown to affect dramatically the amplitude distribution of surface EMGs; thicker subcutaneous tissue and smaller pennation angle result both in more spatially diffused surface EMGs (Farina et al., 2002; Mesin et al., 2011). Current results however did not indicate significant, age differences in gastrocnemius architecture. The lack of anatomical differences between groups leads us to consider the possibility that elderlies activated a larger gastrocnemius volume than young subjects during standing. In spite of recent controversies (Blouin et al., 2016; Vieira et al., 2016), it seems well-accepted that, for the gastrocnemius muscle, EMGs sampled in different proximo-distal regions reflect the activity of different muscle fibers (Vieira et al., 2011). The amplitude of EMGs detected distally and proximally, for example, is associated with the number of active fibers in the muscle distal and proximal regions respectively (Mesin et al., 2011). Given the mean amplitude of EMGs sampled from medial gastrocnemius was similar between groups (**Figure 5B**), the wider skin region from where EMGs with high amplitude were detected (**Figure 5C**) suggests a relatively greater proportion of muscle fibers may have been recruited in the elderlies.

Age differences in the distribution of activity for soleus were not as clear as for gastrocnemius. Since soleus is largely covered by the gastrocnemius muscles, spatial differences in soleus activation were assessed by comparing the amplitude of EMGs detected laterally and medially (**Figure 1C**). Our decision to assess both regions was based on previous evidence showing medio-lateral differences in soleus activation (Staudenmann et al., 2009; Reffad et al., 2014). Given we were here interested in assessing the degree of muscle activity during standing, sampling EMGs unilaterally could provide a biased view on the actual degree of soleus, postural activity. Indeed, even though results in **Figure 5B** indicate EMGs with equal amplitude were detected medio-laterally for both age groups, stating young and aged subjects activate a similar proportion of their soleus muscle in standing is potentially fairly speculative. Considerations on the relevance of spatial differences in soleus activation with age are therefore conditioned to the possibility of sampling EMGs from a greater soleus region (with e.g., intramuscular electrodes) in future investigations.

Future Perspectives and Limitations

Spatial differences in the amplitude of EMGs collected from elderlies and young during standing have methodological and physiological implications. A first crucial point to consider is the localized representation of surface EMG during standing. Here we show that, depending on where a single bipolar EMG is collected from the gastrocnemius muscle, different conclusions maybe drawn on age differences during standing. The local sampling of muscle activity provided by bipolar surface EMGs may indeed contribute to explaining current disparities observed in the literature. While some studies did not report age differences in the degree of plantar flexors' activity during standing at ease (Amiridis et al., 2003; Laughton et al., 2003), others have however documented a significantly higher degree of plantar flexor activation with aging (Nagai et al., 2011; Baudry et al., 2012). Anticipating the differences between studies were due to inappropriate EMG sampling is a statement we strongly discourage. On the other hand, though, our current results suggest that different interpretations may emerge from EMGs detected locally during standing. Of more physiological, applied interest, is the suggestion that elderlies tend to stand with a greater degree of muscle effort than young subjects (**Figures 5A,C**). According to recent evidence, standing with minimal muscular effort while affording some degree of bodily sways may be advantageous; it may reduce the metabolic cost of standing (Bottaro et al., 2008), eliminate motor noise (Loram et al., 2011) and compensate for delays in the feedback loop (Cabrera and Milton, 2002). While acknowledging the value of different protocols so far devised for the balance training (Li et al., 2005; Sayenko et al., 2010), here we suggest that learning to efficiently activate dorsal and plantar flexors during standing could be beneficial for the control of standing posture in aged individuals.

Some additional considerations on the results presented here are necessary. Both young and aged subjects showed a somewhat large variability in the duration of ankle muscles activity (**Figure 5A**). A first possible explanation to such inter-individual variability is the difference in ankle stiffness between subjects (Loram and Lakie, 2002a). Additionally, the inter-individual variability in muscle activation during standing, in particular the duration of tibialis anterior activation in the elderly, may be due to different neural sources. With aging, an assortment of impairments arising at the peripheral and central levels of the nervous system may develop, each impacting detrimentally and differently on the control of the standing posture (Horak et al., 1997). By testing subjects without a sedentary lifestyle we expect to have limited the repertoire of posture-related impairments affecting present results. A final consideration regards whether crosstalk could have affected our results. We believe this possibility is unlikely. First because action potentials were represented locally in the surface EMGs. For example, the fact that action potentials detected from a given gastrocnemius region did not appear in neighbor channels (cf. **Figure 2** and expanded view of EMGs in **Figure 4**) suggest any crosstalk from muscles other than gastrocnemius was relatively marginal. Moreover, the duration of activity of both muscles would be the same if crosstalk from soleus had contributed substantially to EMGs collected from gastrocnemius. In spite of these considerations, our results show the duration and the region of muscle activity, as quantified from surface EMGs, discriminate well-aged from young individuals during standing.

AUTHOR CONTRIBUTIONS

FD and TV were involved with all aspects of the study. TP contributed to acquire, analyse and interpret the data. MG contributed to analyse and interpret the data. All authors contributed to draft the work and revise it critically.

FUNDING

This study was supported by a national research project funded by the Italian Ministry of Education, Universities and Research (Protocol number: 2010R277FT), and cofunded by Compagnia di San Paolo and Fondazione C.R.T. FD is recipient of a scholarship provided by Coordenação de Aperfeiçoamento de Pessoal de Nível Superior / Ciência sem Fronteiras / Processo n° BEX 9404/13-9. TPP is recipient of a scholarship provided by Coordenação de Aperfeiçoamento de Pessoal de Nível Superior / Ciência sem Fronteiras / Processo n° BEX 9130/13-3. The funders had no role in study design, data collection and analysis, decision to publish, or preparation of the manuscript.

ACKNOWLEDGMENTS

The authors wish to acknowledge to Flavia Fontanella for the assistance with data collection.

REFERENCES

Amiridis, I. G., Hatzitaki, V., and Arabatzi, F. (2003). Age-induced modifications of static postural control in humans. *Neurosci. Lett.* 350, 137–140. doi: 10.1016/S0304-3940(03)00878-4

Avancini, C., de Oliveira, L. F., Menegaldo, L. L., and Vieira, T. M. (2015). Variations in the spatial distribution of the amplitude of surface electromyograms are unlikely explained by changes in the length of medial gastrocnemius fibres with knee joint angle. *PLoS ONE* 10:e0126888. doi: 10.1371/journal.pone.0126888

Baudry, S., Lecoeuvre, G., and Duchateau, J. (2012). Age-related changes in the behavior of the muscle-tendon unit of the gastrocnemius medialis during upright stance. *J. Appl. Physiol.* 112, 296–304. doi: 10.1152/japplphysiol.00913.2011

Blouin, J. S., Brown, H. J., Héroux, M. E., Inglis, J. T., and Siegmund, G. P. (2016). Reply from J. S. Blouin, H. J. Brown, M. E. Héroux, J. T. Inglis and G. P. Siegmund. *J. Physiol.* 594, 1955–1955. doi: 10.1113/JP272017

Bottaro, A., Yasutake, Y., Nomura, T., Casadio, M., and Morasso, P. (2008). Bounded stability of the quiet standing posture: an intermittent control model. *Hum. Mov. Sci.* 27, 473–495. doi: 10.1016/j.humov.2007.11.005

Brown, J. M., Wickham, J. B., McAndrew, D. J., and Huang, X. F. (2007). Muscles within muscles: coordination of 19 muscle segments within three shoulder muscles during isometric motor tasks. *J. Electromyogr. Kinesiol.* 17, 57–73. doi: 10.1016/j.jelekin.2005.10.007

Cabrera, J. L., and Milton, J. G. (2002). On-off intermittency in a human balancing task. *Phys. Rev. Lett.* 89:158702. doi: 10.1103/PhysRevLett.89.158702

Chiari, L., Rocchi, L., and Cappello, A. (2002). Stabilometric parameters are affected by anthropometry and foot placement. *Clin. Biomech.* 17, 666–677. doi: 10.1016/S0268-0033(02)00107-9

Di Giulio, I., Maganaris, C. N., Baltzopoulos, V., and Loram, I. D. (2009). The proprioceptive and agonist roles of gastrocnemius, soleus and tibialis anterior muscles in maintaining human upright posture. *J. Physiol.* 587, 2399–2416. doi: 10.1113/jphysiol.2009.168690

Duarte, M., and Zatsiorsky, V. M. (2002). Effects of body lean and visual information on the equilibrium maintenance during stance. *Exp. Brain Res.* 146, 60–69. doi: 10.1007/s00221-002-1154-1

Farina, D., Cescon, C., and Merletti, R. (2002). Influence of anatomical, physical, and detection-system parameters on surface EMG. *Biol. Cybern.* 86, 445–456. doi: 10.1007/s00422-002-0309-2

Farina, D., Leclerc, F., Arendt-Nielsen, L., Buttelli, O., and Madeleine, P. (2008). The change in spatial distribution of upper trapezius muscle activity is correlated to contraction duration. *J. Electromyogr. Kinesiol.* 18, 16–25. doi: 10.1016/j.jelekin.2006.08.005

Gallina, A., Pollock, C. L., Vieira, T. M., Ivanova, T. D., and Garland, S. J. (2016). Between-day reliability of triceps surae responses to standing perturbations in people post-stroke and healthy controls: a high-density surface EMG investigation. *Gait Posture* 44, 103–109. doi: 10.1016/j.gaitpost.2015.11.015

Héroux, M. E., Dakin, C. J., Luu, B. L., Inglis, J. T., and Blouin, J. S. (2014). Absence of lateral gastrocnemius activity and differential motor unit behavior in soleus and medial gastrocnemius during standing balance. *J. Appl. Physiol.* 116, 140–148. doi: 10.1152/japplphysiol.00906.2013

Hodson-Tole, E. F., Loram, I. D., and Vieira, T. M. (2013). Myoelectric activity along human gastrocnemius medialis: different spatial distributions of postural and electrically elicited surface potentials. *J. Electromyogr. Kinesiol.* 23, 43–50. doi: 10.1016/j.jelekin.2012.08.003

Horak, F. B., Henry, S. M., and Shumway-Cook, A. (1997). Postural perturbations: new insights for treatment of balance disorders. *Phys. Ther.* 77, 517–533.

Laughton, C. A., Slavin, M., Katdare, K., Nolan, L., Bean, J. F., Kerrigan, D. C., et al. (2003). Aging, muscle activity, and balance control: physiologic changes associated with balance impairment. *Gait Posture* 18, 101–108. doi: 10.1016/S0966-6362(02)00200-X

Li, F., Harmer, P., Fisher, K. J., McAuley, E., Chaumeton, N., Eckstrom, E., et al. (2005). Tai chi and fall reductions in older adults: a randomized controlled trial. *J. Gerontol. Ser. A Biol. Sci. Med. Sci.* 60, 187–194. doi: 10.1093/gerona/60.2.187

Loram, I. D., Gollee, H., Lakie, M., and Gawthrop, P. J. (2011). Human control of an inverted pendulum: is continuous control necessary? Is intermittent control effective? Is intermittent control physiological? *J. Physiol.* 589, 307–324. doi: 10.1113/jphysiol.2010.194712

Loram, I. D., and Lakie, M. (2002a). Direct measurement of human ankle stiffness during quiet standing: the intrinsic mechanical stiffness is insufficient for stability. *J. Physiol.* 545, 1041–1053. doi: 10.1113/jphysiol.2002.025049

Loram, I. D., and Lakie, M. (2002b). Human balancing of an inverted pendulum: position control by small, ballistic-like, throw and catch movements. *J. Physiol.* 540, 1111–1124. doi: 10.1113/jphysiol.2001.013077

Loram, I. D., Lakie, M., and Gawthrop, P. J. (2009). Visual control of stable and unstable loads: what is the feedback delay and extent of linear time-invariant control? *J. Physiol.* 587, 1343–1365. doi: 10.1113/jphysiol.2008.166173

Loram, I. D., Maganaris, C. N., and Lakie, M. (2005). Human postural sway results from frequent, ballistic bias impulses by soleus and gastrocnemius. *J. Physiol.* 564, 295–311. doi: 10.1113/jphysiol.2004.076307

Masani, K., Sayenko, D. G., and Vette, A. H. (2013). What triggers the continuous muscle activity during upright standing? *Gait Posture* 37, 72–77. doi: 10.1016/j.gaitpost.2012.06.006

McLean, L., and Goudy, N. (2004). Neuromuscular response to sustained low-level muscle activation: within- and between-synergist substitution in the triceps surae muscles. *Eur. J. Appl. Physiol.* 91, 204–216. doi: 10.1007/s00421-003-0967-3

Mesin, L., Merletti, R., and Vieira, T. M. (2011). Insights gained into the interpretation of surface electromyograms from the gastrocnemius muscles: a simulation study. *J. Biomech.* 44, 1096–1103. doi: 10.1016/j.jbiomech.2011.01.031

Nagai, K., Yamada, M., Uemura, K., Yamada, Y., Ichihashi, N., and Tsuboyama, T. (2011). Differences in muscle coactivation during postural control between healthy older and young adults. *Arch. Gerontol. Geriatr.* 53, 338–343. doi: 10.1016/j.archger.2011.01.003

Oliveira, L. F., Simpson, D. M., and Nadal, J. (1996). Calculation of area of stabilometric signals using principal component analysis. *Physiol. Meas.* 17, 305–312. doi: 10.1088/0967-3334/17/4/008

Onambele, G. L., Narici, M. V., and Maganaris, C. N. (2006). Calf muscle-tendon properties and postural balance in old age. *J. Appl. Physiol.* 100, 2048–2056. doi: 10.1152/japplphysiol.01442.2005

Pinsault, N., and Vuillerme, N. (2009). Test-retest reliability of centre of foot pressure measures to assess postural control during unperturbed stance. *Med. Eng. Phys.* 31, 276–286. doi: 10.1016/j.medengphy.2008.08.003

Reffad, A., Mebarkia, K., Vieira, T. M., and Disselhorst-Klug, C. (2014). Effect of contraction force and knee joint angle on the spatial representation of soleus activity using high-density surface EMG. *Biomed. Tech.* 59, 399–411. doi: 10.1515/bmt-2013-0072

Sayenko, D. G., Alekhina, M. I., Masani, K., Vette, A. H., Obata, H., Popovic, M. R., et al. (2010). Positive effect of balance training with visual feedback on standing balance abilities in people with incomplete spinal cord injury. *Spinal Cord* 48, 886–893. doi: 10.1038/sc.2010.41

Staudenmann, D., Kingma, I., Daffertshofer, A., Stegeman, D. F., and van Dieën, J. H. (2009). Heterogeneity of muscle activation in relation to force direction: a multi-channel surface electromyography study on the triceps surae muscle. *J. Electromyogr. Kinesiol.* 19, 882–895. doi: 10.1016/j.jelekin.2008.04.013

Tomioka, K., Iwamoto, J., Saeki, K., and Okamoto, N. (2011). Reliability and validity of the International Physical Activity Questionnaire (IPAQ) in elderly adults: the Fujiwara-kyo Study. *J. Epidemiol.* 21, 459–465. doi: 10.2188/jea.JE20110003

Vieira, T. M., Loram, I. D., Muceli, S., Merletti, R., and Farina, D. (2011). Postural activation of the human medial gastrocnemius muscle: are the muscle units spatially localised? *J. Physiol.* 589, 431–443. doi: 10.1113/jphysiol.2010.201806

Vieira, T. M., Loram, I. D., Muceli, S., Merletti, R., and Farina, D. (2012). Recruitment of motor units in the medial gastrocnemius muscle during human quiet standing: is recruitment intermittent? What triggers recruitment? *J. Neurophysiol.* 107, 666–676. doi: 10.1152/jn.00659.2011

Vieira, T. M., Merletti, R., and Mesin, L. (2010a). Automatic segmentation of surface EMG images: improving the estimation of neuromuscular activity. *J. Biomech.* 43, 2149–2158. doi: 10.1016/j.jbiomech.2010.03.049

Vieira, T. M., Windhorst, U., and Merletti, R. (2010b). Is the stabilization of quiet upright stance in humans driven by synchronized modulations of the activity of medial and lateral gastrocnemius muscles? *J. Appl. Physiol.* 108, 85–97. doi: 10.1152/japplphysiol.00070.2009

Vieira, T. M., Wakeling, J. M., and Hodson-Tole, E. F. (2016). Is there sufficient evidence to claim muscle units are not localised and functionally grouped within the human gastrocnemius? *J. Physiol.* 594, 1953–1954. doi: 10.1113/JP271866

Warnica, M. J., Weaver, T. B., Prentice, S. D., and Laing, A. C. (2014). The influence of ankle muscle activation on postural sway during quiet stance. *Gait Posture* 39, 1115–1121. doi: 10.1016/j.gaitpost.2014.01.019

2

The Neuro-Mechanical Processes that Underlie Goal-Directed Medio-Lateral APA during Gait Initiation

Jean-Louis Honeine [1], Marco Schieppati [1,2], Oscar Crisafulli [1] and Manh-Cuong Do [3]*

[1] *Department of Public Health, Experimental and Forensic Medicine, University of Pavia, Pavia, Italy,* [2] *Centro Studi Attività Motorie (CSAM), Fondazione Salvatore Maugeri (IRCSS), Scientific Institute of Pavia, Pavia, Italy,* [3] *Faculty of Sport Science, Complexité, Innovations, Activités Motrices et Sportives (CIAMS), Université Paris-Saclay, Orsay, France*

Correspondence:
Jean-Louis Honeine
Jeanlouis.honeine@unipv.it

Gait initiation (GI) involves passing from bipedal to unipedal stance. It requires a rapid movement of the center of foot pressure (CoP) towards the future swing foot and of the center of mass (CoM) in the direction of the stance foot prior to the incoming step. This anticipatory postural adjustment (APA) allows disengaging the swing leg from the ground and establishing favorable conditions for stepping. This study aimed to describe the neuro-mechanical process that underlies the goal-directed medio-lateral (ML) APA. We hypothesized that controlled knee flexion of the stance leg contributes to the initial ML displacement of the CoP and to the calibration of the first step. Fourteen subjects initiated gait starting from three different initial stance widths of 15 cm (Small), 30 cm (Medium), and 45 cm (Large). Optoelectronic, force platform and electromyogram (EMG) measurements were performed. During APA, soleus activity diminished bilaterally, while tibialis anterior (TA) activity increased, more so in the stance leg than in the swing leg, and to a larger extent with increasing initial stance width. Knee flexion of the stance leg was observed during APA and correlated with the ML CoP displacement towards the swing leg. ML CoP and CoM displacements during APA increased with increasing stance width. The activity of stance-leg TA was correlated with the degree of knee flexion. Swing-leg tensor fasciae latae (TFL) was also active during APA. Across subjects, when stance-leg tibialis activity was low, TFL activity was large and vice versa. The modulation of the ML CoP position during APA allowed the gravity-driven torque to place the CoM just lateral to the stance foot during step execution. Accordingly, the gravity-driven torque, the ML CoM velocity during step execution, and the step width at foot contact (FC) were lower in the Small and greater in the Large condition. Consequently, the position of the stepping foot at FC remained close to the sagittal plane in all three conditions. Conclusively, coordinated activation of hip abductors and ankle dorsiflexors during APA displaces the CoP towards the swing leg, and sets the contact position for the swing foot.

Keywords: gait initiation, center of pressure, center of mass, frontal plane, knee flexion, ankle dorsiflexor muscles, hip abductor muscles

INTRODUCTION

Gait initiation (GI) is a critical task because it involves transiting from stable bipedal stance to unstable unipedal stance. It requires anticipatory postural adjustments (APA) that reconfigure the position of the center of mass (CoM) with respect to the center of foot pressure (CoP) in order to take advantage of gravity and progress forward (Carlsöö, 1966; Brenière and Do, 1986, 1991; Brenière et al., 1987; Brenière, 2001).

It is well established that the displacement of CoM during APA is achieved by shifting the CoP backwards and in the direction of the swing leg (Jian et al., 1993; Elble et al., 1994; Lepers and Brenière, 1995). The backward shift of the CoP is caused by a reduction in soleus activity and activation of the tibialis anterior (TA; Crenna and Frigo, 1991). During APA, modulation of the antero-posterior distance between the vertical projections to the ground of the CoM and CoP positions generates a torque driven by gravity (henceforth termed disequilibrium torque) that propels the body forward (Lepers and Brenière, 1995; Michel and Do, 2002; Honeine et al., 2013, 2014). In the frontal plane, the initial CoP excursion in the direction of the future swing leg during APA causes gravity to move the CoM closer to the stance leg (Jian et al., 1993; Elble et al., 1994; Lepers and Brenière, 1995; McIlroy and Maki, 1999). By doing so, the nervous system disengages the swing leg from the ground. During the single-support phase of the first step, the distance between CoM and CoP in the frontal plane and the mediolateral (ML) fall of the CoM shape the positioning of the stepping foot at the moment of its contact with the ground (Lyon and Day, 1997, 2005; Caderby et al., 2014).

Carlsöö (1966) and later Winter (1995) stated that the initial displacement of the CoP in the direction of the swing leg is caused by unloading the stance leg and loading the swing leg, which they argued is produced by the hip abductor activity from the swing side. However, this may not be the sole mechanisms underpinning the disengagement of the future swing limb. When standing, the knee joint is extended due to the backward pull of the soleus on the tibia and to the action of gravity (Woodhull et al., 1985) connected with the anterior position of the CoM with respect to the knee. Therefore, the knee acts as a load-bearing joint (Walker and Erkman, 1975; Freeman et al., 1980). Notably, flexion of the knee of the stance leg during single-support is known to occur during gait (Segal et al., 2006; Shamaei et al., 2013). Hence, it may be appropriate to examine whether flexion of the knee also occurs during the APA in order to unload the stance leg during the preparation phase of GI. In this study, we tested the hypothesis that the central nervous system (CNS) employs stance-leg knee flexion as a complementary strategy to swing-leg hip abduction in order to unload the stance leg and displace the CoP in the direction of the swing leg during APA. Furthermore, we postulated that the modulation of the CoP displacement during APA also determines the disequilibrium torque and the lateral fall of the body towards the swing leg during step execution, with the purpose of positioning the stepping foot close to the sagittal plane at its foot contact (FC).

We asked volunteers to start walking from different initial stance widths at their spontaneous forward velocities. Increasing the stance widths prior to step execution has been shown to produce larger CoM and CoP displacements, in order to modulate the distance between CoM and CoP in the frontal plane and consequently the gravity-driven torque during step execution (Lyon and Day, 1997). If our hypothesis is correct, flexion of the knee of the stance leg should occur in the APA phase. The finding of a greater knee flexion of the stance leg accompanied by larger CoM and CoP displacement with a larger initial stance width would corroborate the proposition.

We also expected the ampler CoP displacement, which should occur the larger the initial stance width, to produce a greater gravity-driven torque during step execution. This would in turn increase the velocity of the CoM fall in the frontal plane prompting the stepping foot to land close to the subjects' sagittal plane.

MATERIALS AND METHODS

Participants

Fourteen (11 F) healthy young adults participated in the study. Their mean age, mass and height were 29 years (ranging from 21 to 41), 61 kg (47–80) and 1.68 m (1.58–1.80), respectively. As conformed to the Declaration of Helsinki, subjects provided written informed consent to the experiment, which was approved by the ethics committee of Fondazione Salvatore Maugeri (No. 2056CE).

Tasks and Procedures

Subjects stood with each foot on a distinct force platform (Kistler 9286BA, Winterthur, Switzerland). The position of each heel was equidistant to the border of each platform. Following the start of the acquisition, subjects were instructed to initiate walking in a self-paced mode. This was done to avoid the startle effect on GI, which occurs when subjects are asked to start walking following an acoustic command (Queralt et al., 2010). Subjects were not given any instruction about the speed at which to initiate walking and were left to execute GI at their preferred velocity. They performed three sets of conditions of GI, in which they started from predefined initial stance-widths of 15, 30 and 45 cm, termed Small, Medium and Large, respectively, in the text. There was no explicit instruction about the positioning of the first or successive footsteps. The order of the trials was randomized across subjects. Following GI, subjects were instructed to continue walking for at least six steps. Subjects were not specifically told to execute GI starting from a given leg (Hiraoka et al., 2014), even if in most of the trials subjects initiated gait with the same leg. Subjects performed as many trials as needed in order to achieve at least 12–15 trials per condition, all performed with the same leg. The distribution of the weight over each leg was checked during the experiment so that if the difference exceeded 1 kg before the CoP started moving, the trial was repeated in order to prevent the effects of anticipation on the GI features.

Data Acquisition

Twenty-three reflective markers were positioned on the subjects' body in the following anatomical locations: vertex, acromion, C7, L5 and bilaterally on lateral head, medial epicondyle of the elbow, head of the ulna, anterior superior iliac spine, greater trochanter, lateral epicondyle of the femur (knee), lateral malleolus, heel and 1st metatarsus-phalangeal joint. The Smart-D optoelectronic system (BTS Bioengineering, Italy) employed 12 infrared cameras that measured the position of the body markers with respect to the laboratory global reference. Anthropometric measurements of the segments of the body were made manually. This allowed for the computation of the three-dimensional position of the body's CoM (Winter, 1993). Bipolar electrodes (Freeemg, BTS Bioengineering, Italy) were employed to wirelessly record bilaterally the electromyogram (EMG) of TA, soleus, gastrocnemius medialis, biceps femoris (BF), semitendinosus (ST), semimembranosus (SM), tensor fasciae latae (TFL) and gluteus medius (nine subjects). Skin preparation and electrode placement were performed according to the SENIAM protocol (Merletti and Hermens, 2000). Optoelectronic, force platform and EMG data were recorded synchronously at acquisition frequencies of 140, 560, 1000 Hz, respectively. Data were stored in a computer for off-line analysis using a custom-made program written using Matlab (Mathworks, Natick, MA, USA).

Analysis of Biomechanical Variables

The global ML CoP position was calculated from the output of both force platforms according to Equation 1:

$$CoP_{global} = [(F_1 * CoP_1) + (F_2 * CoP_2)] / (F_1 + F_2) \quad (1)$$

where F_1 and F_2 are the vertical ground reaction forces under each leg, and CoP_1 is the ML position of CoP under one leg while CoP_2 is the ML position of the CoP under the other. The coordinates of CoP_1, CoP_2, CoP_{global} and the positions of each marker were referred to the same laboratory reference system.

The instant at which GI effectively started (t0) was set as the instant at which the ML CoP position exceeded the baseline by three standard deviations. The instant of the first heel-off (HO) was determined when the vertical position of the heel marker of the swing leg exceeded the value at baseline by 1 mm. The instant when the heel marker of the swing-leg reached its lowest vertical position signaled the instant of the successive FC (see **Figure 1**). Both instants were referred to t0. APA was defined as the time-period spanning from t0 to HO. The step execution phase extended from HO until swing foot landing (FC). The velocity of the CoM in the frontal plane was obtained by the derivation of the ML component of CoM position in time. Step length at FC was measured as the distance between the position of the heel of the stepping foot at t0 and at FC in the sagittal plane. Step width at FC was the distance in the frontal plane between the stance-foot heel marker at t0 and stepping-foot heel marker at its FC. The greater trochanter, knee and malleolus markers on both sides were used to calculate the knee angles in the sagittal plane.

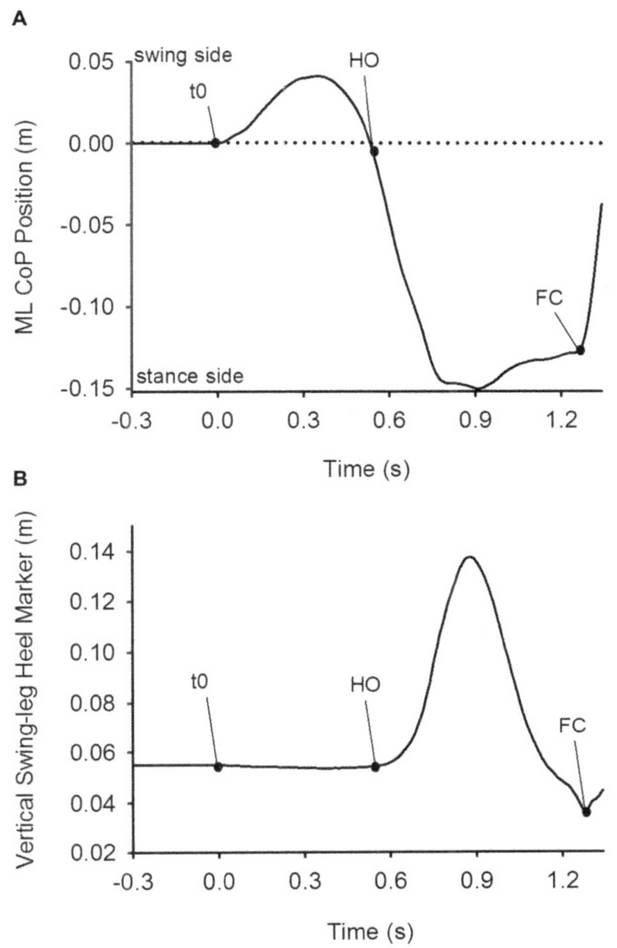

FIGURE 1 | Detection of t0, heel-off (HO) and foot-contact (FC). Panel **(A)** depicts the time-course of the mediolateral (ML) center of foot pressure (CoP) position. Panel **(B)** shows the time-course of the vertical position of the heel marker of the swing leg. Both plots were obtained from a single trial of one subject in the Medium stance-width condition. The dots on the curves indicate the time of initiation of CoF movement (t0), HO and FC. Anticipatory postural adjustment (APA) was defined as the time-period between t0 and HO, and step execution as the time-period between HO and FC.

The unloading of the stance leg was measured as the reduction of vertical ground reaction force at the instant of maximum CoP displacement during APA with respect to that measured at t0. The loading of the swing leg during APA was measured as the amount of increase in vertical ground reaction force at the instant of maximum CoP displacement during APA with respect to that measured prior to t0.

The instantaneous disequilibrium torque acting in the frontal plane was calculated as the product of the vertical ground reaction force and the distance between the ground vertical projection of CoM and CoP in the frontal plane (Equation 2). To calculate the torque, the CoP position and the vertical force were down-sampled to 140 Hz. Due to friction between the foot and the floor, the disequilibrium torque is converted to shear force.

In order to calculate the shear component of the ground reaction force generated by the torque, the latter was divided by the instantaneous height of CoM with respect to CoP (Equation 3):

$$\text{Torque} = \text{d}\,(\text{CoM} - \text{CoP}) * \text{F} \tag{2}$$

$$\text{Shear force} = \text{Torque/h} \tag{3}$$

where d(CoM−CoP) is the distance between CoM and CoP in the frontal plane, F is the vertical force acting on the CoM and h is the vertical position of CoM with respect to the ground. The impulse during APA and during step execution was measured as the product of the average shear force during APA or during step execution and the respective time periods in which the force was applied (Equation 4). The impulse was then normalized by dividing it by the corresponding subject's mass.

$$\text{Impulse} = \text{Shear force}_{\text{Avg}} * \Delta\text{t} \tag{4}$$

Analysis of EMG Activity

To calculate the start and end of EMG activities, the synchrosqueezed wavelet transforms of the raw EMG traces were calculated using the Morlet wavelet (Daubechies et al., 2011; Iatsenko et al., 2015). The final wavelet transform was composed of 125 frequency bins with a bandwidth of about 1.64 Hz ranging from 40 to 244.8 Hz for each time frame. A control-wavelet-coefficient matrix (154 × 1) was then created by averaging the coefficients that were found in the 25th percentile of the coefficient distribution. Multiple single-tailed Student's *t*-test was then used to compare each time-frame of the wavelet transform with the control-wavelet-coefficient matrix. Onset of muscle activation was considered the instant when *p*-value exceeded 0.05 for 50 consecutive time-frames. Offset was considered the instant when *p*-value was inferior to 0.05 for 50 consecutive time-frames (see **Figure 2**). The amplitude of EMG activity was calculated by rectifying the EMG raw traces, low-pass filtering the signal with a second order Butterworth no-lag filter with a cut-off frequency of 25 Hz, and calculating the area under the curve. Maximal EMG isometric activity of all muscles was measured by blocking the pertinent body segment against a rigid frame and asking the subject to exert a maximal isometric contraction against it for about 3–4 s. The peak activity of EMG was detected. The amplitude of the EMG activity during a time-window of 1 s centered around the peak activity was then calculated.

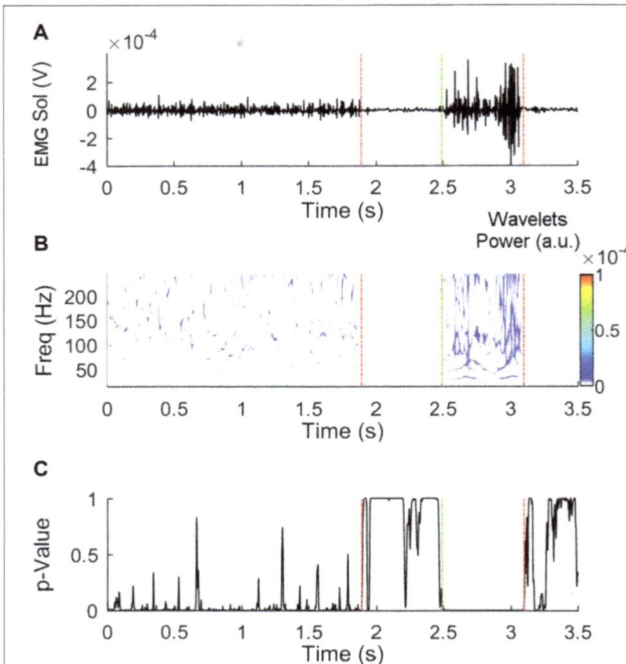

FIGURE 2 | Detection of the beginning and end of electromyogram (EMG) activity. Panel **(A)** shows a raw EMG trace obtained from the soleus muscle of the stance leg during Gait initiation (GI). Panel **(B)** represents the synchrosqueezed transform of the raw trace. The *p*-values of the *t*-test that compares the coefficients in each time-bin with the control-matrix-coefficients are shown in panel **(C)**. Fifty or more consecutive *p*-values inferior to 0.05 indicates that the muscle is active. The vertical dashed lines indicate the instants at which deactivation (red) and activation (green) were detected.

Statistics

We verified the distribution of each parameter by performing a Shapiro-Wilk test. Parameters that did not show a normal distribution were tested using non-parametric methods. Separate repeated-measures ANOVAs were used to test the effect of initial stance-width on the following variables: duration of APA; duration of step execution; anteroposterior (AP) instantaneous velocity of CoM at HO and at FC; maximum distance between CoP and CoM during APA and during step execution; EMG activities of stance-leg soleus, gastrocnemius, TFL and gluteus medius during step execution; position of the swing-leg heel marker at FC; position of the swing-leg hallux marker at FC. Separate 2 (swing − stance) × 3 (Small − Normal − Large) repeated-measures ANOVAs were used to test the statistical difference of the following variables: forward displacement of knee joints during APA; knees flexion during APA. Separate one-way Friedman repeated-measures analyses were used to test, during APA, differences in the amplitude of the swing- and stance leg TA EMG activity; effect of initial stance-width on the activity of the swing-leg TA activity; effect of initial stance-width on the activity of stance-leg tibialis activity; effect of initial stance-width on the activity of the swing-leg TFL. Pearson's method was used to test the linear relationship between the following variables: unloading and loading of the stance and swing legs, respectively, and the maximum displacement of CoP during APA; stance-leg knee forward displacement and stance-leg knee flexion; stance-leg knee flexion and maximum displacement of CoP during APA; amplitude of TA activity and knee flexion of the stance leg during APA; normalized impulse calculated during APA and normalized impulse during step execution; normalized impulse during step execution and ML CoM velocity at FC; normalized impulse during step execution and step width at FC. Hyperbolic fitting was used to determine the relationship between the TFL and TA activity in each of the three conditions. Linear and hyperbolic relationship were done using Sigmaplot (Systat software Inc., San Jose, CA, USA). *Post hoc* analyses of variables following a normal distribution were made by the Fischer's LSD test. The Wilcoxon signed-rank test was used to test non-normally distributed variables. The level of significance in all tests was set at $p < 0.05$. The software Statistica (StatSoft, Tulsa, OK, USA) was used.

RESULTS

Global Kinematics

As expected, prior to stepping, CoP was initially displaced in the direction of the swing leg while CoM moved in the opposite direction. **Figure 3A** shows the time-course of the mean curves of the ML CoP and CoM positions in the three stance-width conditions of a single subject (mean curves were obtained by averaging 15 trials). The instant $t = 0$ s, which is referred to as t0 in the text, indicates the instant at which the ML CoP position starts moving towards the swing leg. As can be seen in the Figure, prior to HO, the CoP is displaced towards the swing leg and the CoM is moved, with a delay, in the direction of the stance leg. Then, the CoP starts moving towards the stance leg. Next, around mid-stance, the CoM lateral excursion peaks and starts moving towards the future stance leg in anticipation of the second step.

The distance between CoP and CoM in the frontal plane was measured at two distinct moments: the instant when CoP lateral excursion peaks during APA and the instant when CoM reaches its maximum displacement during step execution (as indicated by the arrows in **Figure 3A**). Their grand means and standard deviations are shown in **Figures 3B,C**. The ANOVA showed a significant effect of the initial stance-width on the maximal distance between CoP and CoM during APA ($F_{(2,26)} = 156.6$, $p < 0.001$), and on the maximal distance between CoP and CoM during step execution ($F_{(2,26)} = 153$, $p < 0.001$). *Post hoc* analyses showed that the maximal distance between CoP and CoM during APA and during step execution were the lowest in the Small and the greatest in the Large stance-width condition ($p < 0.001$ for all comparisons). The CoP displacement during APA was not significantly correlated with the subjects' height

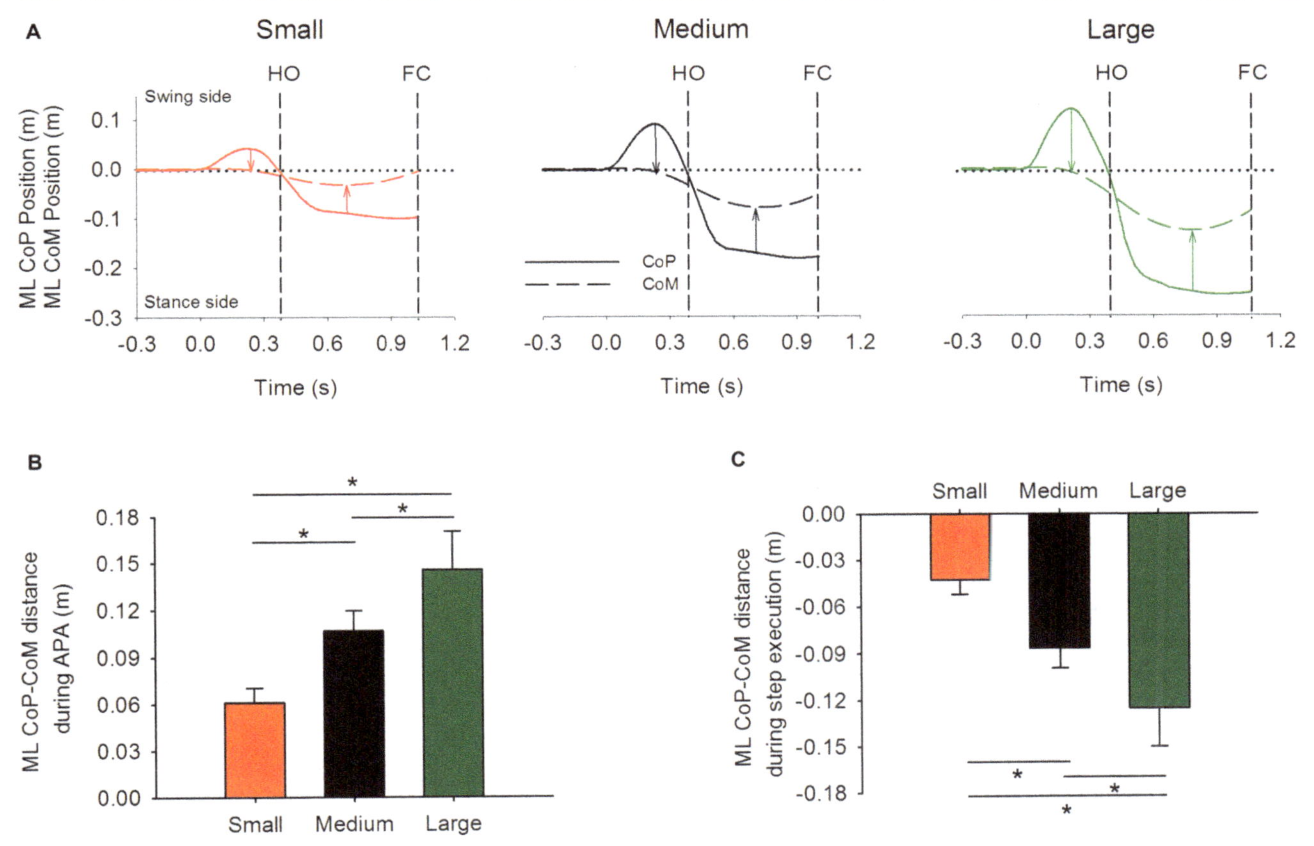

FIGURE 3 | Global kinematics variables in the frontal plane. The average time-course obtained from a single subject of the ML CoP (solid line) and center of mass (CoM) position (dashed line) are shown in panel **(A)**. The vertical dashed lines indicate HO and FC events. Panels **(B,C)** show the grand means and standard deviations of the distance between CoP and CoM at the instant at which CoP displacement peaked during APA (indicated by the leftmost arrows in panel **A**), and of the distance between CoP and CoM at the instant at which CoM displacement peaked during step execution (indicated by the rightmost arrows in panel **A**), respectively. *Indicates significant difference ($p < 0.05$).

TABLE 1 | Global gait initiation (GI) variables.

Condition	Duration of APA (s)	Duration of step execution (s)	CoM velocity at Heel-off (ms^{-1})	CoM velocity at foot-contact (ms^{-1})
Small	0.763 ± 0.06	0.635 ± 0.07	0.12 ± 0.03	0.81 ± 0.14
Medium	0.765 ± 0.05	0.629 ± 0.06	0.12 ± 0.04	0.80 ± 0.14
Large	0.784 ± 0.06	0.581 ± 0.07*	0.11 ± 0.05	0.74 ± 0.16*

**Indicates significant difference, p < 0.05.*

(Small: $r^2 = 0.09$, $p = 0.31$; Medium: $r^2 = 0.04$, $p = 0.48$; Large: $r^2 = 0.06$, $p = 0.41$), or their pelvis width (Small: $r^2 = 0.13$, $p = 0.21$; Medium: $r^2 = 0.07$, $p = 0.36$; Large: $r^2 = 0.01, p = 0.7$).

Table 1 contains the grand mean and standard deviation of the duration of APA, the duration of step execution, the instantaneous forward velocity of the CoM at the time instant of HO, and the forward velocity of CoM at the time instant of FC. Repeated-measures ANOVA showed no effect of initial stance width on the duration of APA ($F_{(2,26)} = 2.5$, $p = 0.1$). The instantaneous forward velocity of CoM measured at the instant of HO was also comparable between the three conditions ($F_{(2,26)} = 1.1$, $p = 0.35$). The ANOVA showed an effect of initial stance width on the duration of step execution ($F_{(2,26)} = 11$, $p < 0.001$) and the instantaneous forward CoM velocity measured at the instant of FC ($F_{(2,26)} = 14.7$, $p < 0.001$). *Post hoc* analysis showed that both duration of step execution and forward velocity of CoM at FC were smaller in the Large stance-width condition with respect to the Small and Medium conditions ($p < 0.001$).

CoP ML Displacement and Flexion of the Knee of the Stance Leg

Figure 4 shows the time-course of the ML CoP position (panel **A**) and the vertical ground reaction force (Panel **B**) under each foot. The traces represent a single trial obtained in each of the three stance-width conditions (Small, Medium and Large). The dots on the curves represent the moment at which the CoP displacement peaked. The loading of the swing and the unloading of the stance leg were accompanied by the displacement of CoP in the direction of the swing leg. **Figure 4C** shows a scatter plot of the maximum displacement of CoP as a function of the sum of the unloading and loading of the stance and swing leg (measured peak to peak). Three distinct linear relationships were obtained between the unloading of the stance leg and the maximum displacement of CoP during APA (Small: $r^2 = 0.66$, Medium: $r^2 = 0.49$, and Large: $r^2 = 0.59$). The relationships diverge because the position of the CoP in the frontal plane is not only caused by the amplitude of the vertical ground reaction force under each leg, but is also dependent on the initial stance width (see Equation 1).

Figure 5A shows a stick diagram of the lower limbs taken at different time-intervals in the sagittal plane. The trial seen in this Figure is the same Medium stance-width trial used in **Figure 4**. **Figures 5B,C** show the time-course of the knee AP position of the stance and swing leg, respectively. **Figures 5D,E** show the time-course of the knee angle of the stance leg and swing leg, respectively. The dots on the curves represent the moment of maximal CoP displacement. As can be seen in the Figure, at t0, i.e., while still standing, both knees are positioned behind the vertical position of CoM, a circumstance that lets gravity extend the knees. Following t0, the stance-leg knee is displaced forward so that it moves anteriorly to the CoM, favoring gravity to flex the knee. Meanwhile, the swing-leg knee is more or less stationary. The stance-leg knee remains anterior to the CoM during APA. Following foot-off of the swing leg, the CoM advancement places the CoM in front of the stance-leg knee so that the action of gravity halts the knee flexion or in some cases extends it slightly.

The grand mean and standard deviation of the AP displacements and flexion angles of the knees at the moment of maximal CoP displacement, relative to the initial position (at t0), are provided in **Figures 5F,G**. The ANOVA showed a difference in the forward displacement between the knees of the stance leg and the swing leg ($F_{(1,13)} = 57$, $p < 0.001$). Knee forward displacement differed across the three conditions ($F_{(2,26)} = 66.2$, $p < 0.001$). A significant interaction between swing- and stance-leg knee forward displacement and initial stance width was also found ($F_{(2,26)} = 14.15$, $p < 0.001$). The knee angle of the swing leg was significantly different from that of the stance leg ($F_{(1,13)} = 210.4$, $p < 0.001$). There was a general effect of condition on knee angle ($F_{(2,26)} = 104.2$, $p < 0.001$). A significant interaction between swing and stance knee angle and initial stance width was also found ($F_{(2,26)} = 42.3$, $p < 0.001$).

Post hoc analysis showed that both forward displacement and the flexion angle of the stance-leg knee were significantly different across conditions ($p < 0.001$). Amplitudes of forward displacement and flexion of the stance-leg were lower for the Small condition and greater for the Large condition compared to Medium ($p < 0.001$). A linear relationship was found between the forward displacement and the flexion angle of the stance-leg knee ($r^2 = 0.52$, **Figure 5H**). Finally, a linear relationship was found between the maximum displacement of CoP and the knee flexion of the stance leg ($r^2 = 0.64$, **Figure 5I**).

EMG Activity During Gait Initiation

Figure 6A shows the time-course of the average traces of the TA, soleus, gastrocnemius medialis, BF, ST, semimenbranosus, TFL and gluteus medius from both legs obtained from one subject during the Medium stance-width condition. The grand mean and standard deviations of the onset and offset of the same muscles (across conditions) are shown by the horizontal bars in **Figure 6B**. When standing, both soleus and BF were

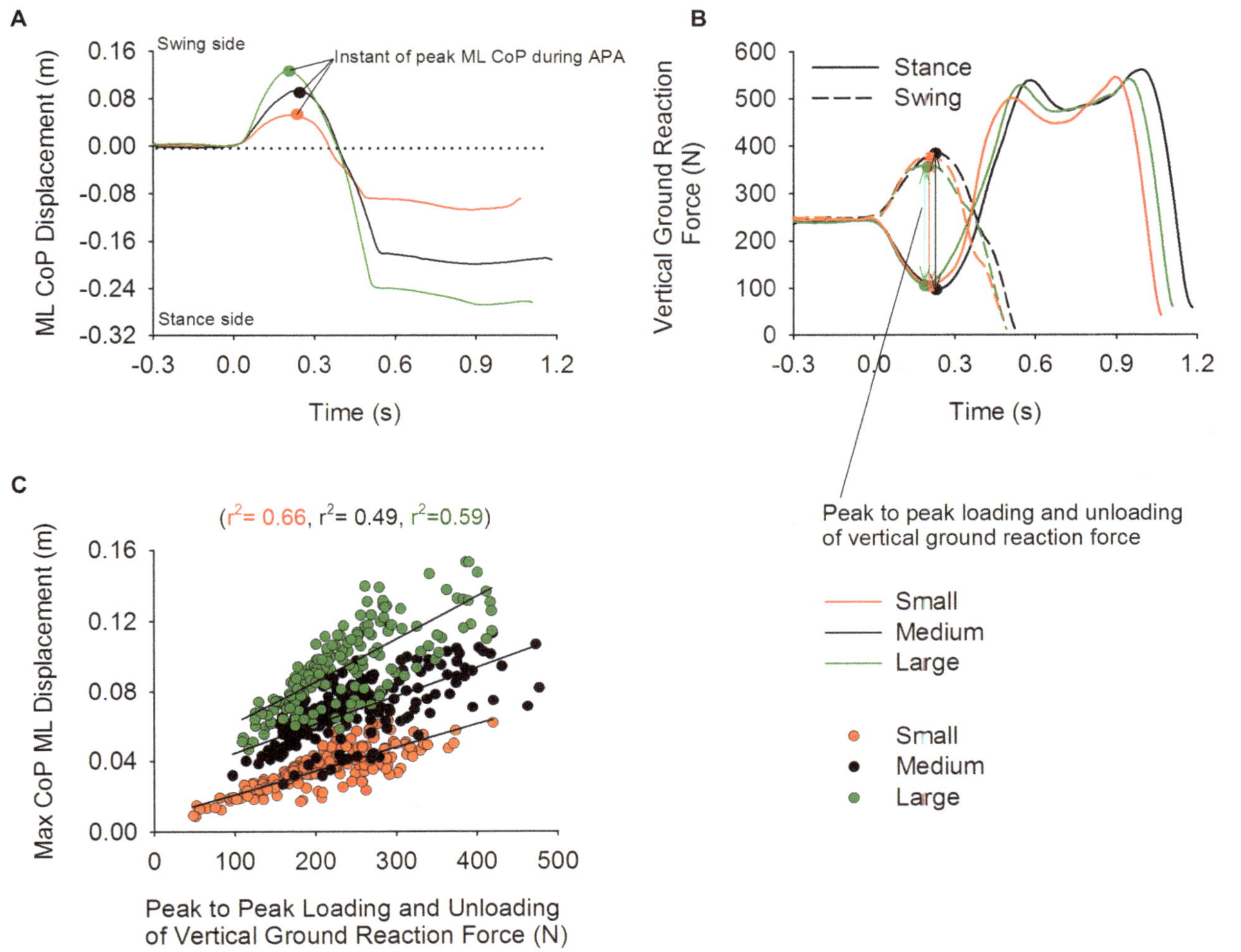

FIGURE 4 | Unloading and loading of the stance and swing leg and CoP displacement during APA. Panels **(A,B)** show the time-course of the CoP displacement and the vertical reaction force under the swing (dashed line) and stance foot (solid line), respectively. The curves were obtained from trials of a single subject from the Small, Medium and Large condition. The small circles on the plot indicate the instant at which the displacement of CoP in the direction of the swing leg peaked during APA. Panel **(C)** shows the three distinct linear relationships (one for each condition) that were found between maximal CoP displacement and the unloading and loading (measured peak to peak) of the stance and swing leg, respectively.

active. About 40 ms prior to t0 both soleus and BF were silenced in both legs while TA was activated bilaterally, concurrently with the swing-leg TFL. The offset of the EMG activity in the stance-leg TA and swing-leg TFL roughly coincided with the moment of HO. Triceps surae and hamstring muscles of the stance leg remained silent throughout the APA phase. The swing-leg TA showed two distinct bursts during the step execution phase that lasted until about 100 ms following FC. A brief increase in EMG activity of the triceps surae, hamstrings and TFL of the swing leg was detected about 100 ms prior to HO and ended around the same time as foot-off. During step execution, the beginning of triceps surae activity of the stance leg was recorded slightly prior to HO and ended about 100 ms following FC. The stance-leg TFL was activated about 150 ms prior to HO and was silenced slightly prior to FC. Finally, hamstrings of the stance leg showed a small burst about 100 ms long following HO that usually ended at about mid-single-stance.

Since hamstrings and gastrocnemius muscles are silent during APA, the only candidate responsible for bringing the stance knee forward and initiate knee flexion is the TA muscle that is active during APA. The time-course of the average traces of TA EMG activity of the swing and stance leg of a single subject is provided in the three upper panels of **Figure 7A**. **Figure 7B** shows the medians and the 25th and 75th percentiles of the amplitude of the EMG activity of the TA activity (with respect to maximum isometric contraction) of the swing leg and stance leg during APA. The Friedman repeated-measures test showed that the activity of TA was in general significantly lower in the swing- than stance-leg during APA ($\chi^2 = 24.4$, $p < 0.001$). The activity of the TA muscle of the swing leg did not differ across the three conditions ($\chi^2 = 1.28$, $p = 0.53$). However, starting to walk

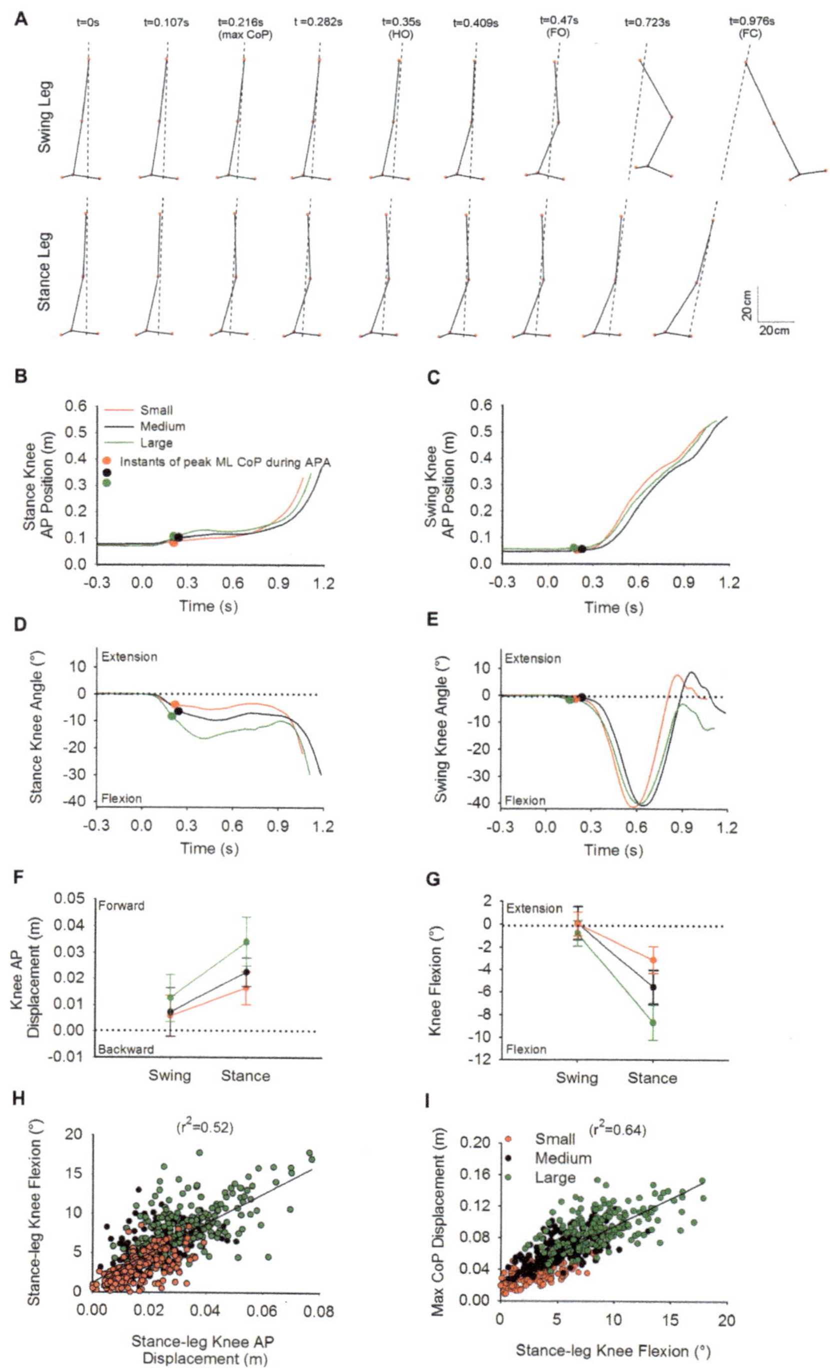

FIGURE 5 | Knee flexion and CoP displacement during APA. Panel **(A)** shows stick diagrams of the swing leg (top) and stance leg (bottom) taken at nine discrete instants in the sagittal plane. The stick diagrams represent the same Medium-condition trial as in **Figure 4**. The dashed lines represent the direction of the CoP-CoM vector. The instants comprise t0, instant of peak ML CoP during APA, HO, foot-off, FC and instants in between. As can be seen at t0, both knees are positioned behind the center of gravity. During APA, the swing-leg knee remains fixed while the ankle joint starts flexing and the stance-leg knee advances ahead of the center of gravity. The time-course of the stance knee position and swing knee position for the three single trials in each condition are found in panels **(B,C)** respectively. Panels **(D,E)** show the time-course of the stance-leg and swing-leg knee angle, respectively. The curves in panels **(B–E)** belong to the same trial. The small circles on the curves indicate the instant at which the maximum displacement of CoP in the direction of the swing leg was reached during APA. Panels **(F,G)** show the grand means and standard deviations of the forward displacement and flexion of the knee of the swing and stance leg, respectively, measured at the instant at which CoP displacement peaked. Panels **(H,I)** portray the linear relationship between the forward displacement of CoP and stance knee flexion, and between the stance-knee flexion and ML CoP displacement, respectively.

from different initial stance width had an effect on the activity of the stance-leg TA muscle ($\chi^2 = 28$, $p < 0.001$). The Wilcoxon matched pair test indicated that the lowest activity of the stance-leg TA muscle was obtained in the Small condition ($p < 0.05$ for both comparisons) while the greatest activity was achieved in the Large condition ($p < 0.05$ for both comparisons).

Figure 7C shows the time-course of the average traces of the TFL of the swing- and stance-leg during GI in a single subject. The medians and the 25 and 75 percentiles of the amplitude of EMG activity (with respect to maximum isometric contraction) of the swing-leg TFL muscle during APA are shown in **Figure 7D**. The Friedman repeated-measures test showed no effect of initial stance width on the amplitude of EMG activity of the swing-leg TFL ($\chi^2 = 4.43$, $p = 0.11$) and gluteus medius ($\chi^2 = 2.6$, $p = 0.09$) during APA. Furthermore, ANOVA showed no difference across conditions in the amplitude of EMG activity during the step execution phase of soleus ($F_{(2,26)} = 0.36$, $p = 0.70$), gastrocnemius ($F_{(2,26)} = 1.02$, $p = 0.37$), TFL ($F_{(2,26)} = 1.97$, $p = 0.16$) and gluteus medius ($F_{(2,16)} = 1.53$, $p = 0.25$) of the stance leg.

We also investigated the complementary contribution of hip abduction of the swing side and of knee flexion of the stance side during APA. **Figure 8** shows the TA activity of the stance leg plotted against that of the swing-leg TFL (both normalized to maximum activity during isometric contraction) during APA in the three conditions. A hyperbolic relationship interpolated the data points in the Small ($r^2 = 0.25$), Medium ($r^2 = 0.23$) and Large condition ($r^2 = 0.24$). By looking closely into **Figure 8**, one can also see that the hyperbolic relationship is partly due to the fact that some subjects preferred the hip abductor activity more than stance-knee flexion and vice versa. **Figure 9** shows a scatter plot of the amplitude of the stance-leg TA activity from onset until the peak of CoP displacement and the stance-leg knee flexion at the peak of CoP displacement. A linear relationship was obtained between tibialis activity and knee flexion ($r^2 = 0.55$).

Disequilibrium Torque During Gait Initiation

Figure 10A shows the average time-course of the shear force calculated by dividing the disequilibrium torque by the instantaneous height of the CoM (black line). For comparison, the gray line indicates the average time-course of the shear force measured by the platform. During APA, the shear force produced by the distance between CoP and CoM in the frontal plane displaced the CoM in the direction of the stance leg (negative values in the Figure). Following HO of the swing leg, the torque started acting in the opposite direction.

The impulse theorem allows to quantify the amount of force generated during a certain time interval. Therefore, the impulse derived from the shear force calculated from the disequilibrium torque (see "Materials and Methods: Analysis of Biomechanical Variables" Section) has been used to describe the effect of the torque during APA and step execution on the kinematics of GI in the frontal plane. A linear relationship was obtained between the impulse values calculated from the shear force during APA and those calculated during step execution ($r^2 = 0.59$; **Figure 10B**). In addition, the impulse calculated during step execution was correlated with the instantaneous velocity of CoM ($r^2 = 0.4$; **Figure 10C**) and step width at FC ($r^2 = 0.46$; see **Figure 10D**).

Figure 10E shows the grand mean and standard deviation of the AP and ML position of the heel and hallux markers at the instants of t0 and FC. The AP position of the markers has been calculated relative to the position of the heel markers at t0 (both feet on ground). The ML position of the markers was computed with respect to the subjects' sagittal plane, calculated as the plane passing between the two anterior superior iliac spines slightly prior to t0. The position of the heel and the hallux markers at FC with respect to the medial line were not different across the three conditions ($F_{(2,26)} = 2.27, p = 0.12$ and $F_{(2,26)} = 0.33, p = 0.72$, respectively). Step length was also comparable across the three conditions ($F_{(2,26)} = 0.21, p = 0.81$).

DISCUSSION

Human gait is a state of controlled disequilibrium, in which anticipating the position of the body with respect to the ground is critical to avoid destabilizing torques (Bauby and Kuo, 2000). It is fragile, because it can be disturbed by many bodily conditions, including even minor degradations of the sensory information or motor output or both (Mazzaro et al., 2005; Nardone et al., 2014), as well as by cognitive tasks (Lajoie et al., 1993). Further, unlike the hopping gait of kangaroos that is characterized by symmetrical leg jumping action, human bipedal gait is asymmetrical and involves alternate single-support and double-support phases. Hence, the asymmetry of human gait requires substantial balance control in the frontal plane in order to prevent lateral falls (Thorstensson et al., 1984; MacKinnon and Winter, 1993; Orendurff et al., 2004; Sozzi et al., 2013; Wang and Srinivasan, 2014).

During GI, the CNS is confronted with the difficult task of transiting between a symmetrical quasi-static state to an asymmetrical dynamic state (Delafontaine et al., 2015). Indeed, to start walking appropriately, the CoM is moved to a position favorable to gait prior to lifting the future swing leg (Carlsöö, 1966; Brenière and Do, 1986; Brenière et al., 1987; Brenière and Do, 1991; Jian et al., 1993; Elble et al., 1994). On the one hand, the backward shift of CoP, which is responsible for the forward movement of the CoM, is caused mainly by activation of TA and decrease in soleus activity (Crenna and Frigo, 1991; Lepers and Brenière, 1995; Brenière, 2001; Honeine et al., 2013, 2014). On the other hand, the initial lateral shift of CoP in the direction of the swing leg causes the CoM to move toward the stance leg. Carlsöö (1966) and Winter (1995) argued that swing-leg abductor activity during APA unloads the stance leg and loads the other which in turn produces a lateral displacement of the CoP. However, flexing the knee of the stance leg during APA can also help unloading the swing leg. It has been already shown that the knee is moderately flexed in the stance leg during walking. This knee flexion prevents higher rate of loading during gait, and translates to attenuated rates of loading and peak vertical ground reaction force in healthy adults (Riskowski et al., 2005; Riskowski,

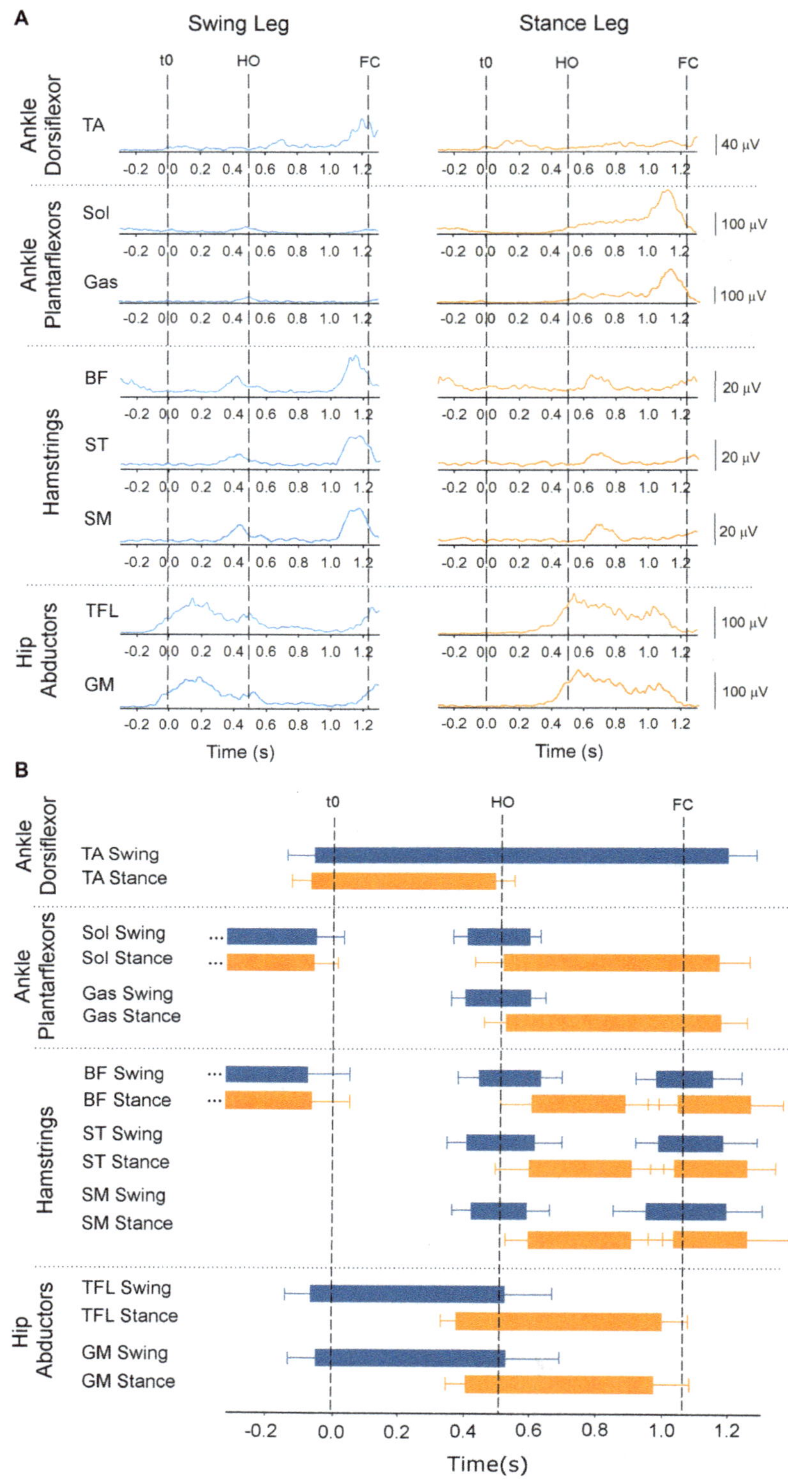

FIGURE 6 | Onset and offset of EMG activity. The figure provides temporal information about the ankle dorsi- and plantar-flexors, knee flexors and hip abductor EMG activity. Panel **(A)** shows the average time-course of one subject (Medium condition) of the rectified and low-pass filtered EMG traces (Fcut = 25 Hz) of the tibialis anterior (TA), soleus (Sol), gastrocnemius medialis (Gas), biceps femoris (BF), semitendinosus (ST), semimembranosus (SM), tensor fasciae latae (TFL) and gluteus medius muscles of the swing side (blue, left) and stance side (orange, right). t0, HO and FC are indicated by the dashed lines. Panel **(B)** shows the grand means and standard deviations of all subjects of the onset and offset across the three conditions of the same muscles' activity calculated with respect to t0.

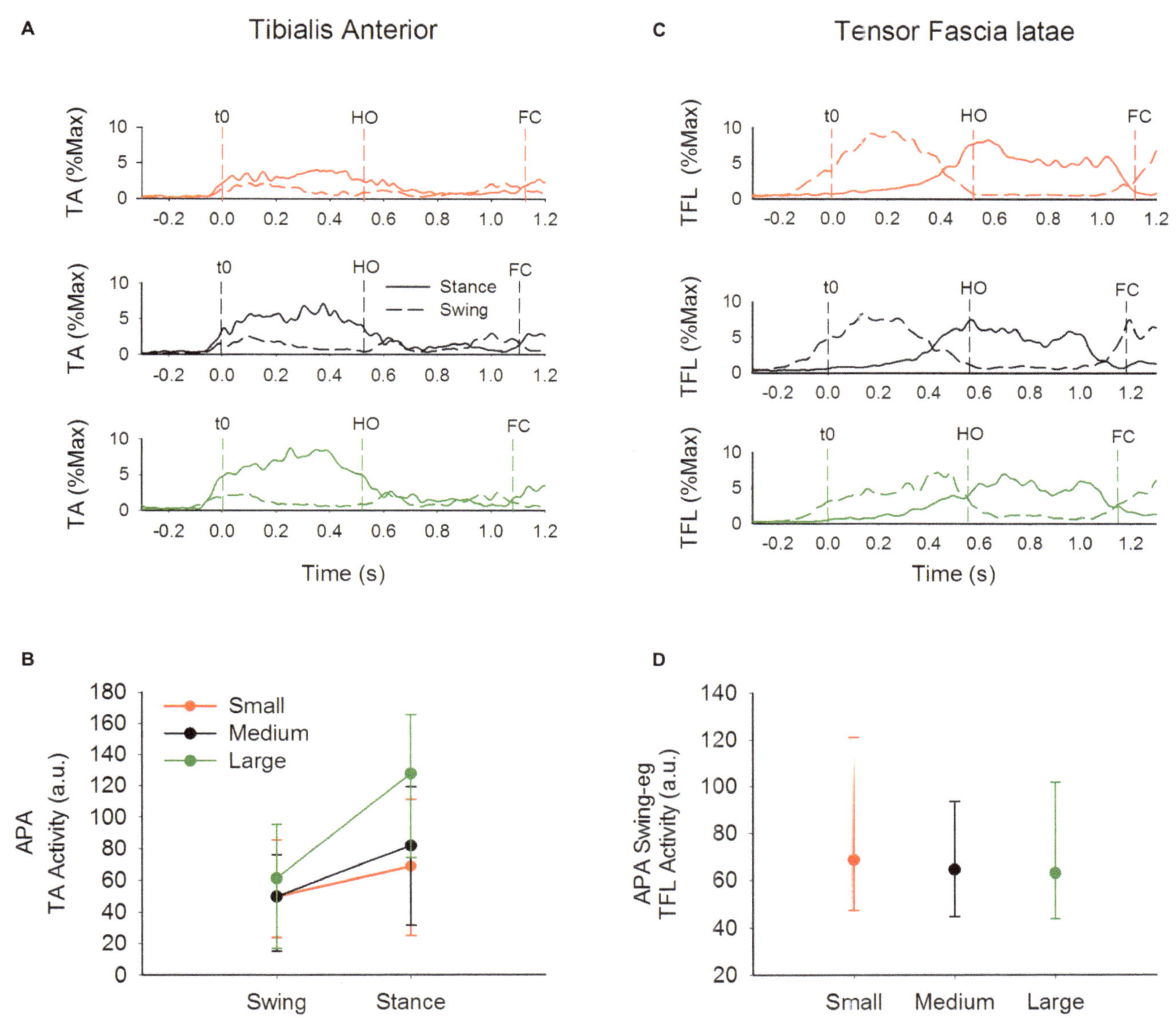

FIGURE 7 | EMG activity of TA and TFL. This figure contains information about the activity of tibialis activity and TFL muscles of both sides during GI. Panels **(A,C)** show the average envelope traces of TA and TFL, respectively, of a single subject in the three conditions (from top to bottom: Small, Medium and Large) of the swing leg (dashed line) and the stance leg (solid line). Panels **(B,D)** show the medians along with the 25th and 75th percentiles of the amplitudes of TA activity of the swing and stance legs and of TFL activity of the swing leg during APA, respectively (values are normalized to maximum isometric contraction). TA activity of the swing leg during APA was not affected by the initial stance width. However, TA activity of the stance leg was larger the greater the initial stance-width. The amplitude of TFL EMG activity was only moderately affected by the initial stance width.

2010). Hence, we hypothesized that the stance-leg knee flexion, which is part of the normal motor program for walking, could also be exploited in order to unload the stance leg during the preparation of GI.

Knee Flexion of the Stance Limb During APA

In line with Lyon and Day (1997), initiating gait at increasing stance widths causes greater displacement of the CoP in the direction of the swing leg and CoM in the opposite direction during APA. Our results also confirm the findings of Carlsöö (1966) and Winter (1995) in that the CoP displacement during APA is caused by unloading and loading the stance and swing legs, respectively (see **Figure 4**). In our hands, the greater excursions of CoP and CoM occurred without significant modifications of the global kinematic variables of GI (see **Table 1**) and most notably the duration of APA. This facilitates the comparisons across conditions without the need to normalize in time.

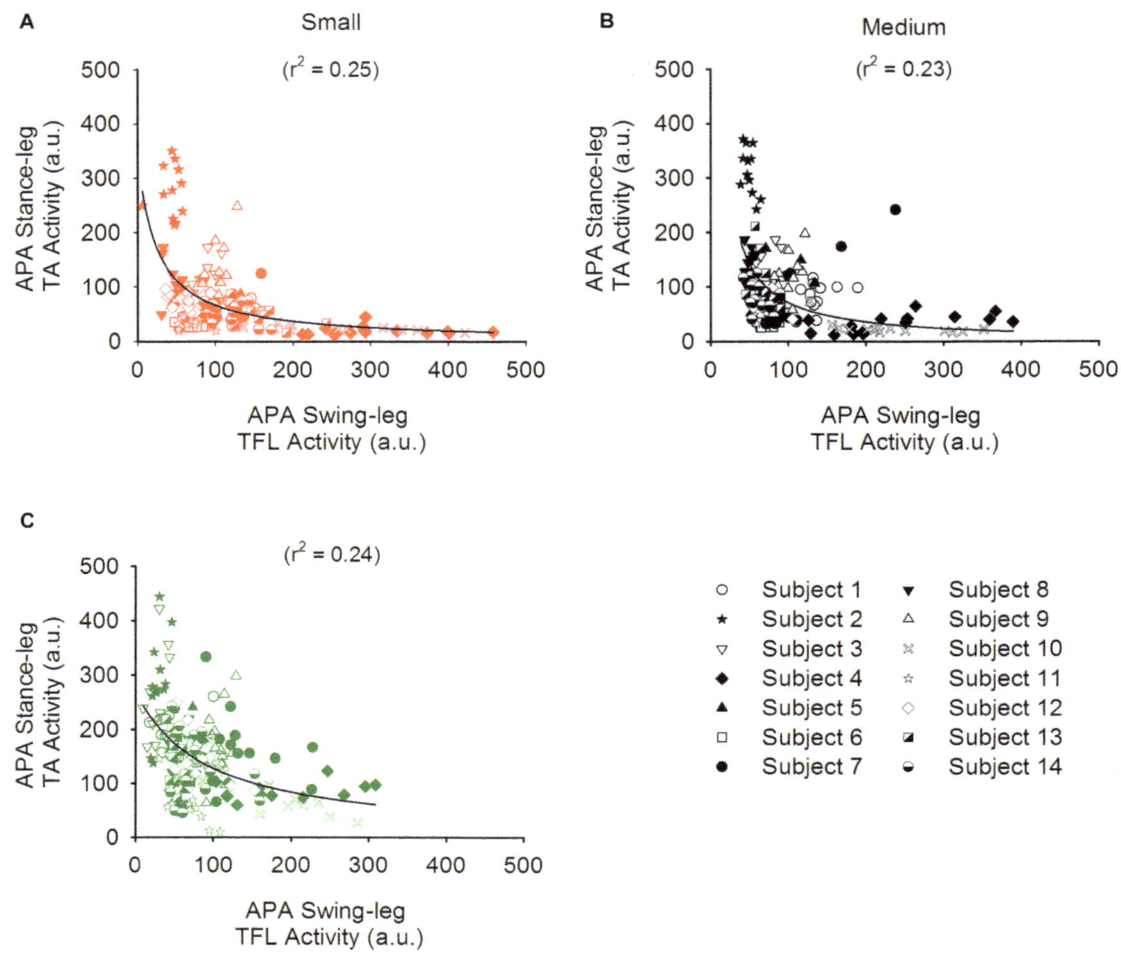

FIGURE 8 | Relationship between the EMG activity of the TA of the stance leg and that of the TFL of the swing leg. Panels **(A–C)** show the amplitude of the stance-leg TA activity plotted against that of the swing-leg TFL for all the trials of all the subjects in the Small (red), Medium (black) and Large (Green) stance-width conditions, respectively. Each subject is symbolized by a different icon. A hyperbolic ($y = ab/(b + x)$) function was found to bind the activity of these muscles.

As can be seen in **Figure 5**, at t0 both knees are placed behind the vertical projection of CoM. However, during APA, the stance knee is displaced forward, placing the joint anterior to the CoM vertical projection in the sagittal plane allowing gravity to participate in flexing the knee. Meanwhile, the swing-leg knee position and angle remain more or less constant. The stance-leg knee forward advancement and flexion augmented with increasing stance width. The amplitude of the flexion of the stance-leg knee was also correlated with the lateral displacement of CoP. The linear relationship between stance-leg knee flexion and lateral displacement of CoP is in line with our hypothesis that stance knee flexion unloads the stance leg and thus participates in shifting the CoP in the direction of the swing leg.

Hamstrings and gastrocnemius activity are associated to knee flexion during the double stance phase of gait (Goldberg et al., 2004). However, none of those muscles were active during flexion of the stance-leg knee in early APA. Moreover, BF that shows tonic activity while standing becomes silent during APA (see **Figure 6**). The reason might be that hamstrings also extend the hip. Hip extension during GI should potentially slightly restrict forward movement and is therefore undesirable. Conversely, the ankle plantarflexion produced by gastrocnemius activation would impede the backward CoP displacement required for generating forward motion. Slightly prior to t0, soleus and BF muscles are silenced bilaterally followed by TA activation (**Figure 6**). As more appropriately stated by Zajac and Gordon (1989), "at times, such as in standing, muscles crossing the ankle extend (soleus) or flex (TA) the knee much more that they flex and extend the ankle". In this study, the amplitude of the TA muscle of the stance leg is greater than that of the swing leg. Furthermore, the amplitude of the stance-leg TA activity increases with larger stance-widths (see **Figure 7**). This result suggests that the reduction in soleus tonic activity and the activation of the TA of the stance leg move the stance-leg knee forward with respect to the CoM position in the sagittal plane, thereby favoring gravity to flex the stance knee. Indeed, a linear relation between the amplitude of EMG activity of TA of the stance leg and flexion of the stance-leg knee is found here (**Figure 9**), strengthening the hypothesis that the stance-leg TA participates in displacing the CoP in the direction of the swing leg during the preparation phase of GI. It is to be noted that feet plantar afferents can influence the activity of TA and soleus during APA when raising one leg quickly (Do and Gilles, 1992). Cutaneous afferents can sense the augmentation in the shear force under the feet (Abbruzzese et al., 1996; Choi et al., 2016) that occurs with increasing stance width (Carmines and MacMahon, 1992). The changes of the cutaneous afferent input, in the different conditions, could have contributed to the modulation of stance-leg TA activity that participates in the lateral displacement of CoP during APA.

Following lift-off of the swing foot, the forward momentum of CoM places the latter anterior to the stance-leg knee, as occurs during the single-support phase of steady-state gait (Liu et al., 2008). This causes gravity to extend the stance knee thereby halting the flexion that occurred during APA. Furthermore, the activity of triceps surae and the hamstring muscles, increases during step execution. Those muscles could also be implicated in checking the knee flexion during single support.

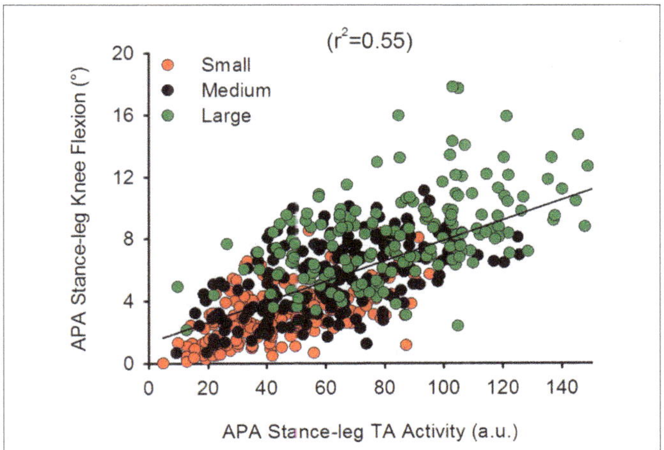

FIGURE 9 | Relationship between stance-leg TA EMG activity and knee flexion. This shows a scatter plot of the stance-leg knee flexion angle plotted against the amplitude of stance-leg TA activity during APA (normalized to maximum isometric contraction). A linear relationship was found to bind the two variables ($y = 0.07x + 1.34$) suggesting that stance-leg knee flexion might be modulated through TA activity of the same leg.

The Complementary Action of Hip Abduction and Stance Knee Flexion

Starting gait with different stance widths has no significant effect on the amplitude of hip abductor EMG activity of the swing leg during APA, albeit a slight tendency of some subjects (9 out of 14) to decrease hip abductor activity was observed when starting gait from a large stance width. Remarkably, a hyperbolic relationship binds the amplitude of stance-leg TA activity with that of the hip abductor muscles of the stance leg in each of the three conditions (see **Figure 8**). Some subjects relied more on swing-leg hip abductor activity and others on stance-leg dorsiflexor activity, while most relied on both rather equally. It is to be noted that the decrease in hip abductor activity in the Large condition of the nine subjects mentioned above is accompanied by a systematic increase in stance-leg knee flexion. A possible explanation is that due to biomechanical constraints, the hip abduction strategy is less efficient when starting from a large stance width. Conclusively, the actions of stance-knee flexion and swing-leg hip abduction appear to be complementary and synergistic in unloading the stance leg and loading the swing leg during APA. The coordination of the two strategies would result in more efficient and flexible ML displacement of the CoP in the direction of the swing leg.

The Effects of Modulation of ML CoP Displacement During APA on the Execution of the First Step

By modulating hip abduction and stance-leg knee flexion during APA, the CNS efficiently controls the distance between CoP and CoM in the frontal plane and consequently the disequilibrium torque during APA. Moreover, due to friction between the floor and the stance foot, the torque is converted into shear force that in turn displaces the CoM and places it just medially with respect to the stance foot during the single-stance phase of the execution of the first step (see **Figure 3**). In line with Lyon and Day (2005), our results show that the subjects modulate the CoP displacement during APA across conditions in order to control the ML distance between CoM and CoP during the step-execution phase. More precisely, the small displacements of CoP during the Small stance-width condition produce a small ML CoM-CoP distance during step execution, while the ample displacements of CoP during the Large stance-width condition produce a greater ML CoM-CoP distance (see **Figure 3**). Consequently, the ML disequilibrium torque and the CoM velocity during step execution are greater when larger the initial stance-width. The greater velocities of the CoM during step execution measured under larger initial stance-width causes the stepping foot to land at a larger distance with respect to the stance foot (Caderby et al., 2014). This causes the foot to be placed close to the subjects' mid-sagittal plane at the FC in all three conditions, so that subjects subsequently progressed easily along their initial straight-ahead line (see **Figure 10**). This result is interesting, because it shows that, already at the first step, subjects tend to place the foot in the appropriate position for performing the next sets, regardless of the initial postural attitude. In Honeine et al. (2014) we showed that by modulating the CoM and CoP distance in the sagittal plane the CNS sets step length, the antero-posterior velocity of CoM and the duration of the first step. Here, we complete those results by showing that by controlling the disequilibrium torque in the frontal plane during APA, the CNS determines also the ML velocity of CoM and the ML position of the swing leg at the instant of first FC.

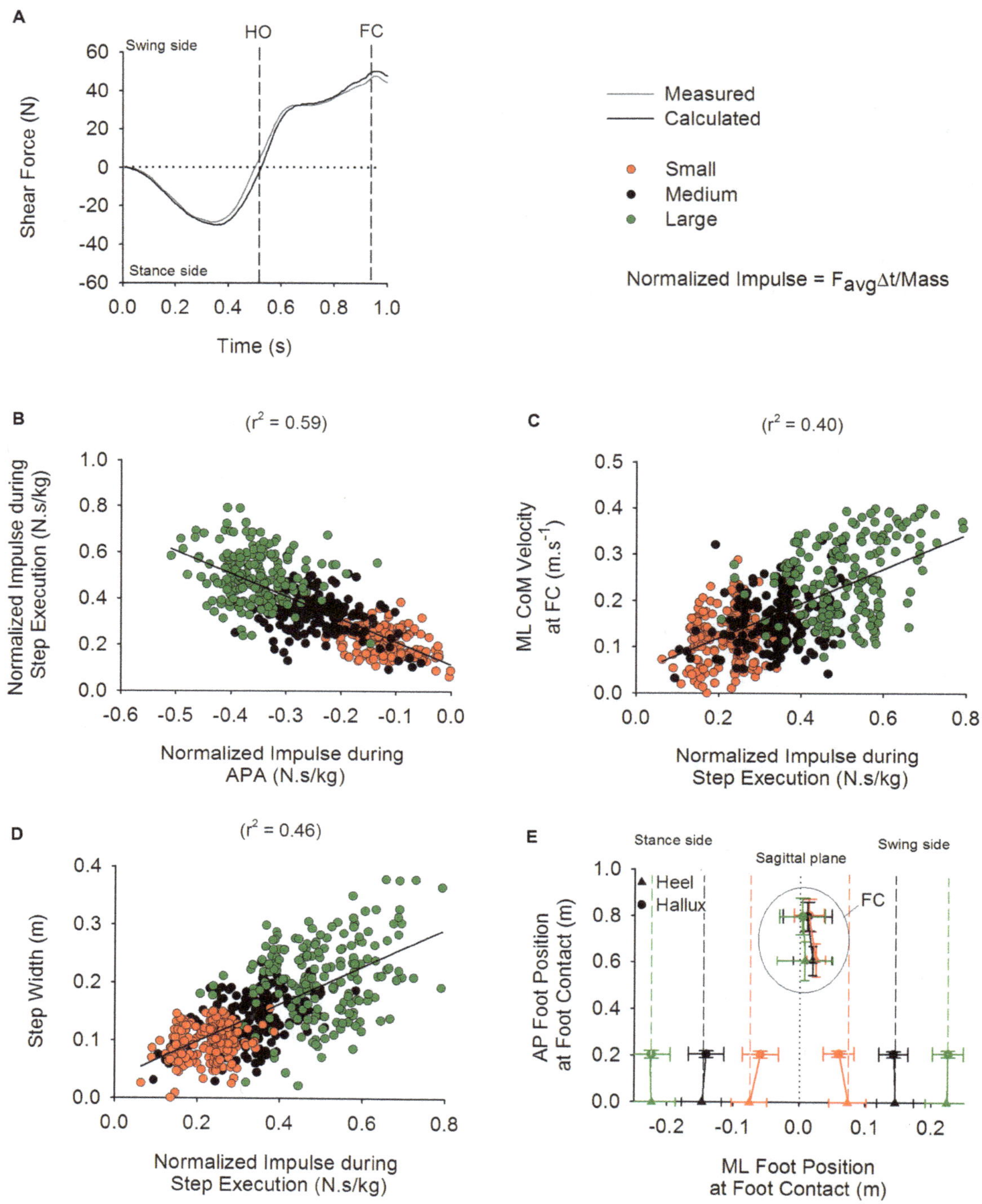

FIGURE 10 | ML disequilibrium torque and step execution parameters. The time-course of the shear force calculated from the disequilibrium torque (black trace) and measured from the platform (gray trace) are shown in panel **(A)** (average of 15 trials). The vertical dashed lines indicate HO and FC events. The negative values during APA indicate that the torque is pushing the body in the direction of the stance side. The positive values during step execution designate that the torque is acting in the direction of the swing leg. Panel **(B)** shows a scatter plot representing a linear relationship between the normalized (divided by mass) impulse calculated during APA and the normalized impulse computed during the step execution ($y = -0.98x + 0.12$). Panel **(C)** shows a scatter plot representing the linear relationship that was found between the normalized impulse during step execution and the instantaneous ML CoM velocity measured at FC ($y = 0.37x + 0.05$). Panel **(D)** shows a scatter plot representing the linear relationship found between the normalized impulse calculated during step execution and step width ($y = 0.32x + 0.03$). Panel **(E)** shows the grand means and standard deviations of the position, with respect to the sagittal plane (dotted line), of the heel and hallux markers in ML and anteroposterior (AP) direction at t0 and at FC in the three conditions. As can be seen, the subjects placed the foot at about the same position and with the same orientation close to the sagittal plane at FC in all three conditions.

Limitations

The initial stance width for each condition (15, 30 and 45 cm) was fixed for all the subjects. Due to anthropometric differences between subjects, a same width of the base of support could provoke different biomechanical constraints on the CoP displacement. Nonetheless, possibly because of the large inter-subject variability, the maximum displacement of the CoP towards the swing leg during APA was not significantly correlated with height or width of the pelvis, measured as the distance between the two anterior superior iliac spines.

Furthermore, the results of this study do not permit to make a quantitative statement about which strategy (hip abduction or stance-leg knee flexion) is mechanically more effective in displacing the CoP towards the swing leg during APA. To do so, in our opinion, this would require the calculation the contribution of the hip abduction and knee flexion torques to the CoP displacement, which is beyond the scope of this current article. One would also consider that different initial stance widths can slightly modify the angle of the tendon insertion between the hip abductors and femur. Therefore, different abduction forces could be generated for the same level of EMG activity, so that comparing EMGs across condition should be done with care.

Final Considerations

Our results support the hypothesis that both hip abduction and stance-leg knee flexion participate in unloading the stance leg and displacing the CoP in the direction of the swing leg during GI. On the one hand, hip abduction is caused by activation of the hip abductors of the swing leg (Carlsöö, 1966; Winter, 1995). On the other hand, stance-leg knee flexion is favored by the activation of TA and silencing of soleus of the same leg. The flexion of the knee during APA could be seen as an adaption of the CNS to facilitate and increase the robustness of the ML balance control process. Consequently, when ML balance control is examined in patients suffering from motor problems during GI, both hip abduction and stance knee flexion should be taken into account, in addition to initial stance width (Goodworth et al., 2014). Knee-flexion control in the frontal plane during APA could be inadequate in patients suffering from gait problems such as cerebral palsy, Parkinson's disease (Hiraoka et al., 2006; Hiraoka and Abe, 2007; Okada et al., 2011a,b; Mazzone et al., 2014), stroke, amputees (Aruin, 2016). For instance, freezing of gait in Parkinsonian patients is associated with knee trembling (Yanagisawa et al., 1991; Ueno et al., 1993; Hausdorff et al., 2003; Schaafsma et al., 2003; Bloem et al., 2004; Moore et al., 2008). Jacobs et al. (2009) found that during GI, knee trembling causes multiple APAs that are observable as a right-left leg loading-unloading cycles. Interestingly, the alternating unloading and loading of the legs was accompanied by similar alternating activation and deactivation of right-left TA (see Figure 2 in Jacobs et al., 2009). Therefore, knee trembling in Parkinson's disease patients might be preventing them from displacing CoM correctly towards the stance leg and thus not allowing them to initiate gait properly. Indeed, the smaller ML CoP displacement during APA and larger step width of the first step at GI have been observed in Parkinson's disease (Okada et al., 2011a,b). This could be in part associated with inappropriate knee flexion. Therefore, correcting the knee flexion angle of the stance leg during APA with a smart orthosis could possibly be an effective solution for enhancing GI and possibly steady-state gait in these patients.

AUTHOR CONTRIBUTIONS

J-LH contributed with project creation, data collection, data analysis and drafted the manuscript. MS contributed with project creation, data analysis. OC contributed in data collection, data analysis. M-CD contributed with project creation and data analysis. All authors discussed the results and participated in the revision of the manuscript.

FUNDING

This study was supported in part by the Ricerca Finalizzata grants (GR-2009-1471033 and RF-2011-02352379) from the Italian Ministry of Health and by the PRIN grants (2009JMMYFZ and 2010MEFNF7) from the Italian Ministry of University.

REFERENCES

Abbruzzese, M., Rubino, V., and Schieppati, M. (1996). Task-dependent effects evoked by foot muscle afferents on leg muscle activity in humans. *Electroencephalogr. Clin. Neurophysiol.* 101, 339–348. doi: 10.1016/0924-980x(96)95682-9

Aruin, A. S. (2016). Enhancing anticipatory postural adjustments: a novel approach to balance rehabilitation. *J. Nov. Physiother.* 6:e144. doi: 10.4172/2165-7025.1000e144

Bauby, C. E., and Kuo, A. D. (2000). Active control of lateral balance in human walking. *J. Biomech.* 33, 1433–1440. doi: 10.1016/s0021-9290(00)00101-9

Bloem, B. R., Hausdorff, J. M., Visser, J. E., and Giladi, N. (2004). Falls and freezing of gait in Parkinson's disease a review of two interconnected, episodic phenomena. *Mov. Disord.* 19, 871–884. doi: 10.1002/mds.20115

Brenière, Y. (2001). Simulation of gait and gait initiation associated with body oscillating behavior in the gravity environment on the moon, mars and Phobos. *Biol. Cybern.* 84, 261–267. doi: 10.1007/s004220000221

Brenière, Y., Cuong, D. M., and Bouisset, S. (1987). Are dynamic phenomena prior to stepping essential to walking? *J. Mot. Behav.* 19, 62–76. doi: 10.1080/00222895.1987.10735400

Brenière, Y., and Do, M. C. (1986). When and how does steady state gait movement induced from upright posture begin? *J. Biomech.* 19, 1035–1040. doi: 10.1016/0021-9290(86)90120-x

Brenière, Y., and Do, M. C. (1991). Control of gait initiation. *J. Mot. Behav.* 23, 235–240. doi: 10.1080/00222895.1991.9942034

Caderby, T., Yiou, E., Peyrot, N., Begon, M., and Dalleau, G. (2014). Influence of gait speed on the control of mediolateral dynamic stability during gait initiation. *J. Biomech.* 47, 417–423. doi: 10.1016/j.jbiomech.2013.11.011

Carlsöö, S. (1966). The initiation of walking. *Acta Anat. (Basel)* 65, 1–9. doi: 10.1159/000142864

Carmines, D. V., and MacMahon, E. B. (1992). Forces and moments on the human leg in the frontal plane during static bipedal stance. *J. Orthop. Res.* 10, 917–925. doi: 10.1002/jor.1100100622

Choi, T. J., Jensen, P., Nielsen, J. B., and Bouyer, L. J. (2016). Error signals driving locomotor adaptation: cutaneous feedback from the foot is used to adapt movement during perturbed walking. *J. Physiol.* doi: 10.1113/jp271996 [Epub ahead of print].

Crenna, P., and Frigo, C. (1991). A motor programme for the initiation of forward-oriented movements in humans. *J. Physiol.* 437, 635–653. doi: 10.1113/jphysiol.1991.sp018616

Daubechies, I., Lu, J., and Wu, H. T. (2011). Synchrosqueezed wavelet transforms: an empirical mode decomposition-like tool. *Appl. Comput. Harmon. Anal.* 30, 243–261. doi: 10.1016/j.acha.2010.08.002

Delafontaine, A., Honeine, J. L., Do, M. C., Gagey, O., and Chong, R. K. (2015). Comparative gait initiation kinematics between simulated unilateral and bilateral ankle hypomobility: does bilateral constraint improve speed performance? *Neurosci Lett.* 603, 55–59. doi: 10.1016/j.neulet.2015.07.016

Do, M. C., and Gilles, M. (1992). Effects of reducing plantar support on anticipatory postural and intentional activities associated with flexion of the lower limb. *Neurosci. Lett.* 148, 181–184. doi: 10.1016/0304-3940(92)90834-t

Elble, R. J., Moody, C., Leffler, K., and Sinha, R. (1994). The initiation of normal walking. *Mov. Disord.* 9, 139–146. doi: 10.1002/mds.870090203

Freeman, M. A. R., Aubriot, J. H., Bryan, R. S., Charnley, J., Coventry, M. B., and Currey, H. L. F., et al. (1980). *Arthritis of the Knee: Clinical Features and Surgical Management.* Berlin, Heidelberg, New York: Springer-Verlag.

Goldberg, S. R., Anderson, F. C., Pandy, M. G., and Delp, S. L. (2004). Muscles that influence knee flexion velocity in double support: implications for stiff-knee gait. *J Biomech.* 37, 1189–1196. doi: 10.1016/j.jbiomech.2003.12.005

Goodworth, A. D., Mellodge, P., and Peterka, R. J. (2014). Stance width changes how sensory feedback is used for multisegmental balance control. *J. Neurophysiol.* 112, 525–542. doi: 10.1152/jn.00490.2013

Hausdorff, J. M., Balash, Y., and Giladi, N. (2003). Time series analysis of leg movements during freezing of gait in Parkinson's disease: akinesia, rhyme or reason? *Physica A Stat. Mech. Appl.* 321, 565–570.doi: 10.1016/s0378-4371(02)01744-2

Hiraoka, K., and Abe, K. (2007). Cortical and spinal control of ankle joint muscles before and during gait initiation. *Somatosens. Mot. Res.* 24, 127–133. doi: 10.1080/10425170701550615

Hiraoka, K., Hatanaka, R., Nikaido, Y., Jono, Y., Nomura, Y., Tani, K., et al. (2014). Asymmetry of anticipatory postural adjustment during gait initiation. *J. Hum. Kinet.* 42, 7–14. doi: 10.2478/hukin-2014-0056

Hiraoka, K., Matuo, Y., Iwata, A., Onishi, T., and Abe, K. (2006). The effects of external cues on ankle control during gait initiation in Parkinson's disease. *Parkinsonism Relat. Disord.* 12, 97–102. doi: 10.1016/j.parkreldis.2005.07.006

Honeine, J. L., Schieppati, M., Gagey, O., and Do, M. C. (2013). The functional role of the triceps surae muscle during human locomotion. *PLoS One* 8:e52943. doi: 10.1371/journal.pone.0052943

Honeine, J. L., Schieppati, M., Gagey, O., and Do, M. C. (2014). By counteracting gravity, triceps surae sets both kinematics and kinetics of gait. *Physiol. Rep.* 2:e00229. doi: 10.1002/phy2.229

Iatsenko, D., McClintock, P. V. E., and Stefanovska, A. (2015). Linear and synchrosqueezed time-frequency representations revisited: overview, standards of use, resolution, reconstruction, concentration and algorithms. *Digit. Signal Process.* 42, 1–26. doi: 10.1016/j.dsp.2015.03.004

Jacobs, J. V., Nutt, J. G., Carlson-Kuhta, P., Stephens, M., and Horak, F. B. (2009). Knee trembling during freezing of gait represents multiple anticipatory postural adjustments. *Exp. Neurol.* 215, 334–341. doi: 10.1016/j.expneurol.2008.10.019

Jian, Y., Winter, D. A., Ishac, M. G., and Gilchrist, L. (1993). Trajectory of the body COG and COP during initiation and termination of gait. *Gait Posture* 1, 9–22. doi: 10.1016/0966-6362(93)90038-3

Lajoie, Y., Teasdale, N., Bard, C., and Fleury, M. (1993). Attentional demands for static and dynamic equilibrium. *Exp. Brain Res.* 97, 139–144. doi: 10.1007/bf00228824

Lepers, R., and Brenière, Y. (1995). The role of anticipatory postural adjustments and gravity in gait initiation. *Exp. Brain. Res.* 107, 118–124. doi: 10.1007/bf00228023

Liu, M. Q., Anderson, F. C., Schwartz, M. H., and Delp, S. L. (2008). Muscle contributions to support and progression over a range of walking speeds. *J. Biomech.* 41, 3243–3452. doi: 10.1016/j.jbiomech.2008.07.031

Lyon, I. N., and Day, B. L. (1997). Control of frontal plane body motion in human stepping. *Exp. Brain Res.* 115, 345–356. doi: 10.1007/pl00005703

Lyon, I. N., and Day, B. L. (2005). Predictive control of body mass trajectory in a two-step sequence. *Exp. Brain Res.* 161, 193–200. doi: 10.1007/s00221-004-2058-z

MacKinnon, C. D., and Winter, D. A. (1993). Control of whole body balance in the frontal plane during human walking. *J. Biomech.* 26, 633–644. doi: 10.1016/0021-9290(93)90027-c

Mazzaro, N., Grey, M. J., Sinkjaer, T., Andersen, J. B., Pareyson, D., and Schieppati, M. (2005). Lack of on-going adaptations in the soleus muscle activity during walking in patients affected by large-fiber neuropathy. *J. Neurophysiol.* 93, 3075–3085. doi: 10.1152/jn.01071.2004

Mazzone, P., Paoloni, M., Mangone, M., Santilli, V., Insola, A., Fini, M., et al. (2014). Unilateral deep brain stimulation of the pedunculopontine tegmental nucleus in idiopathic Parkinson's disease: effects on gait initiation and performance. *Gait Posture* 40, 357–362. doi: 10.1016/j.gaitpost.2014.05.002

McIlroy, W. E., and Maki, B. E. (1999). The control of lateral stability during rapid stepping reactions evoked by antero-posterior perturbation: does anticipatory control play a role? *Gait Posture* 9, 190–198. doi: 10.1016/s0966-6362(99)00013-2

Merletti, M., and Hermens, H. (2000). Introduction to the special issue on the SENIAM European Concerted Action. *J. Electromyogr. Kinesiol.* 10, 283–286. doi: 10.1016/s1050-6411(00)00019-5

Michel, V., and Do, M. C. (2002). Are stance ankle plantar flexor muscles necessary to generate propulsive force during human gait initiation? *Neurosci. Lett.* 325, 139–143. doi: 10.1016/s0304-3940(02)00255-0

Moore, S. T., MacDougall, H. G., and Ondo, W. G. (2008). Ambulatory monitoring of freezing of gait in Parkinson's disease. *J. Neurosci. Methods* 167, 340–348. doi: 10.1016/j.jneumeth.2007.08.023

Nardone, A., Corna, S., Turcato, A. M., and Schieppati, M. (2014). Afferent control of walking: are there distinct deficits associated to loss of fibres of different diameter? *Clin. Neurophysiol.* 125, 327–335. doi: 10.1016/j.clinph.2013.07.007

Okada, Y., Fukumoto, T., Takatori, K., Nagino, K., and Hiraoka, K. (2011a). Abnormalities of the first three steps of gait initiation in patients with Parkinson's disease with freezing of gait. *Parkinsons Dis.* 2011:202937. doi: 10.4061/2011/202937

Okada, Y., Fukumoto, T., Takatori, K., Nagino, K., and Hiraoka, K. (2011b). Variable initial swing side and prolonged double limb support represent abnormalities of the first three steps of gait initiation in patients with Parkinson's disease with freezing of gait. *Front. Neurol.* 2:85. doi: 10.3389/fneur.2011.00085

Orendurff, M. S., Segal, A. D., Klute, G. K., Berge, J. S., Rohr, E. S., and Kadel, N. J. (2004). The effect of walking speed on center of mass displacement. *J. Rehabil. Res. Dev.* 41, 829–834. doi: 10.1682/jrrd.2003.10.0150

Queralt, A., Valls-Solé, J., and Castellote, J. M. (2010). Speeding up gait initiation and gait-pattern with a startling stimulus. *Gait Posture* 31, 185–190. doi: 10.1016/j.gaitpost.2009.10.003

Riskowski, J. L. (2010). Gait and neuromuscular adaptations after using a feedback-based gait monitoring knee brace. *Gait Posture* 32, 242–247. doi: 10.1016/j.gaitpost.2010.05.002

Riskowski, J. L., Mikesky, A. E., Bahamonde, R. E., Alvey, T. V. III, and Burr, D. B. (2005). Proprioception, gait kinematics and rate of loading during walking: are they related? *J. Musculoskelet. Neuronal Interact.* 5, 379–387.

Schaafsma, J. D., Balash, Y., Gurevich, T., Bartels, A. L., Hausdorff, J. M., and Giladi, N. (2003). Characterization of freezing of gait subtypes and the response of each to levodopa in Parkinson's disease. *Eur. J. Neurol.* 10, 391–398. doi: 10.1046/j.1468-1331.2003.00611.x

Segal, A. D., Orendurff, M. S., Klute, G. K., McDowell, M. L., Pecoraro, J. A., Shofer, J., et al. (2006). Kinematic and kinetic comparisons of transfemoral amputee gait using C-Leg and Mauch SNS prosthetic knees. *J. Rehabil. Res. Dev.* 43, 857–870. doi: 10.1682/jrrd.2005.09.0147

Shamaei, K., Sawicki, G. S., and Dollar, A. M. (2013). Estimation of quasi-stiffness of the human knee in the stance phase of walking. *PLoS One* 8:e59993. doi: 10.1371/journal.pone.0059993

Sozzi, S., Honeine, J. L., Do, M. C., and Schieppati, M. (2013). Leg muscle activity during tandem stance and the control of body balance in the frontal plane. *Clin. Neurophysiol.* 124, 1175–1186. doi: 10.1016/j.clinph.2012.12.001

Thorstensson, A., Nilsson, J., Carlson, H., and Zomlefer, M. R. (1984). Trunk movements in human locomotion. *Acta Physiol. Scand.* 121, 9–22. doi: 10.1111/j.1748-1716.1984.tb10452.x

Ueno, E., Yanagisawa, N., and Takami, M. (1993). Gait disorders in parkinsonism. A study with floor reaction forces and EMG. *Adv. Neurol.* 60, 414–418.

Walker, P. S., and Erkman, M. J. (1975). The role of the menisci in force transmission across the knee. *Clin. Orthop. Relat. Res.* 109, 184–192. doi: 10.1097/00003086-197506000-00027

Wang, Y., and Srinivasan, M. (2014). Stepping in the direction of the fall: the next foot placement can be predicted from current upper body state in steady-state walking. *Biol. Lett.* 10:20140405. doi: 10.1098/rsbl.2014.0405

Winter, D. A. (1993). *Biomechanics and Motor Control of Human Movement.* Toronto, ON: Wiley Interscience.

Winter, D. (1995). Human balance and posture control during standing and walking. *Gait Posture* 3, 193–214. doi: 10.1016/0966-6362(96)82849-9

Woodhull, A. M., Maltrud, K., and Mello, B. L. (1985). Alignment of the human body in standing. *Eur. J. Appl. Physiol. Occup. Physiol.* 54, 109–115. doi: 10.1007/bf00426309

Yanagisawa, N., Ueno, E., and Takami, M. (1991). "Frozen gait of Parkinson's disease and parkinsonism. A study with floor reaction forces and EMG," in *Neurobiological Basis of Human Locomotion*, eds M. Shimamura, S. Grillner and V. R. Edgerton (Tokyo: Japan Scientific Societies Press), 291–304.

Zajac, F. E., and Gordon, M. E. (1989). Determining muscle's force and action in multi-articular movement. *Exerc. Sport Sci. Rev.* 17, 187–230. doi: 10.1249/00003677-198900170-00009

3

The Organization and Control of Intra-Limb Anticipatory Postural Adjustments and their Role in Movement Performance

Paolo Cavallari, Francesco Bolzoni, Carlo Bruttini and Roberto Esposti*

Human Motor Control and Posture Lab, Section Human Physiology of the Department of Pathophysiology and Transplantation, Università degli Studi di Milano, Milan, Italy

Correspondence:
Paolo Cavallari
paolo.cavallari@unimi.it

Anticipatory Postural Adjustments (APAs) are commonly described as unconscious muscular activities aimed to counterbalance the perturbation caused by the primary movement, so as to ensure the whole-body balance, as well as contributing to initiate the displacement of the body center of mass when starting gait or whole-body reaching movements. These activities usually create one or more fixation chains which spread over several muscles of different limbs, and may be thus called *inter-limb APAs*. However, it has been reported that APAs also precede voluntary movements involving tiny masses, like a flexion/extension of the wrist or even a brisk flexion of the index-finger. In particular, such movements are preceded by an *intra-limb* APA chain, that involves muscles acting on the proximal joints. Considering the small mass of the moving segments, it is unlikely that the ensuing perturbation could threaten the whole-body balance, so that it is interesting to enquire the physiological role of *intra-limb* APAs and their organization and control compared to *inter-limb* APAs. This review is focused on *intra-limb* APAs and highlights a strict correspondence in their behavior and temporal/spatial organization with respect to *inter-limb* APAs. Hence it is suggested that both are manifestations of the same phenomenon. Particular emphasis is given to *intra-limb* APAs preceding index-finger flexion, because their relatively simple biomechanics and the fact that muscular actions were limited to a single arm allowed peculiar investigations, leading to important conclusions. Indeed, such paradigm provided evidence that by granting a proper fixation of those body segments proximal to the moving one APAs are involved in refining movement precision, and also that APAs and prime mover activation are driven by a shared motor command.

Keywords: intra-limb APAs, precision, motor control, postural control, posturo-focal integration, human

INTRODUCTION

Anticipatory Postural Adjustments (APAs) are commonly described as unconscious muscular activities aiming to maintain the equilibrium of the whole body during various voluntary motor performances (for a review see Massion, 1992; Bouisset and Do, 2008), but they are also known to contribute to initiate the displacement of the body center of mass when starting gait (Brenière et al., 1987) or whole body reaching movements (Stapley et al., 1998, 1999).

However, the importance of APAs is also apparent when considering motion of one single limb (e.g., Belen'kii et al., 1967 for the upper limb; Alexeief and Naidel, 1972 for the lower limb). In the latter context, the main goal of APAs is to minimize the changes in the body center of mass, in order to keep its projection within the support area, and to counteract the self-initiated postural perturbation. These APAs usually spread over several muscles of different limbs, creating one or more fixation chains. For this reason they may be called *inter-limb APA*.

The role of APAs may look less obvious when considering a movement involving little masses, which are not supposed to threaten the whole body postural stability. In this regard, Aoki (1991) reported a pattern of muscular activity in various arm muscles about 50–60 ms before a rapid wrist movement, and showed that this activity is distributed according to the direction of the movement in space. Moreover, Caronni and Cavallari (2009a) found that during index-finger tapping, in which the moving mass is even smaller, an anticipatory postural chain develops in several upper-limb and trunk muscles. These activities, named *intra-limb APAs* since they are distributed to muscles of the same limb in which the movement occurs, precede the onset of the voluntary movement, are polarized according to the task direction in space and adapt to changes in the postural requirement of the task. In other words, they share the same behavioral properties of *inter-limb APA*, as it will be shown as the *first topic* of the present review.

Nevertheless, it is difficult to envisage a postural role for *intra-limb APAs* in the common sense of its acceptation, i.e., preserving the whole body equilibrium or counteracting a self-initiated perturbation that could threaten the body posture. This *intra-limb* APA pattern seems in fact organized so as to preserve the *local equilibrium* of the limb, which, in a behavioral perspective represents a basic requirement for performing precise movements. The involvement of *intra-limb* APAs in setting movement precision will be treated as the *second topic.*

Moreover, the *finger tap* experimental model allowed us to disclose some key aspects of the central organization of voluntary movement and postural actions, aspects that would hardly be revealed by using the classical *whole body* experimental paradigm. Thus, the *last topic* of this review will be about the organization of voluntary and postural actions, either as two different central commands (a focal and a postural component), as classically proposed (Babinski, 1899; Thomas, 1940; Hess, 1943; Gelfand et al., 1966; Cordo and Nashner, 1982; Brown and Frank, 1987) or as a unique motor command as suggested by more recent evidences (Aruin and Latash, 1995; Caronni and Cavallari, 2009b; Petersen et al., 2009; Leonard et al., 2011).

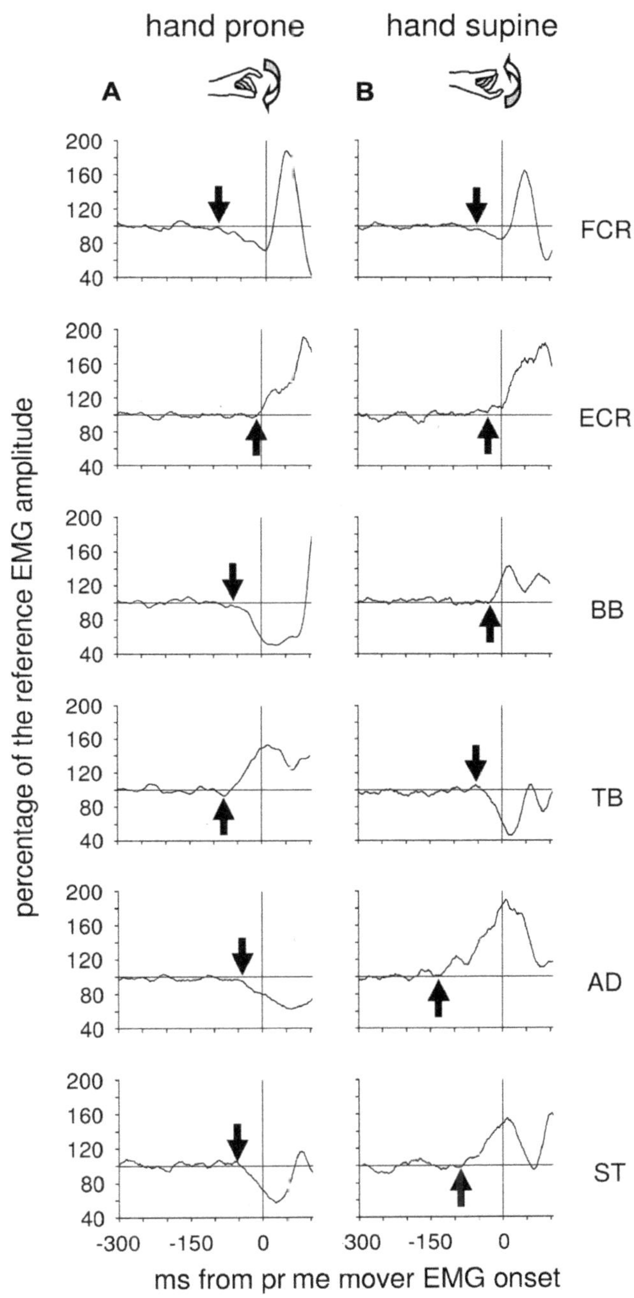

FIGURE 1 | Postural adjustments in upper-limb muscles preceding an index-finger tap with the prone or supine hand. Each graph displays the Anticipatory Postural Adjustments (APA) onset (arrow) and its development on the tonic EMG from different postural muscles of a single representative subject, with the hand resting prone **(A)** or supine **(B)**. Postural muscles: flexor carpi radialis (FCR), extensor carpi radialis (ECR), biceps brachii (BB), triceps brachii (TB), anterior deltoid (AD), superior trapezius (ST). The vertical line at 0 ms marks the onset of the prime mover activity. Note that in the muscles acting at the elbow, the shoulder and the trunk APAs reverts in sign when hand posture changes from prone to supine. EMG is rectified, integrated and averaged (75 trials) and its size expressed in percentage of the mean EMG level recorded 1 s before the go signal.

Brief Historical Background on Posture and Voluntary Movement

To the best of our knowledge, the first to describe the rules governing postural and voluntary movement control was Leonardo da Vinci (1452–1519), in his *Libro A, Trattato della Pittura*, which is now conserved within the *Codex Urbinas*

Latinus. Leonardo wrote: "*I say that if a motionless figure is poised on his feet, and his arm is extended in front of the chest, he will throw backward as much natural weight as the natural and accidental weight which he thrusts forward. And I say the same of each part that projects more than usual beyond the whole*". Moreover, Leonardo stated: "*Never will a weight be lifted and carried by a man, without his extending outside himself more than as much weight as that which he wishes to lift, and he thrust it on the side opposite the one where he lifts the weight*". A couple of centuries later, Giovanni Alfonso Borrelli (1608–1679) followed the pathway of Leonardo in his *De Motu Animalium*, where he described some principles that govern the voluntary movement. In particular, Borelli considered the skeleton as multi-linked system of levers, which can maintain the body balance as long as the center of mass falls within the support base.

After the observation of Leonardo da Vinci and Giovanni Borelli, we had to wait until the end of the 19th century to first clinically observe the importance of correct postural tailoring during voluntary movements in order to execute a successful motor act. Joseph Babinski (1857–1932), in his *De l'asynergie cérebelleuse*, first described the lack of harmonious synergies in cerebellar patients; in particular, he observed the forward displacement of the knees and hips to compensate for the backward displacement of the trunk, neck and head when asking a subject to look upward. Babinski also observed that cerebellar patients, who were asked to perform the same *looking upward* task, were unable to coordinate the upper part of their body to their hip and lower limb, so that they usually fell. However, Babinski did not analyze the temporal relationship between the postural adjustments and the voluntary movement, and therefore he lacked to observe that also an anticipatory postural control, adjusted in a feed-forward manner, is needed when performing a voluntary movement.

In the 20th century, studies about the relationship between posture and voluntary movement stood on the shoulders of three giants of movement physiology: Charles Sherrington (1857–1952, Nobel Prize 1932), Walter Hess (1881–1973, Nobel Prize 1949) and Nikolai Bernstein (1896–1966, Stalin Prize for Science 1948). Sherrington sustained the idea of a dual coordinated control system: one for movement and one for posture. This idea was in agreement with the proposals of Hess, who held the view that without anticipation of postural adaptations (a component of his ereismatic-supporting function system), goal-directed movements were doomed to failure. On the other hand, Bernstein was the first to propose a unique motor command for both posture and voluntary movement: "*movements are not chains of details but structures which are differentiated into details; they are structurally whole*" (Bernstein, 1967). However his ideas did not reach western scientists until several years after his death since his articles and books were only recently translated into English.

SHARED BEHAVIORAL PROPERTIES OF INTER AND INTRA-LIMB APAs

This review deals with *intra-limb* APA, since many other reviews (see "Introduction" Section) have been already devoted to all the features characterizing *inter-limb* APAs. However, it is important to briefly recall (see "Inter-Limb APAs" Section) those specific aspects of *inter-limb* APAs which can be directly compared with *intra-limb* APAs. All other features, like the effects of development, aging and fatigue, extensively studied in *inter-* but not in *intra-limb* APAs, have been thus omitted.

With regard to literature selection, this is a narrative more than a systematic meta-analysis review because in the last decade the *intra-limb* APAs has been mainly treated by our research group (for older studies see "Intra-Limb APAs" Section). However, to avoid missing important literature, *Pubmed®* and *Web of Science®* databases were inquired, by searching for *APAs* or *Anticipatory Postural Action(s)* and verifying item by item whether it was dealing with *inter-* and/or *intra-limb* APAs.

Inter-Limb APAs

These are the most frequently studied APAs. For example, when we intend to move a segment of the upper or the lower limb, a chain of muscular actions develops from that moving segment to the nearest fixation point. These actions precede the primary movement (in the range of tenths ms) and in many cases also the prime mover recruitment, the larger advance being observed in the muscles acting near the fixation point.

These *inter-limb* APAs have been documented for various movements such as: shoulder flexion and extension (Belen'kii et al., 1967; Lee, 1980; Clément et al., 1984; Horak et al., 1984; Bouisset and Zattara, 1987; Maki, 1993 in adults; Riach and Hayes, 1990 in children), shoulder lateral abduction (Aruin and Latash, 1995; Vernazza et al., 1996), elbow flexion (Friedli et al., 1984) and similar movements of the lower limb (Rogers and Pai, 1990; Do et al., 1991; Mouchnino et al., 1991; Nouillot et al., 1992). APAs also accompany movement involving the trunk, when bending it (Oddsson and Thorstensson, 1986; Crenna et al., 1987; Pedotti et al., 1989), during whole body reaching (Stapley et al., 1998), rising up on tiptoe (Houtz and Fischer, 1961; Lipshits et al., 1981; Nardone and Schieppati, 1988) and rocking on the heels (Nardone and Schieppati, 1988). In some experimental situations, it was asked to push or pull a handle with the upper limb, both in normal subjects (Cordo and Nashner, 1982; Lee et al., 1987) and in patients with Parkinson disease (Dick et al., 1986). *Inter-limb APAs* are also associated with movements involving a bimanual load-lifting task, when participants hold an object in one hand and the object is voluntarily lifted by the same person (active lifting) or by an experimenter (passive lifting). In the first case, the voluntary activation of the lifting hand is synchronous with an inhibitory APA in the contralateral biceps brachii (BB), thus avoiding an uncontrolled flexion of the elbow (Hugon et al., 1982) and preserving the upper limb posture. On the contrary, when the object is unexpectedly lifted by the experimenter, the BB inhibition starts about 50 ms after the unloading, showing that is it should have a reflex origin (postural reflex). The described experiment, known as "*the barman task*" allowed to make two conclusions: first, even a movement that does not lead to a whole body imbalance is preceded by APAs, aimed at preserving the single segment's

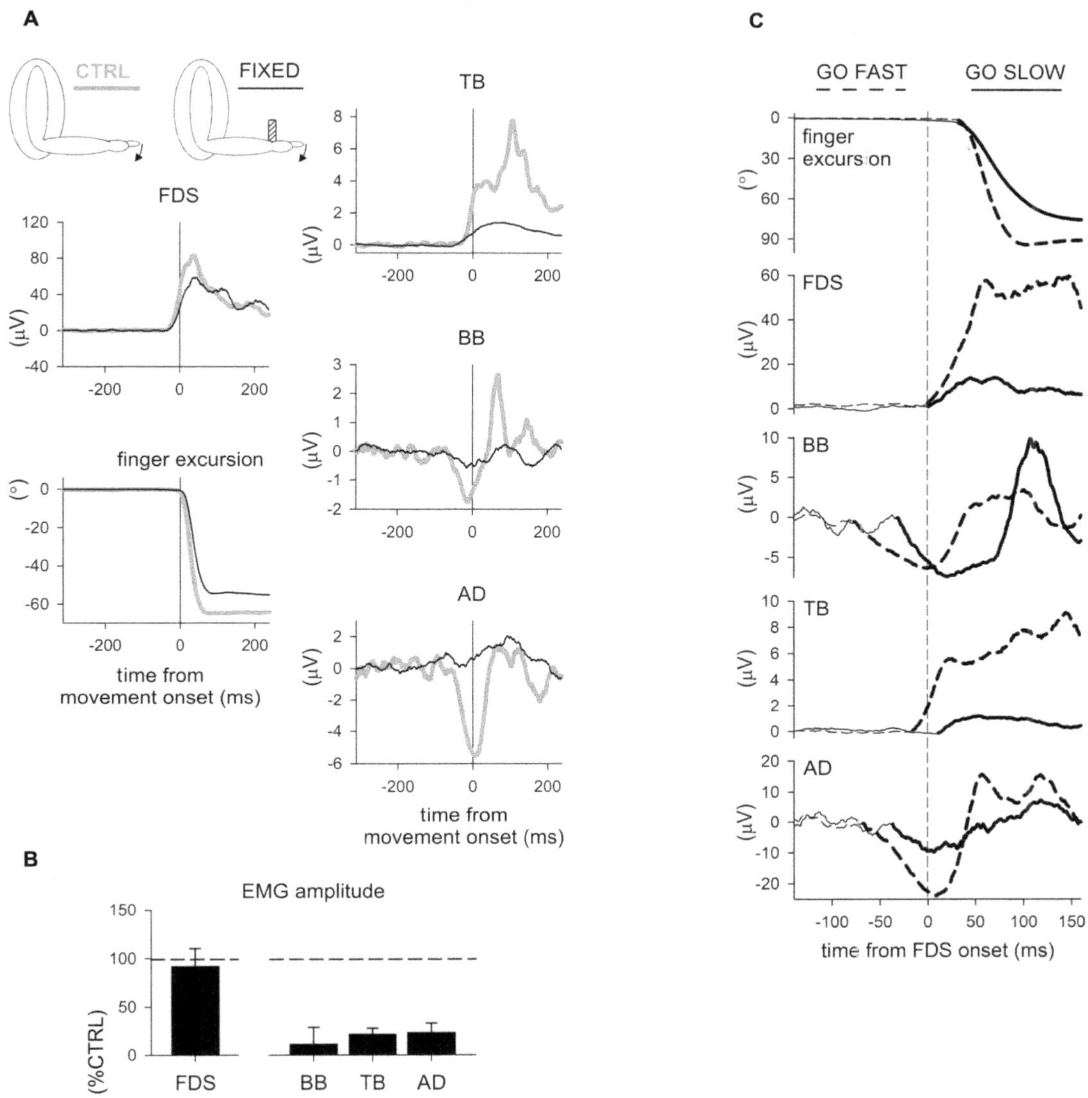

FIGURE 2 | Effects of fixation point and movement velocity on APAs. (A) Recordings of EMG activity in index-finger prime mover and intra-limb APAs in a representative subject, with or without a wrist fixation point. It is evident that both the EMG activity in the prime mover flexor digitorum superficialis (FDS) and the finger movement were comparable both with (FIXED, black) and without (CTRL, gray) the wrist fixation point, while in the FIXED condition APAs were deeply reduced in BB and TB and completely abolished in AD. **(B)** Mean amplitude of pre-movement FDS EMG and of APAs in BB, TB and AD. Values in % of the control sequence (CTRL). A *t*-test showed no CTRL vs. FIXED difference in FDS activation ($t_6 = 0.44$, $p = 0.67$). The average inhibitory effects on BB and AD and excitation in TB revealed a significant reduction in the FIXED condition ($t_6 = 5.01$, $p = 0.002$; $t_6 = 12.41$, $p < 0.0001$; $t_6 = 7.80$, $p = 0.0002$, respectively). *Reproduced from Bruttini et al. (2014), © Springer-Verlag Berlin Heidelberg 2014, with permission of Springer.* **(C)** Go-fast and go-slow movements in a representative subject. Goniometric recording of the index-finger flexion (top panel) and rectified and integrated (25 ms) EMG from the prime mover FDS and from BB, TB and AD. Note that when moving as fast as possible (GO FAST, dashed traces) the prime mover onset was preceded by APAs in BB, TB and AD. APAs (emboldened) were instead clearly delayed when moving at ~50% of maximal speed (GO SLOW, solid traces). Time 0 (vertical dashed line) refers to prime mover EMG onset. *Reproduced from Esposti et al. (2015).*

balance. Second, APAs may develop also in muscles that are not usually considered as *postural muscles*, such as muscles in the upper-limb. Moreover, since the degree of elbow rotation was shown to be lower when the subject unloaded the forearm by himself, the APA mechanism showed a greater efficacy in limb stabilization vs. the reflex mechanisms. The involvement of APAs in controlling the segmental stability was also confirmed for movements affecting the whole body balance (Patla et al., 2002).

Classically, APAs are known to be tuned depending on several kinematic aspects of the primary movement; specifically, the amplitude (Aruin and Shiratori, 2004), the speed

(Horak et al., 1984; Shiratori and Aruin, 2007), the movement direction (Aruin and Latash, 1995; Pozzo et al., 2002) and also the mass of the moving segment (Friedli et al., 1984). Moreover, an increase of APAs was shown when the voluntary movement was performed against resistance (Baldissera et al., 2008).

In addition, the CNS is able to adapt *inter-limb APAs* to changes in the postural demand of the motor task (Belen'kii et al., 1967; Cordo and Nashner, 1982; Aruin and Shiratori, 2004; Shiratori and Aruin, 2007). Clear signs of this adaptative process have been observed even after the very first movement trial (Hall et al., 2010), although they usually develop within few movement repetitions.

Another feature of the APAs is that they overtly develop in those muscles which connect the moving segment(s) to the nearest fixation point (Belen'kii et al., 1967; Marsden et al., 1981; Cordo and Nashner, 1982; for a review see Massion, 1992), while they are correctly shaped, but kept subthreshold, in those muscles in which their action is useless (Baldissera et al., 2002). An indirect issue which is strictly correlated to the above observations is that APAs conform to the adequacy of the fixation point, being smaller and smaller or even disappearing when the fixation point does not guarantee the full discharge of the perturbation (Brenière et al., 1987 balance during locomotion; Nouillot et al., 1992 balance during unipedal stance; Dietz and Colombo, 1996 balance in water; Esposti and Baldissera, 2011 balance with two fixation chains).

Intra-Limb APAs

As explained in the introduction, *intra-limb APAs* are those distributed to muscles of the same limb in which the movement occurs. The first evidence of such APAs dates to 1963, when Hopf and Hufschmidt (1963) observed that the anterior deltoid (AD) activity preceded the voluntary recruitment of BB driving elbow flexion. Later on, Aoki (1991) reported that wrist flexions, performed with the hand prone or supine, were accompanied by APAs in muscles acting at the elbow and that these APAs reverted their pattern in relation to the direction of the movement. In this regard, Chabran et al. (2001), observed also that when providing a support to the elbow the level of postural activity in shoulder muscles was deeply depressed, but the *intra-limb* APAs chronology remained unaffected. Examples of intra-limb APAs were also reported for shoulder and elbow movements by Almeida et al. (1995) and by Gribble and Ostry (1999).

More recently, Caronni and Cavallari (2009a,b) also reported that when only the index-finger is flexed, an APA chain develops in several upper-limb muscles to stabilize the *segmental* equilibrium of the arm. Indeed, these authors described that with the hand prone a brisk finger flexion was preceded by an excitatory burst in Extensor Carpi Radialis (ECR), Triceps Brachii (TB) and Superior Trapezius (ST), while Flexor Carpi Radialis (FCR), BB and AD showed a concomitant inhibition of their tonic activity (**Figure 1A**). The ECR-FCR coupled

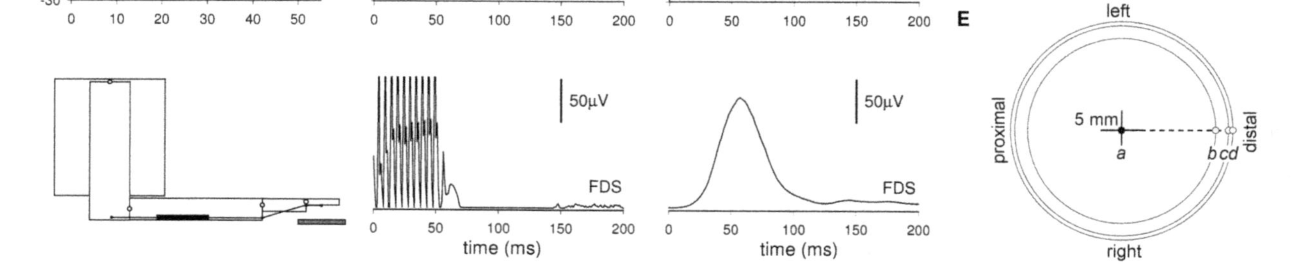

FIGURE 3 | Comparison of arm joint kinematics during a simulated, an *in vivo* evoked and a voluntary finger flexion. Time course of a finger flexion at the metacarpophalangeal (*MP*) joint, and the related changes at wrist (*W*) and elbow (*E*) level, measured in an arm mechanical model (bottom-left inset) when the proximal segments were free to rotate (**A**, dashed lines) or when they were immobilized (**A**, solid lines), so as to produce fictive APAs. Angular displacements of the three joints were also recorded when an index-finger tap was passively evoked *in vivo* by electrical stimulation of the median nerve **(B)** and when it was voluntary performed **(C)** Rectified EMG activity of prime mover FDS in the two lower graphs. Note that the mechanical model well predicts the displacements of the proximal joints both during voluntary (solid lines) and evoked (dashed lines) index-finger tap. Panel **(D)** illustrates the simulated fingertip trajectory when the proximal segments were immobilized (filled circles, fictive APAs), and when they were free to rotate (empty circles). Note that for a vertical displacement of 65 mm, the fingertip hits the table surface (dashed line) more proximally with fictive APAs (*a*) then without them (*d*). Dots *c* and *b* mark the hitting position when the fictive APAs were restrained to the sole shoulder or to shoulder plus elbow, respectively. In the planar graph **(E)** the filled circle is the univocal target position theoretically resulting from a fully expressed APA control. Any disturbance of the APA chain would necessarily lead to impact any other point.

activities were appropriate for contrasting the by-product wrist flexion torque due to the voluntary contraction of the index-finger flexors. At the same time, the TB-BB and ST-AD actions contrasted the elbow and shoulder flexion torques produced by the upward perturbation that the index-finger flexion discharged on the metacarpophalangeal (MP) joint. Interestingly, when the hand posture was changed from prone to supine (**Figure 1B**), the APA pattern reverted in sign in the elbow and shoulder muscles but not in ECR and FCR. This is consistent with the fact that in this condition the perturbation produced on the MP joint was inverted, i.e., downward, but the by-product of recruiting the index-finger flexors was again a wrist flexion torque. These observations witness that APAs are versatile enough to adapt to the mechanical requirements of the postural context. Another proof that *intra-limb* APAs adapt to changes in the postural context within few trials comes from Bruttini et al. (2014) who illustrated that when tapping with the right index-finger, *intra-limb* APAs were deeply reduced (**Figures 2A,B**) if the right forearm was fixated at the wrist, i.e., closer to the voluntary moving segment. Moreover, Esposti et al. (2015) confirmed that also the *intra-limb* APAs adapt to changes in movement speed (**Figure 2C**).

In conclusion, *intra-limb* and *inter-limb* APAs seem to share similar control mechanisms. Indeed, both of them: (1) are distributed to several muscles creating a postural chain aiming to prevent the effects of the interaction torques generated by the voluntary movement; (2) revert in sign when movement direction is reverted; and (3) adapt to changes of the postural context within few trials of movement repetition. Thus, the central nervous system seems to use the same organization of the motor command for controlling both the segmental and the whole-body posture.

APA AND PRECISION

The idea that the precision of a voluntary movement relies on proper APAs was first proposed in relation to *inter-limb* APAs. When pointing toward targets of different sizes, it has been shown that APAs decreased in size as the accuracy demand increased, i.e., when pointing smaller and smaller targets. This feature has been shown both in the upper-limb

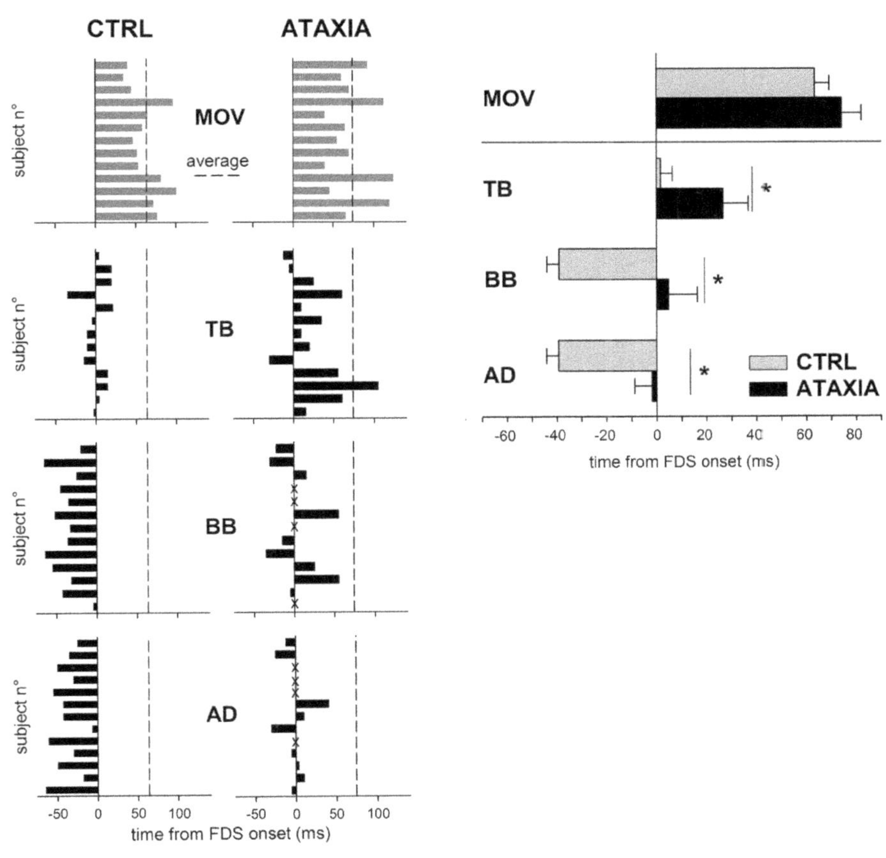

FIGURE 4 | Comparison of the APA chain in healthy (CTRL) and in cerebellar (ATAXIA) subjects. Latencies of finger flexion (MOV) and APA onsets in TB, BB and AD are plotted with respect to the onset of FDS, prime mover. Each single subject is represented. Dashed line marks the average movement latency for either group of subjects. Note that in ATAXIA APAs are delayed or, in some cases absent (marked with X). The right panel shows mean latency (± SE) of the onset of finger flexion and APAs. Asterisks mark significant differences found by the unpaired *t*-test.

(Bonnetblanc et al., 2004; Nana-Ibrahim et al., 2008) and in the lower-limb (Bertucco and Cesari, 2010). Lower limb pointing was also investigated by Duarte and Latash (2007), which have shown that as movement velocity increased, so did APA variability. The relation between movement speed and scattering of the final position around a target was also well described (Schmidt et al., 1979; Fernandez and Bootsma, 2004). All these observations suggest that small and less variable APAs should accompany slow but precise movements. Finally, Berrigan et al. (2006) reported that when pointing is performed towards small targets (i.e., under high accuracy constraints) from an unstable position (i.e., standing vs. sitting), slowing movement speed represents a strategy to reduce the equilibrium disturbance and the associated APAs. However, the above results might simply be an outcome of the relationship between APAs and intended movement speed (Shiratori and Aruin, 2007; Esposti et al., 2015), given the well known inverse relation (Fitts, 1954 law) between target width and movement speed. In order to get rid of such possible bias, Caronni et al. (2013) studied *inter-limb* APAs during an upper limb pointing movement toward a target of fixed dimension, while wearing (or not) prismatic lenses, which shift the binocular eye field and make the subject to miss the target (Redding et al., 2005). Caronni et al. (2013) observed that the focal movement had similar kinematics in the two conditions, but after donning or doffing the lenses appreciable pointing errors occurred. Moreover, when committing such errors, APAs in the lower limb were out of proportion with respect to the recruitment of the upper limb prime mover.

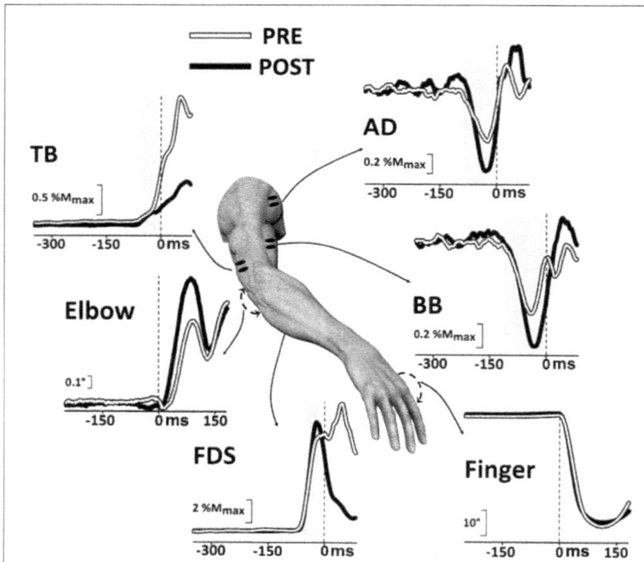

FIGURE 5 | Intra-limb APAs change after short-term immobilization. Average recordings in a representative subject before (PRE, white) and after (POST, black) immobilization. When rapidly flexing the index-finger (prime mover FDS), the arm equilibrium is preserved thanks to APAs (shaded area), which are excitatory in TB and inhibitory in BB and AD. After a 12-h immobilization of the wrist and fingers, FDS activation preceding the movement onset and index-finger movement were unchanged. Instead, inhibitory APAs in BB and AD apparently increased, while excitatory APA in TB was marginally decreased. The changes in the postural chain led to a less effective fixation of the elbow joint, which showed a larger displacement during index-finger acceleration. EMG amplitude was normalized to the maximal motor response (M_{max}) evoked by orthodromic nerve stimulation.

The linkage between APAs and movement precision is also supported by the observation that training induces improvement in the correct tailoring of the APA chain with respect to the prime mover recruitment, both in young adults (Kanekar and Aruin, 2015) and elderly (Kubicki et al., 2012; Aruin et al., 2015). Thus, the increased movement precision observed after training (Hamman et al., 1995; Yang et al., 2013) might be partly due to a more appropriate tuning of the postural adjustments. Other suggestions about the linkage between APAs and precision derive from some motor behaviors in which proper whole-body stabilization is needed to achieve an effective performance. According to shooting coaches and athletes, good postural balance is a vital component of successful shooting. During bipedal standing, top-level rifle shooters stabilized their whole body balance better than naive shooters (Aalto et al., 1990); the capability to reduce the oscillation, especially in the last few seconds before pulling the trigger, expresses better control of posture in athletes and was associated with a better shooting performance (Era et al., 1996; Mononen et al., 2007). More recently, Furuya et al. (2011) demonstrated that professional pianists tended to play using less muscular activity and take greater advantage of shoulder joint rotation during a keystroke than did novice.

In regard to *intra-limb* APAs, Caronni and Cavallari (2009a) suggested that during a brisk index-finger flexion, *intra-limb* APAs not only would guarantee the maintenance of the arm posture, but should also be very important in controlling the trajectory (**Figure 3C**) and thus the final position of the moving segment, i.e., what is clinically indicated as *metria*. Indeed, when simulating an index-finger flexion using a four-joint software mechanical model of the arm (**Figure 3A**), in which only the prime mover was recruited, a clear disturbance of both focal movement and upper-limb posture was observed, with relevant changes at wrist and elbow level. This would affect the final position of the intentional finger movement (**Figures 3D,E**). In the model, the only way to prevent these *collateral effects* was to block all segments but the finger, preventing the proximal joints from rotating (fictive *intra-limb* APAs).

Since this observation was derived from a very simplified system, Caronni and Cavallari (2009a) also looked for a more realistic situation: a finger tap was electrically evoked in a real arm by stimulating the median nerve (**Figure 3B**); such an experiment showed recordings comparable in sign and size to those predicted by the software mechanical model, including the dysmetric motor output. However, both the *software simulation* and the *electrically evoked tap* paradigms did not faithfully represent the *natural dysmetric behavior*, since in the two cases no voluntary command is modeled or generated, respectively. An indirect suggestion of the role of APAs in movement

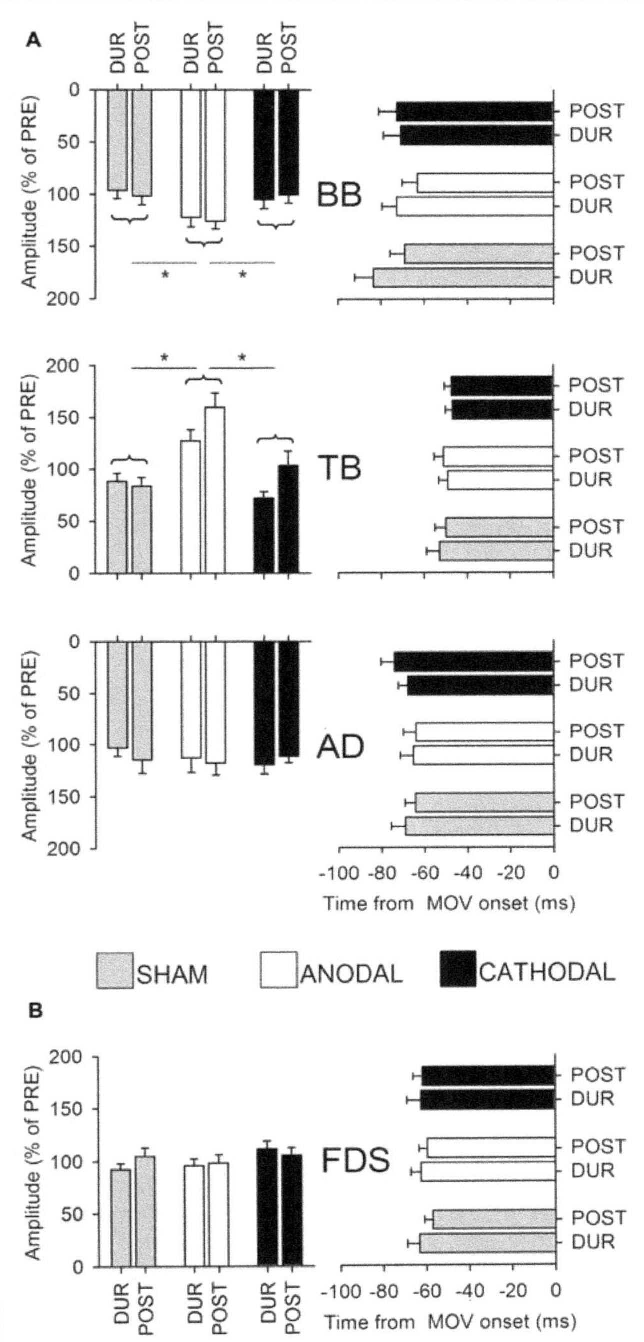

FIGURE 6 | Amplitude and latency of intra-limb APAs (A) and of voluntary recruitment of index-finger prime mover (B). Postural muscles: BB, TB and AD, prime mover FDS. Data were collected from the whole population, in the last 5 min of 1 mA Transcranial Direct Current Stimulation (tDCS) application (DUR) and 20 min after its end (POST). Amplitude data are plotted on the left (expressed as percentage of the amplitude measured before tDCS, % of PRE), latencies referred to movement onset on the right (mean ± SE). Repeated measures *stimulation* × *time* ANOVA, and Tukey *post hoc* (see asterisks), found a significant increase in the amplitude of BB and TB APAs under ANODAL vs. CATHODAL and SHAM stimulation, while the APA in AD was unaffected. No effect of *time* or *interaction* was observed, thus

(Continued)

FIGURE 6 | (Continued)
ANODAL stimulation enhanced APAs in TB and BB with an effect lasting at least 20 min. No significant changes were observed in APAs latency. Note also that tDCS had no effect on the amplitude and latency of FDS activity, witnessing that the increase in BB and TB APAs should not be ascribed to a stronger recruitment of the prime mover. *Reproduced from Bolzoni et al. (2015), © 2015 Elsevier B.V., with permission of Elsevier.*

metria comes from Bruttini et al. (2015), who demonstrated that when performing a brisk index-finger flexion, cerebellar subjects showed a timing-disruption of *intra-limb* APAs (**Figure 4**), while their pattern (excitation in TB; inhibition in BB and AD) was unmodified. These data open the question whether cerebellar dysmetria may stem from an erroneous timing of APAs.

Moreover, considering that a disruption of the APA chain may lead to movement inaccuracy and taking into account that Moisello et al. (2008) demonstrated that 12-h of immobilization are already sufficient in affecting the inter-joint coordination by interfering with the feed-forward mechanisms, Bolzoni et al. (2012) investigated the effect of a short-term immobilization on the *intra-limb* postural control accompanying index-finger flexion. In this article it was shown that 12-h of wrist and finger immobilization effectively modified APAs on elbow and shoulder muscles, without altering the prime mover activation (**Figure 5**). The APA modifications were also paralleled by a less efficient stabilization of the elbow joint. Therefore, these results may shed light on some of the mechanisms underlying the feeling of motor awkwardness and the reduction of the voluntary movement precision that are commonly experienced after the removal of a cast or a splint.

A last apparent evidence in favor of the importance of APAs in movement precision has been recently provided by Bruttini et al. (2016), who illustrated that the different precision observed when comparing pointing movements performed with the preferred vs. non-preferred hand partly stems from changes in the temporal organization of APAs in the two sides. Indeed, APAs were delayed when moving the non-preferred side. This delay was associated to an impaired stability of the elbow joint during the wrist pointing movement. As a result, the focal movement perturbation caused an increased elbow excursion in the non-preferred hand, eventually leading to the diminished movement precision on that side.

Surely, APAs are not the only determinant of movement precision. In fact, it is well known that when a healthy subject points to a target cross, an eventual error in reaching the target derives from an incorrect sensorimotor transformation, from the visual representation of the target to the kinematics representation of the planned trajectory (Soechting and Flanders, 1989a,b; for a review see also Massion, 1992). Indeed, these authors showed that when subjects have to reach a position which has been previously appreciated kinesthetically (thus after having empirically built up the exact transformation), pointing errors dramatically reduce. In particular, several studies showed that the parietal cortices play a critical role in integrating visual and somatic inputs for building up this sensorimotor transformation. Such transformation seems also assisted by the skin receptors, which detect the torsion forces that act on the skin of the feet

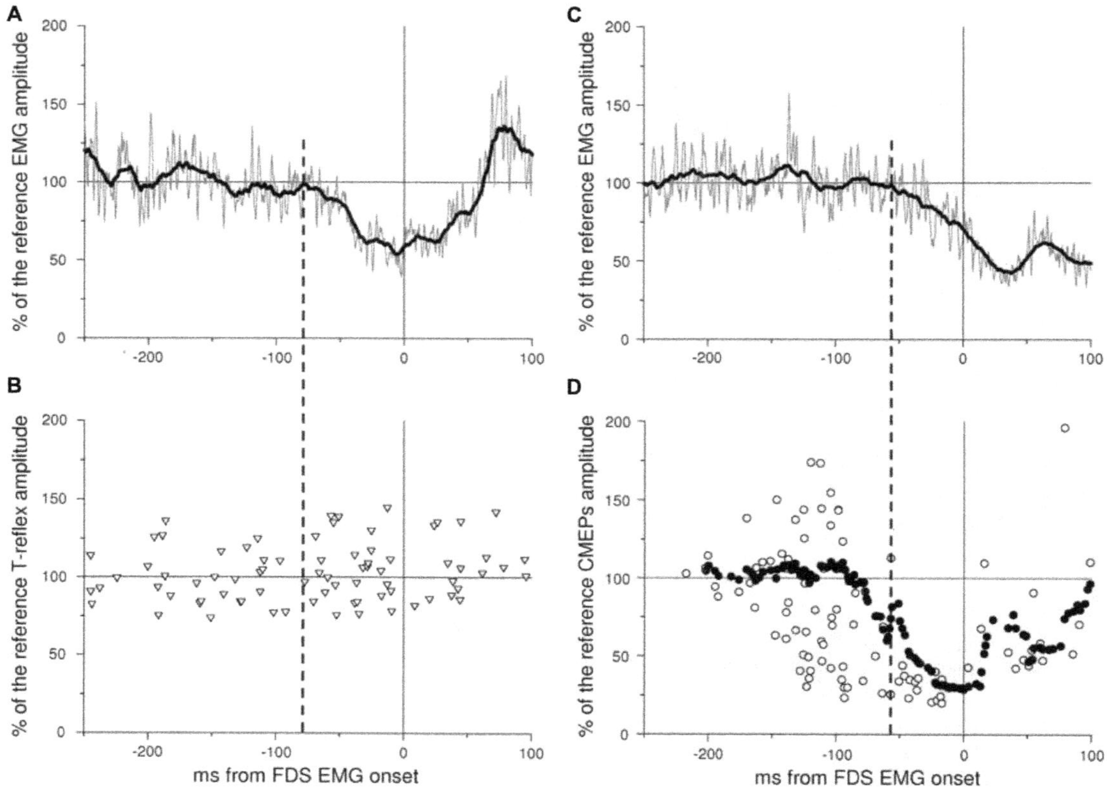

FIGURE 7 | Time course of spinal and cortico-spinal excitability in the resting BB before an index finger flexion. An inhibitory APA (iAPA) occurs in the BB EMG in two representative subjects **(A,C)**: in both cases rectified (gray trace) and integrated (black trace) EMG activity (average of 40 trials) is strongly reduced well in advance to the onset of FDS, taken as time 0. The time course of BB spinal excitability has been tested by means of tendon tap reflexes (T-reflex, triangles in **B)**, while that of BB cortico-spinal excitability by Transcranial Magnetic Stimulation (TMS)-elicited cortical motor-evoked potentials (CMEPs, open circles in **D)**. Each symbol marks amplitude and latency of one single evoked potential. Note that T-reflexes are un-modulated in size in the iAPA window, edged by the iAPA onset (vertical dashed line) and prime mover onset (vertical continuous line), whereas CMEPs are strongly inhibited. To better identify the onset of this inhibitory effect, the CMEPs time course has been integrated with the same time constant used for the EMG (filled circles). Both EMG and evoked potential amplitude are expressed as a percentage of their mean reference amplitude, i.e., that measured before the acoustic go signal.

in contact with the soil (for a review see Kalaska et al., 1997). In this context, it has been also observed (Esposti et al., "APAs associated to reaching movements are programmed according to the availability of visual information", submitted manuscript) that once the target position has been acquired, both visually and kinesthetically, reaching the target while gazing it or in a *blind* condition resulted in similar levels of pointing accuracy; pointing precision was instead significantly impaired in absence of visual information. Finally, these authors suggested that the visuospatial memory may play a key role in movement accuracy, while "active vision" seems to be more engaged in movement precision.

CENTRAL ORGANIZATION OF APAs

Anatomical and Physiological Data

Several studies support the idea that *Supplementary Motor Area* (SMA) is involved in APAs generation. Severe APA impairments were observed in the bimanual load lifting (the so called *barman task*) when the load was held with the forearm contralateral to the lesioned SMA while no APA changes were observed in a patient with normal SMA, but suffering a complete callosal section (Massion et al., 1989; Viallet et al., 1992). This finding supports the idea that coordination between the posture and movement travels through subcortical level. Moreover, a 1-Hz repetitive Transcranial Magnetic Stimulation (TMS) on SMA, which induces an inhibitory effect, reduces the duration of APAs prior to stepping, without affecting their peak amplitude (Jacobs et al., 2009). More recently, Transcranial Direct Current Stimulation (tDCS) over the SMA has been shown to elicit a differential effect on the postural and the focal component of the movement (**Figure 6**), supporting the involvement of SMA in APA programming (Bolzoni et al., 2015).

The role of the *Primary Motor Cortex* in generating APAs has been shown by both human and animal studies. The stimulation of the primary motor cortex in the intact cats was indeed able

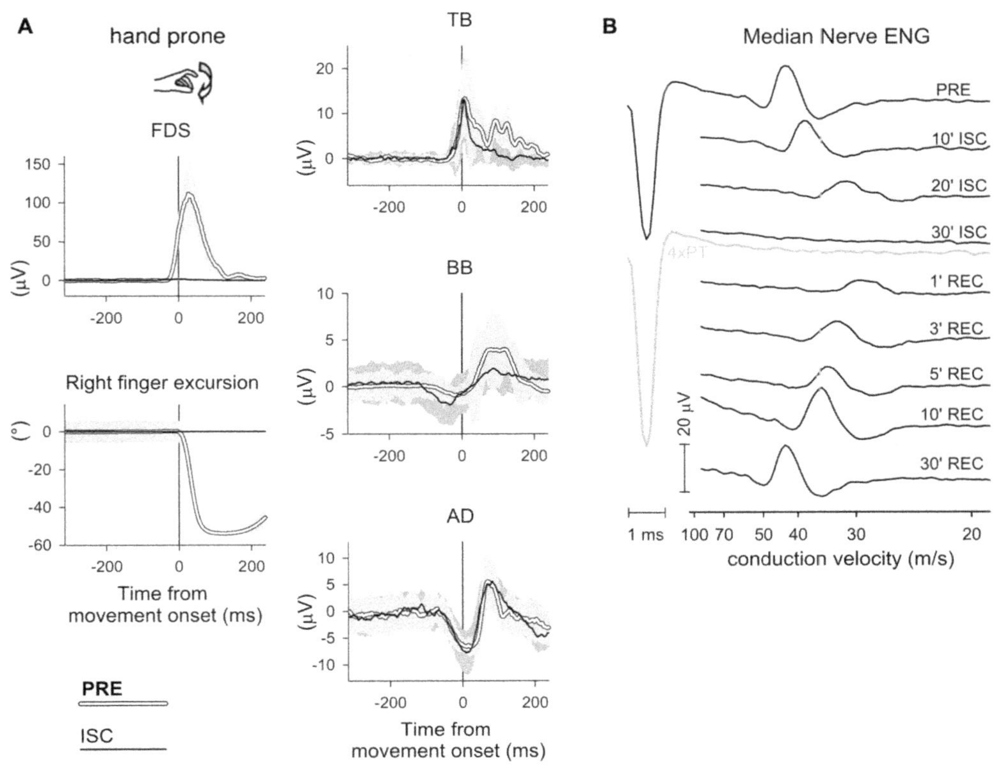

FIGURE 8 | APA persistence under ischemia. (A) Rectified and integrated average recordings of index-finger prime mover EMG and of intra-limb APAs, before and during ischemic block of the median nerve at the forearm. One representative subject. Time 0: movement onset of the left index-finger. When rapidly flexing both index-fingers before ischemia (PRE, white traces, SD in light gray), the right prime mover FDS was activated and the right arm equilibrium was preserved, thanks to an excitatory APA in TB and inhibitory APAs in BB and AD. Under ischemia of the right forearm (ISC, black traces, SD in dark gray), FDS activation and index-finger movement were both suppressed, while excitatory APAs in TB and inhibitory APAs in BB and AD were still evident and qualitatively similar to those recorded in PRE. **(B)** Electroneurogram (ENG) of the right median nerve of one representative subject, showing the effect of ischemia, induced by a pressure cuff, on the afferent volley elicited by electrical stimulation of the index-finger skin (3 × perception threshold, PT). Ischemia progressively reduced the volley amplitude until reaching complete suppression after 30 min (even increasing stimulation to 4 × PT, gray trace, did not elicit a response). After removing the pressure cuff, the effect of ischemia completely recovered in 30 min.

to evoke movement in the contralateral side and APAs in the supporting limbs (Gahéry and Nieoullon, 1978), suggesting that the primary motor cortex in cats is able to control both the voluntary prime mover and the associated postural adjustments. Moreover, in cats, the dynamic of the discharge frequency in pyramidal neurons is time locked and directly proportional with the center of pressure displacement, a key parameter associated to APAs preserving the whole body equilibrium (Yakovenko and Drew, 2009). The role of the primary motor cortex in the anticipatory postural control was also observed in human studies. Indeed, Palmer et al. (1994) used the TMS to induce a silent period in either the left or the right M1 while the subject abducted his left arm, a movement which is known to be preceded by APAs in the contralateral Latissimus Dorsi muscle. Left M1 stimulation produced a delay of the APA onset, while the prime mover timing was unmodified; instead, right M1 stimulation just delayed the prime mover activation. Moreover, it has been shown for both *inter-* (Petersen et al., 2009) and *intra-limb* APAs (Caronni and Cavallari, 2009b) that when a postural muscle is at rest the spinal excitability is un-modulated during the whole period of motor preparation, while when that muscle is recruited in a postural chain the cortical motor action potentials are modulated according to the time course of APAs (**Figure 7**). From one perspective, this indicates that APAs processing involves M1 level, and from another this suggests that APAs and voluntary commands cannot be decoupled, since the former remains subliminal, i.e., it does not produce a mechanical effect, when the muscle is at rest. Although this may appear uneconomical, this result corroborates two previous observations in which the cortical excitability of hand movers has been shown to fluctuate under the threshold for motoneuronal firing when the ipsilateral foot was voluntarily oscillated (Baldissera et al., 2002) and in which the *hidden effect* developed in an overt APA when the hand was recruited in a postural act (Baldissera and Esposti, 2005).

Regarding *Basal Ganglia*, severe APAs impairment in patients with Parkinson's disease were already observed by Viallet et al. (1987). More recently, anticipatory brain activity associated to a bimanual load-lifting task was localized in basal ganglia,

SMA and thalamus, contra lateral to the load-bearing arm (Ng et al., 2013). It is worth noting that these areas are component nodes of the basal ganglia-thalamo-cortical motor network, which is known to be implicated in well-learned finger movements (Boecker et al., 1998). This indicates a superposition of the neural structures for APAs and those for voluntary motor command, and indirectly supports the view of a oneness of the motor command for both posture and primary movement.

The *Cerebellum* is deeply involved in APA regulation. Babinski (1899) reported that a cerebellar lesion disrupted the coordination between voluntary movement and equilibrium stabilization, indicating that the cerebellum is involved in postural control. This view agrees with the idea that the cerebellum contains forward internal models that could predict the consequences of an action (according to the perceived postural context) and can be used to overcome time delays associated with feedback control (Wolpert et al., 1998; Imamizu et al., 2000). Several studies on patients positively concluded for such an involvement. Indeed, patients suffering cerebellar lesions failed to show a normal anticipatory adjustment in grip force when lifting or moving an object (Müller and Dichgans, 1994; Babin-Ratté et al., 1999) and cerebellar lesions abolished APAs plasticity in a bimanual unloading task (Diedrichsen et al., 2005). Congruently, Diener et al. (1992) reported that cerebellar patients produce a normal pattern of APAs, but with abnormalities in their timing relationship with the onset of the prime mover. Finally, as shown in **Figure 4**, Bruttini et al. (2015) demonstrated that when performing a brisk index-finger flexion, cerebellar subjects showed a timing-disruption of *intra-limb* APAs, while their pattern was unmodified. Using functional magnetic resonance imaging, Schmitz et al. (2005) reported that APAs were associated with activation of sensorimotor areas, SMA and the cerebellum. On the contrary, Ng et al. (2013) found no evidence of cerebellar involvement during APAs using magnetoencephalography in a bimanual coordination task. Further support on the role of cerebellum in timing APAs come from animal studies. When reaching a water flask with the mouth, wild type mice showed a clear APA in hind-limb muscles, synchronous to neck muscles, while in transgenic mice with defective cerebellar Purkinje cells the hind-limb activity occurred markedly later than that in neck muscles (Yamaura et al., 2013).

Finally, Schepens and colleagues (Schepens and Drew, 2004; Schepens et al., 2008) emphasized the role of pontomedullary reticular formation (PMRF) in the coordination of posture and movement. In particular, they suggested that PMRF is a site of integration of signals from both cortical and subcortical structures, and that these signals ensure that APAs are appropriately scaled in time and magnitude to the intended movement, contributing to integrate the control of posture and movement, as also illustrated by Toussaint et al. (1998).

In summary, these anatomical and physiological studies show a large superimposition between neural structures governing the voluntary and the postural components of the movement, leaving the question open on whether these two processes are implemented separately or they are an expression of a unique *posturo-focal* command.

Dual vs. Shared Command Hypothesis

According to the classical view, the prime mover activity and the associated postural adjustments result from two different central commands *(dual command hypothesis)*, which are independently dispatched to the prime mover and to the muscles generating the postural chain (Babinski, 1899; Hess, 1943; Cordo and Nashner, 1982; Brown and Frank, 1987). Conversely, a growing body of evidences favors the view that APAs and prime mover recruitment are both controlled by a *shared motor command* (Aruin and Latash, 1995; Stapley et al., 1998, 1999; Caronni and Cavallari, 2009b; Petersen et al., 2009). In this regard, it is interesting to mention the studies of Gritsenko et al. (2009) and Leonard et al. (2011), showing that when correcting an ongoing arm pointing movement, the CNS employs a predictive mode of postural control and consistently adapts the postural muscle activities before modifying the prime mover recruitment. These authors concluded that the postural corrections could be described as being a component of the voluntary movement, rather than ensuring the maintenance of equilibrium. Further, Bruttini et al. (2014) demonstrated that the APA chain associated to a voluntary movement cannot be decoupled from the command driving the focal movement. Indeed, when repeatedly trying to flex the index-finger under forearm ischemia, so that the voluntary command was normally dispatched but the prime mover not able to receive it, significant anticipatory adjustments were clearly visible in BB, TB and AD (**Figure 8**).

In this peculiar condition, in which no postural perturbation is generated, one would have expected that APAs were suppressed since unnecessary and uneconomical, unless the postural and the prime mover muscles obey a "shared" motor command. It is of course apparent that "ischemia" results does not allow to discern whether: (i) one specific neural structure generates both the postural and the voluntary commands; or (ii) two neural structures exist, one for the voluntary and the other for the postural commands, and one of the two acts as a master on the other; or (iii) a third neural structure exists, which simultaneously triggers the two slave "postural" and "voluntary" neural structures. However, from the point of view of the muscles (i.e., the only aspect that such experimental approach allowed to observe), these three ways of organizing the posturo-focal integration are all identical. Given this neural organization, it may be conceived that the system prefers an *economy* in computational terms, rather than in diminishing the number of activated neurons. In this case, one may imagine that any given voluntary command is associated with an arborized pattern of postural commands, forwarded to a number of possible fixation points. Thus, the most useful arborization for providing the actual support would be supraliminarly recruited, while the leftover branches would be still present but kept silent, i.e., under threshold. The amplification of APA transmission to certain targets, and the parallel attenuation towards other targets, could be automatically accomplished by servo-systems like PMRF neurons. This would effectively free the upper centers from the computational demand of adapting the APAs to the postural context. This view is also corroborated by the already cited works of Baldissera et al. (2002) and Baldissera and Esposti (2005), who showed that subliminal *inter-limb* APAs in a resting arm during foot movements become supraliminal when that segment is actively used for postural stabilization. Similar results were also shown for *intra-limb* APAs by Caronni and Cavallari (2009b).

The oneness of postural and voluntary command is also supported by the finding that the APA latency depends on the movement instruction, not on its actual velocity (Esposti et al., 2015). This conclusion was based on two observations. First, no correlation was found between APA latency and movement speed when subjects had to follow a *go fast* instruction (i.e., to move as fast as possible), nor when they had to *go slow* (at half their maximal speed). Second, the maximal speed was variable among subjects, so that minimum movement speeds within the range of *go fast* trials intermingled with maximal movement speeds within the range of *go slow* trials. Despite similar velocities, APAs were earlier in the former and less anticipated in the latter. Thus, APAs looked much more tailored on the expected perturbation than on the real one, favoring the idea of a functionally unique postural and focal command.

CONCLUSIONS

This review shows that *intra-limb* APAs and *inter-limb* APAs share the same organizational and behavioral principles. The simplicity and flexibility of the *finger tap* experimental model has also allowed to shed light on a new general characteristic of the postural control. In fact, APAs not only deal with whole-body equilibrium, segmental posture and movement initiation, but are also involved in providing the correct postural set necessary to obtain precise movements. Finally, this approach has been useful in inspecting the central organization of APAs. In particular, the persistence of APAs after the ischemic block of the prime movers provides a principal piece of evidence in assessing the oneness of the focal and postural commands.

AUTHOR CONTRIBUTIONS

All authors contributed in collecting the literature, critically analyzing it and writing the manuscript. All authors approved the final version and agree to be accountable for all aspects of this work.

ACKNOWLEDGMENTS

We are grateful to Dr. Alex P. Moorhead for his helpful comments on an earlier version of this manuscript and for his precious assistance in improving the writing clarity and English style.

REFERENCES

Aalto, H., Pyykkö, I., Ilmarinen, R., Kähkönen, E., and Starck, J. (1990). Postural stability in shooters. *ORL J. Otorhinolaryngol. Relat. Spec.* 52, 232–238. doi: 10.1159/000276141

Alexeief, M. A., and Naidel, A. V. (1972). The mechanisms of interrelationship between human muscle activity in complex motor tasks. *Zh. Physiol. U.S.S.R.* 58, 1721–1730.

Almeida, G. L., Hong, D. A., Corcos, D., and Gottlieb, G. L. (1995). Organizing principles for voluntary movement: extending single-joint rules. *J. Neurophysiol.* 74, 1374–1381.

Aoki, F. (1991). Activity patterns of upper arm muscles in relation to direction of rapid wrist movement in man. *Exp. Brain Res.* 83, 679–682. doi: 10.1007/bf00229847

Aruin, A. S., Kanekar, N., Lee, Y. J., and Ganesan, M. (2015). Enhancement of anticipatory postural adjustments in older adults as a result of a single session of ball throwing exercise. *Exp. Brain Res.* 233, 649–655. doi: 10.1007/s00221-014-4144-1

Aruin, A. S., and Latash, M. L. (1995). The role of motor action in anticipatory postural adjustments studied with self-induced and externally triggered perturbations. *Exp. Brain Res.* 106, 291–300. doi: 10.1007/bf00241125

Aruin, A. S., and Shiratori, T. (2004). The effect of the amplitude of motor action on anticipatory postural adjustments. *J. Electromyogr. Kinesiol.* 14, 455–462. doi: 10.1016/j.jelekin.2003.12.002

Babin-Ratté, S., Sirigu, A., Gilles, M., and Wing, A. (1999). Impaired anticipatory finger grip-force adjustments in a case of cerebellar degeneration. *Exp. Brain Res.* 128, 81–85. doi: 10.1007/s002210050821

Babinski, J. (1899). De l'asynergie cérebelleuse. *Rev. Neurol.* 7, 806–816.

Baldissera, F., Borroni, P., Cavallari, P., and Cerri, G. (2002). Excitability changes in human corticospinal projections to forearm muscles during voluntary movement of ipsilateral foot. *J. Physiol.* 539, 903–911. doi: 10.1113/jphysiol.2001.013282

Baldissera, F., and Esposti, R. (2005). Postural constraints to coupling of ipsilateral hand-foot movements. *Neuroreport* 16, 1615–1619. doi: 10.1097/01.wnr.0000181586.49130.48

Baldissera, F., Rota, V., and Esposti, R. (2008). Anticipatory postural adjustments in arm muscles associated with movements of the contralateral limb and their possible role in interlimb coordination. *Exp. Brain Res.* 185, 63–74. doi: 10.1007/s00221-007-1131-9

Belen'kii, V. E., Gurfinkel', V. S., and Pal'tsey, E. I. (1967). Control elements of voluntary movements. *Biofizika* 12, 135–141.

Bernstein, N. A. (1967). *The co-ordination and regulation of movements.* Oxford: Pergamon Press.

Berrigan, F., Simoneau, M., Martin, O., and Teasdale, N. (2006). Coordination between posture and movement: interaction between postural and accuracy constraints. *Exp. Brain Res.* 170, 255–264. doi: 10.1007/s00221-005-0210-z

Bertucco, M., and Cesari, P. (2010). Does movement planning follow Fitts' law? Scaling anticipatory postural adjustments with movement speed and accuracy. *Neuroscience* 171, 205–213. doi: 10.1016/j.neuroscience.2010.08.023

Boecker, H., Dagher, A., Ceballos-Baumann, A. O., Passingham, R. E., Samuel, M., Friston, K. J., et al. (1998). Role of the human rostral supplementary motor area and the basal ganglia in motor sequence control: investigations with H_22 ^{15}O PET. *J. Neurophysiol.* 79, 1070–1080.

Bolzoni, F., Bruttini, C., Esposti, R., Castellani, C., and Cavallari, P. (2015). Transcranial direct current stimulation of SMA modulates anticipatory postural adjustments without affecting the primary movement. *Behav. Brain Res.* 291, 407–413. doi: 10.1016/j.bbr.2015.05.044

Bolzoni, F., Bruttini, C., Esposti, R., and Cavallari, P. (2012). Hand immobilization affects arm and shoulder postural control. *Exp. Brain Res.* 220, 63–70. doi: 10.1007/s00221-012-3115-7

Bonnetblanc, F., Martin, O., and Teasdale, N. (2004). Pointing to a target from an upright standing position: anticipatory postural adjustments are modulated by the size of the target in humans. *Neurosci. Lett.* 358, 181–184. doi: 10.1016/j.neulet.2004.01.020

Bouisset, S., and Do, M. C. (2008). Posture, dynamic stability and voluntary movement. *Neurophysiol. Clin.* 38, 345–362. doi: 10.1016/j.neucli.2008.10.001

Bouisset, S., and Zattara, M. (1987). Biomechanical study of the programming of anticipatory postural adjustments associated with voluntary movement. *J. Biomech.* 20, 735–742. doi: 10.1016/0021-9290(87)90052-2

Brenière, Y., Cuong Do, M., and Bouisset, S. (1987). Are dynamic phenomena prior to stepping essential to walking? *J. Mot. Behav.* 19, 62–76. doi: 10.1080/00222895.1987.10735400

Brown, J. E., and Frank, J. S. (1987). Influence of event anticipation on postural actions accompanying voluntary movement. *Exp. Brain Res.* 67, 645–650. doi: 10.1007/bf00247295

Bruttini, C., Esposti, R., Bolzoni, F., and Cavallari, P. (2014). Ischemic block of the forearm abolishes finger movements but not their associated anticipatory postural adjustments. *Exp. Brain Res.* 232, 1739–1750. doi: 10.1007/s00221-014-3866-4

Bruttini, C., Esposti, R., Bolzoni, F., and Cavallari, P. (2016). Higher precision in pointing movements of the preferred vs. non-preferred hand is associated with an earlier occurrence of anticipatory postural adjustments. *Front. Hum. Neurosci.* 10:365. doi: 10.3389/fnhum.2016.00365

Bruttini, C., Esposti, R., Bolzoni, F., Vanotti, A., Mariotti, C., and Cavallari, P. (2015). Temporal disruption of upper-limb anticipatory postural adjustments in cerebellar ataxic patients. *Exp. Brain Res.* 233, 197–203. doi: 10.1007/s00221-014-4103-x

Caronni, A., and Cavallari, P. (2009a). Anticipatory postural adjustments stabilise the whole upper-limb prior to a gentle index-finger tap. *Exp. Brain Res.* 194, 59–66. doi: 10.1007/s00221-008-1668-2

Caronni, A., and Cavallari, P. (2009b). Supra-spinal circuits shape inhibitory postural adjustments anticipating voluntary index-finger flexion. *Exp. Brain Res.* 198, 19–28. doi: 10.1007/s00221-009-1931-1

Caronni, A., Bolzoni, F., Esposti, R., Bruttini, C., and Cavallari, P. (2013). Accuracy of pointing movements relies upon a specific tuning between APAs and prime mover activation. *Acta Physiol. (Oxf)* 208, 111–124. doi: 10.1111/apha.12081

Chabran, E., Maton, B., Ribreau, C., and Fourment, A. (2001). Electromyographic and biomechanical characteristics of segmental postural adjustments associated with voluntary wrist movements. Influence of an elbow support. *Exp. Brain Res.* 141, 133–145. doi: 10.1007/s002210100823

Clément, G., Gurfinkel, V. S., Lestienne, F., Lipshits, M. I., and Pospov, K. E. (1984). Adaptation of postural control to weightlessness. *Exp. Brain Res.* 57, 61–72. doi: 10.1007/bf00231132

Cordo, P. J., and Nashner, L. M. (1982). Properties of postural adjustments associated with rapid arm movements. *J. Neurophysiol.* 47, 287–302.

Crenna, P., Frigo, C., Massion, J., and Pedotti, A. (1987). Forward and backward axial synergies in man. *Exp. Brain Res.* 65, 538–548. doi: 10.1007/bf00235977

Dick, J. P., Rothwell, J. C., Berardelli, A., Thompson, P. D., Gioux, M., Benecke, R., et al. (1986). Associated postural adjustments in Parkinson's disease. *J. Neurol. Neurosurg. Psychiatry* 49, 1378–1385. doi: 10.1136/jnnp.49.12.1378

Diedrichsen, J., Verstynen, T., Lehman, S., and Ivry, R. (2005). Cerebellar involvement in anticipating the consequences of self-produced actions during bimanual movements. *J. Neurophysiol.* 93, 801–812. doi: 10.1152/jn.00662.2004

Diener, H. C., Dichgans, J., Guschlbauer, B., Bacher, M., Rapp, H., and Klockgether, T. (1992). The coordination of posture and voluntary movement in patients with cerebellar dysfunction. *Mov. Disord.* 7, 14–22. doi: 10.1002/mds.870070104

Dietz, V., and Colombo, G. (1996). Effects of body immersion on postural adjustments to voluntary arm movements in humans: role of load receptor input. *J. Physiol.* 497, 849–856. doi: 10.1113/jphysiol.1996.sp021815

Do, M. C., Nouillot, P., and Bouisset, S. (1991). Is balance or posture at the end of a voluntary movement programmed? *Neurosci. Lett.* 130, 9–11. doi: 10.1016/0304-3940(91)90215-f

Duarte, M., and Latash, M. L. (2007). Effects of postural task requirements on the speed-accuracy trade-off. *Exp. Brain Res.* 180, 457–467. doi: 10.1007/s00221-007-0871-x

Era, P., Konttinen, N., Mehto, P., Saarela, P., and Lyytinen, H. (1996). Postural stability and skilled performance—a study on top-level and naive rifle shooters. *J. Biomech.* 29, 301–306. doi: 10.1016/0021-9290(95)00066-6

Esposti, R., and Baldissera, F. G. (2011). Combined recruitment of two fixation chains during cyclic movements of one arm. *Hum. Mov. Sci.* 30, 213–226. doi: 10.1016/j.humov.2010.02.005

Esposti, R., Bruttini, C., Bolzoni, F., and Cavallari, P. (2015). Intended rather than actual movement velocity determines the latency of anticipatory postural adjustments. *Exp. Brain Res.* 233, 397–403. doi: 10.1007/s00221-014-4122-7

Fernandez, L., and Bootsma, R. J. (2004). Effects of biomechanical and task constraints on the organization of movement in precision aiming. *Exp. Brain Res.* 159, 458–466. doi: 10.1007/s00221-004-1964-4

Fitts, P. M. (1954). The information capacity of the human motor system in controlling the amplitude of movement. *J. Exp. Psychol.* 47, 381–391. doi: 10.1037/h0055392

Friedli, W. G., Hallett, M., and Simon, S. R. (1984). Postural adjustments associated with rapid voluntary arm movements 1. Electromyographic data. *J. Neurol. Neurosurg. Psychiatry* 47, 611–622. doi: 10.1136/jnnp.47.6.611

Furuya, S., Goda, T., Katayose, H., Miwa, H., and Nagata, N. (2011). Distinct inter-joint coordination during fast alternate keystrokes in pianists with superior skill. *Front. Hum. Neurosci.* 5:50. doi: 10.3389/fnhum.2011.00050

Gahéry, Y., and Nieoullon, A. (1978). Postural and kinetic coordination following cortical stimuli which induce flexion movements in the cat's limbs. *Brain Res.* 149, 25–37. doi: 10.1016/0006-8993(78)90585-1

Gelfand, I. M., Gurfinkel, V. S., Tsetlin, M. L., and Shik, M. L. (1966). "Problems in analysis of movements," in *Models of the Structural Functional Organization of Certain Biological Systems*, eds I. M. Gelfand, V. S. Gurfinkel, S. V. Fomin and M. L. Tsetlin (Cambridge, MA: MIT Press), 330–345.

Gribble, P. L., and Ostry, D. J. (1999). Compensation for interaction torques during single- and multijoint limb movement. *J. Neurophysiol.* 82, 2310–2326.

Gritsenko, V., Yakovenko, S., and Kalaska, J. F. (2009). Integration of predictive feedforward and sensory feedback signals for online control of visually guided movement. *J. Neurophysiol.* 102, 914–930. doi: 10.1152/jn.91324.2008

Hall, L. M., Brauer, S., Horak, F., and Hodges, P. W. (2010). Adaptive changes in anticipatory postural adjustments with novel and familiar postural support. *J. Neurophysiol.* 103, 968–976. doi: 10.1152/jn.00479.2009

Hamman, R., Longridge, N. S., Mekjavic, I., and Dickinson, J. (1995). Effect of age and training schedules on balance improvement exercises using visual biofeedback. *J. Otolaryngol.* 24, 221–229.

Hess, W. R. (1943). Teleokinetisches und ereismatisches Kraftesystem in Biomotorik. *Helv. Physiol. Pharmacol. Acta* 1, C62–C63.

Hopf, H. C., and Hufschmidt, H. J. (1963). Coordination of adjoining muscles in simple voluntary movements. *Dtsch. Z. Nervenheilkd.* 185, 191–202.

Horak, F. B., Esselman, P., Anderson, M. E., and Lynch, M. K. (1984). The effects of movement velocity, mass displaced and task certainty on associated postural adjustments made by normal and hemiplegic individuals. *J. Neurol. Neurosurg. Psychiatry* 47, 1020–1028. doi: 10.1136/jnnp.47.9.1020

Houtz, S. J., and Fischer, F. J. (1961). Function of leg muscles acting on foot as modified by body movements. *J. Appl. Physiol.* 16, 597–605.

Hugon, M., Massion, J., and Wiesendanger, M. (1982). Anticipatory postural changes induced by active unloading and comparison with passive unloading in man. *Pflugers Arch.* 393, 292–296. doi: 10.1007/bf00581412

Imamizu, H., Miyauchi, S., Tamada, T., Sasaki, Y., Takino, R., Pütz, B., et al. (2000). Human cerebellar activity reflecting an acquired internal model of a new tool. *Nature* 403, 192–195. doi: 10.1038/35003194

Jacobs, J. V., Lou, J. S., Kraakevik, J. A., and Horak, F. B. (2009). The supplementary motor area contributes to the timing of the anticipatory postural adjustment during step initiation in participants with and without Parkinson's disease. *Neuroscience* 164, 877–885. doi: 10.1016/j.neuroscience.2009.08.002

Kalaska, J. F., Scott, S. H., Cisek, P., and Sergio, L. E. (1997). Cortical control of reaching movements. *Curr. Opin. Neurobiol.* 7, 849–859. doi: 10.1016/s0959-4388(97)80146-8

Kanekar, N., and Aruin, A. S. (2015). Improvement of anticipatory postural adjustments for balance control: effect of a single training session. *J. Electromyogr. Kinesiol.* 25, 400–405. doi: 10.1016/j.jelekin.2014.11.002

Kubicki, A., Petrement, G., Bonnetblanc, F., Ballay, Y., and Mourey, F. (2012). Practice-related improvements in postural control during rapid arm movement in older adults: a preliminary study. *J. Gerontol. A Biol. Sci. Med. Sci.* 67, 196–203. doi: 10.1093/gerona/glr148

Lee, W. A. (1980). Anticipatory control of postural and task muscles during rapid arm flexion. *J. Mot. Behav.* 12, 185–196. doi: 10.1080/00222895.1980.10735219

Lee, W. A., Buchanan, T. S., and Rogers, M. W. (1987). Effects of arm acceleration and behavioral conditions on the organization of postural adjustments during arm flexion. *Exp. Brain Res.* 66, 257–270. doi: 10.1007/bf00243303

Leonard, J. A., Gritsenko, V., Ouckama, R., and Stapley, P. J. (2011). Postural adjustments for online corrections of arm movements in standing humans. *J. Neurophysiol.* 105, 2375–2388. doi: 10.1152/jn.00944.2010

Lipshits, M. I., Mauritz, K., and Popov, K. E. (1981). Quantitative analysis of anticipatory postural components of a complex voluntary movement. *Hum. Physiol.* 7, 165–173.

Maki, B. E. (1993). Biomechanical approach to quantifying anticipatory postural adjustments in the elderly. *Med. Biol. Eng. Comput.* 31, 355–362. doi: 10.1007/bf02446688

Marsden, C. D., Merton, P. A., and Morton, H. B. (1981). Human postural responses. *Brain* 104, 513–534. doi: 10.1093/brain/104.3.513

Massion, J. (1992). Movement, posture and equilibrium: interaction and coordination. *Prog. Neurobiol.* 38, 35–56. doi: 10.1016/0301-0082(92)90034-c

Massion, J., Viallet, F., Massarino, R., and Khalil, R. (1989). The supplementary motor area is implicated in the coordination between posture and movement in man. *C. R. Acad. Sci. III* 308, 417–423.

Moisello, C., Bove, M., Huber, R., Abbruzzese, G., Battaglia, F., Tononi, G., et al. (2008). Short-term limb immobilization affects motor performance. *J. Mot. Behav.* 40, 165–176. doi: 10.3200/jmbr.40.2.165-176

Mononen, K., Konttinen, N., Viitasalo, J., and Era, P. (2007). Relationships between postural balance, rifle stability and shooting accuracy among novice rifle shooters. *Scand. J. Med. Sci. Sports* 17, 180–185. doi: 10.1111/j.1600-0838.2006.00549.x

Mouchnino, L., Aurenty, R., Massion, J., and Pedotti, A. (1991). Strategies for simultaneous control of the equilibrium and of the head position during the raising movement of a leg. *C. R. Acad. Sci. III* 312, 225–232.

Müller, F., and Dichgans, J. (1994). Impairments of precision grip in two patients with acute unilateral cerebellar lesions: a simple parametric test for clinical use. *Neuropsychologia* 32, 265–269. doi: 10.1016/0028-3932(94)90012-4

Nana-Ibrahim, S., Vieilledent, S., Leroyer, P., Viale, F., and Zattara, M. (2008). Target size modifies anticipatory postural adjustments and subsequent elementary arm pointing. *Exp. Brain Res.* 184, 255–260. doi: 10.1007/s00221-007-1178-7

Nardone, A., and Schieppati, M. (1988). Postural adjustments associated with voluntary contraction of leg muscles in standing man. *Exp. Brain Res.* 69, 469–480. doi: 10.1007/bf00247301

Ng, T. H., Sowman, P. F., Brock, J., and Johnson, B. W. (2013). Neuromagnetic brain activity associated with anticipatory postural adjustments for bimanual load lifting. *Neuroimage* 66, 343–352. doi: 10.1016/j.neuroimage.2012.10.042

Nouillot, P., Bouisset, S., and Do, M. C. (1992). Do fast voluntary movements necessitate anticipatory postural adjustments even if equilibrium is unstable? *Neurosci. Lett.* 147, 1–4. doi: 10.1016/0304-3940(92)90760-5

Oddsson, L., and Thorstensson, A. (1986). Fast voluntary trunk flexion movements in standing: primary movements and associated postural adjustments. *Acta Physiol. Scand.* 128, 341–349. doi: 10.1111/j.1748-1716.1986.tb07987.x

Palmer, E., Cafarelli, E., and Ashby, P. (1994). The processing of human ballistic movements explored by stimulation over the cortex. *J. Physiol.* 481, 509–520. doi: 10.1113/jphysiol.1994.sp020459

Patla, A. E., Ishac, M. G., and Winter, D. A. (2002). Anticipatory control of center of mass and joint stability during voluntary arm movement from a standing posture: interplay between active and passive control. *Exp. Brain Res.* 143, 318–327. doi: 10.1007/s00221-001-0968-6

Pedotti, A., Crenna, P., Deat, A., Frigo, C., and Massion, J. (1989). Postural synergies in axial movements: short and long-term adaptation. *Exp. Brain Res.* 74, 3–10. doi: 10.1007/bf00248275

Petersen, T. H., Rosenberg, K., Petersen, N. C., and Nielsen, J. B. (2009). Cortical involvement in anticipatory postural reactions in man. *Exp. Brain Res.* 193, 161–171. doi: 10.1007/s00221-008-1603-6

Pozzo, T., Stapley, P. J., and Papaxanthis, C. (2002). Coordination between equilibrium and hand trajectories during whole body pointing movements. *Exp. Brain Res.* 144, 343–350. doi: 10.1007/s00221-002-1052-6

Redding, G. M., Rossetti, Y., and Wallace, B. (2005). Applications of prism adaptation: a tutorial in theory and method. *Neurosci. Biobehav. Rev.* 29, 431–444. doi: 10.1016/j.neubiorev.2004.12.004

Riach, C. L., and Hayes, K. C. (1990). Anticipatory postural control in children. *J. Mot. Behav.* 22, 250–266. doi: 10.1080/00222895.1990.10735513

Rogers, M. W., and Pai, Y.-C. (1990). Dynamic transitions in stance support accompanying leg flexion movements in man. *Exp. Brain Res.* 81, 398–402. doi: 10.1007/bf00228132

Schepens, B., and Drew, T. (2004). Independent and convergent signals from the pontomedullary reticular formation contribute to the control of posture and movement during reaching in the cat. *J. Neurophysiol.* 92, 2217–2238. doi: 10.1152/jn.01189.2003

Schepens, B., Stapley, P., and Drew, T. (2008). Neurons in the pontomedullary reticular formation signal posture and movement both as an integrated behavior and independently. *J. Neurophysiol.* 100, 2235–2253. doi: 10.1152/jn.01381.2007

Schmidt, R. A., Zelaznik, H., Hawkins, B., Frank, J. S., and Quinn, J. T. Jr. (1979). Motor-output variability: a theory for the accuracy of rapid motor acts. *Psychol. Rev.* 47, 415–451.

Schmitz, C., Jenmalm, P., Westling, G., Ehrsson, H., and Forssberg, H. (2005). Anticipatory postural adjustments in a bimanual load-lifting task: central aspects. *Gait Posture* 21:S50. doi: 10.1016/S0966-6362(05)80165-1

Shiratori, T., and Aruin, A. (2007). Modulation of anticipatory postural adjustments associated with unloading perturbation: effect of characteristics of a motor action. *Exp. Brain Res.* 178, 206–215. doi: 10.1007/s00221-006-0725-y

Soechting, J. F., and Flanders, M. (1989a). Sensorimotor representations for pointing to targets in three-dimensional space. *J. Neurophysiol.* 62, 582–594.

Soechting, J. F., and Flanders, M. (1989b). Errors in pointing are due to approximations in sensorimotor transformations. *J. Neurophysiol.* 62, 595–608.

Stapley, P. J., Pozzo, T., Cheron, G., and Grishin, A. (1999). Does the coordination between posture and movement during human whole-body reaching ensure center of mass stabilization? *Exp. Brain Res.* 129, 134–146. doi: 10.1007/s002210050944

Stapley, P., Pozzo, T., and Grishin, A. (1998). The role of anticipatory postural adjustments during whole body forward reaching movements. *Neuroreport* 9, 395–401. doi: 10.1097/00001756-199802160-00007

Thomas, A. (1940). *Équilibre et équilibration.* Paris: Masson.

Toussaint, H. M., Michiesm, M., Faber, M. N., Commissaris, D. A., and van Dieën, J. H. (1998). Scaling anticipatory postural adjustments dependent on confidence of load estimation in a bi-manual whole-body lifting task. *Exp. Brain Res.* 120, 85–94. doi: 10.1007/s002210050380

Vernazza, S., Cincera, M., Pedotti, A., and Massion, J. (1996). Balance control during lateral arm raising in humans. *Neuroreport* 7, 1543–1548. doi: 10.1097/00001756-199607080-00002

Viallet, F., Massion, J., Massarino, R., and Khalil, R. (1987). Performance of a bimanual load-lifting task by parkinsonian patients. *J. Neurol. Neurosurg. Psychiatry* 50, 1274–1283. doi: 10.1136/jnnp.50.10.1274

Viallet, F., Massion, J., Massarino, R., and Khalil, R. (1992). Coordination between posture and movement in a bimanual load lifting task: putative role of a medial frontal region including the supplementary motor area. *Exp. Brain Res.* 88, 674–684. doi: 10.1007/bf00228197

Wolpert, D. M., Miall, R. C., and Kawato, M. (1998). Internal models in the cerebellum. *Trends Cogn. Sci.* 2, 333–347. doi: 10.1016/S1364-6613(98)01221-2

Yakovenko, S., and Drew, T. (2009). A motor cortical contribution to the anticipatory postural adjustments that precede reaching in the cat. *J. Neurophysiol.* 102, 853–874. doi: 10.1152/jn.00042.2009

Yamaura, H., Hirai, H., and Yanagihara, D. (2013). Postural dysfunction in a transgenic mouse model of spinocerebellar ataxia type 3. *Neuroscience* 243, 126–135. doi: 10.1016/j.neuroscience.2013.03.044

Yang, W. W., Liu, Y. C., Lu, L. C., Chang, H. Y., Chou, P. P., and Liu, C. (2013). Performance enhancement among adolescent players after 10 weeks of pitching training with appropriate baseball weights. *J. Strength Cond. Res.* 27, 3245–3251. doi: 10.1519/JSC.0b013e31828ddfeb

4

Sample Entropy, Univariate and Multivariate Multi-Scale Entropy in Comparison with Classical Postural Sway Parameters in Young Healthy Adults

Clint Hansen[1], *Qin Wei*[2], *Jiann-Shing Shieh*[3*], *Paul Fourcade*[4], *Brice Isableu*[5] *and Lina Majed*[6]

[1] Research Department, Aspetar Qatar Orthopaedic and Sports Medicine, Doha, Qatar, [2] School of Information Engineering, Wuhan University of Technology, Wuhan, China, [3] Department of Mechanical Engineering, Yuan Ze University, Chung-Li, Taiwan, [4] URCIAMS – Motor Control and Perception Team, University Paris-Sud, Orsay, France, [5] PSYCLE, Aix Marseille University, Aix-en-Provence, France, [6] Sport Science Program, College of Arts and Science, Qatar University, Doha, Qatar

***Correspondence:**
Jiann-Shing Shieh
jsshieh@saturn.yzu.edu.tw

The present study aimed to compare various entropy measures to assess the dynamics and complexity of center of pressure (COP) displacements. Perturbing balance tests are often used in healthy subjects to imitate either pathological conditions or to test the sensitivity of postural analysis techniques. Eleven healthy adult subjects were asked to stand in normal stance in three experimental conditions while the visuo-kinesthetic input was altered. COP displacement was recorded using a force plate. Three entropy measures [Sample Entropy (SE), Multi-Scale Entropy (MSE), and Multivariate Multi Scale Entropy (MMSE)] describing COP regularity at different scales were compared to traditional measures of COP variability. The analyses of the COP trajectories revealed that suppression of vision produced minor changes in COP displacement and in the COP characteristics. The comparison with the reference analysis showed that the entropy measures analysis techniques are more sensitive in the incremented time series compared to the classical parameters and entropy measures of original time series. Non-linear methods appear to be an additional valuable tool for analysis of the dynamics of posture especially when applied on incremental time series.

Keywords: center of pressure, sample entropy, multi-scale entropy, multivariate multi-scale entropy, visuo-kinesthetic effect

INTRODUCTION

Postural control is of paramount importance to ensure safe completion of complex tasks such as locomotion or simpler tasks such as standing. Postural control in healthy subjects is strongly affected by spatial orientation (Isableu et al., 1998) which in turn is based on both vestibulo-proprioceptive and visual cues (Asch and Witkin, 1948). Some subjects show an increased visual dependency (Guerraz et al., 2001) and therefore closing the eyes or introducing distorted visual feedback (e.g., wearing translucent goggles) increases the difficulty of standing tasks (Bronstein, 1986). A diminished postural control may result in a loss of equilibrium and consequently in falling (Carroll and Freedman, 1993; Collins and De Luca, 1993). This diminution may either be due to normal ageing (Pascolo et al., 2005, 2006) or due to a neurodegenerative disorder such as Parkinson's disease (Sabatini, 2000; Duarte and Zatsiorsky, 2001).

Usually, the quantification of postural control is included in clinical assessments but this strongly depends on the technology available. Either the postural control is rated based on clinical rating scales (Bloem et al., 2016) e.g., Tinetti Balance Scale, Rating Scale for Gait Evaluation, or on specific equipment such as force plates (Yamada, 1995; Newell et al., 1997) to measure body sway. The displacement of the center of pressure (COP) (the point of application of the vertical resultant force acting on the body from the supporting surface, dos Santos, 2008) is commonly measured when evaluating the postural control of a person (Carroll and Freedman, 1993; Collins and De Luca, 1993). The COP is highly irregular and non-stationary which has led multiple studies to characterize the functional effects of conditions such as disease, aging, cognitive task and visual perception on the postural stability (Ramdani et al., 2009).

Techniques for quantifying the displacement of the COP vary from descriptive measures (mean or standard deviation) to techniques taken from signal processing (root-mean-square and frequency analyses). The non-linear deterministic methods allow for the exploration of the randomness or predictability of the COP fluctuations. Those methods were used in studies investigating the deterministic features of COP dynamics (Myklebust et al., 1995; Riley et al., 1999; Doyle, 2004; Doyle et al., 2005), and their potentially chaotic behavior (Cavanaugh, 2005; Costa et al., 2005; Roerdink et al., 2006; Cavanaugh et al., 2007) but also on the quantification of the complexity of COP time series (Ramdani et al., 2009). Entropy family, as a non-linear measure of time series, has been widely applied to study features of COP displacement in different situations.

Entropy family quantifies the regularity (predictability) of a signal, with predictable (e.g., periodic) signals resulting in low entropy, or completely unpredictable signals, resulting in high entropy. A more regular COP pattern indicates that the postural behavior is more rigid (Donker et al., 2007), suggesting that the regularity of COP displacements and the amount of attention paid to postural control are dependent (Donker et al., 2007; Vuillerme and Nafati, 2007). Complexity on the other hand is associated with meaningful structural richness (Grassberger, 1991) incorporating correlations over multiple spatio-temporal scales. A decrease of complexity is related with a functional decline; and a more rigid postural behavior results in dysfunctional balance control during perturbations (Schniepp et al., 2013).

For instance, the Sample Entropy (SE) (Roerdink et al., 2006) has been used to investigate the effect of visual perception (Sabatini, 2000), cerebral concussion (Cavanaugh, 2005; Cavanaugh et al., 2007) and cognitive tasks (Wei et al., 2012) on postural dynamics. Multi-scale Entropy (MSE) and Multivariate Multi-Scale Entropy (MMSE) (Ahmed and Mandic, 2011) are both able to represent the complexity of non-linear time series in different scales (Ahmed and Mandic, 2011). They measure and quantify the intrinsic complexity (Costa et al., 2005) of single and multi-channel signals and then provide a meaningful measure of regularity in biological signals as e.g., COP measurements (Ahmed and Mandic, 2012).

To extract additional features of the COP displacement, the analysis of incremented time series of original signals may be useful (Ramdani et al., 2009) and this approach provides extra information compared to other approaches (Huang et al., 2013). Incremented time series, equivalent to the velocity of the COP displacements have been shown to be effective in the analysis of physiological signals (Costa et al., 2007). In this study two types of incremented time series were computed and studied, the relationship between anterior-posterior (A/P) and medio-lateral (M/L) COP displacement while using univariate and bivariate entropy measures. Although previous studies (Costa et al., 2007; Ramdani et al., 2009) applied incremental time series in their COP analysis, no proof has been provided to determine its performance and advantage.

The working hypothesis was to test if non-linear entropy family methods quantify COP displacement better when using incremented time series during three standing conditions with varying visuo-kinesthetic input. In addition to the entropy measures, classical posturographic methods were also used to assess the COP displacement. The classical methods were then compared with the entropy measures of the original time series.

METHODS EXPERIMENTS AND SUBJECTS

Eleven healthy subjects (Mean age: 25.6 years; Mean bodyweight 73.76 kg) voluntarily participated in the experiment after signing a statement of informed consent as required by the Helsinki declaration and the Paris-Saclay STAPS (Sciences and Techniques of Sports and Physical Activities) local Ethics Committee. Subjects stood upright looking forward, on a force plate (AMTI OR6001200, Watertown, MA, USA) with their arms hanging loosely by their sides and feet separated by a self-selected distance (typically approximately 10 cm) for 30 s. Foot position was marked with an erasable marker to ensure the position was maintained if subjects needed to step off the force plate between trials or conditions. Subjects performed three trials of stationary bipedal standing in three different sensory conditions, eyes open (EO), eyes closed (EC) and perturbed vision (PV) by wearing translucent goggles, resulting in a total of nine trials. The trials for each condition were averaged accordingly.

In the PV condition, even though the eyes were opened, the visual input did not constitute a valid and meaningful source (i.e., neither self-motion nor self-orientation cues) of spatial referencing for postural balance, and cannot be integrated together with proprioception in an optimal manner (Jeka et al., 2000; Oie et al., 2001). Conditions were presented in a random order for each participant. Subjects were instructed to stand as still as possible with either the eyes open, eyes closed or wearing translucent goggles. The COP trajectories were recorded in both A/P and M/L directions at a sampling frequency of 250 Hz as shown in **Figure 1**. Rest periods of 60 s were provided between trials. The resulting data was low-pass filtered at 5 Hz using an 8th order Butterworth filter with a zero-phase digital filter (filtfilt.m) in the Matlab (MathWorks, Inc., USA) environment.

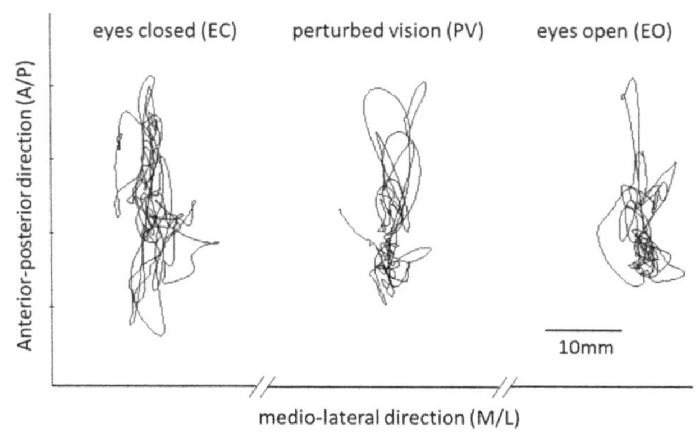

FIGURE 1 | This figure shows representative time series of COP data in each of the three experimental conditions (EO, EC, PV). Differences between conditions are explored using both classical parameters and entropy based methods.

ANALYSIS

Classical Methods

To quantify differences between the conditions (EC, PV, EO), the following variables were calculated from the postural sway: the root-mean square (RMS), mean velocity (MV), path length (PL), mean frequency (MF) and the surface area (SA) of COP displacements in A/P and M/L directions. The RMS was defined as the quadratic mean and is a measure of the postural sway displacement in both the A/P and M/L directions [mm]. The mean velocity defines the mean velocity of the postural sway representing the path length divided by the trial duration [mm/s]. The path length was defined as the length of the COP trajectory displacements on the platform surface [mm]. The MF is the mean frequency of the power spectrum of the postural sway in both the A/P and M/L directions. The SA is the surface area given by the 95% confidence ellipse representing the smallest ellipse that covers 95% of the points of the postural sway [mm^2] (Paillard et al., 2006).

Non-linear Methods

Three non-linear methods were used to measure the regularity of COP signals and compare their sensitivity between the incremented time series and the original time series. Sample Entropy is essentially a negative logarithm of conditional probability of the sequences of a data vector. If a vector of length N has repeated itself in tolerance γ for m points, it will also do so for m+1 points. The conditional probability means the ratio of counts of repeated time of m+1 points to that of m points. Thereby, high SE arises from a low probability of repeated sequences in the data. Higher SE means lower regularity and more complexity in the data. On the basis of SE, MSE is a method to evaluate the complexity of signals over different time-scales while MMSE generalizes the analysis to the multivariate case (Wei et al., 2012).

The SE is mathematically computed as follows:

First, from a vector $X_N = \{x_1, x_2, \cdots, x_N\}$, two sequences of m consecutive points $X_m(i) = \{x_i, \ldots, x_{i+m-1}\}$ and $X_m(j) = \{x_j, \ldots, x_{j+m-1}\}$ $(i, j \in [1, N-m], i \neq j)$ are selected to compute the maximum distance and compared to tolerance γ for repeated sequences counting, according to Equation (1). For the sequence $X_m(i)$, its count is defined as $B_i^m(\gamma)$.

$$d\left[X_m(i), X_m(j)\right] = \max[|x_{i+k}, x_{j+k}|] \leq \gamma(k \in [0, m-1], \gamma \geq 0) \quad (1)$$

1 where the tolerance γ equals to 0.1~0.2*SD (Richman and Moorman, 2000), SD is the standard deviation of X_N.

$B^m(\gamma)$ is the average amount of $B_i^m(\gamma)$ for $i \in [1, N-m]$, and $B^{m+1}(\gamma)$ is the average of m +1 consecutive points. Thus, SE is obtained using the Equation (2).

$$SE(N, m, \gamma) = -ln\left[\frac{B^{m+1}(\gamma)}{B^m(\gamma)}\right] = -ln\left[\frac{(N-m-1)^{-1}\sum_{i=1}^{N-m-1} B_i^{m+1}(\gamma)}{(N-m)^{-1}\sum_{i=1}^{N-m} B_i^m(\gamma)}\right] \quad (2)$$

MSE has a coarse-grain procedure for the data vector X_N before SE computation, which is the main computation difference between MSE and SE. Due to this procedure, MSE is able to measure the distribution of complexity on multiple time-scales, which is fundamentally different from SE. The coarse-grain procedure averages each τ points to generate a new sequence from the data. It is similar to a non-overlapping mean filter with a window length τ. Changing τ leads to sequences in different time-scales. Higher τ means lower frequency components in the sequences. MSE generates the complexity distribution of the data through the sequences in different time-scales, and MSE is equal to SE when $\tau = 1$. The parameter m is the length of repeated mode in the data vector, which is defined by the data itself; and the tolerance γ decides the limitation condition of repeated mode. In biological time-series analysis, m is typically set at 2 or 3 and γ is 0.15*standard deviation (SD) (X_N) (Costa et al., 2005).

To calculate MSE, the following steps have to be computed: the first step is to form a sequence $y_j^{(\tau)}$ based on the scale factor τ, which can be found using the Equation (3):

$$y_j^{(\tau)} = \frac{1}{\tau}\sum_{i=(j-1)\tau+1}^{j\tau} x_i \quad (3)$$

The equation to compute MSE can be expressed as follows:

$$MSE(N, m, \tau, \gamma) = -\ln\left[\frac{A^{m+1}(\gamma)}{A^m(\gamma)}\right] \quad (4)$$

where both $A^m(\gamma)$ and $A^{m+1}(\gamma)$ are the average repeated amount of two *sequences* $Y_m(i)$ and $Y_{m+1}(i)$ [see Equations (1, 2)] to calculate $B_i^m(\gamma)$) and tolerance γ is also for the formed sequences $y_j^{(\tau)}$ with the length $N' = N/\tau \in [10^m, 30^m]$ (Pincus and Goldberger, 1994). Therefore, τ is defined by length of N of X_N and m. For example, N = 10,000 and m = 2,500 as the median of $[10^2, 30^2]$ could be selected to calculate the τ_{max} = 10,000/500 = 20 and $\tau \in [1, 20]$.

MMSE provides a complexity distribution too, not for a data vector but for the matrix vector from multichannel or multivariate data, which is more adaptive to multi-dimension or multi-parameter time series that are routinely measured in experimental and biological systems.

Given the matrix $X(p, N)$, p is the number of channels or variates, N is the original length, so that the first step for this matrix is just transforming it into a new matrix $X'(p, N')$, based on scale factor τ regardless of m, which gives the new matrix in a new time scale like the coarse-grain procedure in MSE. In the second step, m and ε are extended to an embedding vector and a time lag vector for a p -variate embedded reconstruction respectively. For the consistence of each variate in the matrix, the values of m and ε are identical, e.g., $m = [3,3,3]$; $\varepsilon = [1, 1, 1]$. That means three MSE computations with the embedding dimension $m = 3$ for three variates and the time delay $\varepsilon = 1$. The time delay $\varepsilon = 1$ is the best choice when the minimum embedding dimension for each of the time series is 3 (Cao et al., 1998).

In practice its first step is to define temporal scales of the increased length by coarse-graining the *p-variate* $\{x_{k,i}\}_{i=1}^{N}, k = 1, 2, \ldots, p$. For a scale factor τ, the multivariate coarse-grained time series $y_{k,j}^{(\tau)}$ is calculated [see Equation (5)], where $1 \leq j \leq N/\tau$.

$$y_{k,j}^{(\tau)} = \frac{1}{\tau} \sum_{i=(j-1)\tau+1}^{j\tau} x_{k,i} \tag{5}$$

In order to obtain the MMSE, the multivariate embedded vectors $Y_m(i) \in \mathbb{R}^p$ must be constructed firstl, which is shown as:

$$\begin{aligned} Y_m(i) = {} & [y_{1,i}, y_{1,i+\varepsilon_1}, \ldots, y_{1,i+(m_1-1)\varepsilon_1}, y_{2,i}, y_{2,i+\varepsilon_2}, \ldots, \\ & y_{2,i+(m_2-1)\varepsilon_2}, \ldots, y_{p,i}, y_{p,i+\varepsilon_p}, \ldots, y_{p,i+(m_p-1)\varepsilon_p}] \end{aligned} \tag{6}$$

where $1 \leq i \leq N' - n$ and $N' = N/\tau$, $n = max\{M\} \times max\{\varepsilon\}$. $M = [m_1, m_2, \ldots, m_p] \in \mathbb{R}^p$ is the embedding vector, while $\varepsilon = [\varepsilon_1, \varepsilon_1, \ldots, \varepsilon_p]$ is the time lag vector and $M = \sum_{k=1}^{p} m_k$. Then the maximum norm is defined by Chebyshev distance between any two composite delay vectors $Y_m(i)$ and $Y_m(j)$, that is expressed as:

$$\begin{aligned} d[Y_m(i), Y_m(j)] = {} & max_{l=1,\ldots,m} \\ & \{|y(i + l - 1) - y(j + l - 1)|\} \end{aligned} \tag{7}$$

where $j \in [1, N' - n], j \neq i$. For a given $Y_m(i)$, P_i is the number of vector pairs that meets $d[Y_m(i), Y_m(j)] \leq \gamma$, so that $A_i^m(\gamma) = P_i/(N' - n - 1)$, where $n = max\{M\} \times max\{\tau\}$. And for all i, $A^m(\gamma) = (N' - n)^{-1} \sum_{i=1}^{N'-n} A_i^m(\gamma)$.

Finally, the average similarity $A^m(\gamma)$ over all $i \in [1, N' - n]$ and the $A^{m+1}(\gamma)$ over all $i \in [1, p * (N' - n)]$ are used to gain the MMSE, as shown in Equation (8).

$$MMSE(N', M, \tau, \gamma) = -ln \left[\frac{A^{m+1}(\gamma)}{A^m(\gamma)} \right] \tag{8}$$

where γ is the tolerance level and N' is the length of the time series $y_{k,j}^{(\tau)}$.

The embedding vector $M = [m_1, m_2, \ldots, m_p] \in \mathbb{R}^p$ and the tolerance level γ in MMSE have the equivalent values with parameters m and γ in MSE (Wei et al., 2012).

The three non-linear entropy methods are effective to measure complexity of time series, specifically the SE for the univariate vector, MSE for the univariate vector in multiple time-scale, and MMSE for the multivariate matrix in multiple time-scale respectively. Moreover, it is crucial to have the original time series filtered as all entropy methods are extremely sensitive to random noise. Therefore, our COP data was filtered by a low-pass filter before the computation of entropy.

Incremental Time Series

The postural sway was analyzed in the A/P and the M/L direction, COP (A/P) and COP (M/L) respectively. Additional to the original COP data, its increments were calculated 2-fold: First $\Delta_{inc}x = [x(t + 1) - x(t - 1)]$, defined as the ***Increment***; second $\Delta_{diff}x = [x(t + 1) - x(t)]$, defined as ***Difference***. Since mean velocity is a classical parameter of COP estimation, the increments of original COP data, as its equivalent velocity, were created from the original data to remove long-range correlations and avoid potential masking of the complexity of the COP time series.

Simulation

In the simulation, both the original and incremental time series are used to evaluate differences by means of SE, MSE, and MMSE. White noise and 1/f noise are prominent signals to test entropy family measures because of their short-term and long-term correlated properties (Richman and Moorman, 2000; Costa et al., 2005; Ahmed and Mandic, 2011; Wei et al., 2012). To illustrate the behavior of incremental time series and its influence on entropy measures, we considered six time series with a length of $N = 20{,}000$ (meeting the range minimum $10^m \times \tau_{max}$ when $m = 3$ and $\tau_{max} = 20$) of each data vector corresponding to 80 s (near to the sum of 30 s in trail and 60 s in rest) of data acquisition at 250 Hz: 1/f noise, 1/f noise ***Increment***, 1/f noise ***Difference***, white noise, white noise ***Increment***, white noise ***Difference***. ***Increment*** and ***Difference*** are computed from both the 1/f noise and the white noise data through $\Delta_{inc}x = [x(t+1) - x(t-1)]$ and $\Delta_{diff}x = [x(t + 1) - x(t)]$ respectively. MSE and MMSE were calculated with m = 2 and 3, $\gamma = 0.15$*SD (Costa et al., 2005) and a scale factor of $\tau = 1$ to 20 (**Figure 2**) (meeting the range minimum, Richman and Moorman, 2000).

The results of the simulations show decreasing complexity with increasing scale factor except for the 1/f noise series. To understand the differences between $m = 2$ & 3 on the entropy values, **Table 1** shows individual differences as a function of the scale factor for the six considered time series. The simulation results show differences between scale factors 11 and 15 with an absolute deviation of 0.01, indicating that SE is more sensitive on a larger scale with a pattern length of $m = 3$ (**Figure 2**). The MMSE analysis of bivariate time series shows similar patterns but larger entropy values in the correlated bivariate time series (**Figure 3**). When computing MSE and MMSE for short-term

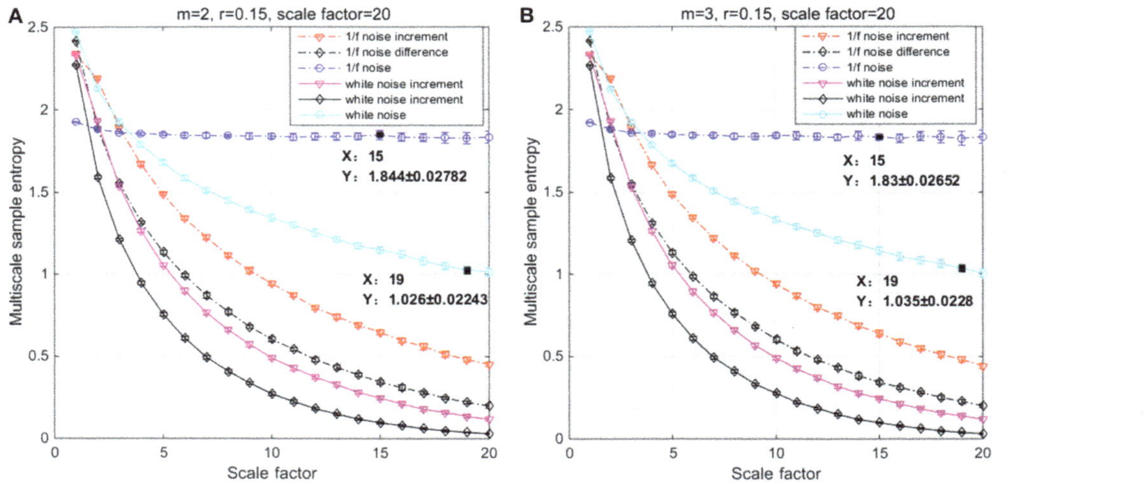

FIGURE 2 | Multiscale entropy (MSE) analysis of white noise, 1/f noise and their Increment and Difference using (A) $m = 2$, $r = 0.15$, and $\tau = 20$ and **(B)** $m = 3$, $r = 0.15$, and $\tau = 20$. Each channel has 20 000 data points, and the plots represent an average of 20 independent groups and error bars the standard deviation (SD).

TABLE 1 | Differences between the SE calculated with $m = 2$ and $m = 3$ for different scales and noises.

Scale factor	1/f noise			White noise		
	Original	Increment	Difference	Original	Increment	Difference
1	0.0010	0.0020	0.0010	0.0000	0.0010	0.0050
2	−0.0020	0.0010	0.0010	0.0010	0.0020	0.0070
3	0.0010	0.0000	−0.0015	0.0010	0.0060	0.0060
4	−0.0020	0.0050	0.0020	0.0010	−0.0010	0.0013
5	0.0020	0.0000	0.0020	0.0040	0.0000	−0.0036
6	−0.0020	−0.0050	0.0057	0.0000	0.0038	0.0010
7	−0.0030	0.0050	0.0045	0.0040	−0.0024	−0.0030
8	0.0020	0.0010	0.0025	0.0080	−0.0010	−0.0025
9	0.0050	0.0010	−0.0027	0.0030	0.0042	0.0056
10	−0.0030	0.0019	0.0000	0.0011	−0.0021	−0.0052
11	−0.0070	0.0028	0.0074	−0.0091	0.0028	0.0017
12	0.0000	−0.0039	−0.0011	−0.0010	0.0000	−0.0046
13	0.0080	−0.0064	0.0000	0.0050	0.0070	−0.0020
14	−0.0010	0.0038	0.0035	−0.0050	0.0018	0.0010
15	0.0140	0.0051	−0.0090	0.0030	−0.0040	−0.0024
16	0.0090	0.0059	−0.0080	0.0015	−0.0070	0.0093
17	−0.0060	0.0010	−0.0019	−0.0030	−0.0050	−0.0022
18	−0.0030	0.0030	−0.0045	−0.0013	0.0022	0.0020
19	0.0030	−0.0070	−0.0059	−0.0090	−0.0035	−0.0038
20	0.0000	0.0011	−0.0017	0.0010	−0.0016	−0.0020

correlated signals (white noise), a reduction in complexity occurs with larger scale factors in contrast to long-term correlated signals (1/f noise).

When computing MSE and MMSE for incremented time series with white noise and 1/f noise, reductions of complexity with increasing scales occur. The incremental time series removes the long-term correlated components from the original time series and represent short-term complexity. Compared to the MSE, the MMSE analysis shows lower entropy values per scale and seems to detect signal divergence faster and can, therefore, be considered more suitable for complexity detection.

Based on the simulation results indicating that SE is more sensitive on larger scales, while m was set to three, $\gamma = 0.15$*SD and a scale factor ranging from 1 to 20. A larger scale factor

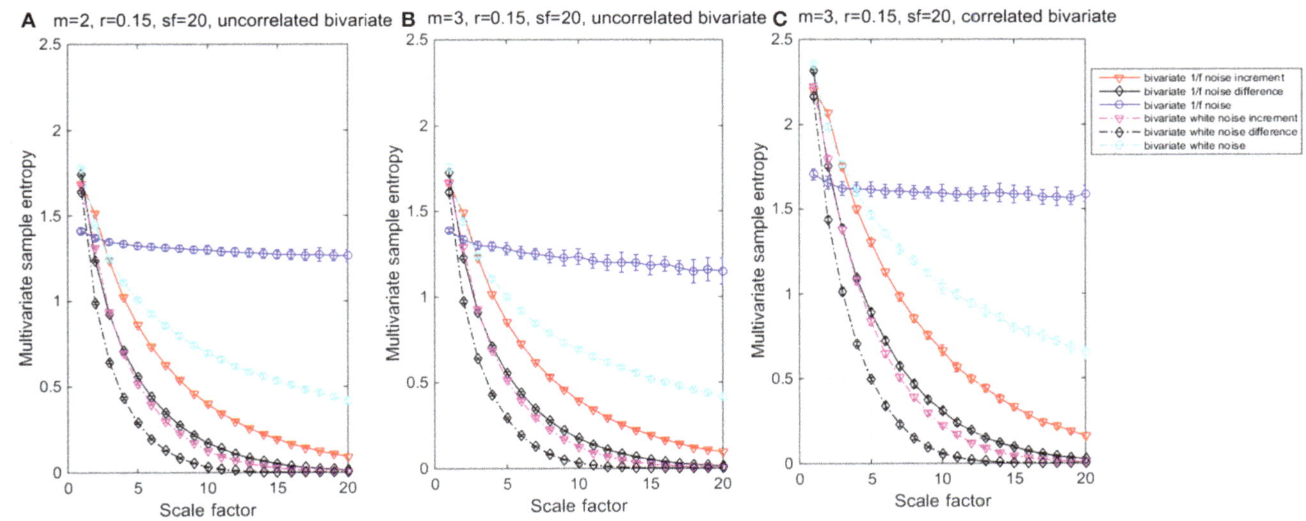

FIGURE 3 | Multivariate multiscale entropy (MMSE) analysis for uncorrelated bivariate 1/f noise, white noise and their Increment and Difference within $m = 2$ (A) and 3 **(B)** respectively; and for **(C)** correlated bivariate 1/f noise, white noise and their Increment and Difference within $m = 3$.

provides a higher resolution of complexity in the time domain and visuo-vestibular regulation is related to low frequencies (0–0.5 Hz) of the COP displacement (Dichgans et al., 1976; Paillard et al., 2006).

Statistical Analysis

Friedman tests were used to examine the effect of condition (i.e., EO, EC, PV) on all postural parameters. The complexity index (CI), defined as the integral of the MSE or MMSE curve, was used for the statistical analysis of the entropy measures (MSE, MMSE). The normality of the data sets was verified using the Kolmogorov-Smirnov test. *Post-hoc* pairwise comparisons (between-conditions) were performed when needed using Wilcoxon's tests with a Bonferroni adjustment. The effect size values were described by the magnitude of change expressed as Cliff's delta ($|r|$). All tests were performed using IBM SPSS Statistics version 16 with a level of significance set at $p < 0.05$.

RESULTS

The Kolmogorov-Smirnov tests indicated non-parametric distribution of the data sets and therefore the data is reported using median (*Med*) and inter-quartile range (*IQR*). For the classical parameters, Friedman tests indicated significant differences in path length, mean velocity and mean frequency (A/P), depending on the condition (**Table 2**). The *post-hoc* Wilcoxon's analyses revealed a statistically significant difference between the EO and EC conditions for path length, [EC ($Med = 230.95$, $IQR = 120.52$) and EO ($Med = 184.19$, $IQR = 53.62$), $z = 2.934$, $p \leq 0.01$], mean velocity [EC ($Med = 7.7$, $IQR = 4.02$) and EO ($Med = 6.14$, $IQR = 1.78$), $z = 2.934$, $p \leq 0.01$], and mean frequency [EC ($Med = 0.52$, $IQR = 0.31$) and EO ($Med = 0.45$, $IQR = 0.30$), $z = 2.934$, $p \leq 0.01$]. The small effect size calculation for the tree parameters with Cliff's delta values ($r < 0.35$) suggests minimal practical significance. For the 95% confidence ellipse, mean frequency (M/L), root-mean-square in A/P, or M/L direction (**Table 2**) no differences were found.

The analysis for ***Original*** time series showed a significant effect of condition on CI_MSE (A/P) and CI_MMSE (**Table 2**). The *post-hoc* Wilcoxon's analyses revealed a statistically significant difference between the EO and PV conditions for CI_MMSE, [EO ($Med = 13.98$, $IQR = 1.15$) and PV ($Med = 13.58$, $IQR = 1.12$), $z = 2.401$, $p \leq 0.05$]. The large effect size calculation with a Cliff's delta value ($r > 0.80$) suggests high practical significance.

For the ***Incremented*** time series, significant differences between conditions were found in three of the five parameters (**Table 2**). The *post-hoc* Wilcoxon's analyses revealed a statistically significant difference between the EC and EO conditions for CI_MSE (A/P) [EC ($Med = 18.91$, $IQR = 1.14$) and EO ($Med = 17.99$, $IQR = 1.73$), $z = 2.934$, $p \leq 0.01$], CI_MSE (M/L) [EC ($Med = 20.29$, $IQR = 1.37$) and EO ($Med = 19.00$, $IQR = 0.95$), $z = 2.490$, $p \leq 0.05$], and CI_MMSE [EC ($Med = 9.03$, $IQR = 0.40$) and EO ($Med = 8.46$, $IQR = 0.71$), $z = 2.934$, $p \leq 0.01$]. The small effect size calculation for the tree parameters with Cliff's delta values ($r < 0.35$) suggests minimal practical significance.

When comparing the EC and PV conditions, the *post-hoc* Wilcoxon's analyses revealed a statistically significant differences for CI_MSE (A/P) [EC ($Med = 18.91$, $IQR = 1.14$) and PV ($Med = 18.29$, $IQR = 1.35$), $z = 2.401$, $p \leq 0.05$], CI_MSE (M/L) [EC ($Med = 20.29$, $IQR = 1.37$) and PV ($Med = 19.94$, $IQR = 0.84$), $z = 2.701$, $p \leq 0.01$], and CI_MMSE [EC ($Med = 9.03$, $IQR = 0.40$) and PV ($Med = 8.83$, $IQR = 0.43$), $z = 2.667$, $p \leq 0.01$]. The large effect size calculation for the three parameters with Cliff's delta values ($r > 0.95$) suggests large practical significance.

When comparing the PV and EO conditions, the *post-hoc* Wilcoxon's analyses revealed statistically significant differences for CI_MSE(A/P) [PV ($Med = 18.29$, $IQR = 1.35$) and EO (Med

TABLE 2 | Results of non-parametric statistical tests (median ± IQR) on differences between the three experimental conditions (EC, PV, EO) on classical and non-linear complexity parameters.

	Classical parameters				Friedman tests		Wilcoxon's *post-hoc* comparisons					
							EC vs. EO		EC vs. PV		PV vs. EO	
	EC	PV	EO	Trend	$\chi^2(2)$	*p*	*z*	|r|	*z*	|r|	*z*	|r|
Path Length	230.95 ± 120.52	208.14 ± 76.33	184.19 ± 53.62		14.73	**0.001**	2.934	0.273**				
Mean Velocity	7.7 ± 4.02	6.94 ± 2.54	6.14 ± 1.78		14.73	**0.001**	2.934	0.273**				
Confidence Ellipse	75.77 ± 61.27	84.32 ± 120.52	77.81 ± 43.34		0.55	0.761						
Mean Frequency (A/P)	0.52 ± 0.31	0.42 ± 0.33	0.45 ± 0.3		10.36	**0.006**	2.934	0.339**				
Mean Frequency (M/L)	0.26 ± 0.13	0.2 ± 0.08	0.15 ± 0.11		5.09	0.078						
RMS (A/P)	1.11 ± 0.66	1.19 ± 0.85	1.3 ± 0.5		0.55	0.761						
RMS (M/L)	3.79 ± 2.22	3.34 ± 2.38	4.4 ± 2.44		0.55	0.761						
		Original time series			$\chi^2(2)$	*p*	*z*	|r|	*z*	|r|	*z*	|r|
SE (A/P)	1.28 ± 0.16	1.30 ± 0.15	1.32 ± 0.13		0.55	0.761						
SE (M/L)	0.76 ± 0.28	0.72 ± 0.16	0.77 ± 0.46		2.91	0.234						
CI_MSE (A/P)	18.99 ± 2.4	19.4 ± 2.26	19.14 ± 1.47		6.73	**0.035**						
CI_MSE (M/L)	12.49 ± 4.26	11.46 ± 2.09	11.07 ± 6.13		1.27	0.529						
CI_MMSE	13.98 ± 1.15	13.58 ± 1.12	14.17 ± 0.56		6.73	**0.035**					2.401	0.818*
		Incremented time series			$\chi^2(2)$	*p*	*z*	|r|	*z*	|r|	*z*	|r|
SE (A/P)	2.35 ± 0.02	2.34 ± 0.01	2.34 ± 0.01		5.09	0.078						
SE (M/L)	2.36 ± 0.01	2.35 ± 0.01	2.35 ± 0.02		4.55	0.103						
CI_MSE (A/P)	18.91 ± 1.14	18.29 ± 1.35	17.99 ± 1.73		18.727	**0.000**	2.934	−0.025**	2.401	1.000*	2.934	0.669**
CI_MSE (M/L)	20.29 ± 1.37	19.94 ± 0.84	19 ± 0.95		8.419	**0.015**	2.490	0.124*	2.701	0.950**		
CI_MMSE	9.03 ± 0.4	8.83 ± 0.43	8.46 ± 0.71		14.727	**0.001**	2.934	0.008**	2.667	0.967**	2.578	0.752*
		Difference time series			$\chi^2(2)$	*p*	*z*	|r|	*z*	|r|	*z*	|r|
SE (A/P)	2.27 ± 0.01	2.27 ± 0.01	2.27 ± 0.01		7.47	**0.024**						
SE (M/L)	2.27 ± 0.01	2.27 ± 0.01	2.26 ± 0.01		3.82	0.148						
CI_MSE (A/P)	12.29 ± 0.84	11.94 ± 0.85	11.62 ± 1.14		17.636	**0.001**	2.934	−0.074**			2.934	0.686**
CI_MSE (M/L)	13.2 ± 0.99	12.88 ± 0.69	12.03 ± 0.65		8.727	**0.013**	2.534	−0.074*	2.667	0.950**		
CI_MMSE	5.24 ± 0.23	5.15 ± 0.19	5 ± 0.23		16.233	**0.000**	2.934	−0.091**	2.497	1.000*	2.801	0.669**

*EC, eyes closed condition; PV, perturbed vision; EO, eyes open condition. A/P, anterior-posterior; M/L, medio-lateral. SE, Sample Entropy; CI_MSE, complexity index of Multi-Scale Entropy; CI_MMSE, complexity index of Multivariate Multi-Scale Entropy. *$p < 0.05$ (after Bonferroni correction, $p < 0.017$), **$p < 0.01$. Bold values shows significantly different among three conditions.*

= 17.99, $IQR = 1.73$), $z = 2.934$, $p \leq 0.01$], and CI_MMSE [PV ($Med = 7.7$, $IQR = 4.02$) and EO ($Med = 6.14$, $IQR = 1.78$), $z = 2.578$, $p \leq 0.05$]. The medium effect size calculation for the two parameters with Cliff's delta values ($r > 0.65$) suggests high practical significance.

In the ***Difference*** time series, four of the five non-linear parameters significantly changed between conditions (**Table 1**). The *post-hoc* Wilcoxon's analyses revealed statistically significant differences between the EO and EC conditions for CI_MSE (A/P) [EC ($Med = 12, 29$ $IQR = 0.84$) and EO ($Med = 11.62$, $IQR = 1.14$), $z = 2.934$, $p \leq 0.01$], CI_MSE (M/L) [EC ($Med = 13.20$, $IQR = 0.99$) and EO ($Med = 12.03$, $IQR = 0.65$), $z = 2.534$, $p \leq 0.05$], and CI_MMSE [EC ($Med = 5.24$, $IQR = 0.23$) and EO ($Med = 5.00$, $IQR = 0.23$), $z = 2.934$, $p \leq 0.01$]. The small effect size calculation for the tree parameters with Cliff's delta values ($r < 0.35$) suggests minimal practical significance.

When comparing the EC and PV conditions, the *post-hoc* Wilcoxon's analyses revealed a statistically significant differences for CI_MSE (M/L), [EC ($Med = 13.20$, $IQR = 0.99$) and PV ($Med = 12.88$ $IQR = 0.69$), $z = 2.667$, $p \leq 0.01$], and CI_MMSE [EC ($Med = 5.24$, $IQR = 0.23$) and PV ($Med = 5.15$, $IQR = 0.19$), $z = 2.497$, $p \leq 0.05$]. The large effect size calculation for the three parameters with Cliff's delta values ($r > 0.90$) suggests large practical significance.

When comparing the PV and EO conditions, the *post-hoc* Wilcoxon's analyses revealed statistically significant differences for CI_MSE (A/P), [PV ($Med = 11.94$, $IQR = 0.85$) and EO ($Med = 11.62$, $IQR = 1.14$), $z = 2.934$, $p \leq 0.01$], and CI_MMSE [PV ($Med = 5.15$, $IQR = 0.19$) and EO ($Med = 5.00$, $IQR = 0.23$), $z = 2.801$, $p \leq 0.01$]. The medium to large effect size calculation for the two parameters with Cliff's delta values ($r > 0.60$) suggests large practical significance.

DISCUSSION

In this experiment, classical parameters were tested against non-linear complexity parameters to reveal differences between the COP displacements during three standing conditions. Non-linear entropy family methods resulted in better uncovering of postural displacement differences when compared to the classical posturographic methods. Only three of the seven classical parameters [i.e., PL, MV, MF (A/P)] were able to differentiate between conditions (EO, EC, PV). Amongst the five studied entropy measures, only two showed significant differences between conditions [i.e., CI_MSE (A/P) and CI_MMSE] using the ***Original*** time series, and in the ***Incremented*** and ***Difference*** time series CI_MSE (A/P), CI_MSE (M/L) and CI_MMSE showed higher sensitivity to the condition effect. Between-conditions differences in the ***Original*** time series were only revealed for the CI_MMSE parameter. In the ***Increment*** and ***Difference*** time series between-conditions differences were found for CI_MSE (A/P), CI_MSE (M/L) and CI_MMSE parameters. The most consistent parameter for the three time series is the CI_MMSE and could therefore be considered as the most reliable parameter in detecting between-conditions differences.

For visual feedback, the results show that the complexity quantified by MSE, and MMSE statistic in ***Increment*** and ***Difference*** is lower in the EC condition compared to EO and PV. Even though the statistical analysis has not shown significant differences on the COP displacement related to the effect of visual feedback, the entropy values for SE (A/P) of the ***Original*** is lowest in the EC condition. Higher entropy values are related to more irregularity, something that may be associated with a functional decline of the postural control system resulting in maladaptive responses to perturbations and thereby destabilizing the balance control (Vaillancourt and Newell, 2002; Schniepp et al., 2013). This finding is consistent with previous research (Roerdink et al., 2011) showing that physical and physiological visual parameters affect postural control during quiet standing and therefore the COP displacement (cf. Stins et al., 2009; Vuillerme and Pinsault, 2009). The sample size and the choice of young healthy participants that were recruited from the Sports Science department may have influenced the results as they may have higher postural capacities compared to age matched subjects. Working with healthy young adults increases the difficulty to distinguish between EO and EC compared to older adults (Prieto et al., 1996). Taking this into account the relation between COP regularity and the amount of attention invested in posture (Donker et al., 2007; Stins et al., 2009), are in line with the findings of our study. The COP regularity in the ***Original*** time series showed no differences between conditions by means of sample entropy while in the ***Difference*** time series such differences were uncovered. This confirms previous work showing that a decrease of the complexity of the physiological and behavioral systems is observed when the kinesthetic cues are reduced (Newell et al., 1997) but also that incremented time series provide short-term correlated components containing more information about the non-linear system (Ramdani et al., 2009).

Using entropy measures allows us to deal with highly irregular and variable signals like postural sway (Prieto et al., 1996). However, limitations of the particular parameters and properties of the entropy measures have to be discussed. MSE is an entropy measure for univariate time series and MMSE is extended to multivariate cases. Even though the results of MSE and multivariate MSE analysis are promising, some problems still have to be resolved when working with postural data. Entropy measures assess the complexity of physiological time series signals rather than measure motor performance. The creation of one complexity index summing all twenty scales needs to be addressed in future research as it is currently unknown which time-scale is more important or related to postural control. Data length affects entropy measures but it depends on the experiment and therefore a high sampling rate of 250 Hz was chosen to obtain the necessary data length. The COP signal does not contain high frequency signals and the use of a low-pass filter (cut-off 5 Hz) is common. This may create an oversampling issue and the first several scales may not have physiological meaningful information related to dynamical COP changes. Furthermore, the coarse-graining procedure reduced the input data length to half its original size for each successive data scale and therefore potentially changed the intrinsic dynamical scales defined by the signal-generating system.

The reduction of MSE with increasing time-scale is based on the tolerance settings (i.e., constant fraction of the variance of the original time series) and the conventional γ*SD tolerance could be replaced by the variance of each coarse grained time series (Humeau-Heurtier, 2015).

Previous research from our laboratory has shown those MSE characteristics and a possible solution could be the use of diverse empirical mode decomposition techniques (Shih et al., 2015). Decomposing the ***Original*** time series into intrinsic mode functions when testing different combinations of frequency bands with relevant complexity indexes has been shown to be efficient and promising in studies on elderly subjects exposed to slight vibrations under their feet (Wei et al., 2012). Empirical mode decomposition and Hilbert–Huang transformation can also be used to observe the physiological signals in instantaneous frequency and instantaneous amplitude through intrinsic mode functions, and then transformed inversely into the time domain to observe the changes in different conditions (Shih et al., 2015). However, the ***Increment*** and ***Difference*** time series approaches also seem appropriate as they removed trends from the original time series and showed changes in the COP displacements. Other approaches (Yeh et al., 2016) such as the above-mentioned empirical mode decomposition also provide useful data-driven scale factor and intrinsic entropy calculation of complex time series showing the possibility to explore the dynamical complexity of postural control in the future by combining incremented time series and empirical mode decomposition methods.

CONCLUSIONS

The current work supports the notion that some measures of non-linear entropy discriminate postural displacement better than classical measures when using incremented time series. Future studies should look to extend applied methods by examining other populations with impaired motor control. We also suggest that future research should consider empirical mode decomposition in combination with incremented time series across different clinical conditions to establish the reliability and validity of this new approach.

AUTHOR CONTRIBUTIONS

CH, LM, PF, and BI designed and conducted the experiment, QW and JS conducted the analysis and simulations, CH, QW, and JS wrote the manuscript.

ACKNOWLEDGMENTS

This research was supported by the Innovation Center for Big Data and Digital Convergence, Yuan Ze University, Taoyuan, Chung-Li, Taiwan which is sponsored by Ministry of Education. Also, it was supported by Ministry of Science and Technology (Grant Number: NSC 102-2221-E-155-028-MY3).

REFERENCES

Ahmed, M. U., and Mandic, D. P. (2011). Multivariate multiscale entropy: a tool for complexity analysis of multichannel data. *Phys. Rev. E Stat. Nonlin. Soft Matter Phys.* 84(6 Pt 1):061918. doi: 10.1103/physreve.84.061918

Ahmed, M. U., and Mandic, D. P. (2012). Multivariate multiscale entropy analysis. *IEEE Signal. Process. Lett.* 19, 91–94. doi: 10.1109/LSP.2011.2180713

Asch, S. E., and Witkin, H. A. (1948). Studies in space orientation. II. Perception of the upright with displaced visual fields and with body tilted. *J. Exp. Psychol.* 38, 455–475. doi: 10.1037/h0054121

Bloem, B. R., Marinus, J., Almeida, Q., Dibble, L., Nieuwboer, A., Post, B., et al. (2016). Measurement instruments to assess posture, gait, and balance in Parkinson's disease: critique and recommendations. *Mov. Disord.* 31, 1342–1355. doi: 10.1002/mds.26572

Bronstein, A. M. (1986). Suppression of visually evoked postural responses. *Exp. Brain Res.* 63, 655–658. doi: 10.1007/bf00237488

Cao, L. Y., Mees, A., and Judd, K. (1998). Dynamics from multivariate time series. *Phys. D. Nonlin. Phenomena* 121, 75–88. doi: 10.1016/S0167-2789(98)00151-1

Carroll, J. P., and Freedman, W. (1993). Nonstationary properties of postural sway. *J. Biomech.* 26, 409–416. doi: 10.1016/0021-9290(93)90004-X

Cavanaugh, J. T. (2005). Detecting altered postural control after cerebral concussion in athletes with normal postural stability. *Br. J. Sports Med.* 39, 805–811. doi: 10.1136/bjsm.2004.015909

Cavanaugh, J. T., Mercer, V. S., and Stergiou, N. (2007). Approximate entropy detects the effect of a secondary cognitive task on postural control in healthy young adults: a methodological report. *J. Neuroeng. Rehabil.* 4:42. doi: 10.1186/1743-0003-4-42

Collins, J. J., and De Luca, C. J. (1993). Open-loop and closed-loop control of posture: a random-walk analysis of center-of-pressure trajectories. *Exp. Brain Res.* 95, 308–318. doi: 10.1007/BF00229788

Costa, M., Goldberger, A. L., and Peng, C. K. (2005). Multiscale entropy analysis of biological signals. *Phys. Rev. E* 71:021906. doi: 10.1103/physreve.71.021906

Costa, M., Priplata, A. A., Lipsitz, L. A., Wu, Z., Huang, N. E., Goldberger, A. L., et al. (2007). Noise and poise: enhancement of postural complexity in the elderly with a stochastic-resonance–based therapy. *Europhys. Lett.* 77:68008. doi: 10.1209/0295-5075/77/68008

Dichgans, J., Mauritz, K. H., Allum, J. H., and Brandt, T. (1976). Postural sway in normals and atactic patients: analysis of the stabilising and destabilizing effects of vision. *Agressologie* 17, 15–24.

Donker, S. F., Roerdink, M., Greven, A. J., and Beek, P. J. (2007). Regularity of center-of-pressure trajectories depends on the amount of attention invested in postural control. *Exp. Brain Res.* 181, 1–11. doi: 10.1007/s00221-007-0905-4

dos Santos, A. D. (2008). *Multi-muscle Coordination in Postural Tasks.* ProQuest Dissertations & Theses Global, 304508614.

Doyle, T. L. A. (2004). Discriminating between elderly and young using a fractal dimension analysis of centre of pressure. *Int. J. Med. Sci.* 11, 11–20. doi: 10.7150/ijms.1.11

Doyle, T. L., Newton, R. U., and Burnett, A. F. (2005). Reliability of traditional and fractal dimension measures of quiet stance center of pressure in young, healthy people. *Arch. Phys. Med. Rehabil.* 86, 2034–2040. doi: 10.1016/j.apmr.2005.05.014

Duarte, M., and Zatsiorsky, V. M. (2001). Long-range correlations in human standing. *Phys. Lett. A* 283, 124–128. doi: 10.1016/S0375-9601(01)00188-8

Grassberger, P. (1991). "Information and complexity measures in dynamical systems," *Information Dynamics*, eds H. Atmanspacher and H. Scheingraber (New York, NY: Plenum Press), 15–33.

Guerraz, M., Yardley, L., Bertholon, P., Pollak, L., Rudge, P., Gresty, M. A., et al. (2001). Visual vertigo: symptom assessment, spatial orientation and postural control. *Brain* 124, 1646–1656. doi: 10.1093/brain/124.8.1646

Huang, L., Zhuang, J., and Zhang, Y. (2013). The application of computer musculoskeletal modeling and simulation to investigate compressive tibiofemoral force and muscle functions in obese children. *Comput. Math. Methods Med.* 2013, 1–10. doi: 10.1155/2013/698395

Humeau-Heurtier, A. (2015). The multiscale entropy algorithm and its variants: a review. *Entropy* 17, 3110–3123. doi: 10.3390/e17053110

Isableu, B., Ohlmann, T., Cremieux, J., and Amblard, B. (1998). How dynamic visual field dependence-independence interacts with the visual contribution to postural control. *Hum. Mov. Sci.* 17, 367–391. doi: 10.1016/S0167-9457(98)00005-0

Jeka, J., Oie, K. S., and Kiemel, T. (2000). Multisensory information for human postural control: integrating touch and vision. *Exp. Brain Res.* 134, 107–125. doi: 10.1007/s002210000412

Myklebust, J. B., Prieto, T., and Myklebust, B. (1995). Evaluation of nonlinear dynamics in postural steadiness time series. *Ann. Biomed. Eng.* 23, 711–719. doi: 10.1007/BF02584470

Newell, K. M., Slobounov, S. M., Slobounova, E. S., and Molenaar, P. C. M. (1997). Stochastic processes in postural center-of-pressure profiles. *Exp. Brain Res.* 113, 158–164. doi: 10.1007/BF02454152

Oie, K. S., Kiemel, T., and Jeka, J. J. (2001). Human multisensory fusion of vision and touch: detecting non-linearity with small changes in the sensory environment. *Neurosci. Lett.* 315, 113–116. doi: 10.1016/S0304-3940(01)02348-5

Paillard, T., Noe, F., Riviere, T., Marion, V., Montoya, R., and Dupui, P. (2006). Postural performance and strategy in the unipedal stance of soccer players at different levels of competition. *J. Athl. Train.* 41, 172–176.

Pascolo, P., Barazza, F., and Carniel, R. (2006). Considerations on the application of the chaos paradigm to describe the postural sway. *Chaos Solitons Fractals* 27, 1339–1346. doi: 10.1016/j.chaos.2005.04.111

Pascolo, P. B., Marini, A., Carniel, R., and Barazza, F. (2005). Posture as a chaotic system and an application to the Parkinson's disease. *Chaos Solitons Fractals* 24, 1343–1346. doi: 10.1016/j.chaos.2004.09.062

Pincus, S. M., and Goldberger, A. L. (1994). Physiological time-series analysis: what does regularity quantify? *Am. J. Physiol. Heart Circ. Physiol.* 266, 1643–1656.

Prieto, T. E., Myklebust, J. B., Hoffmann, R. G., Lovett, E. G., and Myklebust, B. M. (1996). Measures of postural steadiness: differences between healthy young and elderly adults. *IEEE Trans. Biomed. Eng.* 43, 956–966. doi: 10.1109/10.532130

Ramdani, S., Seigle, B., Lagarde, J., Bouchara, F., and Bernard, P. L. (2009). On the use of sample entropy to analyze human postural sway data. *Med. Eng. Phys.* 31, 1023–1031. doi: 10.1016/j.medengphy.2009.06.004

Richman, J., and Moorman, J. (2000). Physiological time series analysis using approximate entropy and sample entropy. *Am. J. Physiol.* 278, H2039–H2049.

Riley, M., Balasubramaniam, R., and Turvey, M. (1999). Recurrence quantification analysis of postural fluctuations. *Gait Posture* 9, 65–78. doi: 10.1016/S0966-6362(98)00044-7

Roerdink, M., De Haart, M., Daffertshofer, A., Donker, S. F., Geurts, A. C. H., and Beek, P. J. (2006). Dynamical structure of center-of-pressure trajectories in patients recovering from stroke. *Exp. Brain Res.* 174, 256–269. doi: 10.1007/s00221-006-0441-7

Roerdink, M., Hlavackova, P., and Vuillerme, N. (2011). Center-of-pressure regularity as a marker for attentional investment in postural control: a comparison between sitting and standing postures. *Hum. Mov. Sci.* 30, 203–212. doi: 10.1016/j.humov.2010.04.005

Sabatini, A. M. (2000). Analysis of postural sway using entropy measures of signal complexity. *Med. Biol. Eng. Comput.* 38, 617–624. doi: 10.1007/BF023 44866

Schniepp, R., Wuehr, M., Pradhan, C., Novozhilov, S., Krafczyk, S., Brandt, T., et al. (2013). Nonlinear variability of body sway in patients with phobic postural vertigo. *Front. Neurol.* 4:115. doi: 10.3389/fneur.2013.00115

Shih, M.-T., Doctor, F., Fan, S.-Z., Jen, K.-K., and Shieh, J.-S. (2015). Instantaneous 3D EEG signal analysis based on empirical mode decomposition and the hilbert–huang transform applied to depth of anaesthesia. *Entropy* 17, 928–949. doi: 10.3390/e17030928

Stins, J. F., Michielsen, M. E., Roerdink, M., and Beek, P. J. (2009). Sway regularity reflects attentional involvement in postural control: effects of expertise, vision and cognition. *Gait Posture* 30, 106–109. doi: 10.1016/j.gaitpost.2009.04.001

Vaillancourt, D. E., and Newell, K. M. (2002). Changing complexity in human behavior and physiology through aging and disease. *Neurobiol. Aging* 23, 1–11. doi: 10.1016/S0197-4580(01)00247-0

Vuillerme, N., and Nafati, G. (2007). How attentional focus on body sway affects postural control during quiet standing. *Psychol. Res.* 71, 192–200. doi: 10.1007/s00426-005-0018-2

Vuillerme, N., and Pinsault, N. (2009). Experimental neck muscle pain impairs standing balance in humans. *Exp. Brain Res.* 192, 723–729. doi: 10.1007/s00221-008-1639-7

Wei, Q., Liu, D. H., Wang, K. H., Liu, Q., Abbod, M., Jiang, B., et al. (2012). Multivariate multiscale entropy applied to center of pressure signals analysis: an effect of vibration stimulation of shoes. *Entropy* 14, 2157–2172. doi: 10.3390/e14112157

Yamada, N. (1995). Chaotic swaying of the upright posture. *Hum. Mov. Sci.* 14, 711–726. doi: 10.1016/0167-9457(95)00032-1

Yeh, J. R., Peng, C. K., and Huang, N. E. (2016). Scale-dependent intrinsic entropies of complex time series. *Philos. Trans. R. Soc. Math. Phys. Eng. Sci.* 374:20150204. doi: 10.1098/rsta.2015.0204

5

Effect of Experimentally-Induced Trunk Muscular Tensions on the Sit-to-Stand Task Performance and Associated Postural Adjustments

Alain Hamaoui[1,2]* *and Caroline Alamini-Rodrigues*[2]

[1]Laboratoire de Physiologie de la Posture et du Mouvement, Centre universitaire de formation et de recherche Jean-François Champollion, Albi, France, [2]Laboratoire Mouvement, Equilibre, Performance, Santé (EA 4445), Université de Pau et des Pays de l'Adour, Tarbes, France

***Correspondence:**
Alain Hamaoui
alain.hamaoui@univ-jfc.fr

It has been shown that increased muscular activity along the trunk is likely to impair body balance, but there is little knowledge about its consequences on more dynamic tasks. The purpose of this study was to determine the effect of unilateral and bilateral increases of muscular tension along the trunk on the sit-to-stand task (STS) performance and associated anticipatory postural adjustments (APAs). Twelve healthy females (23 ± 3 years, 163 ± 0.06 cm, 56 ± 9 kg), free of any neurological or musculoskeletal disorders, performed six trials of the STS at maximum speed, in seven experimental conditions varying the muscular tension along each side of the trunk, using a specific bimanual compressive load paradigm. A six-channel force plate was used to calculate the coordinates of the center of pressure (CP) along the anterior-posterior and medial-lateral axes, and the kinematics of the head, spine and pelvis, were estimated using three pairs of uni-axial accelerometers. The postural and focal components of the task were assessed using three biomechanical parameters calculated from CP signals: the duration and magnitude of APAs, and the duration of focal movement (dFM). Results showed that beyond a given level, higher muscular tension along the trunk results in longer APAs, but with a stable duration of the focal movement. In addition, no significant variation of APAs and FM parameters was found between bilateral and unilateral increases of muscular tension. It was suggested that restricted mobility due to higher muscular tension along the trunk requires an adaptation of the programming of APAs to keep the same level of performance in the STS task. These findings may have implications in treatment strategies aimed at preserving functional autonomy in pathologies including a rise of muscular tension.

Keywords: muscular tension, mobility, trunk, sit-to-stand, focal movement, postural adjustments

INTRODUCTION

According to the seminal work of Bouisset and Zattara (1981), voluntary movement induces a perturbation to balance, and a counter-perturbation must be developed for the movement to be performed efficiently. This counter-perturbation starts prior to the onset of the voluntary movement, and serves to create in the rest of the body a movement whose forces of inertia would, when the times comes, balance the inertia forces due to the voluntary movement. This early postural activity, termed anticipatory postural adjustments (APAs), is organized according to a reproducible pattern for a given movement and for every subject (Bouisset and Zattara, 1981, 1983). According to the hypotheses developed by Gelfand et al. (1966), the voluntary movement may be broken up into two components, one focal and one postural. The former refers to the voluntary movement itself, and the latter to the associated stabilizing activity of the body (Bouisset and Do, 2008). These two components require the mobility of a focal and a postural chain, which are usually located in distinct parts of the musculo-skeletal system. For example, the antepulsion of the upper limb is preceded by an acceleration of the shank (Bouisset and Zattara, 1983), and a bimanual isometric push task involves the mobility of the pelvis (Le Bozec and Bouisset, 2004). Consequently, restricted mobility of the bony chain may impair motor performance, even though its source is located in a part remote from the focal movement (FM).

According to Bouisset and Le Bozec (2002), postural chain dynamic mobility results from anatomical and physiological factors. The former ones refer to the structural properties of the bony chain (ligaments, bony stops...) which determine the articular range of motion, and can be considered as inherently passive. The latter and active factors are related to the pattern of muscular excitation, which can either generate or restrict bony segment displacements, depending on the agonist or antagonist function of the active muscles, respectively. In a pathological context, it has been assumed that a pain-related rise in muscular tension in low back pain is likely to impair the dynamic mobility capacity of the postural chain through a slowing-down effect (Hamaoui et al., 2004). Still for this pathology, it has also been shown an alteration of the APAs when performing upper limbs movements (Hodges and Richardson, 1999).

To date, a number of experiments have explored the effect of passive restrictions of postural chain mobility on voluntary movements. For example, a lower performance was shown to be associated with restricted pelvis mobility in a pointing task (Lino and Bouisset, 1994), in isometric pushing efforts (Le Bozec and Bouisset, 2004), or in the sit-to-stand task (STS; Diakhaté et al., 2013). However, few data are available on the influence of higher muscular tensions, although they represent a frequent symptom in a number of pathologies (hemiplegia, Parkinson's disease, back pain, muscular spasms in sports medicine...). Based on different bimanual isometric pushing paradigms varying muscular activity along the trunk while seated (Hamaoui et al., 2007) and standing (Hamaoui et al., 2011; Hamaoui and Le Bozec, 2014), a number of studies support the view that muscular tension impairs body balance when it exceeds a given level, with a more significant effect in case of asymmetrical tensions. In line with these studies, the present work is aimed at exploring the effect of increased muscular tension along the trunk when performing a usual voluntary movement, the STS task. The STS task is considered as a very common daily activity (Burdett et al., 1985; Riley et al., 1991; Roebroeck et al., 1994), which is required for independent living (Inkster and Eng, 2004). It is defined as moving the mass center of the body upward, from a sitting to a standing position, without losing balance (Roebroeck et al., 1994). The STS involves a transition from an intrinsically stable three-point support to a dynamically stable two-point support and is considered in some respects as the most mechanically demanding functional task routinely undertaken during daily activities (Riley et al., 1991). Different strategies of kinematic and muscular patterns are possible (Doorenbosch et al., 1994; Rodrigues-de-Paula Goulart and Valls-Solé, 1999), with sagittal plane motion dominant (Shepherd and Gentile, 1994). Based on the above mentioned literature on postural chain mobility and muscular tension, it is hypothesized that higher muscular tensions along the trunk may cause the focal and postural components of the task to vary. This assumption will be explored using a biomechanical analysis of the STS task in different conditions varying muscular tension level and symmetry along the trunk.

MATERIALS AND METHODS

Participants

Twelve healthy female subjects (age: 23 ± 3 years; weight: 56 ± 9 kg; height: 163 ± 0.05 cm, body mass index, BMI: 21 ± 3 kg/m^2), free of any neurological or musculoskeletal disease took part in this study. To avoid any variation of muscular strength and spine mobility related to gender differences, we did not include male participants.

This study was carried out in accordance with the recommendations of the local "Ethics Committee for Human Movement Analysis". All subjects gave written informed consent in accordance with the Declaration of Helsinki.

Experimental Set-Up

Force Plate

A six-channel force plate (Bertec Corp., ref. 6012-15, Columbus, OH, USA), which collected the ground reaction forces and moments applied at its top surface was used to calculate the coordinates of the center of pressure (CP) along the anterior-posterior (Xp) and medial-lateral (Yp) axes, with the following formulas: Xp = My/Rz Yp = Mx/Rz (Rz is the vertical ground-reaction force; Mx and My are the moments around the anterior-posterior and medial-lateral axes, respectively).

A stool (height = 48 cm; depth = 39 cm) with four legs and a round wooden top (diameter = 30 cm) was screwed on to the force plate and used for the experiments (**Figure 1**). To keep constant the friction forces between the stool top and the surface contact of the body, all participants wore the same kind of shorts.

Pressure Sensor

A pressure sensor was placed under the left front leg of the stool to determine the "seat off" instant.

Accelerometers

Three pairs of mono-axial accelerometers (FGP sensors, ref XA1010-B, ±10 g, Les Clayes Sous Bois, France), were used to assess the local accelerations of the pelvis and trunk. Each pair was screwed on to a customized cube (length = 2 cm) with the two active axes located along the anterior-posterior and the vertical

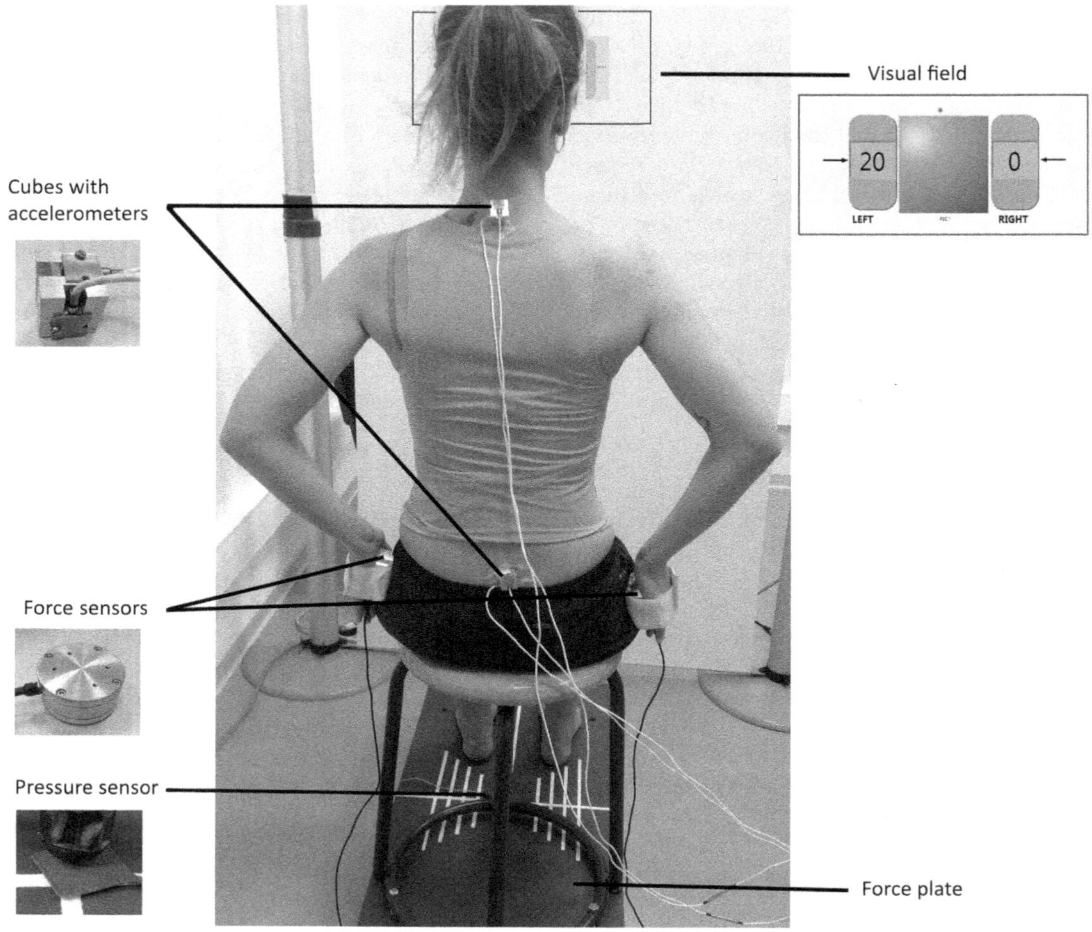

FIGURE 1 | Experimental set-up with the subject applying a unilateral compressive load at 20% of the maximum voluntary contraction (MVC).

axes. The cubes were adhered to the skin with double-sided tape at the level of the first sacral vertebra and first thoracic vertebra (**Figure 1**).

Force Sensors

Two cylindrical load cells (FN 2114 model, FGP Sensors, Les Clayes Sous Bois, France) were used to set the active muscular tension at different levels alongside the torso when performing a bimanual compressive load paradigm (**Figure 1**). They were equipped with adjustable Velcro bands designed to keep each sensor in contact with the hand palm, and preventing it from falling.

Visual Field

The subject's visual field consisted of a frontal white board, located 72 cm apart from the stool. A panel representing the tension generated on each load cell was screened on the board at the subject's eye level, using a video-projector (**Figure 1**). The signals were displayed as a percentage of the maximum voluntary contraction (MVC) in a left and a right numerical indicator representing each sensor, and designed in Labview software (National Instruments). The background color of these indicators changed from red to green when the subject reached the required value, enriching the basic feedback by a specific indication of the task to perform. The experimentation room was lit with artificial lighting to obtain constant brightness.

Data Acquisition System

Data collected by the force plate, the pressure sensor, and the load cells were sampled at 200 Hz with a 16-bit A/D converter board (model CompactDAQ with 9215 modules, National Instruments, Austin, TX, USA), controlled by a custom code written in Labview software (National Instruments).

Procedure

The participants sat on the platform with hips and knees approximately flexed to 90°, barefoot and feet apart. Adhesive tape was put around the feet outline in order to keep the same positioning for every trial. The load cells were positioned against hands palms and applied on the sides of the pelvis against the lateral surface of the trochanter major, with shoulders abducted to 35° (**Figure 1**). Subjects were asked to focus their gaze on the numerical indicators screened on the visual field and representing the load applied on the force sensors. This bimanual compressive load paradigm, which has been extensively described in a previous study (Hamaoui and Le Bozec, 2014) was considered as a reliable tool to control the active muscular tension along each side of the torso. Using an extensive surface EMG analysis, the authors found that the main muscles of this isometric task were latissimus dorsi, pectoralis major and thoracic erector spinae, while secondary muscles were identified as lumbar erector spinae, trapezius pars ascendez and obliquus externus abdominis. The mean EMG of the main muscles was reported to increase with the compressive load level, with a negligible activity toward the non-active side in unilateral loads.

Two 3-s trials in bilateral maximum compressive load were first performed to determine the MVC. Subjects had next to achieve the STS transfer while performing a compressive load in seven conditions varying the load level (0%, 20% and 40% of the MVC) and side (left, right, bilateral). It must be noted that for a compressive load at 0% (no force applied) the experimental instructions were the same for left, right and bilateral loads, and only one condition was considered. For each condition, the participants had to reach the requested compressive load parameters before starting the STS transfer and to keep them constant during the task, using the feedback screened on the visual field. This way, the variations of the muscular pattern that may be associated with the task completion were minimized.

The "STS" paradigm consisted in rising from the stool to reach the standing position as fast as possible, in response to a "Go" signal. A training period was used to familiarize the subjects with the paradigm before recording. Six 3-s runs were performed in every condition, with six additional runs in 0% for subsequent statistical analysis. The rest period was 30 s between runs and 1 min between series.

The order of the experimental condition was randomly assigned to avoid any order effect.

Data Analysis

A careful visual inspection of CP curves along the anterior-posterior and medial-lateral axes was first performed for qualitative assessment (general time-course, curve shape). It was followed by a quantitative analysis of the APAs and FM of the STS. These two distinct phases were considered to be separated by the seat-off instant, for which the curve of the pressure sensor starts its fall towards zero. Three parameters were calculated from CP signals along the anterior- posterior axis:

- Duration of APAs (*dAPAs*): delay between the instant of seat-off and the first inflexion of the CP curve.
- Magnitude of APAs (ΔXp): difference between the maximum and the minimum values of CP during the APAs phase.
- Duration of the focal movement (*dFM*): delay between the seat-off instant and the stabilization of the CP curve (beginning of the plateau region).

Data from the accelerometers were used to ensure that the head and trunk were kept still before the « Go » signal, and to discard trials in which the participants anticipated the instructions of the experimenter.

All parameters were calculated using a customized program written in MatLab software (The MathWorks, Inc., Natick, MA, USA).

Statistical analysis was performed using the Statistical Package for Social Sciences (SPSS) software V22 (Chicago, IL, USA). Normality of data distribution and the condition of sphericity were first checked using Shapiro-Wilk and Mauchly tests, respectively. A two-way repeated measures analysis of variance (ANOVA) was conducted for each dependent variable, with compressive load intensity (0%, 20% and 40% of the MVC) and laterality (bilateral, unilateral) as within-subjects factors. Values for the unilateral level were calculated from the mean between the left and right trials, as this study did not focus on specific left and right variations that might have resulted from handedness. When statistical significance was reached for compressive load intensity, the ANOVA was followed by a within-subjects analysis of contrasts (difference contrast) to compare the three levels of the independent variable. The level of statistical significance was set at $p < 0.05$.

RESULTS

Qualitative Assessment of CP Curves

The CP time course along the anterior-posterior axis revealed a typical shape which always starts with an almost linear backward displacement (beginning of the APAs), followed by a forward displacement with a steeper slope, and which ends with a less regular stabilization phase preceding the plateau (end of the FM; **Figure 2**). This pattern, which is consistent with data displayed in previous experiments (e.g., Schenkman et al., 1990; Diakhaté et al., 2013) was reproducible across subjects and conditions.

No such typical trace was found along the medial-lateral axis, with a high variability of CP displacements during APAs and FM. In addition, the scale of the signal was about ten times lower than along the anterior-posterior axis, and no specific lateral slope was found in relation to the side of the compressive load (left or right) in unilateral conditions.

Quantitative Assessment of APAs and Focal Movement

The ANOVA revealed that increased compressive load level was associated with a longer duration of the APAs, with a significant main effect ($p < 0.05$). Subsequent contrast analysis showed a significant variation between a compressive load at 40% (comp40) and at the two other levels, namely 0% (comp0) and 20% (comp20), but no substantial difference between comp0 and comp20 conditions (**Table 1**, **Figure 3**). However APAs magnitude (ΔXp) and focal movement duration (dFM) were not sensitive to the level of the applied load (**Table 1**, **Figure 4**). These results were visible in CP traces, which exhibited longer APAs duration for comp40 and relative to comp20 and comp0,

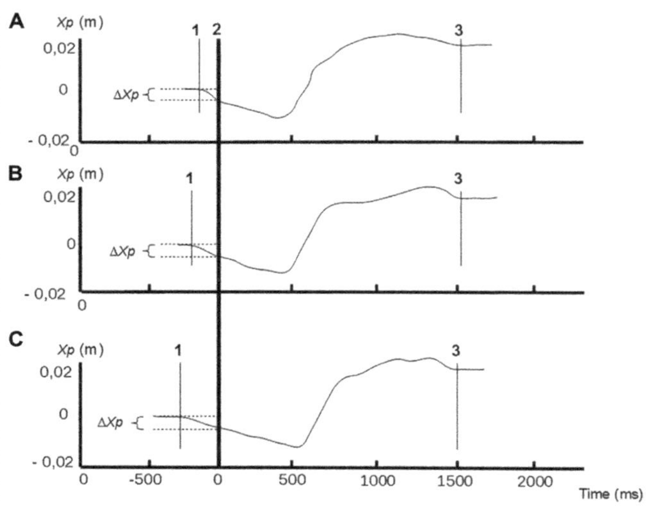

FIGURE 2 | Center of pressure (CP) traces along the anterior-posterior axis (Xp) of a representative subject, in different conditions of bilateral compressive load: no compression (A) compressive load at 20% of the MVC **(B)**, compressive load at 40% of the MVC **(C)**. Line 1: CP onset; line 2: instant of « seat-off »; line 3: CP stabilization. Anticipatory postural adjustments (APAs) phase is between lines 1 and 2, and focal phase between lines 2 and 3. ΔXp represents the amplitude of the APAs.

whereas APAs magnitude and FM duration remained stable (**Figure 2**).

Compared to bilateral loads, unilateral loads resulted in smaller mean duration of APAs and longer mean duration of FM, but with no significant variation (**Figures 3, 5, Table 1**).

DISCUSSION

Increased Muscular Tension Along the Torso Induces a Reorganization of the APAs

According to the analysis of dAPAs, higher muscular tension along the trunk resulted in longer APAs, with significant variations when the compressive load reached 40% of the MVC (comp40 relative to comp20 and comp0). This variation may be interpreted as a reorganization of the motor pattern, aimed at compensating for the lower capacity to generate counter-disturbing movements due to higher active muscular tension. It has already been assumed that postural chain muscular stiffening may slow down the counter-perturbing movements necessary to keep the body stable, and make them less efficient (Hamaoui et al., 2007). In a more conceptual point of view, it was also suggested that active muscular stiffening along the torso, when it exceeds a given level, is likely to alter the posturo-kinetic capacity (PKC; Hamaoui et al., 2011), which is defined as the ability to develop a counter-perturbation to the posture perturbation induced by segmental movement (Bouisset and Le Bozec, 1999). This reorganization of the APAs, which become longer but retains a similar magnitude, can be considered as efficient enough to keep constant the performance of the FM, as no variation was observed for FM duration. Longer APAs would allow more time to generate the inertia forces, which are necessary to balance the disturbing effect of the FM when the time comes, as hypothesized by Bouisset and Zattara (1981). With respect to the STS, it may favor the generation of the early propulsive impulse in the sagittal plane, which is an essential requirement of the task (Pai et al., 1994).

This variation of APAs duration has already been described in a previous study using the paradigm of shoulder flexion at maximum velocity, in different conditions varying the support base surface (Zattara and Bouisset, 1992). The authors showed that restricted support base surface induced longer APAs, which were in this case associated with a decrease of FM performance. Therefore, it can be hypothesized that the restriction of the PKC induced by increased muscular tension along the trunk in the present study, was relatively moderate and likely to be compensated for a reorganization of the APAs. This adaptability of the APAs has been described since the early works, with a variation of their duration and magnitude according to additional inertia loads (Bouisset and Zattara, 1981, 1983), support base configuration (Zattara and Bouisset, 1992; Lino and Bouisset, 1994; Yiou et al., 2007), and pelvic mobility (Le Bozec and Bouisset, 2004; Diakhaté et al., 2013).

TABLE 1 | Anticipatory postural adjustments (APAs) and focal movement (FM) parameters as a function of compressive load parameters.

		COMP 0	COMP 20	COMP 40	*p(Comp main)*	*p(Comp 20/ Comp 0)*	*p(Comp 40/ previous)*	*p(Lat main)*
dAPAs (ms)	BILAT	98 ± 46	106 ± 50	123 ± 69	0.042	NS	0.048	NS
	UNILAT	99 ± 42	99 ± 44	107 ± 57				
ΔXP (m)	BILAT	0.043 ± 0.024	0.041 ± 0.020	0.044 ± 0.020	NS	NS	NS	NS
	UNILAT	0.046 ± 0.024	0.041 ± 0.018	0.040 ± 0.021				
dFM (ms)	BILAT	1693 ± 161	1641 ± 218	1593 ± 196	NS	NS	NS	NS
	UNILAT	1694 ± 190	1662 ± 222	1608 ± 150				

Mean ± SD of APAs duration (dAPAs, in ms), APAs magnitude (ΔXp, in m) and focal movement duration (dFM, in ms) are presented in bilateral (BILAT) and unilateral (UNILAT) compressive loads, at 0% (COMP 0), 20% (COMP 20) and 40% (COMP 40) of the maximum voluntary contraction (MVC). Results of statistical analysis display the main effect of the analysis of variance (ANOVA) for compressive load intensity (Comp main) and laterality (Lat main), and the contrast analysis for compressive load intensity (Comp 20 and Comp 40 relative to previous levels). NS: non significant.

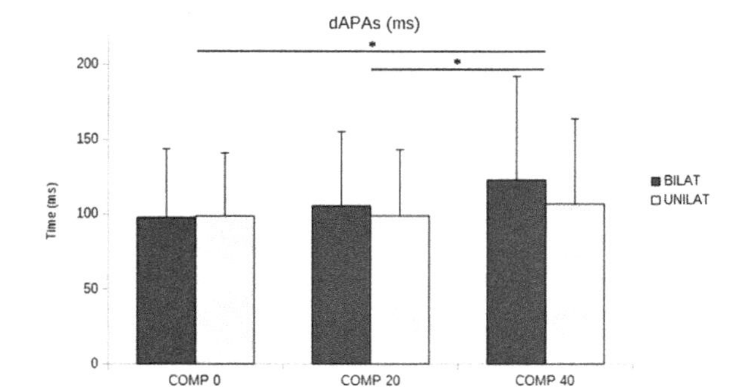

FIGURE 3 | Duration of APAs (dAPAs, in ms) as a function of the compressive load: means and standard deviations (error bars) are presented in unilateral (UNILAT) and bilateral (BILAT) compressive load, at 0% (COMP 0), 20% (COMP 20) and 40% (COMP 40) of the MVC. $^*p < 0.05$.

Unilateral and Bilateral Compressive Loads Did Not Impair the Focal Component of the STS

In contrast with previous studies describing lower body balance in case of increased trunk muscular tension in seated (Hamaoui et al., 2007) or standing (Hamaoui et al., 2011) postures, no variation of FM duration, and thus of performance, was observed in the present experiment. This difference might be attributed to the high levels of motor muscles activity (Rodrigues-de-Paula Goulart and Valls-Solé, 1999) and range of motion (Roebroeck et al., 1994) associated with the STS task, as compared to the low levels required for postural maintenance. Indeed, joint movements have been reported to be less than 1° while standing (Hodges et al., 2002), with a postural activity below 10% of the MVC (Okada, 1973). This low activity might be sensitive to postural muscles tensions, even limited by the maximum compressive load at 40% of the MVC. In contrast, the very dynamic displacements of the articulated chain required for the STS task, may overcome the slowing down effect induced by the compressive load paradigm.

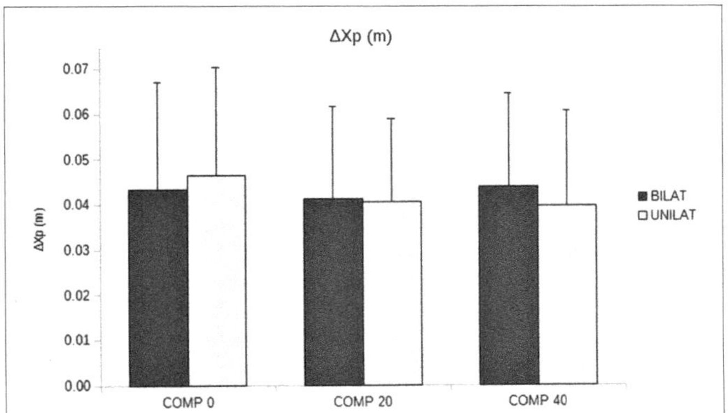

FIGURE 4 | Amplitude of APAs (ΔXp, in m) as a function of the compressive load: means and standard deviations (error bars) are presented in unilateral (UNILAT) and bilateral (BILAT) compressive loads, at 0% (COMP 0), 20% (COMP 20) and 40% (COMP 40) of the MVC.

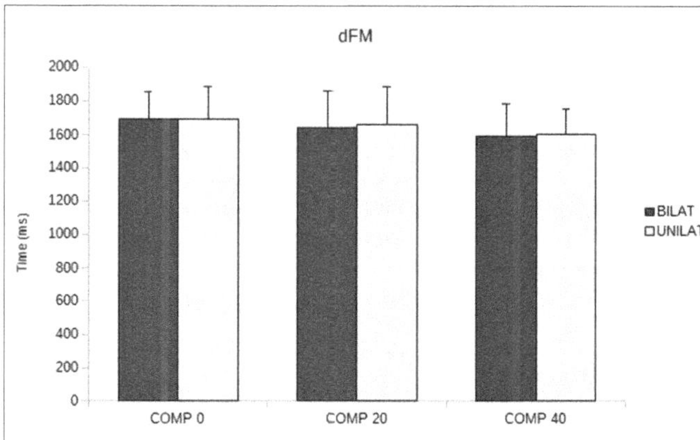

FIGURE 5 | Duration of focal movement (dFM, in ms) as a function of the compressive load: means and standard deviations (error bars) are presented in unilateral (UNILAT) and bilateral (BILAT) compressive loads, at 0% (COMP 0), 20% (COMP 20) and 40% (COMP 40) of the MVC.

Still in contrast with a study carried out during postural maintenance (Hamaoui and Le Bozec, 2014), the performance did not appear lower for unilateral loads, with similar FM duration between unilateral and bilateral conditions. Likewise, APAs duration and magnitude did not present any significant variation between the two conditions, suggesting a similar PKC. This result might first be explained by a lesser net muscular activity along the whole trunk in unilateral conditions, as the load is only applied on one side. It can also be assumed that the inherently sagittal characteristics of the STS kinematics and kinetics (Shepherd and Gentile, 1994), attested in this study by the absence of a typical CP along the medial lateral axis, may limit its sensitivity to a left-right asymmetry of muscular tension. Finally, it can also be hypothesized that the CNS has integrated the asymmetry of postural muscles activity, which was set before the « Go » signal, in the programming of the task, and tuned the postural adjustments accordingly. All these hypotheses need further experiments to be tested and refined.

Increased Muscular Tension in a Clinical Context May Require a Reorganization of the STS Motor Program

As increased active muscular tension is a very frequent symptom in various pathologies of the musculo-skeletal (muscular spasms in sports medicine or in degenerative diseases of the joints) and central nervous (hemiplegia, Parkinson's disease) systems, the results from this study are worth being interpreted in a clinical perspective. It can first be assumed that a pathological increase of trunk muscular tension, when it exceeds a given level, may require an adaptation of the APAs pattern in order to keep the same level of performance in the STS task. It can also be considered that a limited asymmetry of trunk muscular tension may induce a negligible effect on the STS task performance. However, as increased tension was experimentally induced on healthy participants in this study, it is necessary to take into account the possible interaction with other symptoms in a pathological context, which may lead to more prominent effects. This might be the case in Parkinson's disease or stroke, which are both associated with other deficits and have proved to impair STS task performance (Inkster and Eng, 2004; Boukadida et al., 2015). Therefore, treating pathological muscular tensions, by means of drugs or physiotherapy, might reduce the necessity for APAs reprogramming and favor STS performance in some pathologies.

Limitation

There were some methodological limitations of the study which need to be acknowledged. First, we used a model of increased muscular tension based on voluntary contractions performed in healthy subjects, which intrinsically differ from pathological variations related to deficits of the nervous or musculo-skeletal systems. Second, the STS task was performed at maximum velocity in young adults, whereas slower movements are frequently observed in a pathological population, with possible variations of the focal and postural components of the task. Third, we only used participants with a normal BMI, whereas the STS task requires the generation of high propulsive forces that may lead to different strategies in subjects presenting high BMI. For these reasons, future experiments are needed to confirm our hypotheses in a more realistic context, including different pathologies and classes of participants.

CONCLUSION

The findings of this study support the view that experimentally increased muscular tension along the trunk requires an adaptation of the APAs, which become longer, to maintain the same level of performance in the STS. This effect, which might be more prominent in a clinical context where it is bound be associated with other symptoms, may have some implications in treatment strategies intended to improve functional autonomy.

AUTHOR CONTRIBUTIONS

AH contributed with project creation, data analysis, and drafted the manuscript. CA-R contributed with project creation, data collection and data analysis. AH and CA-R discussed the results and revised the manuscript.

FUNDING

This work was funded by University JF Champollion and Conseil Régional Occitanie, France.

ACKNOWLEDGMENTS

The authors thank Vérane Faure for her valuable help in the analysis of the results.

REFERENCES

Bouisset, S., and Do, M.-C. (2008). Posture, dynamic stability, and voluntary movement. *Neurophysiol. Clin.* 38, 345–362. doi: 10.1016/j.neucli.2008.10.001

Bouisset, S., and Le Bozec, S. (1999). "Body balance stability and postural adjustments associated with voluntary movement," in *Motor Control: Today and Tomorrow*, eds G. N. Gantchev, S. Mori and J. Massion (Sofia: Academic Publishing House), 275–291.

Bouisset, S., and Le Bozec, S. (2002). "3 Chapter - Posturo-kinetic capacity and postural function in voluntary movement," in *Progress in Motor Control: Structure-Function Relations in Voluntary Movements*, ed. M. L. Latash (Champaign, IL: Human Kinetics), 25–52.

Bouisset, S., and Zattara, M. (1981). A sequence of postural movements precedes voluntary movement. *Neurosci. Lett.* 22, 263–270. doi: 10.1016/0304-3940(81)90117-8

Bouisset, S., and Zattara, M. (1983). "Anticipatory postural movements related to a voluntary movement," in *Space Physiology* (Toulouse: Cepadues Editions) 137–141.

Boukadida, A., Piotte, F., Dehail, P., and Nadeau, S. (2015). Determinants of sit-to-stand tasks in individuals with hemiparesis post stroke: a review. *Ann. Phys. Rehabil. Med.* 58, 167–172. doi: 10.1016/j.rehab.2015.04.007

Burdett, R. G., Habasevich, R., Pisciotta, J., and Simon, S. R. (1985). Biomechanical comparison of rising from two types of chairs. *Phys. Ther.* 65, 1177–1183.

Diakhaté, D. G., Do, M. C., and Le Bozec, S. (2013). Effects of seat-thigh contact on kinematics performance in sit-to-stand trunk flexion tasks. *J. Biomech.* 46, 879–882. doi: 10.1016/j.jbiomech.2012.12.022

Doorenbosch, C. A., Harlaar, J., Roebroeck, M. E., and Lankhorst, G. J. (1994). Two strategies of transferring from sit-to-stand; the activation of monoarticular and biarticular muscles. *J. Biomech.* 27, 1299–1307. doi: 10.1016/0021-9290(94)90039-6

Gelfand, I. M., Gurfinkel, V. S., Tsetlin, M. L., and Shik, M. L. (1966). "Problems in analysis of movements," in *Models of the Structural Functionnal Organization of Certain Biological Systems* (Amer. translation, 1971), eds I. M. Gelfand, V. S. Gurfinkel, S. V. Fomin and M. L. Tsetlin (Cambridge, MA: MIT Press), 330–345.

Hamaoui, A., Do, M. C., and Bouisset, S. (2004). Postural sway increase in low back pain subjects is not related to reduced spine range of motion. *Neurosci. Lett.* 357, 135–138. doi: 10.1016/j.neulet.2003.12.047

Hamaoui, A., Friant, Y., and Le Bozec, S. (2011). Does increased muscular tension along the torso impair postural equilibrium in a standing posture? *Gait Posture* 34, 457–461. doi: 10.1016/j.gaitpost.2011.06.017

Hamaoui, A., and Le Bozec, S. (2014). Does increased muscular tension along the torso disturb postural equilibrium more when it is asymmetrical? *Gait Posture* 39, 333–338. doi: 10.1016/j.gaitpost.2013.07.131

Hamaoui, A., Le Bozec, S., Poupard, L., and Bouisset, S. (2007). Does postural chain muscular stiffness reduce postural steadiness in a sitting posture? *Gait Posture* 25, 199–204. doi: 10.1016/j.gaitpost.2006.03.012

Hodges, P. W., Gurfinkel, V. S., Brumagne, S., Smith, T. C., and Cordo, P. C. (2002). Coexistence of stability and mobility in postural control: evidence from postural compensation for respiration. *Exp. Brain Res.* 144, 293–302. doi: 10.1007/s00221-002-1040-x

Hodges, P. W., and Richardson, C. A. (1999). Altered trunk muscle recruitment in people with low back pain with upper limb movement at different speeds. *Arch. Phys. Med. Rehabil.* 80, 1005–1012. doi: 10.1016/s0003-9993(99)90052-7

Inkster, L. M., and Eng, J. J. (2004). Postural control during a sit-to-stand task in individuals with mild Parkinson's disease. *Exp. Brain Res.* 154, 33–38. doi: 10.1007/s00221-003-1629-8

Le Bozec, S., and Bouisset, S. (2004). Does postural chain mobility influence muscular control in sitting ramp pushes? *Exp. Brain Res.* 158, 427–437. doi: 10.1007/s00221-004-1918-x

Lino, F., and Bouisset, S. (1994). Is velocity of a pointing movement performed in a sitting posture increased by upper body instability? *J. Biomech.* 27:733. doi: 10.1016/0021-9290(94)91153-3

Okada, M. (1973). An electromyographic estimation of the relative muscular load in different human postures. *J. Hum. Ergol. (Tokyo)* 1, 75–93.

Pai, Y.-C., Naughton, B. J., Chang, R. W., and Rogers, M. W. (1994). Control of body centre of mass momentum during sit-to-stand among young and elderly adults. *Gait Posture* 2, 109–116. doi: 10.1016/0966-6362(94)90100-7

Riley, P. O., Schenkman, M. L., Mann, R. W., and Hodge, W. A. (1991). Mechanics of a constrained chair-rise. *J. Biomech.* 24, 77–85. doi: 10.1016/0021-9290(91)90328-k

Rodrigues-de-Paula Goulart, F., and Valls-Solé, J. (1999). Patterned electromyographic activity in the sit-to-stand movement. *Clin. Neurophysiol.* 110, 1634–1640. doi: 10.1016/s1388-2457(99)00109-1

Roebroeck, M. E., Doorenbosch, C. A. M., Harlaar, J., Jacobs, R., and Lankhorst, G. J. (1994). Biomechanics and muscular activity during sit-to-stand transfer. *Clin. Biomech.* 9, 235–244. doi: 10.1016/0268-0033(94)90004-3

Schenkman, M., Berger, R. A., Riley, P. O., Mann, R. W., and Hodge, W. A. (1990). Whole-body movements during rising to standing from sitting. *Phys. Ther.* 70, 638–648.

Shepherd, R. B., and Gentile, A. M. (1994). Sit-to-stand: functional relationship between upper body and lower limb segments. *Hum. Mov. Sci.* 13, 817–840. doi: 10.1016/0167-9457(94)90020-5

Yiou, E., Hamaoui, A., and Le Bozec, S. (2007). Influence of base of support size on arm pointing performance and associated anticipatory postural adjustments. *Neurosci. Lett.* 423, 29–34. doi: 10.1016/j.neulet.2007.06.034

Zattara, M., and Bouisset, S. (1992). "Influence of a reduction of postural base configuration on the velocity of unilateral and bilateral upper limbs movements," in *Proceedings of VIIIth Meeting of the European Society of Biomechanics* (Rome: Bellotti P and Cappozzo A), 226.

6

Effects of Muscle Fatigue, Creep and Musculoskeletal Pain on Neuromuscular Responses to Unexpected Perturbation of the Trunk

Jacques Abboud[1]*, *Arnaud Lardon*[2,3], *Frédéric Boivin*[3], *Claude Dugas*[3] and *Martin Descarreaux*[3]

[1] *Département D'anatomie, Université du Québec à Trois-Rivières, Trois-Rivières, QC, Canada,* [2] *Pôle Recherche Clinique Chiropratique, Institut Franco-Européen de Chiropraxie, Ivry-Sur-Seine, France,* [3] *Département des Sciences de L'activité Physique, Université du Québec à Trois-Rivières, Trois-Rivières, QC, Canada*

Correspondence:
Jacques Abboud
jacques.abboud@uqtr.ca

Introduction: Trunk neuromuscular responses have been shown to adapt under the influence of muscle fatigue, as well as spinal tissue creep or even with the presence of low back pain (LBP). Despite a large number of studies exploring how these external perturbations affect the spinal stability, characteristics of such adaptations remains unclear.

Aim: The purpose of this systematic review was to assess the quality of evidence of studies investigating trunk neuromuscular responses to unexpected trunk perturbation. More specifically, the targeted neuromuscular responses were trunk muscle activity reflex and trunk kinematics under the influence of muscle fatigue, spinal creep, and musculoskeletal pain.

Methods: A research of the literature was conducted in Pubmed, Embase, and Sport-Discus databases using terms related to trunk neuromuscular reflex responses, measured by electromyography (baseline activity, reflex latency, and reflex amplitude) and/or trunk kinematic, in context of unexpected external perturbation. Moreover, independent variables must be either trunk muscle fatigue or spinal tissue creep or LBP. All included articles were scored for their electromyography methodology based on the "Surface Electromyography for the Non-Invasive Assessment of Muscles (SENIAM)" and the "International Society of Electrophysiology and Kinesiology (ISEK)" recommendations whereas overall quality of articles was scored using a specific quality checklist modified from the Quality Index. Meta-analysis was performed on reflex latency variable.

Results: A final set of 29 articles underwent quality assessments. The mean quality score was 79%. No effect of muscle fatigue on erector spinae reflex latency following an unexpected perturbation, nor any other distinctive effects was found for back muscle fatigue and reflex parameters. As for spinal tissue creep effects, no alteration was found for any of the trunk reflex variables. Finally, the meta-analysis revealed an increased erector spinae reflex latency in patients with chronic LBP in comparison with healthy controls following an unexpected trunk perturbation.

Conclusion: The literature provides some evidence with regard to trunk adaptions in a context of spinal instability. However, most of the evidence was inconclusive due to a high methodological heterogeneity between the studies.

Keywords: electromyography, kinematics, reflex, spinal stability, low back pain, fatigue, ceep

INTRODUCTION

Postural balance is constantly challenged, sometimes unexpectedly, by mechanical forces applied in different directions and continuously triggering postural adjustments. In expected conditions, prior to any movement, the central nervous systems triggers muscles activation/deactivation, and then a movement occurs after a short period of a few milliseconds. These pre-planned adjustments are considered anticipatory postural adjustments (Belen'kii et al., 1967; Bouisset and Do, 2008). For instance, trunk postural adjustments can be represented by early muscle activations (Bouisset and Zattara, 1981; Hodges and Richardson, 1997), as well as increases in muscle activity prior to any external perturbation (Lavender et al., 1993; Cresswell et al., 1994; Moseley et al., 2003) that are believed to contribute to spinal stability. On the other hand, when subjected to unexpected external perturbations of the trunk, muscle activation is delayed (Eriksson Crommert and Thorstensson, 2009), leaving the spine with reduced stability for few milliseconds. Spinal stability is defined as the harmonious cohesion between active muscles surrounding the spine, passive spinal tissues, and neuromuscular control (Panjabi, 1992).

When one or more of these spinal stability components are challenged, adaptations in the trunk system occurs in order to maintain a certain performance level in everyday functional motor tasks. Over the past decades, fundamental research efforts have focused on the quantification of these adaptations through the analysis of trunk muscle activity recordings and trunk kinematic data. Challenges to spinal stability have been commonly investigated using muscle fatigue, spinal tissue creep but also by studying patients with low back pain (LBP). Challenging trunk stability using muscle fatigue has been associated with adaptations in muscle activity recruitment patterns, such as trunk flexor and extensor co-contraction phenomena (Allison and Henry, 2001). Reorganization in spatial low back muscle activity have also been described as a potential strategy to offset muscle fatigue effects (Tucker et al., 2009; Abboud et al., 2014). Moreover, the observation of an altered coordination of trunk muscle activation, a decreased control of trunk movements (Boucher et al., 2012), and alterations in lumbopelvic dynamics have been reported under the influence of muscle fatigue (Descarreaux et al., 2010). Similar trunk neuromuscular adaptations have been observed when passive tissue components of spinal stability are challenged. Active or passive prolonged deep flexions of the trunk, which is believed to generate spinal tissue creep, are usually followed by an increase in trunk flexion range of motion (Rogers and Granata, 2006; Howarth et al., 2013; Olson, 2014). Moreover, an increase in back muscle activity has also been described as a compensating mechanism for the reduced contribution of passive tissues to spinal stability (Olson et al., 2004; Shin et al., 2009; Abboud et al., 2016). Neuromuscular control of the trunk, such as trunk coordination and trunk muscle activation, is commonly altered in patients with chronic LBP (Hodges, 2011; Hodges and Tucker, 2011; Abboud et al., 2014). For example, patients with chronic LBP show longer time-delay of trunk muscle activation during a predictable perturbation (Hodges and Richardson, 1998). Overall, challenges to spinal stability components have been associated with numerous alterations in trunk neuromuscular control.

To investigate neuromuscular adaptations to unexpected trunk perturbations, most studies report adaptations in electromyography (EMG) recordings based on the analysis of baseline activity, reflex latency, and reflex amplitude. However, high heterogeneity in EMG reflex variable analyses led to conflicting results and an incomplete understanding of stabilizing responses to unexpected trunk perturbations. Indeed, most of the studies report different criteria to detect spinal reflex parameters. For instance, baseline activity, also called pre-activation level, is calculated from different time windows ranging from 50-ms to 3-s prior to the onset of an unexpected trunk perturbation (Newcomer et al., 2002; Granata et al., 2004, 2005; Herrmann et al., 2006; Rogers and Granata, 2006; Stokes et al., 2006; Mawston et al., 2007; Grondin and Potvin, 2009; Dupeyron et al., 2010; Lariviere et al., 2010; Ramprasad et al., 2010; Bazrgari et al., 2011; Hendershot et al., 2011; Jacobs et al., 2011; Jones et al., 2012a; Liebetrau et al., 2013; Miller et al., 2013; Muslim et al., 2013; Olson, 2014). The onset of EMG reflex, also called reflex latency, is generally calculated, using the standard deviation method proposed by Hodges and Bui (1996). Although, two standard deviations (SD) seems to be the most used reflex onset detection method (Granata et al., 2004, 2005; Herrmann et al., 2006; Rogers and Granata, 2006; Dupeyron et al., 2010; Lariviere et al., 2010; Ramprasad et al., 2010; Bazrgari et al., 2011; Hendershot et al., 2011; Toosizadeh et al., 2013; Olson, 2014), few others studies used alternate standard deviations values, such as 1.4 SD (Radebold et al., 2000, 2001; Cholewicki et al., 2002), 1.5 SD (Reeves et al., 2005), 3 SD (Stokes et al., 2006; Gao et al., 2014; Akbari et al., 2015), and 4 SD (Liebetrau et al., 2013). Sometimes, the EMG reflex onset is also determined by visual inspection of EMG signals (Newcomer et al., 2002; Mawston et al., 2007; Sanchez-Zuriaga et al., 2010). Maximal amplitude value is usually the predominant method to determine reflex amplitude (Granata et al., 2004, 2005;

Herrmann et al., 2006; Rogers and Granata, 2006; Grondin and Potvin, 2009; Dupeyron et al., 2010; Sanchez-Zuriaga et al., 2010; Liebetrau et al., 2013; Olson, 2014). However, a few studies have also examined reflex amplitude through EMG time windows of various duration (i.e., 10- to 75-ms windows; MacDonald et al., 2010; Ramprasad et al., 2010; Jacobs et al., 2011; Jones et al., 2012a,b; Shenoy et al., 2013). Finally, and perhaps of utmost importance, authors seems to disagree on what should be consider as reflex responses or voluntary movements. Indeed, some authors consider that muscle activity responses longer than 120-ms should be considered non-reflexive (Granata et al., 2005; Herrmann et al., 2006; Rogers and Granata, 2006; Dupeyron et al., 2010; Jacobs et al., 2011) while other authors included responses occurring between the perturbation onset and 150-ms (Lariviere et al., 2010; Bazrgari et al., 2011; Toosizadeh et al., 2013; Olson, 2014), 200-ms (Liebetrau et al., 2013), 250-ms (Cholewicki et al., 2002), and 300-ms (Radebold et al., 2001).

While there is no doubt that spinal reflexes play a major role in spinal stability mechanisms (Moorhouse and Granata, 2007), well-standardized measurement protocols enabling a better understanding of neurophysiological adaptations to unexpected trunk perturbation are still lacking. Consequently, the main purpose of this study was to systematically assess the quality of evidence of studies investigating neuromuscular responses to unexpected trunk perturbation. More specifically, the targeted neuromuscular responses were trunk muscle activity reflex and trunk kinematics under the influence of muscle fatigue, spinal creep, and musculoskeletal pain. This review also addresses two fundamental questions: What are the most relevant EMG and kinematic variables to properly observe and study neuromuscular adaptions to unexpected loading of the trunk? Are neuromuscular adaptations to unexpected perturbations similar under the influence of erector spinae muscle fatigue, musculoskeletal LBP and spinal creep deformation? We believe that the results of this review will guide future research in the field of trunk neuromuscular control. Moreover, this review may have some potential applications in the development of standardized functional spinal evaluation and biomedical engineering diagnostic tools, as well as progress in ergonomic risk assessment strategies.

MATERIALS AND METHODS

Registration

This review protocol was registered in PROSPERO International Prospective Register of Systematic Reviews on May 27, 2016 (CRD42016039374).

Search Strategy

Searches were performed in Pubmed, Embase, and Sport-Discus databases in May 2016 without any time limit. A systematic search of the literature was conducted using the following keywords and search terms alone and in combination: (Perturbation OR Unexpected perturbation OR Postural perturbation OR Sudden release OR Sudden loading OR Quick release OR External load) AND (Back OR Spine OR Spinal OR Trunk OR Lumbar) AND (Muscle fatigue OR Fatigue OR Muscle endurance OR Back pain OR Lumbar impairment OR Stretch OR Creep OR Viscoelastic deformation OR Passive tissue OR Paraspinal tissue OR Prolonged flexion OR Tension–relaxation OR Stiffness OR Static flexion OR Cyclic movement OR Flexion OR Passive movement). Additional data sources included the authors' pre-existing knowledge of the literature, manual review of reference lists of laboratory studies and forward citation tracking. Search strategy is presented in the Appendix A in Supplementary Material.

Eligibility Criteria

Only experimental studies in a controlled environment were selected for this review. Letters, editorials, commentaries, unpublished manuscripts, books and book chapters, conference proceedings, cost analyses, narrative reviews, systematic reviews, clinical practice guidelines were excluded from the study. Studies measuring the effects of any intervention program on trunk stabilization (wearing a lifting belt, rehabilitation, exercise, pharmacology...) were excluded as well. The search strategy was restricted to English and French publications.

Studies were included for subsequent methodological quality assessments if the following criteria were all satisfied: (1) postural perturbation was unexpected; (2) one or more trunk muscle response to postural perturbation was studied; (3) main outcome measure was either trunk muscle reflex recorded with EMG or trunk movement following perturbation; (4) independent variables were erector spinae muscle fatigue or spinal tissue creep or non-specific LBP; (5) human adults participants were tested.

Study Selection

Two independent reviewers (JA, AL) screened citation titles and abstracts to identify the potential eligible articles. A third reviewer (MD) was consulted to resolve any disagreement between the reviewers. Once this first step was done, the relevant full texts were assessed by three independent reviewers (JA, FB, AL) to verify if they could be included in the review according to the five inclusion criteria described previously. In case of disagreement, the two others authors (CD and MD) were consulted. The flowchart of the study has been reported in **Figure 1**. Excluded articles and the reasons for exclusion were explained in this figure.

Tools Used in the Risk of Bias Assessment

To our knowledge, no validated assessments checklists are available to evaluate the quality of laboratory studies including EMG. Therefore, a custom quality checklist adapted from the Quality Index developed by Downs and Black (Downs and Black, 1998) for the first part and based on the "Surface Electromyography for the Non-Invasive Assessment of Muscles (SENIAM)" (Hermens et al., 1999) and the "International Society of Electrophysiology and Kinesiology (ISEK)" (Merletti, 1999) recommendations for the EMG quality assessment for the second part was created in relation to the specific needs of the objectives of this review.

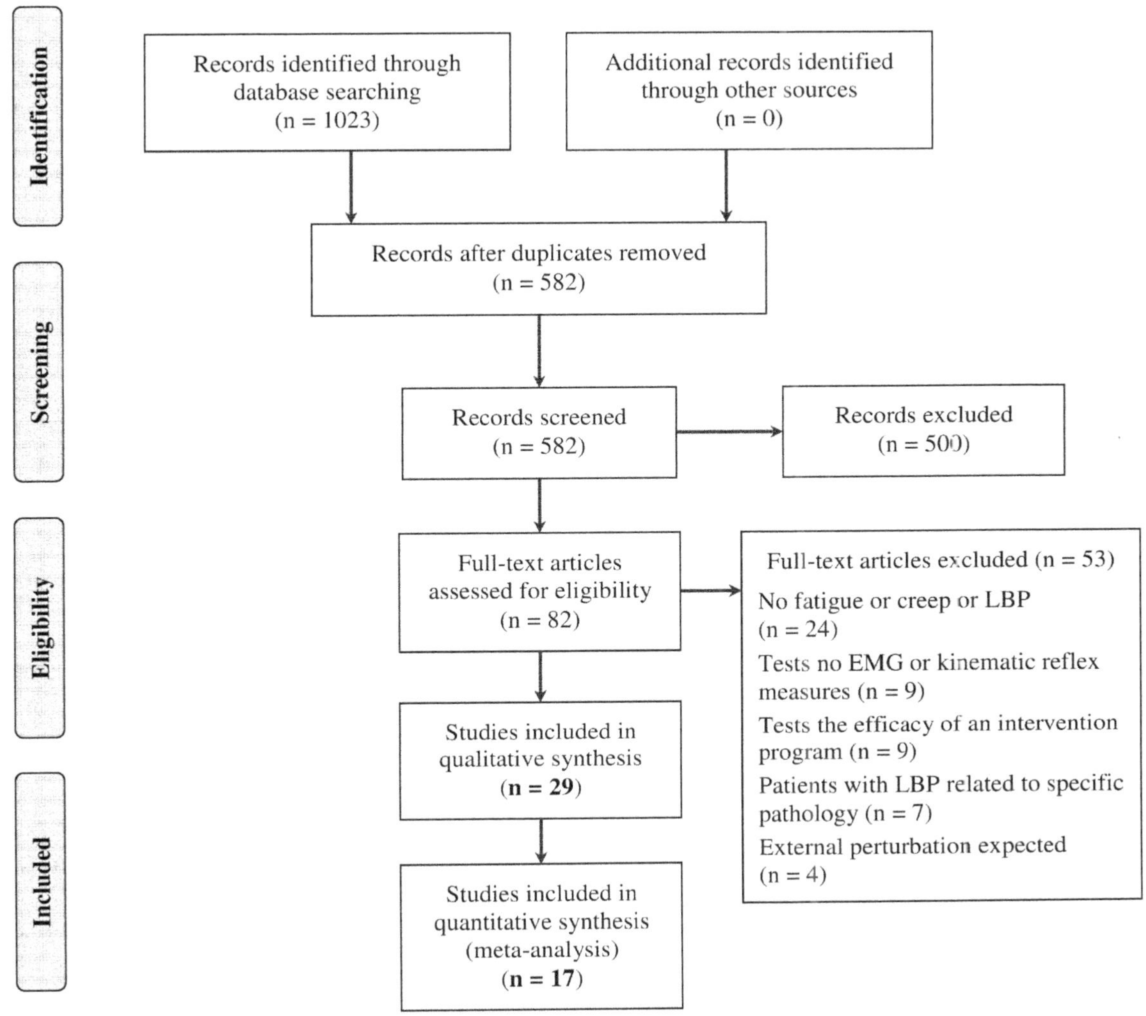

FIGURE 1 | Preferred Reporting Items for Systematic Reviews and Meta-Analyses (PRISMA) flowchart of the literature search.

Quality Index

The Quality Index is a 27-item checklist for assessing the methodological quality of both randomized and non-randomized studies of health care interventions (Downs and Black, 1998). This tool has been extensively used in the literature and presents a good test-retest reliability ($r = 0.88$) as well as a good inter-rater reliability ($r = 0.75$). From the original 27 items, it was decided during a consensus meeting to create a modified version of the Quality Index using 10 items which were deemed relevant in the assessment of the selected studies (for more details of each items, see Appendix B in Supplementary Material). From the initial Quality Index, 7 items were selected from the category "*reporting part*" (Items 1, 2, 3, 4, 6, 7, 10). Those items assessed if the information provided by the authors allow the reader to have an unbiased view of the study findings. Among the "*external validity*" category, which assesses the overall generalizability of the results, only one item was selected (item 12). Finally, 2 of the 6 items (Items 16, 18) for "*Internal validity—Bias*" were also selected. Each item was scored 0 or 1. When applicable, item 4 "*are the interventions of interest clearly described?*" was divided in two subcategories (item 4.1: description of the perturbation protocol and item 4.2: description of either the muscle fatigue protocol, or the spinal creep protocol). Both of these subcategories were also scored 0 or 1 when applicable. The total maximum score was either 10 cr 11 for this section of the checklist.

EMG

Electromyography was the main outcome from all the studies included in this review. Based on SENIAM (Hermens et al., 1999) and ISEK (Merletti, 1999) recommendations, the assessment checklist quality was divided in 4 main categories: (1) Surface EMG sensors: 1.1: inter electrode distance, 1.2: material (Ag/AgCl), and 1.3: construction (bipolar). (2) Sensor placement and location: 2.1: Skin preparation, 2.2: placement, and fixation, 2.3: reference electrode and orientation on muscle. (3) Signal processing: 3.1: Filters (type, kind, bandwidth, and order), 3.2: rectification method (full wave, half wave), 3.3: sampling (manufacturer/type of analogue-to digital (A/D) conversion board, sampling frequency, number of bits, input amplitude range), 3.4: amplitude processing (smoothing, average rectified value, root mean square, integrated EMG), and (4) normalization. Each main categories was scored 0 or 1. For the first three main categories, a score of 1 was only attributed when a minimum of 2 items of each category was reported. On the contrary, a score of 0 was attributed. When normalization item was not applicable (i.e., only reflex latency outcome), the total EMG quality score was 3.

Quality Total Score

Depending of the item 4 and normalization scoring, the total maximum quality score was either 13, 14, or 15. The total quality score for each study was expressed as percentage to facilitate comparison between them.

Risk of Bias Assessment

Three of the authors (JA, AL, FB) independently assessed the quality of included studies. Assessments were then compared during a formal meeting. Two others authors (CD, MD) were involved in resolving any disagreement between the three first authors when a consensus was not reach after the meeting. If additional information was required to complete the assessment, the corresponding authors of the included studies were contacted.

Data Extraction and Synthesis

The first authors (JA) extracted data from the selected studies and completed the evidence table (Appendix C in Supplementary Material).

Statistical Analyses

Inter-rater reliability of the methodological quality checklist was assessed using Fleiss's Kappa statistic with divisions suggested by Landis and Koch (<0.00, poor; 0.00–0.20, slight; 0.21–0.40, fair; 0.41–0.60, moderate; 0.61–0.80, substantial, 0.81–1.00, almost perfect; Landis and Koch, 1977). Meta-analysis could only be performed on reflex latency results because all the authors reported their results with the same unit (ms) while for the other EMG variables, authors reported their results using different units (% of MVC, μV with or without normalization) and it was not possible to pool these outcomes variables together in the same statistical model. To perform the meta-analysis, a random effect model was used since the samples of the included studies did not emanate from the same underlying study population. Meta-analysis were performed using Stata statistical software (College Station, TX: StataCorp LP. 2013). The heterogeneity across the studies was reported as the I^2 (Higgins et al., 2003). It was decided to report a large heterogeneity that was found instead of not reporting the results of the existing evidence.

RESULTS

Search Results

A total of 582 articles were identified from the literature search and 29 articles fulfilled selection criteria. A summary of the search results is presented in **Figure 1**.

Inter-Rater Reliability

The inter-rater reliability, measured by Kappa values, of all items from the quality checklist and EMG quality checklist ranged from moderate to almost perfect (0.52–1.00). As for the % of disagreement, the highest values were found for checklist items 1 (objectives clearly described) and 2 (EMG reflex outcomes clearly described) with 17% of disagreement, item 4a (perturbation protocol clearly described), 6 (EMG reflex response clearly described), and EMG 2.4 (electrode orientation on muscle) with 14% of disagreement (**Table 1**). General agreement among raters was at 90% or more for all other methodological quality checklist items. Item 18 (statistical tests appropriate) was excluded from the inter-rater analysis since, an external assessor helped the three authors (JA, AL, FB) assess this item for most of the included studies. A consensus was reached for each article.

Quality Assessment

Results of the adapted version of the Quality Index are presented in **Table 2**. The mean score obtained from all

TABLE 1 | Inter-rater reliability of quality checklist items [Kappa (95% Confidence interval) and % of disagreement].

	Items	Fleiss's Kappa (95% CI)	% disagreement
Quality index checklist	1	0.66 (0.45–0.87)	17
	2	0.52 (0.31–0.73)	17
	3	0.82 (0.61–1.03)	14
	4a	0.58 (0.37–0.79)	7
	4b	1.00	0
	6	0.55 (0.34–0.76)	14
	7	1.00	0
	10	0.85 (0.64–1.06)	10
	12	0.80 (0.59–1.01)	10
	16	1.00	0
EMG quality checklist	1.1	1.00	0
	1.2	0.94 (0.72–1.15)	3
	1.3	0.91 (0.70–1.12)	3
	2.1	1.00	0
	2.2	0.74 (0.53–0.95)	3
	2.3	1.00	0
	2.4	0.78 (0.57–0.99)	14
	3.1	1.00	0
	3.2	0.91 (0.70–1.12)	3
	3.3	1.00	0
	3.4	0.58 (0.37–0.79)	7
	4	0.86 (0.63–1.09)	7

TABLE 2 | Quality Index assessment scores (*Studies investigated the effect of low back pain were rated using a 10 point scale).

Authors (year)	1	2	3	4a	4b	6	7	10	12	16	18	Score (/10* or /11)	Score (%)
Akbari et al., 2015	0	1	1	1	n/a	1	1	1	0	1	0	7*	70
Bazrgari et al., 2011	1	0	1	1	1	1	1	1	0	1	1	9	81.8
Dupeyron et al., 2010	1	1	0	1	1	1	1	0	0	1	1	8	72.7
Gao et al., 2014	1	0	1	1	n/a	1	1	1	1	1	1	9*	90
Granata et al., 2001	1	0	0	1	1	0	1	0	0	1	1	6	54.6
Granata et al., 2005	1	1	0	1	1	1	1	1	0	1	1	9	81.8
Granata et al., 2004	1	1	0	0	1	1	1	0	0	1	0	6	54.6
Grondin and Potvin, 2009	1	1	0	1	1	1	1	0	0	1	1	8	72.7
Hendershct et al., 2011	1	1	1	1	1	1	1	1	0	1	1	10	90.9
Herrmann et al., 2006	0	1	0	1	1	1	1	1	0	1	1	8	72.7
Jacobs et al., 2011	1	1	1	1	n/a	1	1	1	1	1	1	10*	100
Jones et al., 2012a	1	1	1	1	n/a	1	1	0	1	1	0	8*	80
Jones et al., 2012b	1	1	1	1	n/a	1	1	1	1	1	1	10*	100
Lariviere et al., 2010	1	1	1	1	n/a	1	1	1	0	1	1	9*	90
Liebetrau et al., 2013	0	1	0	1	n/a	1	1	0	0	1	1	6*	60
MacDonald et al., 2010	1	1	1	1	n/a	1	1	1	0	1	1	9*	90
Mawston et al., 2007	1	1	0	1	1	1	1	1	0	1	1	9	81.8
Muslim et al., 2013	1	1	1	1	1	1	1	1	0	1	1	10	90.9
Newcomer et al., 2002	1	1	1	1	n/a	1	1	1	0	1	1	9*	90
Olson, 2014	1	1	0	1	1	1	1	1	0	1	1	9	81.8
Radebold et al., 2000	1	1	0	1	n/a	1	1	0	0	1	0	6*	60
Radebold et al., 2001	1	1	1	1	n/a	1	1	0	0	1	0	7*	70
Ramprasad et al., 2010	1	0	0	1	n/a	0	1	0	1	1	0	5*	50
Reeves et al., 2005	0	1	1	1	n/a	1	1	1	0	1	1	8*	80
Rogers and Granata, 2006	1	1	0	1	1	1	1	1	0	1	1	9	81.8
Sanchez-Zuriaga et al., 2010	1	1	0	1	1	1	1	1	0	1	1	9	81.8
Shenoy et al., 2013	1	0	0	1	n/a	0	1	0	0	0	0	3*	30
Stokes et al., 2006	1	1	0	1	n/a	1	1	0	1	1	0	7*	70
Toosizadeh et al., 2013	1	1	1	1	1	1	1	1	0	1	1	10	90.9

the included studies was 75% (ranging from 30 to 100%). Item 3, which relates to the characteristics of participants generally scored poorly. Only 15 studies were considered to provide sufficient information about the inclusion and/or exclusion criteria of their recruited participants. Item 12 relating to the external validity was the one with the lowest score and in only eight studies, authors have identified the source population or recruitment procedure for their participants.

As for the EMG quality, the assessment yielded a mean score of 86% (express as percentage, obtained from all the included studies ranging from 50 to 100%; **Table 3**).

The total quality score, including the Quality Index and EMG, was 79% (ranging from 43 to 100%; **Table 4**).

Muscle Fatigue

A total of 7 studies investigated the effect of erector spinae muscle fatigue and neuromuscular adaptations following unexpected perturbation of the trunk (Granata et al., 2001, 2004; Herrmann et al., 2006; Mawston et al., 2007; Grondin and Potvin, 2009; Dupeyron et al., 2010; Sanchez-Zuriaga et al., 2010). **Figure 2** provides an overview of results drawn from these studies.

Baseline Activity

Among these studies, results for erector spinae muscle baseline activity prior to an unexpected perturbation was increase after a fatigue task (Granata et al., 2001, 2004; Grondin and Potvin, 2009), while three others studies found no impact on erector spinae baseline activity under the influence of muscle fatigue (Herrmann et al., 2006; Mawston et al., 2007; Dupeyron et al., 2010). As for abdominal muscles, baseline activity results were also mixed. Baseline activity was found to increase after an erector spinae muscle fatigue task for external obliquus in 3 studies (Granata et al., 2001, 2004; Grondin and Potvin, 2009), and for internal obliquus in 2 studies (Granata et al., 2001; Grondin and Potvin, 2009). Conversely 2 other studies found no difference for external obliquus (Mawston et al., 2007; Dupeyron et al., 2010) and internal obliquus muscles (Granata et al., 2004; Mawston et al., 2007). Finally, two studies reported a higher rectus abdominis baseline activity under the

TABLE 3 | EMG quality assessment scores (*When normalization was not necessary, studies were rated on 3 point scale).

Authors (year)	1.1	1.2	1.3	2.1	2.2	2.3	2.4	3.1	3.2	3.3	3.4	4	Score (/3* or /4)
Akbari et al., 2015	1	1	0	1	1	0	1	1	0	1	1	1	4
Bazrgari et al., 2011	0	1	1	0	1	0	0	1	0	1	1	0	2
Dupeyron et al., 2010	0	1	1	1	1	1	1	1	1	1	1	1	4
Gao et al., 2014	0	0	0	1	1	1	1	1	0	1	1	1	3
Granata et al., 2001	0	0	1	1	1	0	1	1	1	1	1	1	3
Granata et al., 2005	0	0	1	0	1	0	0	1	1	1	1	1	2
Granata et al., 2004	0	0	1	0	1	0	1	1	1	1	1	1	3
Grondin and Potvin, 2009	1	1	1	1	1	1	1	1	1	1	0	1	4
Hendershot et al., 2011	0	1	1	1	1	0	0	1	1	1	1	0	3
Herrmann et al., 2006	1	1	0	1	1	0	1	1	1	1	1	1	4
Jacobs et al., 2011	1	1	1	1	1	0	1	1	1	1	1	1	4
Jones et al., 2012a	1	1	1	1	1	0	1	1	1	1	1	1	4
Jones et al., 2012b	1	1	1	1	1	0	1	1	1	1	1	1	4
Lariviere et al., 2010	0	0	0	1	1	1	1	1	1	1	1	1	3
Liebetrau et al., 2013	1	1	1	1	1	1	1	1	1	1	1	0	3
MacDonald et al., 2010	1	1	1	n/a	1	1	1	1	1	1	1	0	3
Mawston et al., 2007	1	1	1	1	1	0	1	1	1	1	1	1	4
Muslim et al., 2013	0	1	1	1	1	0	0	1	0	1	1	0	3
Newcomer et al., 2002	1	0	1	1	1	0	0	1	0	1	1	n/a	3*
Olson, 2014	1	1	1	1	1	1	1	1	1	1	1	1	4
Radebold et al., 2000	1	1	1	1	1	0	1	1	1	1	1	n/a	3*
Radebold et al., 2001	1	1	1	1	1	0	1	1	1	1	1	n/a	3*
Ramprasad et al., 2010	1	1	1	1	1	1	1	1	1	1	1	1	4
Reeves et al., 2005	1	1	1	0	1	0	0	1	1	1	1	n/a	2*
Rogers and Granata, 2006	1	1	1	0	1	1	0	1	1	1	1	1	4
Sanchez-Zuriaga et al., 2010	1	1	0	1	1	1	1	1	1	1	1	0	3
Shenoy et al., 2013	1	0	1	1	1	1	1	1	1	1	1	0	3
Stokes et al., 2006	1	1	1	1	1	1	1	1	1	1	1	1	4
Toosizadeh et al., 2013	0	1	1	0	1	0	0	1	1	1	1	1	3

influence of erector spinae muscle fatigue (Granata et al., 2001, 2004).

Reflex Latency

In the presence of lower back muscle fatigue, reflex latency of erector spinae muscles was not affected in the majority of studies (Granata et al., 2004; Herrmann et al., 2006; Dupeyron et al., 2010; Sanchez-Zuriaga et al., 2010). One study indicated that the reflex latency was significantly decreased after a fatigue protocol involving erector spinae muscles (Mawston et al., 2007). Following an unexpected perturbation, reflex latency of the internal (Granata et al., 2004; Mawston et al., 2007) and external obliquus (Granata et al., 2004; Dupeyron et al., 2010) and rectus abdominis (Granata et al., 2004) was found to be unchanged in the presence of muscle fatigue. In opposition, one study showed a decrease external obliquus reflex latency after erector spinae muscles fatigue (Mawston et al., 2007). Altogether, results of the meta-analysis shows that there is no effect of muscle fatigue on reflex latency of erector spinae muscles [Standardized mean difference (SMD) $= 0.54$; 95%CI: -0.71, 1.78; $I^2 = 86.5\%$; **Figure 3**].

Reflex Amplitude

In 3 studies, reflex amplitude of the erector spinae was similar with or without muscle fatigue (Granata et al., 2004; Grondin and Potvin, 2009; Sanchez-Zuriaga et al., 2010), while 2 studies found an increased reflex amplitude with fatigue (Herrmann et al., 2006; Dupeyron et al., 2010). External and internal obliquus (Granata et al., 2004; Grondin and Potvin, 2009) and rectus abdominis (Granata et al., 2004) reflex amplitude were not affected by the presence of erector spinae muscle fatigue.

Kinematics

Only 2 studies investigated trunk kinematic behavior in response to a sudden perturbation with erector spinae muscle fatigue. These studies did not observe a difference in kinematics between pre and post fatigue condition (Granata et al., 2004; Mawston et al., 2007).

TABLE 4 | Quality total score (#Studies investigated the effect of low back pain when normalization was not necessary were rated using a 13 point scale; *Studies investigated the effect of low back pain were rated using a 14 point scale).

Authors (year)	Score quality index (/10* or /11)	Score EMG (/3* or /4)	Total score (/13# or /14* or /15)	Note (%)
Akbari et al., 2015	7*	4	11*	78.6
Bazrgari et al., 2011	9	2	11	73.3
Dupeyron et al., 2010	8	4	12	80
Gao et al., 2014	9*	3	12*	85.7
Granata et al., 2001	6	3	9	60
Granata et al., 2005	9	2	11	73.3
Granata et al., 2004	6	3	9	60
Grondin and Potvin, 2009	8	4	12	80
Hendershot et al., 2011	10	3	13	86.7
Herrmann et al., 2006	8	4	12	80
Jacobs et al., 2011	10*	4	14*	100
Jones et al., 2012a	8*	4	12*	85.7
Jones et al., 2012b	10*	4	14*	100
Lariviere et al., 2010	9*	3	12*	85.7
Liebetrau et al., 2013	6*	3	9*	64.3
MacDonald et al., 2010	9*	3	12*	85.7
Mawston et al., 2007	9	4	13	86.7
Muslim et al., 2013	10	3	13	86.7
Newcomer et al., 2002	9*	3*	12#	92.3
Olson, 2014	9	4	13	86.7
Radebold et al., 2000	6*	3*	9#	69.2
Radebold et al., 2001	7*	3*	10#	76.9
Ramprasad et al., 2010	5*	4	9*	64.3
Reeves et al., 2005	8*	2*	10#	76.9
Rogers and Granata, 2006	9	4	13	86.7
Sanchez-Zuriaga et al., 2010	9	3	12	80
Shenoy et al., 2013	3*	3	6*	42.9
Stokes et al., 2006	7*	4	11*	78.6
Toosizadeh et al., 2013	10	3	13	86.7

Spinal Creep

A total of 8 studies reported on the effect of spinal tissue creep and neuromuscular adaptations following unexpected perturbation of the trunk (Granata et al., 2005; Rogers and Granata, 2006; Sanchez-Zuriaga et al., 2010; Bazrgari et al., 2011; Hendershot et al., 2011; Muslim et al., 2013; Toosizadeh et al., 2013; Olson, 2014). **Figure 4** provides an overview of results from these studies.

Baseline Activity

Prior to an unexpected perturbation, baseline activity remained unchanged under the influence of spinal tissue creep for the majority of studies and for all trunk muscles (Granata et al., 2005; Rogers and Granata, 2006; Bazrgari et al., 2011; Hendershot et al., 2011; Muslim et al., 2013; Olson, 2014). Only one study found a decrease in external obliquus baseline activity following creep deformation (Rogers and Granata, 2006).

Reflex Latency

Two studies showed that, under the influence of spinal tissue creep, reflex latency of the erector spinae muscles increased (Sanchez-Zuriaga et al., 2010; Toosizadeh et al., 2013). Conversely, one study reported that erector spinae reflex latency was shorter in the presence of spinal tissue creep (Muslim et al., 2013). Finally, four studies did not observe significant changes in reflex latency between pre- and post-creep conditions for erector spinae muscles (Granata et al., 2005; Bazrgari et al., 2011; Hendershot et al., 2011; Olson, 2014), as well as for the external obliquus and the rectus abdominis muscles (Olson, 2014). Results of the meta-analysis shows that creep does not have an effect on reflex latency (SMD $= -0.26$; 95%CI: $-0.83, 0.31$; $I^2 = 69.1\%$) of erector spinae muscles (**Figure 3**).

Reflex Amplitude

Following an unknown perturbation, erector spinae muscle reflex amplitude are generally unaffected by the presence of creep (Granata et al., 2005; Sanchez-Zuriaga et al., 2010; Olson, 2014). One study also found no impact of spinal tissue creep for the external obliquus and the rectus abdominis muscles reflex amplitude following a sudden perturbation (Olson, 2014). Only one study found lower reflex amplitude values following creep deformation for paraspinal muscles (Rogers and Granata, 2006).

Kinematics

As for trunk kinematics behavior following an unexpected perturbation under spinal creep condition, two studies found no difference between pre- and post-creep conditions (Rogers and Granata, 2006; Olson, 2014), while one study reported decreased trunk kinematic gain following a creep deformation (Granata et al., 2005).

Clinical LBP

A total of 15 studies investigated the effect of LBP and neuromuscular adaptations following unexpected trunk perturbation (Radebold et al., 2000, 2001; Newcomer et al., 2002; Reeves et al., 2005; Stokes et al., 2006; Lariviere et al., 2010; MacDonald et al., 2010; Ramprasad et al., 2010; Jacobs et al., 2011; Jones et al., 2012a,b; Liebetrau et al., 2013; Shenoy et al., 2013; Gao et al., 2014; Akbari et al., 2015). Among these studies, two recruited participants with acute/episodic LBP (Stokes et al., 2006; Jones et al., 2012b) while all other included participants with chronic LBP. **Figure 5** provides an overview of results drawn from these studies.

Baseline Activity

Prior to an unexpected perturbation, patients with chronic LBP demonstrated, in most cases, a significant increase of baseline activity of erector spinae muscles (Lariviere et al., 2010; Jacobs et al., 2011; Jones et al., 2012a). An increase in erector spinae baseline activity was also found in patients with acute LBP (Stokes et al., 2006). Nevertheless, three studies failed to identify differences in back muscle baseline activity between healthy participants and patients with chronic LBP (MacDonald et al., 2010; Liebetrau et al., 2013) or acute LBP (Jones et al., 2012b). As for trunk flexor muscles, three different studies did

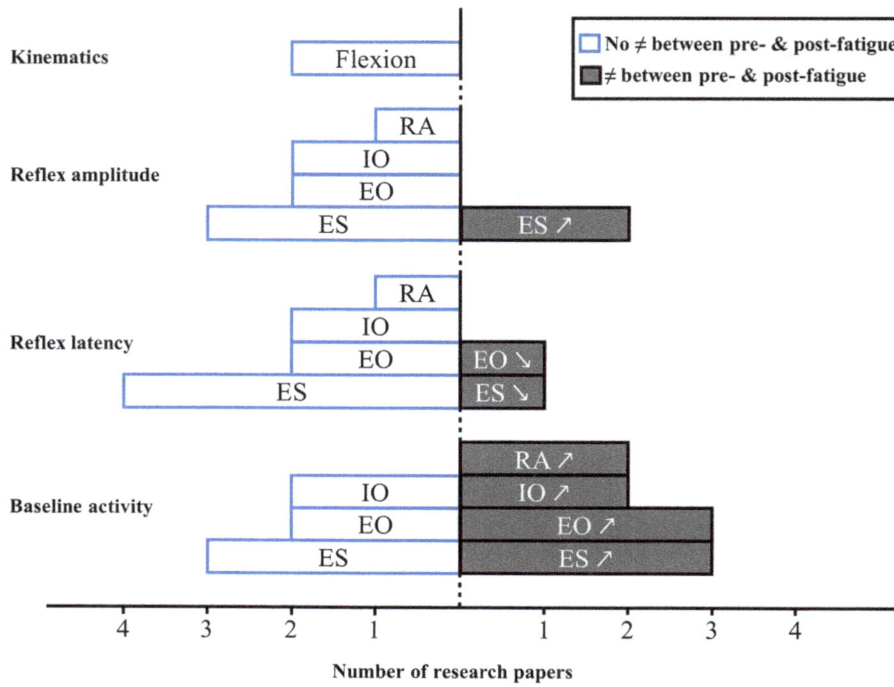

FIGURE 2 | Muscle activity reflex responses to unexpected postural perturbation of the trunk under the influence of muscle fatigue expressed in number of research papers (↗, higher value with muscle fatigue; ↘, lower value with muscle fatigue; RA, rectus abdominis; IO, internal obliquus; EO, external obliquus; ES, erector spinae).

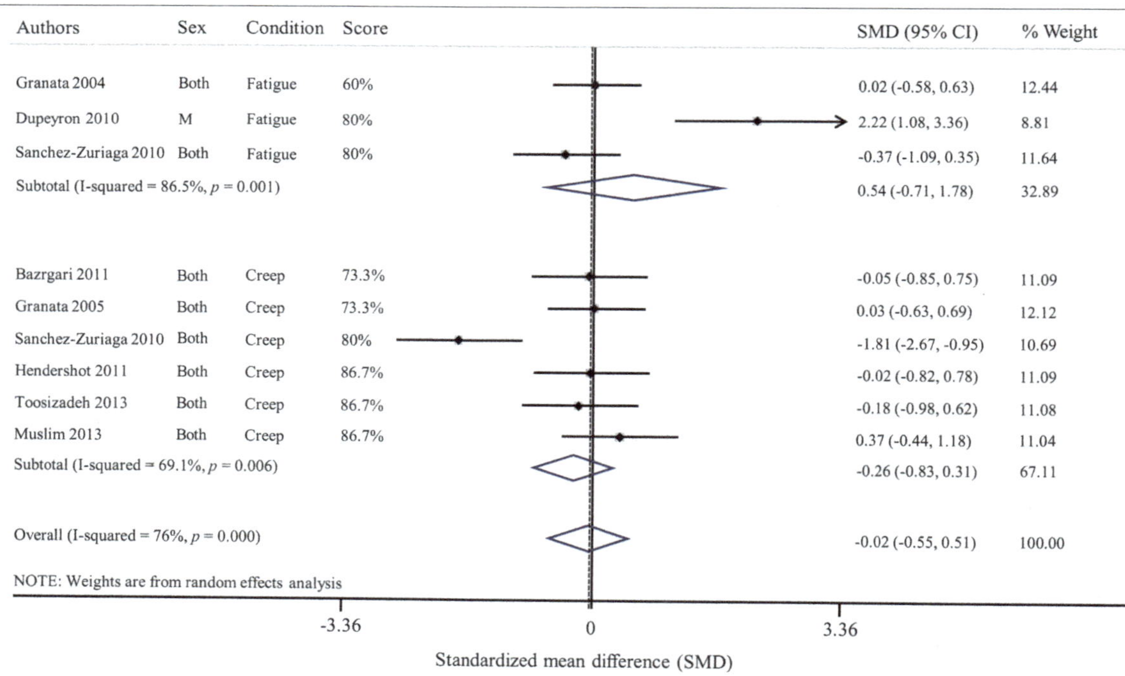

FIGURE 3 | Forest plot of erector spinae reflex latencies under the influence of muscle fatigue and spinal tissue creep (SMD, Standardized mean difference).

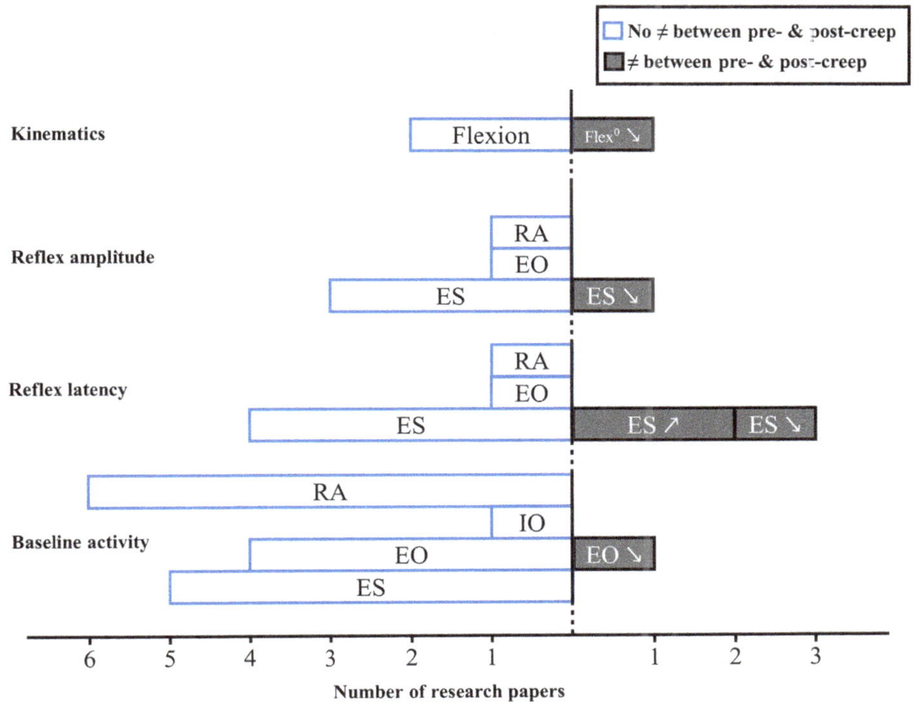

FIGURE 4 | Muscle activity reflex responses to unexpected postural perturbation of the trunk under the influence of spinal tissue creep expressed in number of research papers (↗, higher value with creep; ↘, lower value with creep; RA, rectus abdominis; IO, internal obliquus; EO, external obliquus; ES, erector spinae).

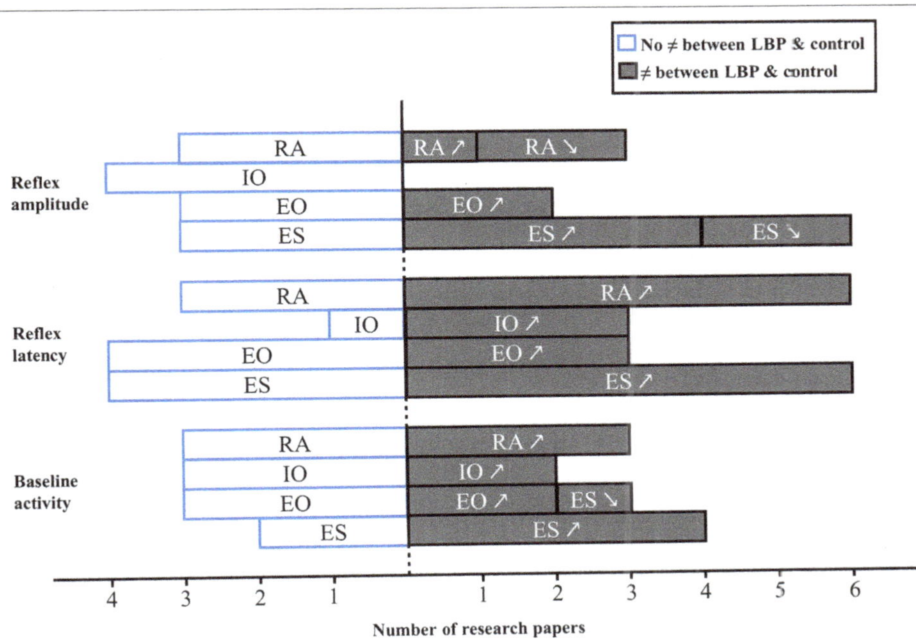

FIGURE 5 | Muscle activity reflex responses to unexpected postural perturbation of the trunk in patient with LBP expressed in number of research papers (↗, higher value in LBP group; ↘, lower value in LBP group; RA, rectus abdominis; IO, internal obliquus; EO, external obliquus; ES, erector spinae).

not report any difference between patients with chronic LBP (Lariviere et al., 2010; Liebetrau et al., 2013) or acute LBP (except for the external obliquus baseline activity which decreased in patients; Jones et al., 2012a) and healthy participants, while two studies reported an increase in baseline activity in patients with chronic (Jones et al., 2012a) or acute LBP (Stokes et al., 2006).

Reflex Latency

Among all studies investigating erector spinae reflex latency in patients with LBP, six studies found longer latencies in patients vs. healthy participants (Radebold et al., 2000, 2001; Reeves et al., 2005; Ramprasad et al., 2010; Shenoy et al., 2013; Gao et al., 2014), while four studies did not find significant differences between those two populations (Newcomer et al., 2002; Lariviere et al., 2010; Liebetrau et al., 2013; Akbari et al., 2015). As for external obliquus reflex latencies, results from three different studies showed longer latencies (Radebold et al., 2000, 2001; Reeves et al., 2005), while four studies did not find differences between patients with chronic LBP and healthy participants (Lariviere et al., 2010; Liebetrau et al., 2013; Gao et al., 2014; Akbari et al., 2015). Three studies reported increased internal obliquus reflex latencies in patients with LBP (Radebold et al., 2000, 2001; Liebetrau et al., 2013), while one did not (Akbari et al., 2015). Lastly, patients with LBP exhibited significantly longer reflex latencies over the rectus abdominis muscles in a majority of studies (Radebold et al., 2000, 2001; Reeves et al., 2005; Ramprasad et al., 2010; Liebetrau et al., 2013; Shenoy et al., 2013). However, three studies failed to identify differences between LBP patients and controls (Newcomer et al., 2002; Lariviere et al., 2010; Akbari et al., 2015). Overall, results of the meta-analysis showed that erector spinae reflex latency was increased in patients with LBP vs. healthy participants (SMD = 0.53; 95%CI: 0.19, 0.87; $I^2 = 62.3\%$; **Figure 6**).

Reflex Amplitude

Erector spinae reflex amplitude behavior in response to a sudden perturbation seemed in most cases to be increased in patients with chronic LBP (Lariviere et al., 2010; Jones et al., 2012a; Gao et al., 2014) as well as in patients with acute LBP (Jones et al., 2012b). However, two studies reported a decreased erector spinae muscle reflex amplitude in patients with chronic LBP (Ramprasad et al., 2010; Shenoy et al., 2013), while two others studies failed to identify differences between patients with chronic LBP and healthy controls (Jacobs et al., 2011; Liebetrau et al., 2013). Moreover, one study has found that the superficial multifidus reflex amplitude decreased in patients with chronic LBP compared to controls (MacDonald et al., 2010), while one study failed to found a difference between patients with chronic LBP and controls (Liebetrau et al., 2013). As for trunk flexors reflex amplitude, no difference were reported for internal obliquus muscle in people with acute or chronic LBP as compared to asymptomatic participants. External obliquus reflex amplitude was found to be increased in patients with chronic (Jones et al., 2012a) or acute LBP (Jones et al., 2012b), whereas three studies did not observed any difference (Jacobs et al., 2011; Liebetrau et al., 2013; Gao et al., 2014). Finally, no difference were reported for the rectus abdominis reflex amplitude response to a sudden perturbation between healthy participants and patients with chronic (Jacobs et al., 2011; Liebetrau et al., 2013) or acute LBP (Jones et al., 2012b).

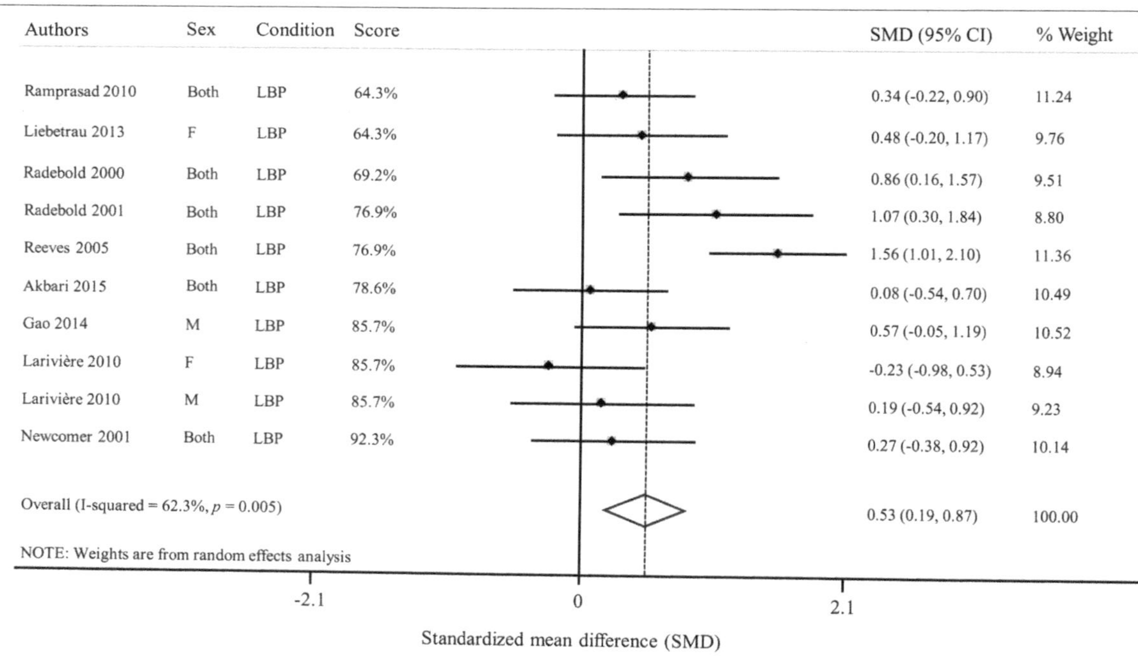

FIGURE 6 | Forest plot of erector spinae reflex latencies in patients with low back pain (SMD, Standardized mean difference).

DISCUSSION

To our knowledge, this is the first systematic review that explores the quality of evidence related to muscle activity reflex in response to unexpected trunk perturbation. Since a high heterogeneity was present among the selected studies, our ability to pool data and draw conclusions was limited.

Quality Assessment

The total score of the methodological quality assessment was 79%, with only one study scoring below 50% (Shenoy et al., 2013). Overall, it seems reasonable to suggest that the quality of the included studies was good. However, when quality checklist items are considered individually, some methodological weaknesses emerge. The characteristics of the participants included in the studies were clearly described in only half of the studies. Most studies only mentioned if their participants were healthy participants or patients with LBP without any further clinical details. In most cases, the description of the control group was limited to "healthy" and when a group of LBP was included, the duration and nature of LBP, or any other medical condition were often omitted in inclusion/exclusion criteria. Lack of specific inclusion and exclusion criteria may lead to inherent heterogeneity in patients responses to perturbation as it is known, that patients with acute or chronic LBP can exhibit various neuromuscular adaptations and that such adaptation may be influence by patient's clinical characteristics (Hodges and Tucker, 2011). Another significant methodological weakness identified was external validity. Indeed, only 6/29 studies identified the source population for the recruited participants. This suggest that the overall generalizability of results to the related population is limited. Furthermore, eight studies had small sample size, with fifteen or less participants included. Having such small sample sizes may lead to statistical power issues, which could potentially lead to type II error (Cohen, 1992). Finally, the lack of information concerning the p-values was identified in the methodological assessment. The absence of true p-value ($p \leq 0.05$) can lead to the misinterpretation of significant differences and overall interpretation of study results (i.e., $p = 0.049$ vs. $p = 0.011$). Moreover, even if not considered as a criteria of the Quality Index developed by Downs and Black, the 95% confidence interval should also be presented but was reported in only 3 of the included studies.

On the other hand, high methodological quality was found for the descriptions of sudden external perturbation experimental protocols. Moreover, descriptions of the fatigue and/or creep protocols were also appropriately detailed. This indicates that these experimental protocols would be replicable. Unfortunately, a high heterogeneity between experimental protocols makes the interpretation of the original study results difficult. Indeed, sudden external perturbations were applied in different positions (standing and semi-sitting) with different magnitudes, and sometimes using a familiarization perturbation protocol. As for EMG assessment, the overall quality was good. However, three items drawn from ISEK and SENIAM recommendations were absent in most of the studies: description of the inter electrode distance, the reference electrode and the normalization procedures. The inter electrode distance could influence data recording, due crosstalk effects (Hermens et al., 1999; De Luca et al., 2012), whereas the absence of normalization may lead to misinterpretation of results when comparing the amplitude of muscle activity (reflex amplitude or baseline activity prior to perturbation) between participants (Merletti, 1999).

Baseline Activity

Experiencing an unexpected perturbation limits the nervous system capacity to anticipate and preprogram a motor response. Yet, baseline muscle activity, was one of the most reported variable in studies that evaluated the effect of unexpected perturbation (19/29 of the included studies). Despite the absence of feedforward strategies, small changes in baseline activity have been described under muscle fatigue or in the presence of LBP, while baseline activity is not modified under the influence of spinal creep. Anxiety can also affect postural stability (Wada et al., 2001; Stambolieva and Angov, 2010) and therefore potentially modulate baseline activity while "waiting" for an external perturbation to happen. However, there is not enough evidence to strongly propose that baseline activity can be influenced by the varying perturbation delays. Indeed, this review could not reach any definite conclusion with regard to baseline activity since the included articles did not report specific perturbation delays. Most articles reported a variation of time delay (i.e., between 1 and 10 s) or they did not report any details.

Muscle Fatigue Effects on Spinal Stability

The relationship between muscle fatigue and spinal stability remains unclear. Despite the varying reflex latency values between studies, this review suggests that trunk muscle reflex response latencies do not change under the influence of back muscles fatigue. This suggest that, in order to stabilize the spine, the central nervous system generates earlier postural muscle adjustments similarly regardless of muscle fatigue presence. The results from the metanalysis should, however, be interpreted with caution. An I square superior to 80% suggests the presence of a substantial heterogeneity between those studies. As for baseline activity and reflex amplitude of erector spinae muscles, surprisingly, no consensus was found in this review. Since the presence muscle fatigue is usually characterized by an increase in the EMG amplitude signal in submaximal muscle contractions (De Luca, 1997), a higher trunk muscle EMG amplitude was expected, especially in muscles targeted by the fatigue protocol. The flexor muscle baseline activity and reflex amplitude did not seem to be affected by the presence of back muscle fatigue in most studies and only the rectus abdominis baseline activity increased prior to an unknown perturbation in the presence of muscle fatigue. However, these results should be interpreted with caution since only two studies reported such responses to muscle fatigue. This note of caution can also apply to trunk kinematic behaviors since the lack of any effect of erector spinae muscle fatigue on trunk kinematics was reported in very few studies. Overall, it could be hypothesized that muscle fatigue has a negligible impact on spinal stability. A previous study showed that even in the presence of upper limb muscle fatigue, movement accuracy with external perturbation remains constant (Takahashi et al., 2006). Moreover, the lack of trunk movement changes in a fatiguing state could be explained by the trunk muscle system's redundancy which offers various adaptation possibilities to achieve a similar goal (Latash and Anson, 2006). Investigating neuromuscular strategies such as variability in muscle activity recruitment pattern should shed some light on the effects of trunk muscle fatigue during unexpected trunk perturbations.

Spinal Tissue Creep Effects on Spinal Stability

Overall, the presence of spinal tissue creep does not seem to affect spinal stability in a context of unexpected perturbation. Indeed, this review revealed that trunk muscle baseline activity prior to a perturbation does not change following either an active or a static deformation of passive spinal tissues. Following an unknown perturbation, participants showed similar trunk muscle reflex amplitude. Again, active vs. passive deformation do not yield distinct effects on reflex amplitude. Such result is surprising since it is expected that creep deformation will lead to an increase muscle activity amplitude (Olson et al., 2009; Abboud et al., 2016), which is believed to act as a spinal stabilization mechanism. Interesting new findings have shown that following a prolonged intermittent trunk flexion of 1 h, an increase of trunk stiffness is observed (Voglar et al., 2016). This observation confirms previous findings suggesting that in the first 30 min of cyclic trunk flexion, a decrease in intrinsic stiffness occurs, whereas, the following 30 min, spinal stiffness increases (Parkinson et al., 2004). Since spinal stiffness has been associated with spinal stability (Graham and Brown, 2012), it can be hypothesized that no adjustment of reflex amplitude is needed when intrinsic stiffness increases. However, studies included in this review cannot support this hypothesis, since spinal creep deformation lasting from 15 min to 1 h did not modify the reflex amplitude. As for reflex latency, no distinct effect of spinal tissue creep could be identified in the meta-analysis. In most cases, reflex latency did not change in the presence of spinal tissue creep. Once again, the results drawn from the metanalysis should be interpreted with caution due to the heterogeneity between the included studies ($I^2 = 69\%$). Overall, this review suggest that spinal tissue creep had no or only minor effects on trunk neuromuscular adaptations to unexpected perturbation. Moreover, no definite conclusion can be drawn for trunk kinematics since only three studies investigated the effect of spinal tissue creep and reported conflicting results. It seems reasonable to suggest that, in a context of spinal instability, the impact of transient spinal tissue deformation can be counteracted by recruiting other muscle groups and using alternate neuromuscular strategies. Indeed, it has already been proposed that the loss of viscoelastic tissues of ligaments, discs, and joint capsules properties can be counteracted by adjusting the co-contraction levels of agonist and antagonist muscles (Solomonow et al., 1999).

Musculoskeletal LBP Effects on Spinal Stability

The effect of LBP on spinal stability was the most common topic identified in the current review. Despite the number of studies available, no definite conclusion could be drawn. Results for most EMG reflex variables included in this review were found to be conflicting across studies. More studies found differences between a healthy population and populations of patients with chronic LBP than studies that did not, especially for the trunk muscles baseline activity. Similar observations were found in patients with acute or episodic LBP. On the other hand, studies investigating the effects of acute clinical LBP induced by experimental LBP, consistently reported no change in trunk muscle baseline activity prior to an unexpected perturbation (Gregory et al., 2008; Boudreau et al., 2011; Miller et al., 2013). Despite the overall conflicting observations, results from the meta-analysis showed a moderate effect indicating a longer reflex latency for erector spinae muscles in patients with chronic LBP compared to healthy participants. However, the meta-analysis results for reflex latency should be interpreted with care since the analysis was conducted using reflex latency values that were drawn directly from the article or provided by the authors. Although, no meta-analysis was conducted for reflex amplitude, erector spinae muscle reflex amplitude was found to be significantly higher in patients with acute or chronic LBP in most studies while two studies reported a decrease in the same population. It should be noted that, these two latter studies reporting a lower erector spinae reflex amplitude in patients with chronic LBP were among the studies with the lowest quality score (see **Table 4**). It is known that patients with LBP are highly heterogeneous and many studies have attempted to identify subgroups (O'sullivan, 2005; Fersum et al., 2010). Patients described in the included studies differed, from a study to another, with regard to their respective pain scores (2–4.7/10 on numerical pain scale), their disability scores (very low to moderate), as well as in the pain duration (3 months to several years). If these subgroups exist, one typical neuromuscular response could be associated with one typical subgroup. The heterogeneity of the results reported in this review highlights the importance of standardized and well described inclusion and exclusion criteria in experimental studies investigating patients' populations.

Limitations

Since no validated assessment checklist was available to evaluate the quality of laboratory studies using EMG assessments, a custom made quality checklist was adapted from an already validated existing checklist (Downs and Black, 1998). However, to improve the validity and reliability of our checklist, three independent assessors completed the quality checklist and showed a high level of agreement. A methodological limitation of this review is that only one author have extracted the data (Appendix C in Supplementary Material). Another limitation of this review is the limited number of studies investigating muscle fatigue, spinal tissue creep, and musculoskeletal pain effects. Diverse sensorimotor and biomechanical external perturbation, such as vibration (Arashanapalli and Wilson, 2008; Santos et al., 2008; Arora and Grenier, 2013; MacIntyre and Cort, 2014) and delayed onset muscle soreness (Hjortskov et al., 2005), were identified during the preliminary search. However, an insufficient number of studies was available to consider these topics in the review.

This systematic review assessed the overall quality of the included articles. However, due to the large number of included studies, it was not feasible to contact all the authors of articles who omitted methodological details, such as inclusion/exclusion recruitment criterion, electrode placement, etc. Moreover, in order to guide future research, this review was designed to highlight the lack of standardization and information characterizing this type of study. This review did not assess the reliability and validity of the main outcomes. Besides, almost all studies did not provide data about EMG reflex variable reliability and/or validity, we decided not to penalize study who did not report theses information since EMG was already proven to be valid and reliable assessment tool in many studies. Instead, it was chosen to focus on the quality of EMG data acquisition and analyses which are considered key factors in the value and interpretation of results (De Luca, 1997). A final limitation of this review was the incapacity to conduct meta-analysis on variables other than reflex latency. Unfortunately, the use of different units (% of MVC, μV, normalized EMG with no unit, etc.) to express reflex amplitude or baseline activity made the meta-analysis virtually impossible.

Research Recommendations

It is clear that standardization for conducting and reporting EMG fundamental studies should be a priority in future research. The development of an adapted checklist for EMG fundamental and clinical studies may be a helpful tool to achieve such a goal. Moreover, future studies should establish the reliability of the EMG reflex variables. Despite the presence of a good reliability in the determination of reflex latency using SD methods (Hodges and Bui, 1996), reliability or validity of reflex amplitude and baseline activity have not been assessed in most studies. Given the various reflex outcomes studied and the overall heterogeneity of the studies included in this systematic review, determining how physical and physiological reflex responses adapt in various spinal instability conditions should remain an active domain of research. Future research should also consider exploring the impact of spinal instability on trunk kinematic behavior in the presence of expected and unexpected external perturbations.

AUTHOR CONTRIBUTIONS

Substantial contributions to the conception or design of the work; or analysis, or interpretation of data for the work: JA, AL, FB, CD, MD. Drafting the work and revising it critically for important intellectual content: JA, AL, FB, CD, MD. Final approval of the version to be published: JA, AL, FB, CD, MD. Agreement to be accountable for all aspects of the work in ensuring that questions related to the accuracy or integrity of any part of the work are appropriately investigated and resolved: JA, AL, FB, CD, MD.

FUNDING

This study was funded through the Natural Sciences and Engineering Research Council of Canada in the form of both a scholarship and discovery grant.

REFERENCES

Abboud, J., Nougarou, F., and Descarreaux, M. (2016). Muscle activity adaptations to spinal tissue creep in the presence of muscle fatigue. *PLoS ONE* 11:e0149076. doi: 10.1371/journal.pone.0149076

Abboud, J., Nougarou, F., Page, I., Cantin, V., Massicotte, D., and Descarreaux, M. (2014). Trunk motor variability in patients with non-specific chronic low back pain. *Eur. J. Appl. Physiol.* 114, 2645–2654. doi: 10.1007/s00421-014-2985-8

Akbari, M., Sarrafzadeh, J., Maroufi, N., and Haghani, H. (2015). Changes in postural and trunk muscles responses in patients with chronic nonspecific low back pain during sudden upper limb loading. *Med. J. Islam. Repub. Iran* 29, 265.

Allison, G. T., and Henry, S. M. (2001). Trunk muscle fatigue during a back extension task in standing. *Man. Ther.* 6, 221–228. doi: 10.1054/math.2001.0412

Arashanapalli, M., and Wilson, S. E. (2008). Paraspinal muscle vibration alters dynamic motion of the trunk. *J. Biomech. Eng.* 130, 021001. doi: 10.1115/1.2898734

Arora, N., and Grenier, S. G. (2013). Acute effects of whole body vibration on directionality and reaction time latency of trunk muscles: the importance of rest and implications for spine stability. *J. Electromyogr. Kinesiol.* 23, 394–401. doi: 10.1016/j.jelekin.2012.10.018

Bazrgari, B., Hendershot, B., Muslim, K., Toosizadeh, N., Nussbaum, M. A., and Madigan, M. L. (2011). Disturbance and recovery of trunk mechanical and neuromuscular behaviours following prolonged trunk flexion: influences of duration and external load on creep-induced effects. *Ergonomics* 54, 1043–1052. doi: 10.1080/00140139.2011.614357

Belen'kii, V. E., Gurfinkel, V. S., and Pal'tsev, E. I. (1967). [Control elements of voluntary movements]. *Biofizika* 12, 135–141.

Boucher, J. A., Abboud, J., and Descarreaux, M. (2012). The influence of acute back muscle fatigue and fatigue recovery on trunk sensorimotor control. *J. Manipulative Physiol. Ther.* 35, 662–668. doi: 10.1016/j.jmpt.2012.10.003

Boudreau, S., Farina, D., Kongstad, L., Buus, D., Redder, J., Sverrisdottir, E., et al. (2011). The relative timing of trunk muscle activation is retained in response to unanticipated postural-perturbations during acute low back pain. *Exp. Brain Res.* 210, 259–267. doi: 10.1007/s00221-011-2629-8

Bouisset, S., and Do, M. C. (2008). Posture, dynamic stability, and voluntary movement. *Neurophysiol. Clin.* 38, 345–362. doi: 10.1016/j.neucli.2008.10.001

Bouisset, S., and Zattara, M. (1981). A sequence of postural movements precedes voluntary movement. *Neurosci. Lett.* 22, 263–270. doi: 10.1016/0304-3940(81)90117-8

Cholewicki, J., Greene, H. S., Polzhofer, G. K., Galloway, M. T., Shah, R. A., and Radebold, A. (2002). Neuromuscular function in athletes following recovery from a recent acute low back injury. *J. Orthop. Sports Phys. Ther.* 32, 568–575. doi: 10.2519/jospt.2002.32.11.568

Cohen, J. (1992). A power primer. *Psychol. Bull.* 112, 155–159. doi: 10.1037/0033-2909.112.1.155

Cresswell, A. G., Oddsson, L., and Thorstensson, A. (1994). The influence of sudden perturbations on trunk muscle activity and intra-abdominal pressure while standing. *Exp. Brain Res.* 98, 336–341. doi: 10.1007/BF00228421

De Luca, C. J. (1997). The use of surface electromyography in biomechanics. *J. Appl. Biomech.* 13, 135–163. doi: 10.1123/jab.13.2.135

De Luca, C. J., Kuznetsov, M., Gilmore, L. D., and Roy, S. H. (2012). Inter-electrode spacing of surface EMG sensors: reduction of crosstalk contamination during voluntary contractions. *J. Biomech.* 45, 555–561. doi: 10.1016/j.jbiomech.2011.11.010

Descarreaux, M., Lafond, D., and Cantin, V. (2010). Changes in the flexion-relaxation response induced by hip extensor and erector spinae muscle fatigue. *BMC Musculoskelet. Disord.* 11:112. doi: 10.1186/1471-2474-11-112

Downs, S. H., and Black, N. (1998). The feasibility of creating a checklist for the assessment of the methodological quality both of randomised and non-randomised studies of health care interventions. *J. Epidemiol. Community Health* 52, 377–384. doi: 10.1136/jech.52.6.377

Dupeyron, A., Perrey, S., Micallef, J. P., and Pelissier, J. (2010). Influence of back muscle fatigue on lumbar reflex adaptation during sudden external force perturbations. *J. Electromyogr. Kinesiol.* 20, 426–432. doi: 10.1016/j.jelekin.2009.05.004

Eriksson Crommert, A. E., and Thorstensson, A. (2009). Trunk muscle reactions to sudden unexpected and expected perturbations in the absence of upright postural demand. *Exp. Brain Res.* 196, 385–392. doi: 10.1007/s00221-009-1860-z

Fersum, K. V., Dankaerts, W., O'sullivan, P. B., Maes, J., Skouen, J. S., Bjordal, J. M., et al. (2010). Integration of subclassification strategies in randomised controlled clinical trials evaluating manual therapy treatment and exercise therapy for non-specific chronic low back pain: a systematic review. *Br. J. Sports Med.* 44, 1054–1062. doi: 10.1136/bjsm.2009.063289

Gao, Y., Shi, J. G., Ye, H., Liu, Z. R., Zheng, L. B., Ni, Z. M., et al. (2014). Adaptation of muscles of the lumbar spine to sudden imbalance in patients with lower back pain caused by military training. *J. Spinal Cord Med.* 37, 774–781. doi: 10.1179/2045772313Y.0000000170

Graham, R. B., and Brown, S. H. (2012). A direct comparison of spine rotational stiffness and dynamic spine stability during repetitive lifting tasks. *J. Biomech.* 45, 1593–1600. doi: 10.1016/j.jbiomech.2012.04.007

Granata, K. P., Orishimo, K. F., and Sanford, A. H. (2001). Trunk muscle coactivation in preparation for sudden load. *J. Electromyogr. Kinesiol.* 11, 247–254. doi: 10.1016/S1050-6411(01)00003-7

Granata, K. P., Rogers, E., and Moorhouse, K. (2005). Effects of static flexion-relaxation on paraspinal reflex behavior. *Clin. Biomech.* 20, 16–24. doi: 10.1016/j.clinbiomech.2004.09.001

Granata, K. P., Slota, G. P., and Wilson, S. E. (2004). Influence of fatigue in neuromuscular control of spinal stability. *Hum. Factors* 46, 81–91. doi: 10.1518/hfes.46.1.81.30391

Gregory, D. E., Brown, S. H., and Callaghan, J. P. (2008). Trunk muscle responses to suddenly applied loads: do individuals who develop discomfort during prolonged standing respond differently? *J. Electromyogr. Kinesiol.* 18, 495–502. doi: 10.1016/j.jelekin.2006.12.005

Grondin, D. E., and Potvin, J. R. (2009). Effects of trunk muscle fatigue and load timing on spinal responses during sudden hand loading. *J. Electromyogr. Kinesiol.* 19, e237–e245. doi: 10.1016/j.jelekin.2008.05.006

Hendershot, B., Bazrgari, B., Muslim, K., Toosizadeh, N., Nussbaum, M. A., and Madigan, M. L. (2011). Disturbance and recovery of trunk stiffness and reflexive muscle responses following prolonged trunk flexion: influences of flexion angle and duration. *Clin. Biomech. (Bristol Avon).* 26, 250–256. doi: 10.1016/j.clinbiomech.2010.09.019

Hermens, H. J., Commission Des Communautés, E., Biomedical, and Health Research, P. (1999). *SENIAM: European Recommendations for Surface Electromyography: Results of the SENIAM Project.* Enschede: Roessingh Research and Development.

Herrmann, C. M., Madigan, M. L., Davidson, B. S., and Granata, K. P. (2006). Effect of lumbar extensor fatigue on paraspinal muscle reflexes. *J. Electromyogr. Kinesiol.* 16, 637–641. doi: 10.1016/j.jelekin.2005.11.004

Higgins, J. P., Thompson, S. G., Deeks, J. J., and Altman, D. G. (2003). Measuring inconsistency in meta-analyses. *BMJ* 327, 557–560. doi: 10.1136/bmj.327.7414.557

Hjortskov, N., Essendrop, M., Skotte, J., and Fallentin, N. (2005). The effect of delayed-onset muscle soreness on stretch reflexes in human low back muscles. *Scand. J. Med. Sci. Sports* 15, 409–415. doi: 10.1111/j.1600-0838.2004.00438.x

Hodges, P. W. (2011). Pain and motor control: from the laboratory to rehabilitation. *J. Electromyogr. Kinesiol.* 21, 220–228. doi: 10.1016/j.jelekin.2011.01.002

Hodges, P. W., and Bui, B. H. (1996). A comparison of computer-based methods for the determination of onset of muscle contraction using electromyography. *Electroencephalogr. Clin. Neurophysiol.* 101, 511–519. doi: 10.1016/S0013-4694(96)95190-5

Hodges, P. W., and Richardson, C. A. (1997). Feedforward contraction of transversus abdominis is not influenced by the direction of arm movement. *Exp. Brain Res.* 114, 362–370. doi: 10.1007/PL00005644

Hodges, P. W., and Richardson, C. A. (1998). Delayed postural contraction of transversus abdominis in low back pain associated with movement of the lower limb. *J. Spinal Disord.* 11, 46–56. doi: 10.1097/00002517-199802000-00008

Hodges, P. W., and Tucker, K. (2011). Moving differently in pain: a new theory to explain the adaptation to pain. *Pain* 152, S90–S98. doi: 10.1016/j.pain.2010.10.020

Howarth, S. J., Kingston, D. C., Brown, S. H., and Graham, R. B. (2013). Viscoelastic creep induced by repetitive spine flexion and its relationship to dynamic spine stability. *J. Electromyogr. Kinesiol.* 23, 794–800. doi: 10.1016/j.jelekin.2013.04.002

Jacobs, J. V., Henry, S. M., Jones, S. L., Hitt, J. R., and Bunn, J. Y. (2011). A history of low back pain associates with altered electromyographic activation patterns in response to perturbations of standing balance. *J. Neurophysiol.* 106, 2506–2514. doi: 10.1152/jn.00296.2011

Jones, S. L., Henry, S. M., Raasch, C. C., Hitt, J. R., and Bunn, J. Y. (2012a). Individuals with non-specific low back pain use a trunk stiffening strategy to maintain upright posture. *J. Electromyogr. Kinesiol.* 22, 13–20. doi: 10.1016/j.jelekin.2011.10.006

Jones, S. L., Hitt, J. R., Desarno, M. J., and Henry, S. M. (2012b). Individuals with non-specific low back pain in an active episode demonstrate temporally altered torque responses and direction-specific enhanced muscle activity following unexpected balance perturbations. *Exp. Brain Res.* 221, 413–426. doi: 10.1007/s00221-012-3183-8

Landis, J. R., and Koch, G. G. (1977). The measurement of observer agreement for categorical data. *Biometrics* 33, 159–174. doi: 10.2307/2529310

Lariviere, C., Forget, R., Vadeboncoeur, R., Bilodeau, M., and Mecheri, H. (2010). The effect of sex and chronic low back pain on back muscle reflex responses. *Eur. J. Appl. Physiol.* 109, 577–590. doi: 10.1007/s00421-010-1389-7

Latash, M. L., and Anson, J. G. (2006). Synergies in health and disease: relations to adaptive changes in motor coordination. *Phys. Ther.* 86, 1151–1160.

Lavender, S. A., Marras, W. S., and Miller, R. A. (1993). The development of response strategies in preparation for sudden loading to the torso. *Spine (Phila Pa 1976)* 18, 2097–2105. doi: 10.1097/00007632-199310001-00029

Liebetrau, A., Puta, C., Anders, C., De Lussanet, M. H., and Wagner, H. (2013). Influence of delayed muscle reflexes on spinal stability: model-based predictions allow alternative interpretations of experimental data. *Hum. Mov. Sci.* 32, 954–970. doi: 10.1016/j.humov.2013.03.006

MacDonald, D., Moseley, G. L., and Hodges, P. W. (2010). People with recurrent low back pain respond differently to trunk loading despite remission from symptoms. *Spine (Phila Pa 1976)* 35, 818–824. doi: 10.1097/BRS.0b013e3181bc98f1

MacIntyre, D., and Cort, J. A. (2014). Neuromuscular response of the trunk to inertial based sudden perturbations following whole body vibration exposure. *J. Electromyogr. Kinesiol.* 24, 977–985. doi: 10.1016/j.jelekin.2014.08.001

Mawston, G. A., McNair, P. J., and Boocock, M. G. (2007). The effects of prior warning and lifting-induced fatigue on trunk muscle and postural responses to sudden loading during manual handling. *Ergonomics* 50, 2157–2170. doi: 10.1080/00140130701510139

Merletti, R. (1999). Standards for reporting EMG data. *J. Electromyogr. Kinesiol.* 9, 3–4.

Miller, E. M., Bazrgari, B., Nussbaum, M. A., and Madigan, M. L. (2013). Effects of exercise-induced low back pain on intrinsic trunk stiffness and paraspinal muscle reflexes. *J. Biomech.* 46, 801–805. doi: 10.1016/j.jbiomech.2012.11.023

Moorhouse, K. M., and Granata, K. P. (2007). Role of reflex dynamics in spinal stability: intrinsic muscle stiffness alone is insufficient for stability. *J. Biomech.* 40, 1058–1065. doi: 10.1016/j.jbiomech.2006.04.018

Moseley, G. L., Hodges, P. W., and Gandevia, S. C. (2003). External perturbation of the trunk in standing humans differentially activates components of the medial back muscles. *J. Physiol.* 547, 581–587. doi: 10.1113/jphysiol.2002.024950

Muslim, K., Bazrgari, B., Hendershot, B., Toosizadeh, N., Nussbaum, M. A., and Madigan, M. L. (2013). Disturbance and recovery of trunk mechanical and neuromuscular behaviors following repeated static trunk flexion: influences of duration and duty cycle on creep-induced effects. *Appl. Ergon.* 44, 643–651. doi: 10.1016/j.apergo.2012.12.004

Newcomer, K. L., Jacobson, T. D., Gabriel, D. A., Larson, D. R., Brey, R. H., and An, K. N. (2002). Muscle activation patterns in subjects with and without low back pain. *Arch. Phys. Med. Rehabil.* 83, 816–821. doi: 10.1053/apmr.2002.32826

Olson, M. W. (2014). Comparison of trunk muscle reflex activation patterns between active and passive trunk flexion-extension loading conditions. *Hum. Mov. Sci.* 34, 12–27. doi: 10.1016/j.humov.2014.03.004

Olson, M. W., Li, L., and Solomonow, M. (2004). Flexion-relaxation response to cyclic lumbar flexion. *Clin. Biomech. (Bristol, Avon).* 19, 769–776. doi: 10.1016/j.clinbiomech.2004.05.007

Olson, M. W., Li, L., and Solomonow, M. (2009). Interaction of viscoelastic tissue compliance with lumbar muscles during passive cyclic flexion-extension. *J. Electromyogr. Kinesiol.* 19, 30–38. doi: 10.1016/j.jelekin.2007.06.011

O'sullivan, P. (2005). Diagnosis and classification of chronic low back pain disorders: maladaptive movement and motor control impairments as underlying mechanism. *Man. Ther.* 10, 242–255. doi: 10.1016/j.math.2005.07.001

Panjabi, M. M. (1992). The stabilizing system of the spine. Part I. Function, dysfunction, adaptation, and enhancement. *J. Spinal Disord.* 5, 383–389. discussion: 397. doi: 10.1097/00002517-199212000-00001

Parkinson, R. J., Beach, T. A., and Callaghan, J. P. (2004). The time-varying response of the *in vivo* lumbar spine to dynamic repetitive flexion. *Clin. Biomech. (Bristol, Avon).* 19, 330–336. doi: 10.1016/j.clinbiomech.2004.01.002

Radebold, A., Cholewicki, J., Panjabi, M. M., and Patel, T. C. (2000). Muscle response pattern to sudden trunk loading in healthy individuals and in patients with chronic low back pain. *Spine* 25, 947–954. doi: 10.1097/00007632-200004150-00009

Radebold, A., Cholewicki, J., Polzhofer, G. K., and Greene, H. S. (2001). Impaired postural control of the lumbar spine is associated with delayed muscle response times in patients with chronic idiopathic low back pain. *Spine* 26, 724–730. doi: 10.1097/00007632-200104010-00004

Ramprasad, M., Shenoy, D. S., Singh, S. J., Sankara, N., and Joseley, S. R. (2010). The magnitude of pre-programmed reaction dysfunction in back pain patients: experimental pilot electromyography study. *J. Back Musculoskelet. Rehabil.* 23, 77–86. doi: 10.3233/BMR-2010-0254

Reeves, N. P., Cholewicki, J., and Milner, T. E. (2005). Muscle reflex classification of low-back pain. *J. Electromyogr. Kinesiol.* 15, 53–60. doi: 10.1016/j.jelekin.2004.07.001

Rogers, E. L., and Granata, K. P. (2006). Disturbed paraspinal reflex following prolonged flexion-relaxation and recovery. *Spine (Phila Pa 1976)* 31, 839–845. doi: 10.1097/01.brs.0000206361.53451.c7

Sanchez-Zuriaga, D., Adams, M. A., and Dolan, P. (2010). Is activation of the back muscles impaired by creep or muscle fatigue? *Spine (Phila Pa 1976)* 35, 517–525. doi: 10.1097/BRS.0b013e3181b967ea

Santos, B. R., Lariviere, C., Delisle, A., Plamondon, A., Boileau, P. E., and Imbeau, D. (2008). A laboratory study to quantify the biomechanical responses to whole-body vibration: the influence on balance, reflex response, muscular activity and fatigue. *Int. J. Ind. Ergon.* 38, 626–639. doi: 10.1016/j.ergon.2008.01.015

Shenoy, S., Balachander, H., and Sandhu, J. S. (2013). Long latency reflex response of superficial trunk musculature in athletes with chronic low back pain. *J. Back Musculoskelet. Rehabil.* 26, 445–450. doi: 10.3233/BMR-130404

Shin, G., D'souza, C., and Liu, Y. H. (2009). Creep and fatigue development in the low back in static flexion. *Spine (Phila Pa 1976)* 34, 1873–1878. doi: 10.1097/BRS.0b013e3181aa6a55

Solomonow, M., Zhou, B. H., Baratta, R. V., Lu, Y., and Harris, M. (1999). Biomechanics of increased exposure to lumbar injury caused by cyclic loading: Part 1. Loss of reflexive muscular stabilization. *Spine (Phila Pa 1976)* 24, 2426–2434. doi: 10.1097/00007632-199912010-00003

Stambolieva, K., and Angov, G. (2010). Balance control in quiet upright standing in patients with panic disorder. *Eur. Arch. Otorhinolaryngol.* 267, 1695–1699. doi: 10.1007/s00405-010-1303-2

Stokes, I. A., Fox, J. R., and Henry, S. M. (2006). Trunk muscular activation patterns and responses to transient force perturbation in persons with self-reported low back pain. *Eur. Spine J.* 15, 658–667. doi: 10.1007/s00586-005-0893-7

Takahashi, C. D., Nemet, D., Rose-Gottron, C. M., Larson, J. K., Cooper, D. M., and Reinkensmeyer, D. J. (2006). Effect of muscle fatigue on internal model formation and retention during reaching with the arm. *J. Appl. Physiol. (1985)* 100, 695–706. doi: 10.1152/japplphysiol.00140.2005

Toosizadeh, N., Bazrgari, B., Hendershot, B., Muslim, K., Nussbaum, M. A., and Madigan, M. L. (2013). Disturbance and recovery of trunk mechanical and neuromuscular behaviours following repetitive lifting: influences of flexion angle and lift rate on creep-induced effects. *Ergonomics* 56, 954–963. doi: 10.1080/00140139.2013.785601

Tucker, K., Falla, D., Graven-Nielsen, T., and Farina, D. (2009). Electromyographic mapping of the erector spinae muscle with varying load and during sustained contraction. *J. Electromyogr. Kinesiol.* 19, 373–379. doi: 10.1016/j.jelekin.2007.10.003

Voglar, M., Wamerdam, J., Kingma, I., Sarabon, N., and Van Dieën, J. H. (2016). Prolonged intermittent trunk flexion increases trunk muscles reflex gains and trunk stiffness. *PLoS ONE* 11:e0162703. doi: 10.1371/journal.pone.0162703

Wada, M., Sunaga, N., and Nagai, M. (2001). Anxiety affects the postural sway of the antero-posterior axis in college students. *Neurosci. Lett.* 302, 157–159. doi: 10.1016/S0304-3940(01)01662-7

7

Calibration of the Leg Muscle Responses Elicited by Predictable Perturbations of Stance and the Effect of Vision

Stefania Sozzi [1]***, Antonio Nardone*** [2,3] ***and Marco Schieppati*** [1,4]*******

[1] Centro Studi Attività Motorie (CSAM), Fondazione Salvatore Maugeri (IRCCS), Pavia, Italy, [2] Posture and Movement Laboratory, Physical Medicine and Rehabilitation, Fondazione Salvatore Maugeri (IRCCS), Veruno, Italy, [3] Department of Translational Medicine, University of Eastern Piedmont, Novara, Italy, [4] Department of Public Health, Experimental and Forensic Medicine, University of Pavia, Pavia, Italy

***Correspondence:**
Marco Schieppati
marco.schieppati@unipv.it

Motor adaptation due to task practice implies a gradual shift from deliberate control of behavior to automatic processing, which is less resource- and effort-demanding. This is true both for deliberate aiming movements and for more stereotyped movements such as locomotion and equilibrium maintenance. Balance control under persisting critical conditions would require large conscious and motor effort in the absence of gradual modification of the behavior. We defined time-course of kinematic and muscle features of the process of adaptation to repeated, predictable perturbations of balance eliciting both reflex and anticipatory responses. Fifty-nine sinusoidal (10 cm, 0.6 Hz) platform displacement cycles were administered to 10 subjects eyes-closed (EC) and eyes-open (EO). Head and Center of Mass (CoM) position, ankle angle and Tibialis Anterior (TA) and Soleus (Sol) EMG were assessed. EMG bursts were classified as reflex or anticipatory based on the relationship between burst amplitude and ankle angular velocity. Muscle activity decreased over time, to a much larger extent for TA than Sol. The attenuation was larger for the reflex than the anticipatory responses. Regardless of muscle activity attenuation, latency of muscle bursts and peak-to-peak CoM displacement did not change across perturbation cycles. Vision more than doubled speed and the amount of EMG adaptation particularly for TA activity, rapidly enhanced body segment coordination, and crucially reduced head displacement. The findings give new insight on the mode of amplitude- and time-modulation of motor output during adaptation in a balancing task, advocate a protocol for assessing flexibility of balance strategies, and provide a reference for addressing balance problems in patients with movement disorders.

Keywords: moving platform, balancing behavior, adaptation, kinematics, EMG, reflex and anticipatory response, vision

---

Abbreviations: A-P, antero-posterior; CC, cross-correlation; CoM, center of mass; EC, eyes closed; EO, eyes open; FPR, fall preventing response; LLR, long latency response; MLR, medium latency response; PAR, proactive response; SLR, short latency response; Sol, Soleus; TA, Tibialis Anterior.

INTRODUCTION

Practice improves movement kinematics and diminishes the accompanying metabolic and cognitive cost. Motor adaptation implies a gradual shift from a more conscious control of behavior to automatic processing, which is less resource- and effort-demanding, and produces a gradual modification of the behavior that makes it more fit under the conditions of its environment (Shadmehr et al., 2010). Adaptation is common to both voluntary movements, where repetition and task practice improve performance (Lotze et al., 2003), and movements in which automatism prevails (Saling and Phillips, 2007) as in locomotor (Prokop et al., 1995) and postural tasks (Nashner, 1976). Balance perturbations can be of very different nature, from displacement of the base of support (Nashner, 1976; Horak and Nashner, 1986) to vibratory proprioceptive (De Nunzio and Schieppati, 2007; De Nunzio et al., 2008) and galvanic vestibular stimulation (Fransson et al., 2007; Tjernström et al., 2010a). Berger et al. (1992) and Dietz et al. (1993) described leg muscle activity and biomechanical patterns in subjects standing on an unstable support basis, such as a treadmill moving backward and forward. Their pioneer study suggested that the aim of the control process is to stabilize the position of the body's center of gravity relative to the feet, while the forces acting on the body during the treadmill movements are minimized.

Balance perturbations delivered by repeated sinusoidal translations of the support base have been employed frequently in both control subjects and patients, in order to investigate balancing behavior under dynamic conditions, as opposed to quiet stance. Within the frame of a reproducible general pattern, an ample range of variability has been observed for successive cycles of the same perturbation, suggesting flexibility of dynamic postures (Schieppati et al., 2002; Cappa et al., 2008; Kennedy et al., 2012). Clear-cut differences in balancing behavior have also been observed in the presence or absence of vision (Buchanan and Horak, 1999; Corna et al., 1999; Fujiwara et al., 2006; Schmid et al., 2011). For instance, when vision is gradually degraded experimentally, good visual acuity strongly reinforces a "head-fixed-in-space" behavior, while poor vision and no vision rather produce a "head-moving-with-platform" displacement (Schmid et al., 2007, 2008). Notably, aging is associated with reduced head stabilization in the absence of vision, particularly for high-frequency platform translations (Nardone et al., 2000). The balancing behavior is fairly resistant to abnormal proprioceptive noise obtained by postural muscle vibration (De Nunzio et al., 2005) and is hardly affected in patients with neuropathy and with Parkinson's disease (Nardone and Schieppati, 2006; Nardone et al., 2006, 2007), pointing to significant intervention of feed-forward mechanisms.

In the above cited reports, the first few cycles of the sequence of oscillations were deliberately excluded from the analysis in order to get rid of the initial large EMG activation bursts and body movements elicited by the supposed startling effect of the onset of the perturbation (Nonnekes et al., 2015), and to describe and measure the adapted behavior at steady state. The question of the initial EMG adaptation had been addressed with a sequence of discrete impulsive perturbations by Keshner et al. (1987), who suggested that adaptation is due to a generalized habituation in the postural control system. Fujiwara et al. (2007) described adaptation of the balancing strategy to continuous floor oscillation. By recording event-related potentials, reflecting cortical activation by sensory information related to the postural disturbance, they suggested that attention to information processing decreases with adaptation (Fujiwara et al., 2012, 2016). Mierau et al. (2015) also reported adaptation of the negative cortical potential and reduced muscle co-contraction during a prolonged balancing task under critical standing-balance condition. Notably, at the beginning of the perturbation series, the extra facilitatory effect from higher centers on the spinal motoneuronal pools gradually vanishes as automatisms prevail (Solopova et al., 2014).

Siegmund et al. (2008) advised that the large muscle response to a novel transient perturbation consists of combined postural and startle responses. On the other hand, Oude Nijhuis et al. (2009) and Allum et al. (2011) reported on the response to the first perturbing trial of a sequence, and compared that response to a startle reaction elicited by an acoustic stimulus. They highlighted the substantial differences between the "true" startle reaction and the response to the first trial of a balance perturbation, and concluded that future studies should no longer discard the latter response, but routinely include it in the analysis (Tang et al., 2012).

Short- and long-latency leg muscle reflexes are elicited by the displacement of the body segments, and produce balance correcting effects (Horak et al., 1989; Nardone et al., 1990). Proactive strategies (Massion, 1992; Bouisset and Do, 2008) are also produced to counteract the balance perturbations elicited by the platform displacement reversal (Rogers et al., 2003; Jacobs and Horak, 2007). These anticipatory postural adjustments may not necessarily be optimally tuned to the complex combination of active and passive body movements from the beginning of the perturbation sequence (Aruin et al., 1998, 2015). In the assumption that both reflex responses and proactive strategies are contributing to the balancing behavior on the continuously translating platform (Laessoe and Voigt, 2008) and that both undergo adaptation with the repetition of the perturbation cycles (Dietz et al., 1993; Taube et al., 2007; Kennedy et al., 2012), we set out to record activity of the leg flexor and extensor postural muscles and body kinematics. Our attempt was to better identify the muscle responses and the potentially different adaptation pattern thereof, and to assess any relationship between the adaptation of muscle activity and the balancing behavior by using support surface translation stimuli. We expected to get an answer to the following questions. What is the time course of adaptation? Is adaptation common to both muscles acting on the ankle joint? Is this process accompanied by modulation of co-contraction rate of both antagonist muscles? Is it similar for muscle activities having a presumed different origin (reflex vs. proactive)? Does adaptation imply amplitude modulation of EMG bursts, or does their latency also change over time? Is there a correspondence between adaptation of leg muscle activity and changes in the position of the center of mass (CoM)? To what extent does vision affect adaptation? What are the functional advantages of adaptation?

MATERIALS AND METHODS

Subjects and Task

Ten healthy subjects (5 males and 5 females, mean age 30.8 years ± 6.3 SD, height 173.7 cm ± 5.3 SD, weight 66.2 kg ± 10.9 SD) stood with bare feet spaced about 10 cm apart on a mobile platform, translating in a sinusoidal way in the antero-posterior (A-P) direction at 0.6 Hz and 10 cm amplitude. They were not aware of the onset of the movement of the platform, which started pseudo-randomly within 5–10 s from the acquisition onset (known to the subjects). Subjects wore soundproof earphones in order to mask the noise made by the platform. Each acquisition was composed of three parts: subjects stood on the still platform (5–10 s); the platform made 59 consecutive oscillation cycles (total duration 100 s); the platform stopped and subjects stood on the still platform for 5 s more. Subjects performed one single such trial with the eyes closed (EC), and one trial with the eyes open (EO) in a separate session after 5–7 days. Felt-tip pen marks on the skin helped to place the electrodes in the same position during the two test conditions. No randomization was performed. In parallel experiments, a second group of naive subjects was studied (n = 10; 4 males and 6 females, mean age 25.5 years ± 2.9 SD, height 171.8 cm ± 9.2 SD, weight 68.6 kg ± 16.3 SD), to which EO condition only was administered. This allowed checking any persistence of adapted behavior due to the EC trial preceding the EO trial in the former group of subjects. All subjects were naive to the experimental procedures or to any balance-oriented experiments and all succeeded in performing the trials. Experiments were performed in accordance with the Declaration of Helsinki. The institutional ethics committee (Central Ethics Committee, Fondazione Salvatore Maugeri, approval number # 905 CEC) specifically approved the study and the consent procedures, which were carried out with the adequate understanding and written informed consent.

Data Acquisition

Kinematic data were recorded by means of an optoelectronic device (Smart-D, BTS, Italy). For computation of CoM and orientation in space of the body segments, 19 reflective markers were placed bilaterally on these body positions (Winter, 2009): vertex and lateral head, acromion, C7, L5, anterior superior iliac spinae, greater trochanter, lateral epicondyle of the femur, lateral malleolus, heel and forefoot (dorsally, about over the 1st metatarso-phalangeal joint). Subjects' arms were folded not to interfere with marker capture. The marker positions in space were recorded by 12 cameras at 140 Hz and stored in a PC for off-line analysis. For subsequent analysis, the kinematic data were resampled at a frequency of 1000 Hz after linear interpolation by the BTS proprietary software, in order to display both kinematic and EMG data on the same scale.

EMG was recorded by pairs of surface electrodes placed, for both legs, over the muscle bellies of Tibialis Anterior (TA) on the anterior aspect of the upper third of the leg, and of Soleus (Sol) posteriorly, 5 cm below the insertion of the gastrocnemii in the Achilles' tendon. The distance between the recording leads was 1.5 cm. EMGs were wirelessly recorded (Freeemg, BTS, Italy) at 1000 Hz. Signals were filtered with a high-pass filter (cut-off 50 Hz), full-wave rectified and then filtered with a low-pass filter with a cut-off frequency of 200 Hz. EMG signals were acquired through the same Smart-D system, and were synchronized with the kinematic data.

The EMGs of TA and Sol of both legs were also recorded in each subject during *ad hoc* trials in which subjects produced bursts of maximal activity, for each muscle separately, before each EC and EO trial. For each muscle and leg, three maximal isometric contraction efforts, each lasting 2–4 s, were performed. For TA, during standing, the foot was blocked to the ground preventing foot dorsiflexion. For Sol, while subjects were sitting on a chair, the knee was blocked against a resistance to keep ankle and knee angles at about 90°. The level of EMGs activity recorded during the balancing trials were expressed as percent of the maximal voluntary activity of the respective muscles.

Data Analysis

EMG Activity and Burst Identification

We offline separated the cycles of the platform perturbation by a software developed using Labview (National Instruments, Austin, TX, USA), where each cycle began with the platform forward translation. For a clearer representation of what happened during each cycle, in the **Figures 4–9** a time-window starting 0.2 s before the initial forward movement of the platform and lasting 2.5 s is depicted, whereas the analyses were made on a time-window having a duration equal to the oscillation cycle (1.7 s) starting from the backward-most platform position.

The mean value of TA and Sol activity within each of the successive cycles was calculated in each subject. In addition, the traces of the rectified TA and Sol activity of all consecutive cycles were averaged. Different bursts of activity were regularly present on the TA and Sol mean traces. The time-windows, in which TA or Sol bursts were consistently present, are highlighted by shaded areas in **Figure 4**. For TA, we classified: (a) a reflex response, the first part of which occurred at about 80 ms after the beginning of the forward translation of the platform and lasted about 100 ms; this response was named medium-latency response (MLR), following Schieppati and Nardone (1995) and Nardone and Schieppati (1998); (b) a second part of the reflex response occurred at about 200 ms after the forward platform translation and lasted about 100 ms; this was the long-latency response (LLR; Nardone et al., 1990); (c) a burst just around the anterior platform turn-around point, starting about 700 ms after the forward translation and lasting about 200 ms, was arbitrarily named fall-preventing response (FPR) and (d) a burst roughly in correspondence with the period of backward platform movement, starting at around 1.2 s after the forward translation and lasting around 300 ms; this was arbitrarily named proactive response (PAR), since it brakes the CoM backward displacement just prior to the forward platform movement of the subsequent cycle. For Sol, the bursts were almost superimposable to those of TA when the Sol trace was shifted by $\frac{1}{2}$ cycle, so that stretch and anticipatory responses would match the corresponding platform displacement (forward for TA and backward for Sol). Hence, following the same criteria used for TA and referring to the onset of forward translation, we identified: (a) a burst before the peak of the forward excursion, starting about 300 ms after forward translation and lasting about 300 ms (PAR), this response mainly occurs during Sol shortening, and would correspond to the TA PAR; (b) a double-peak reflex response, occurring at about 800 ms after the forward translation (at the beginning of the backward platform displacement) and lasting about 100 ms; in the Sol, a short-latency stretch response is evoked immediately prior to the MLR (hence, this burst was named SLR + MLR); (c) a burst in correspondence with the backward platform movement, starting at around 1.1 s after the forward translation and lasting around 100 ms (LLR); and (d) a burst after the peak of backward excursion, starting about 1.5 s after the forward translation and lasting about 100 ms (FPR). Then, for each cycle of each subject, the actual onset and termination of each response was visually identified by means of a custom-made Labview software on the display of each EMG trace. The response identification was aided by the superimposition of the traces of the homonymous muscles of both legs. Two experimenters (SS and MS) agreed on the identification of the burst onset and termination. In the subsequent analysis, the onset latency of each TA response was referred to the onset of platform forward movement, and for Sol to the onset of platform backward movement.

The area (time-integral) of the rectified TA and Sol muscle EMG measured within the time-interval defined by onset and end of each response was expressed as a percentage of the area of the EMG corresponding to the maximal voluntary contraction, calculated on an equal time-interval as the individual response bursts. The area of the TA and Sol bursts were plotted against the ankle angular velocity measured 50 ms before the onset of the respective TA or Sol burst in order to check the hypothesis that the response is related to muscle stretch and represents a short-latency response to muscle lengthening. The 50 ms interval was arbitrarily selected for all responses, based on the presumed "average" latency of the TA and Sol reflex activation by muscle stretch, and assuming that the muscles had no slack due to their background activation.

Kinematics

The CoM was computed according to the Winter (2009) protocol by a software developed in Matlab (MathWorks Inc., Natick, MA, USA). In order to infer changes in muscle length and velocity occurring during the perturbation cycles, the ankle angle of both legs was computed from the position in space of the markers placed on the lateral femoral condyle, lateral malleolus and forefoot. The changes in foot dorsum deformation were estimated from the height of the marker placed on malleolus. The marker traces were filtered with a low-pass filter (cut-off 3 Hz). The velocity of ankle angular variation was the derivative of the ankle angle. Positive velocities corresponded to TA stretch (or Sol lengthening).

For each subject, the standard deviation of all the values of the A-P displacement trace of CoM and head vertex was calculated for the entire duration of the platform perturbation, and considered a global index of displacement amplitude (small and large standard deviations pointing to stable and unstable segment position in space, respectively; Corna et al., 1999). For each subject and oscillation cycle, a cross-correlation (CC) analysis was performed between the traces of platform and CoM A-P displacement (both referred to the laboratory space). The CC coefficient (*R*) at time lag = 0 s was calculated by means of the CC routine of the software Origin (OriginLab Corporation, Northampton, MA, USA). A positive coefficient indicates in-phase displacement of CoM and platform, a negative coefficient indicates anti-phase displacement. The time lag was the time interval at which the absolute value of R was maximum. The 95% confidence interval of the highest CC value was used to assess if the time lag between platform and CoM displacement was statistically significant (Li and Caldwell, 1999). A positive time lag indicates that CoM movement lagged the platform movement.

The CoM back-and-forth displacement with respect to the malleolus was also plotted against the ankle angle and the coefficient of determination (r^2) of the regression line was calculated for each subject and successive cycle.

Adaptation Rate Assessed by Exponential Fit

In order to grossly quantify the adaptation process, we fitted the relevant data with an exponential function ($y = A + Be^{-t/\tau}$). To this aim, the exponential-fit routine of the software Origin was used, τ (tau) being the time-constant, A the value at steady state (asymptote), A + B the intercept with the ordinate (Sozzi et al., 2011). A, B and τ parameters were computed by using the Levenberg-Marquardt algorithm. Using this procedure, we fitted over time the mean CoM A-P position, the time lags between platform and CoM displacement The changes in the relationship between CoM displacement and ankle angle identified by the r^2 coefficient of the regression lines were also fitted in the same way. The mean EMG activity of TA and Sol of each cycle was plotted as a function of the successive cycles: these values generally exhibited a rapid initial variation and a trend to plateau with time. Of note, the exponential fit was made on the entire sequence of cycles, including the first one. The time, at which steady state was reached, was estimated by 3 * τ, which corresponds to a reduction to less than 5% of the initial value.

In addition, we fitted a double exponential function ($y = Ae^{-t/\tau 1} + Be^{-t/\tau 2} + C$) to the area data of the identified bursts of the successive cycles in order to take into account the possibility that a dual process (Huberdeau et al., 2015) featuring a complex evolution over time underpins the adaptation of both reflex and proactive bursts. τ_1 and τ_2 were the time-constants (expressed in cycle number), C the value at steady state, A + B + C the intercept with the ordinate. The values of the asymptote and of the intercept at the second oscillation cycle of the fitted exponentials (therefore excluding the "first-trial effect") served to assess the amplitude adaptation of the EMG responses. When the software did not converge to the imposed exponential, we simply interpolated the data with a linear fit, and estimated the amplitude of adaptation by the difference between the values of the fitted line at the second and last cycle.

Assessment of the TA-Sol Co-Contraction Pattern

In order to quantify the possible co-contraction of TA and Sol muscles and its variation over time, for each cycle the instantaneous rectified EMG activity of the two muscles of the right leg was plotted one against the other. For each subject and cycle, we defined a co-contraction index as follows: each value of the level of TA activity was multiplied by the corresponding value of Sol activity, and all products were averaged. Each co-contraction index of each cycle was then identified by a variable k (the mean value of all products within the cycle). Hence, for each subject, the k values across all successive cycles were fitted with the exponential function $y = A + Be^{-t/\tau}$, in order to assess any change over time of the co-contraction pattern.

Statistical Analysis

Statistical computations are listed below in the order of appearance in the "Results" section. All variables had normal distribution, as tested by the Kolmogorov-Smirnov test. Systematic effects (EO vs. EC, TA vs. Sol) often produced substantially different data variability, as tested by Levene's test. However, since the coefficients of variations were remarkably constant across conditions, the log transformation was applied (Lison, 1960) prior to applying parametric statistics.

The mean activity across cycles of TA and Sol was compared by a 3-way repeated measures ANOVA with muscles (TA and Sol), visual condition (EC and EO) and leg (right and left) as factors. Across subjects, the time-constants of the mean activity values of TA and Sol were compared by a 2-way repeated measures ANOVA, with muscles and visual condition as factors. The mean EMG activities at steady state (the asymptotic value of the exponential fit) were compared by a 2-way repeated measures ANOVA, with muscle and visual condition as factors.

The time-constants of EMG adaptation (TA and Sol) between the group that received the EO perturbations only and the group that received the EO after the EC perturbations were compared, separately for the two muscles, with a Student's t-test.

Three-way repeated-measures ANOVAs, with muscle, vision, response type (MLR or SLR + MLR, LLR, FPR and PAR) as factors, were used to compare: onset latency, duration and area of TA and Sol response bursts, and ankle angular velocities. Four one-way ANOVA were used to assess differences in the mean latencies of various TA EC responses across cycles.

The changes in the area of TA and Sol responses across the successive cycles were interpolated with a double exponential function. When the algorithm converged to the exponential model, the time-constants thus obtained (τ_1 and τ_2) were compared by a 4-way repeated-measures ANOVA with τ_1 and τ_2, muscle, visual condition, response type (MLR or SLR + MLR, LLR, FPR and PAR) as factors.

To estimate the adaptation in burst amplitude, the differences between the intercept values at the second oscillation cycle and the asymptotic values were compared with a 4-way repeated-measures ANOVA with EMG level at second cycle and steady-state, muscle, visual condition and response type as factors.

The standard deviations of CoM and of head periodic displacement (arbitrarily taken as a global index of segment instability) were compared with a 2-way repeated measures ANOVA with variables (CoM and head) and visual condition (EC and EO) as factors.

The time-constants obtained by fitting the exponential functions to the CC coefficients and to the time-lag between CoM and platform across cycles were compared between EO and EC by paired Student's t-test. The time-constant of the changes over the successive cycles of the r^2 coefficient of the lines best fitting CoM against ankle angle and that of the parameter k (indicating co-contraction) were compared with a 2-way repeated measures ANOVA with variables (time-constants of r^2 and k) and visual conditions as factors. For all ANOVAs, the *post hoc* analyses were made with the Fisher's LSD test. The software package used was Statistica (StatSoft, Tulsa, OK, USA).

RESULTS

Changes in EMG and Kinematics Over Time

Figure 1 illustrates the adaptation phenomenon: the top trace **(A,B)** is the platform periodic displacement, identical for the EC and EO condition. Figures **(C–F)** show the grand mean (of the 10 subjects, who performed the EO after the EC trial) of the rectified traces of the TA and Sol muscle activity over the entire perturbation period. Displacements of CoM and head vertex are reported for EC and EO in **(G–J)**, respectively. A progressive reduction in the TA activity was obvious with EC **(C)**. Sol activity diminished rapidly to then remain sustained until the end of the acquisition period **(E)**. TA activity was much smaller under EO than EC condition, both at the beginning and at steady-state **(D)**, which was reached within very few cycles. Conversely, the level of Sol activity with EO **(F)** was broadly similar to that recorded with EC. CoM displacement was consistent from the beginning to the end of the translation cycles, and was similar under EC and EO condition. Still, the head back-and-forth displacement was much larger and more variable for EC than EO. Overall, these patterns of EMG and kinematic changes were common to all subjects.

TA and Sol Activity Across Successive Cycles: Levels and Time-Constants

The mean activity of TA and Sol was averaged cycle by cycle across subjects, for EC and EO. It was similar between right and left leg, both EC (gray bars in **A** and **E**) and EO (white bars in **A** and **E**) ($F_{(1,9)} = 2.16$, $p = 0.17$; **Figure 2**). Hence,

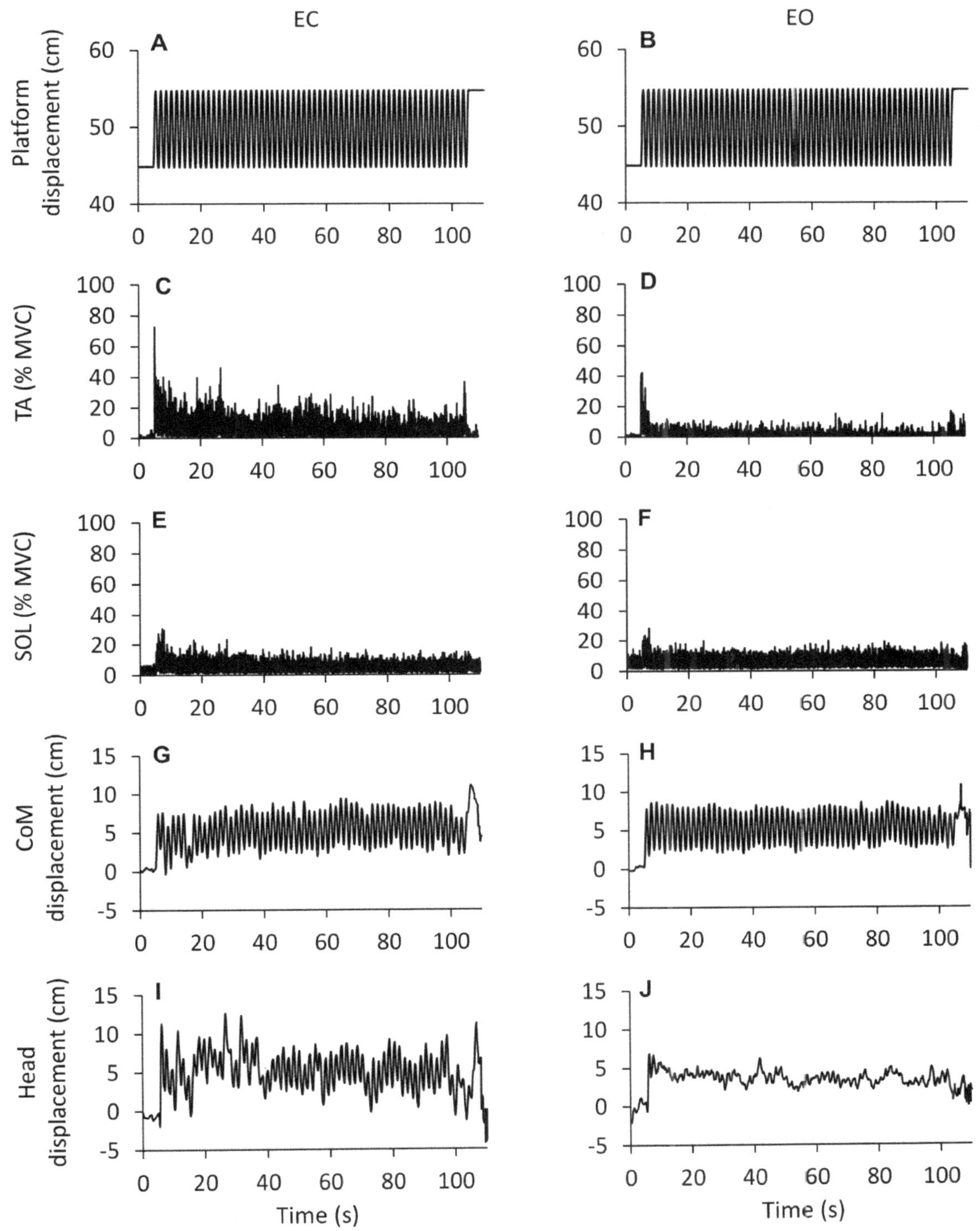

FIGURE 1 | Changes in EMG and kinematics over time. Grand mean ($n = 10$ subjects) of the traces recorded during eyes closed (EC) and eyes open (EO) conditions. **(A,B)** show the platform sinusoidal translation (10 cm, 0.6 Hz) in the antero-posterior (A-P) direction (forward upwards). The first cycle begins after 5 s from the acquisition onset, the last cycle ends at 105 s. **(C–F)** show the grand mean of the rectified EMG traces of the Tibialis Anterior (TA) and Soleus (Sol) expressed as percent of the maximal voluntary contraction. There is a progressive reduction in muscle activity EC and EO. TA activity is much smaller EO than EC (not so for Sol). **(G,H)** Displacement of center of mass (CoM). **(I,J)** Displacement of head (marker on the vertex). The CoM back-and-forth displacement is similar EC and EO, whereas the head back-and-forth displacement is larger EC than EO. The larger deflections of the EMG and kinematic traces at the very end of the acquisition are connected with the sudden halt of the platform.

further analysis was performed on the mean EMG values of the two legs. **Figure 2** also shows the grand mean of the EMG activity of each of the successive perturbation cycles, for TA (**B,C**) and Sol (**F,G**) during the EC and EO conditions. With EC, a gradual decrease in TA activity is obvious (**B**). The exponential curve fitted to the data points has a time-constant of about 5 cycles ($\tau = 5.1$ cycles); therefore, after about 15 cycles ($\sim 3 * \tau$), i.e., about 25 s considering that each cycle lasts 1.7 s, TA activity reached a value close to the asymptotic value (steady-state). A gradual decrease was also present for Sol activity with EC (**F**, $\tau = 4.3$ cycles). The mean values of the time-constants of the exponentials fitted to the profiles of TA and Sol activity of each subject were 6.5 ± 4.8 cycles (TA) and 5.9 ± 5.6 cycles (Sol) (not shown in Figure). With EO, both TA (**C**) and Sol (**G**) activities diminished rapidly and reached steady state very quickly ($\tau = 1.1 \pm 0.7$ cycles, TA; 3.4 ± 3.7 cycles, Sol). ANOVA on the time-constants of TA and Sol, after log transformation, showed a difference between visual conditions ($F_{(1,9)} = 23.75$, $p < 0.001$), no difference between muscles ($F_{(1,9)} = 3.23$, $p = 0.1$) and an interaction between muscles and vision ($F_{(1,9)} = 11.46$, $p < 0.01$). The time-constants of TA EO were just smaller than those of Sol EO (*post hoc*, $p < 0.01$), while there was no difference between TA and Sol in the EC condition (*post hoc*, $p = 0.36$). Moreover, there was no difference in the time-constant of Sol between EC and EO (*post hoc*, $p = 0.1$).

At the end of the perturbation cycles (**Figure 2D**), there was a difference in the mean level of EMG activity between TA and Sol ($F_{(1,9)} = 11.4$, $p < 0.01$). This was due to their different behavior as a function of the visual condition. There was a difference between EC and EO ($F_{(1,9)} = 16.37$, $p < 0.01$) and an interaction between muscles (TA and Sol) and visual condition ($F_{(1,9)} = 8.9$, $p < 0.05$). TA activity at steady state was smaller with EO than EC (*post hoc*, $p < 0.01$), while the level of Sol activity was not affected by vision ($p = 0.99$).

Also in the 10 subjects who performed the EO condition only, TA and Sol reached steady state very quickly ($\tau = 1.50 \pm 1.0$, TA, and 3.3 ± 6.3, Sol). Overall, there was no difference in the mean time-constants between the two groups (Student's t-test, $p > 0.3$, for TA and Sol muscles, separately analyzed). Therefore, for simplicity and for exploiting repeated-measures tests, we analyzed the findings pertaining to EC and EO behavior only in the group that performed EC before EO.

Co-Activation Turns to Reciprocal Activation During Adaptation

Not only did muscle activity decrease over time, but there was also a change in the pattern of recruitment of the antagonist TA and Sol muscles. For all cycles, the TA activity profile was plotted against that of Sol in order to detect any prevalent activation pattern (reciprocal activation or co-activation). Each individual symbol of (**A**) to (**C**) of **Figure 3** corresponds to one TA and Sol EMG sample (1000 Hz) recorded during three non-consecutive cycles in a representative subject (the cycles were arbitrarily chosen as examples of the pattern of activity recorded during the first (1st to 20th cycle) and third (41th to 59th cycle) segment of the entire sequence, see **Figure 4**). The value (k) of TA and Sol co-contraction index (see "Materials and Methods" Section) diminished over the cycles. The lower panels (**D**, EC and **E**, EO) show the grand means of k of all subjects over cycles, featuring a progressive reduction of the k value, therefore a shift from co-activation to reciprocal activation. For each subject, the k value was then plotted as a function of the successive cycles and fitted with an exponential function. The average time-constant of the adaptation of k (panel **F**) was

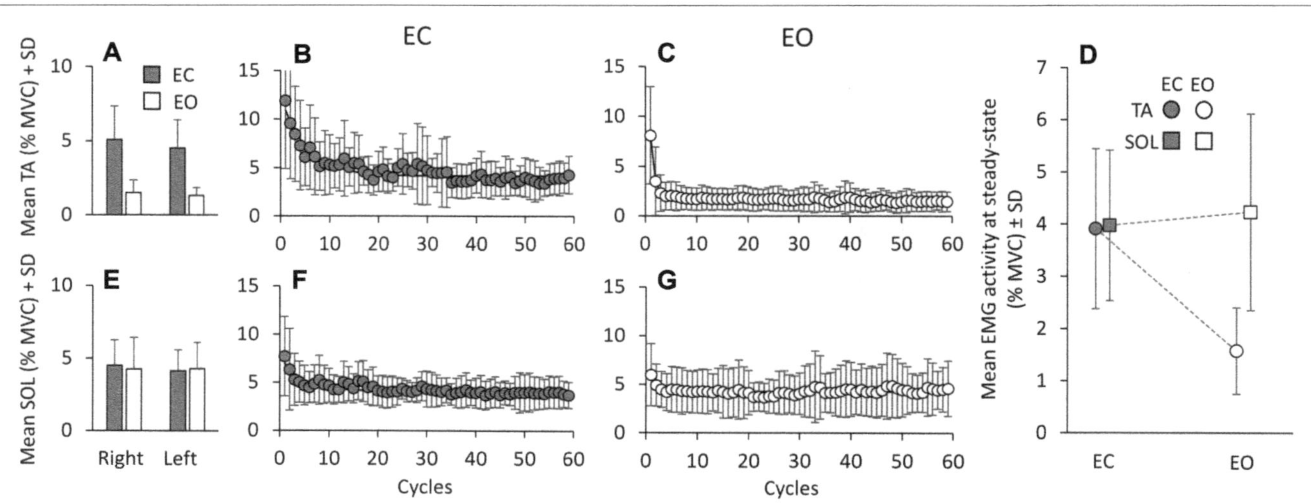

FIGURE 2 | Mean TA and Sol activity. Mean muscle activities, across cycles and subjects in EC (gray bars) and EO (white bars) conditions, are almost the same between legs, for TA **(A)** and Sol **(E)**. The mean activity of TA **(B,C)** and Sol **(F,G)** are calculated for each platform cycle, EC and EO. With EC, both TA and Sol activities gradually decrease to steady state. The exponential functions fitted to the EC data are $y = 4.15 + 6.77e^{-t/5.1}$ for TA and $y = 4.09 + 2.87e^{-t/4.3}$ for Sol. With EO, both TA and Sol activities reach steady state very soon. The functions best fitting the mean muscle activities with EO are: $y = 1.63 + 6.42e^{-t/0.8}$ for TA and $y = 4.26 + 1.71e^{-t/0.97}$ for Sol. **(D)** shows that the mean Sol activity level at steady state is similar EC and EO, while TA is greatly reduced EO.

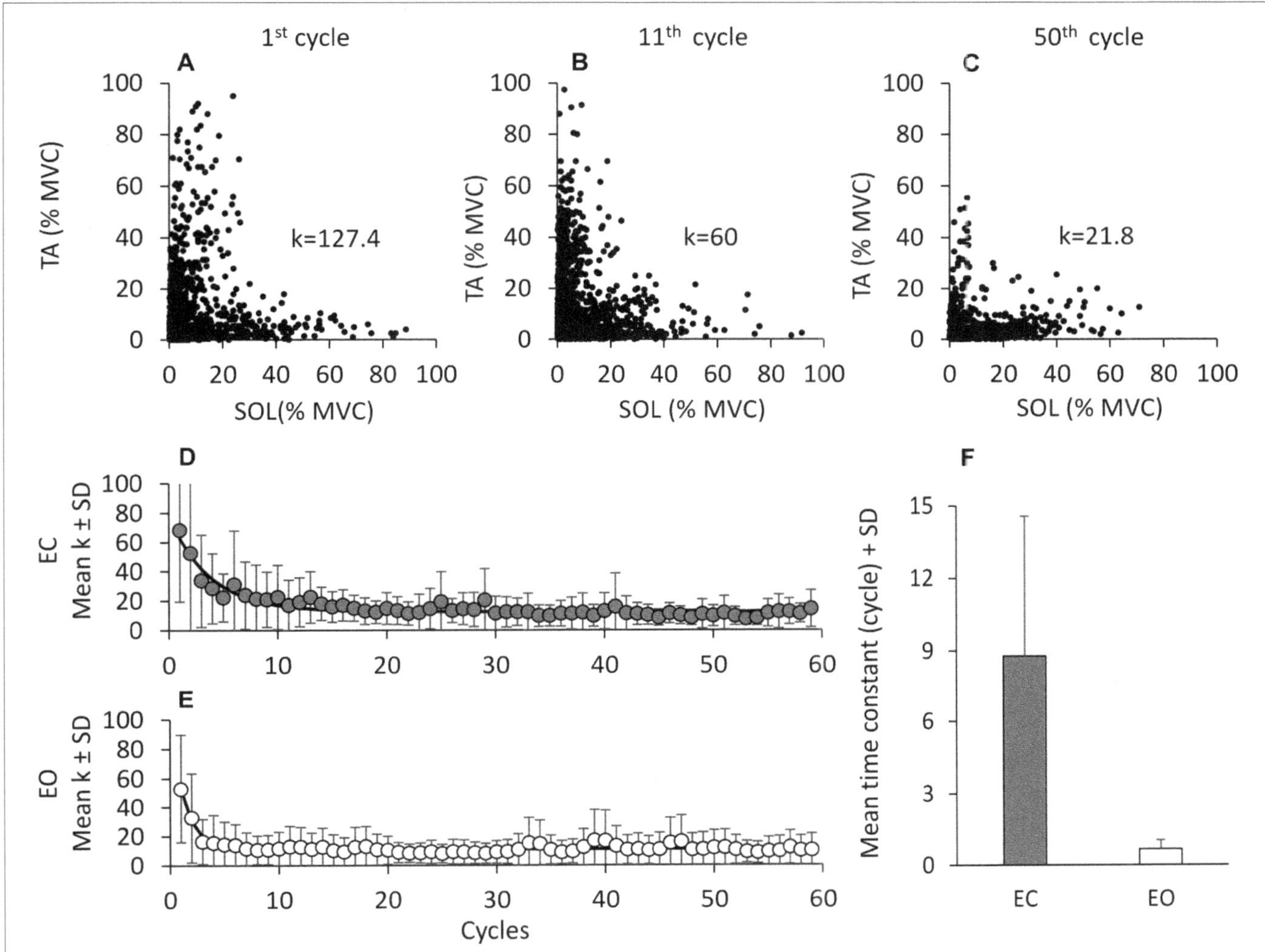

FIGURE 3 | Reciprocal activation of TA and Sol. In **(A–C)**, TA activity is plotted against that of Sol for three non-consecutive cycles in one subject to show the progressive decrease in the co-activation pattern. The value of *k* (the TA and Sol co-contraction index) diminishes with cycle repetition. **(D,E)** show the grand means of k, obtained by averaging the *k* of each subject for each subsequent cycle, EC **(D)** and EO **(E)**. The exponential functions fitted to the data points are $y = 12.4 + 50.4e^{-t/4.2}$, EC; and $y = 8.5 + 34.8e^{-t/1.2}$, EO. **(F)** show the mean time-constants obtained by fitting an exponential function to the data points of each subject and of each condition. The time-constant of the "co-activation" adaptations is much longer EC (gray bar) than EO (white bar).

much larger with EC (8.8 cycles ± 5.8 cycles) than EO (0.6 cycles ± 0.4 cycles; *post hoc*, $p < 0.001$), indicating that the initial co-activation patterns disappeared much more rapidly for EO than EC. Overall, it appears that co-contraction of the antagonist leg muscles promptly subsides with adaptation, more or less rapidly as a function of visual condition, to give way to reciprocal activation.

Reflex and Anticipatory Responses

TA and Sol bursts showed consistent features across perturbation cycles. The bursts were easily identified in the successive cycles, both EC and EO. This is obvious in **Figure 4**, showing the grand mean of the rectified EMGs obtained by averaging the traces across subjects and cycles. The gray traces refer to the TA **(C,D)** and Sol burst **(E,F)** recorded during the first cycle. The three superimposed colored traces are the result of averaging the EMG traces of the same muscles recorded during the cycles from 2nd to 20th, 21th to 40th and 41th to 59th (black to green in that order). Activity was much larger in the first cycle (particularly for TA) under both EC and EO condition. The bursts took place within the same time-windows from the beginning to the end of the perturbation cycles. In spite of their diminishing amplitude, TA and Sol profiles were almost reciprocal, underlining the conclusion of the previous paragraph. The four bottom panels of **Figure 4** show the grand means of the changes in the ankle angle **(G,H)** and in its angular velocity **(I,J)**. The ankle angle had an average range of about 2°, which would have produced minor, but not negligible changes in length of the muscles around the joint. The angular velocity was overall positive (ankle angle increases and TA lengthens/Sol shortens) during the

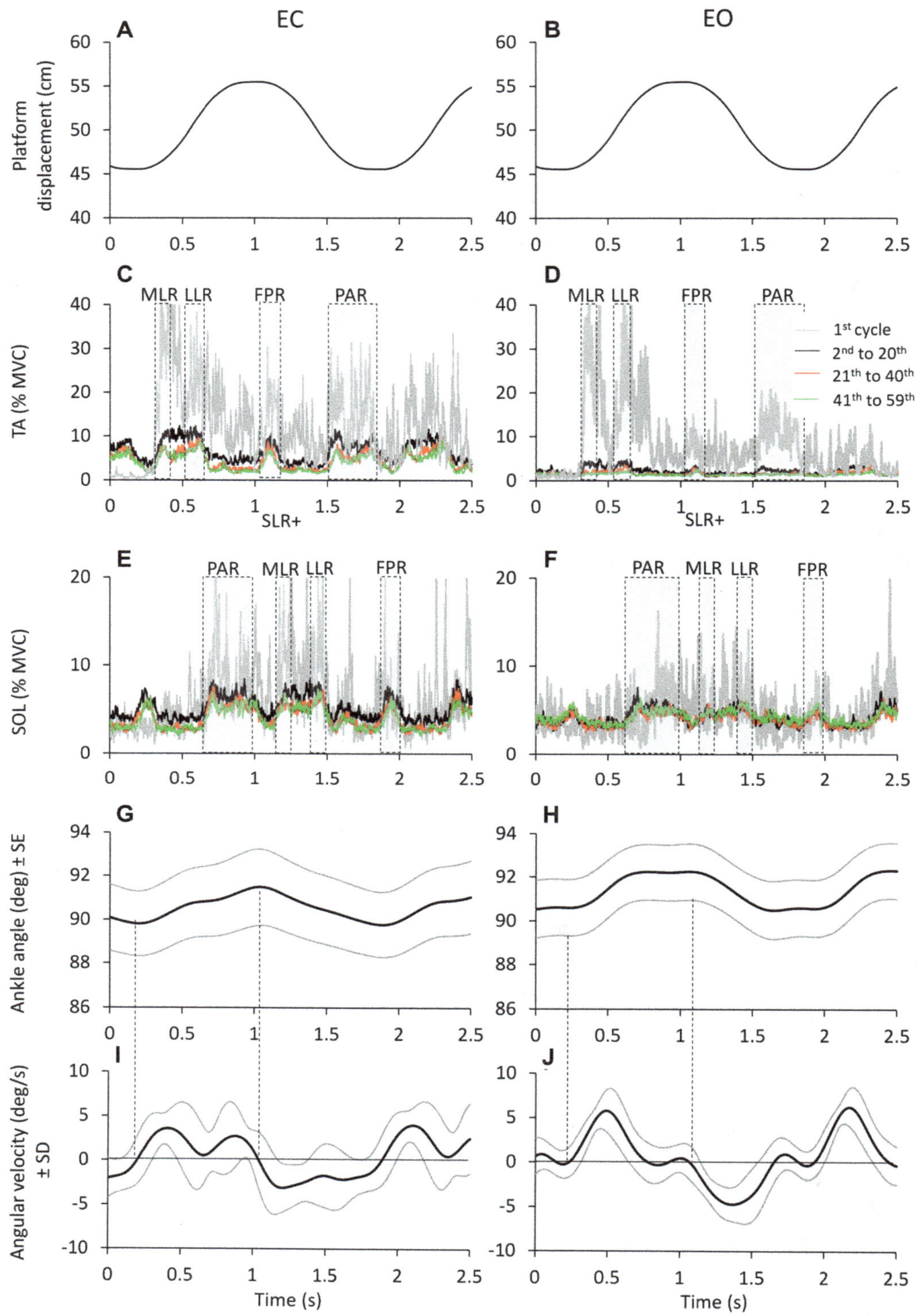

FIGURE 4 | Time windows of TA and Sol bursts. Platform displacement **(A,B)**. Mean across subjects of TA **(C,D)** and Sol **(E,F)** EMG of the first cycle (gray traces) 2nd to 20th cycle (black traces), 21th to 40th (red traces) and 41th to 59th (green traces), EC (left panels) and EO (right panels). TA and Sol EMG are almost reciprocal and segmented in different bursts. These bursts rise and decrease sharply as a sign of high synchronization and consistency across subjects. The different time windows of activation of TA and Sol are highlighted by gray dashed boxes. **(G,H)** show the grand averages of the ankle angle changes (subjects and cycles collapsed) and **(I,J)** show the corresponding changes in angular velocity. The black lines refer to the grand mean of ankle angle and angular velocity changes; the gray lines show the standard error for the ankle angular changes and the standard deviation for the angular velocity changes.

platform forward translation and negative (ankle angle decreases and TA shortens/Sol lengthens) during the platform backward translation.

Figure 5 shows that these bursts had a remarkably constant latency throughout the successive cycles, in spite of the mentioned changes in size. Latencies were measured from the onset of the forward translation of each cycle for the TA (**A**, one subject) and from the onset of the backward translation for Sol (**C**). We compared the onset latencies of the four identified TA bursts (EC) across cycles and subjects. ANOVA showed no significant effect of the cycle number on the mean latencies (MLR: $F_{(1,58)} = 0.75$, $p = 0.9$; LLR $F_{(1,58)} = 1.3$, $p = 0.08$; FPR: $F_{(1,58)} = 1.07$, $p = 0.4$; PAR: $F_{(1,58)} = 1.28$, $p = 0.09$). Moreover, the *post hoc* analysis showed no difference in the mean latencies among the first 5 cycles ($p > 0.05$, for all responses). Not only the latencies were consistent within each subject, but they were almost superimposed in all the subjects, as shown by the small standard deviation of the bars reporting the mean latency values for each burst (**B** and **D**). Furthermore, the mean latencies were not different between EC and EO ($F_{(1,9)} = 0.04$, $p = 0.85$).

To account for the variability in the latency of the reflex or PARs, for each subject the standard deviation of the onset latency of the various TA burst (EC) were calculated and compared across responses by the Levene's test ($F_{(3,36)} = 8.89$, $p < 0.001$). The variability of PAR response proved to be significantly larger than that of the other bursts (*post hoc*, $p < 0.01$ for the four comparisons), while there was no difference across the other responses (*post hoc*, $p > 0.3$).

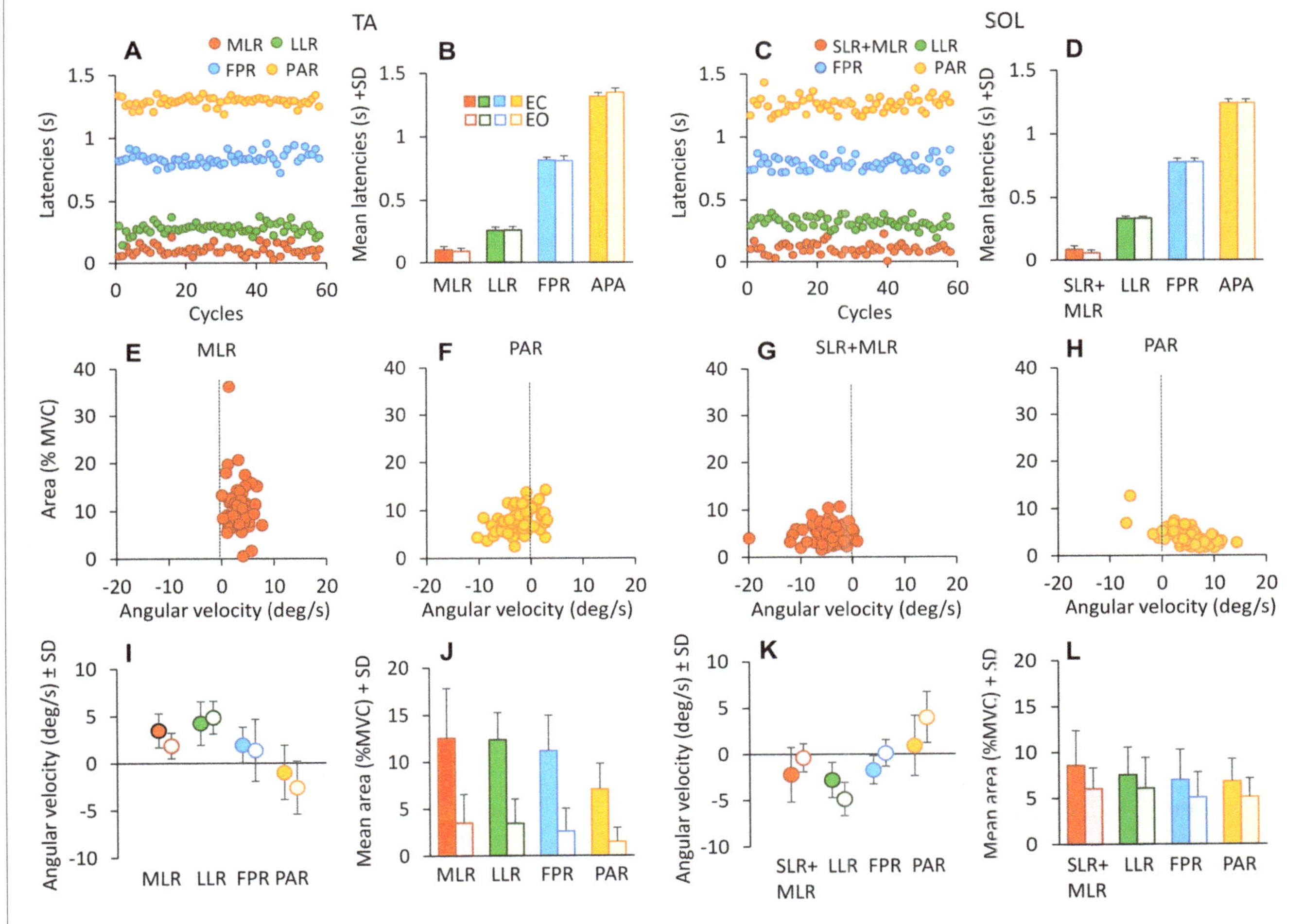

FIGURE 5 | Latencies of TA and Sol bursts. These are expressed with respect to the onset of platform forward movement (TA, left panels), and to the onset of backward movement for Sol (right panels). **(A,C)** show the onset latencies for TA and Sol bursts, in one subject cycle by cycle and for all response types (red medium-latency response (MLR) or SLR + MLR, green long-latency response (LLR), blue fall-preventing response (FPR) and yellow proactive response (PAR)). The grand means of the onset latencies of TA **(B)** and Sol **(D)** responses are reported. There are no differences in burst latencies between EC and EO, for both TA and Sol. **(E–H)** show TA (MLR, **E**; PAR, **F**) and Sol (SLR + MLR, **G**; PAR, **H**) burst areas against the corresponding ankle angular velocities for all cycles in one subject EC. TA and Sol reflex responses occur during muscle lengthening (positive ankle velocity for TA, negative for Sol), whereas PAR responses do not, for either TA or Sol. **(I,K)** show the grand means of ankle angular velocities preceding TA **(I)** and Sol **(K)** bursts EC and EO. Velocities are similar between EC and EO, but not across responses. **(J,L)** show the grand means of TA **(J)** and Sol **(L)** response area EC and EO. Bursts are smaller EO than EC for all responses. TA activity diminishes more than Sol activity passing from EC to EO.

The mean duration of the bursts across subjects (not shown in the Figure) ranged from about 60 ms (MLR) to about 250 ms (PAR) for TA and from about 65 ms (SLR + MLR) to about 360 ms (PAR) for Sol. For each response, the mean duration of the bursts was not different between EC and EO conditions ($F_{(1,9)} = 0.075$, $p = 0.79$), but was different between muscles ($F_{(1,9)} = 87.9$, $p < 0.01$). There was also an interaction between muscle and vision ($F_{(1,9)} = 38.3$, $p < 0.01$), since durations were generally longer with EO for Sol and with EC for TA, but significantly so only for PAR and FPR response (*post hoc*, $p < 0.05$, for all comparisons).

Figures 5E–H also show the result of the attempt to correlate the size of the bursts to the angular velocity of the ankle angle, in order to identify reflex and non-reflex responses. Some burst proved to be directly connected to stretch of the homonymous muscle, while others were not. The TA bursts at the beginning of each platform forward translation (MLR) were associated with the increase in ankle angle (positive angular velocities in **E**), while other bursts occurred in the absence of consistent positive angular velocity or even with negative velocity (for instance, TA PAR was often present when the ankle angle decreased, corresponding to TA shortening, see **F**). A similar pattern occurred for Sol (**G,H**; note that negative velocities stand here for the reduction in ankle angle, therefore Sol lengthening). The third row (**I** and **K**) summarizes this finding, where the successive points belong to reflex or anticipatory responses within a cycle. Each response occurred at different mean ankle angular velocity, for both TA ($F_{(3,24)} = 12.88$, $p < 0.001$) and Sol ($F_{(3,27)} = 16.03$, $p < 0.001$). In particular, for TA, across subjects and cycles, the mean angular velocities were positive for MLR, LLR and FPR and negative for PAR (there was a difference between the ankle angular velocity for PAR and for the other three responses, *post hoc* $p < 0.001$ for the three comparisons). **Figures 5J,L** show that burst area was smaller with EO than EC for all TA and Sol responses ($F_{(1,9)} = 32.35$, $p < 0.001$). There was an interaction between muscle and vision ($F_{(1,9)} = 17.81, p < 0.01$), since with EO, TA area was much smaller than Sol area, for all responses (*post hoc*, $p < 0.005$). There was a difference between response types ($F_{(3,27)} = 10.11$, $p < 0.001$), and an interaction between the response and vision ($F_{(3,27)} = 3.17$, $p < 0.05$).

Figure 6 shows the change over time in the mean values of the area of the reflex burst (MLR, A and SLR + MLR, B), of the FPR (**C,D**) and of the PAR (**E,F**) for both TA and Sol, EC. For each subject, the decay of the areas of the bursts was described by exponential functions with two time-constants. The mean time-constants for the various responses of all subjects are reported in panels (**G,H**) for TA and SOL, EC and EO. Both TA and Sol showed an initial rapid decrease (τ_1); then, the EMG activity of both muscles continued to decrease more slowly (τ_2). The fitting algorithm did not converge to the exponential model for $n = 4$ bursts of TA PARs (EO condition only) and for $n = 17$ bursts of Sol (comprising both EC and EO proactive and reflex responses), since the amplitude of those bursts proved to be almost constant from the beginning to the end of the perturbation sequence. On averaging the valid time-constant values, τ_1 proved to be shorter than τ_2 ($F_{(1,115)} = 106.5$, $p < 0.001$). All time-constant collapsed, there was a difference between TA and Sol (TA longer than Sol, $F_{(1,115)} = 6.98, p < 0.05$) and between visual condition (τ_1 and τ_2 were longer with EC than EO, $F_{(1,115)} = 59.96$, $p < 0.001$). There was an interaction between τ_1 and τ_2, muscles and vision, since vision decreased τ_1 and τ_2 to a larger extent in TA than Sol ($F_{(1,115)} = 4.89$, $p < 0.05$). Vision significantly decreased τ_2 for all TA bursts (*post hoc*, $p < 0.05$ for the four comparisons). All types of response (reflex or proactive) decreased over time with similar time-constants in both muscles ($F_{(3,115)} = 1.7, p = 0.17$). This was true both for τ_1 and for τ_2 (interaction between time-constants and type of response, $F_{(3,115)} = 0.9$, $p = 0.44$). With EC, the TA reflex responses exhibited the shortest initial rapid decrease (τ_1, MLR $= 0.7 \pm 0.5$ cycles, TA LLR $= 1.1 \pm 0.1$ cycles) suggesting that the "first trial effect" had vanished already at the 2nd cycle. τ_1 was instead just longer for the proactive than the reflex responses (1.7 ± 0.2 cycles for FPR and 2.3 ± 0.1 cycles for PAR) but not significantly so (*post hoc* $p > 0.10$ for all comparisons).

In order to assess the amount of reduction in the burst area during adaptation, for each burst we calculated the difference between the values of the burst at the second oscillation cycle and the asymptotic value, based on the exponential fit. **Figures 6I,J** report the amount of reduction calculated for the different responses, for TA (**I**) and Sol (**J**). A great difference between the value of a response at the second oscillation cycle and the asymptotic value points to a large response adaptation. Conversely, short histogram bars (e.g., (**J**), EO data) point to minimal amplitude adaptation. Under EO condition, in six subjects, TA responses disappeared in the final perturbation cycles and in two subjects the TA FPR response was never present. The entity of the reduction in amplitude was larger with EC than EO ($F_{(1,9)} = 8.54$, $p < 0.05$) for all the responses and greater for TA than for SOL ($F_{(1,9)} = 13.88$, $p < 0.01$). There was also a difference between type of response ($F_{(3,27)} = 12.7$, $p < 0.001$) and an interaction between type of response and muscles ($F_{(3,27)} = 13.48$, $p < 0.001$). For TA, both under EC and EO condition, the entity of adaptation of the reflex responses (MLR and LLR) was larger than that of the PARs (FPR and PAR; *post hoc*, $p < 0.05$, for all comparisons).

Head and CoM A-P Behavior During the Entire Perturbation Period

The value of the standard deviation of the entire trace of the head and CoM displacements was calculated (not shown) to get a global index of the segment oscillation amplitude. This mean across-subjects oscillation index was for the CoM: 3.1 ± 0.8 cm (EC), and 2.3 ± 0.8 cm (EO), and for the head: 5.1 ± 2.0 cm (EC), and 2.3 ± 0.7 cm (EO). ANOVA showed an effect of vision on the oscillation indexes ($F_{(1,9)} = 34.25$, $p < 0.001$), a difference between head and CoM index ($F_{(1,9)} = 7.74, p < 0.05$), and an interaction with vision ($F_{(1,9)} = 94.92$, $p < 0.001$).

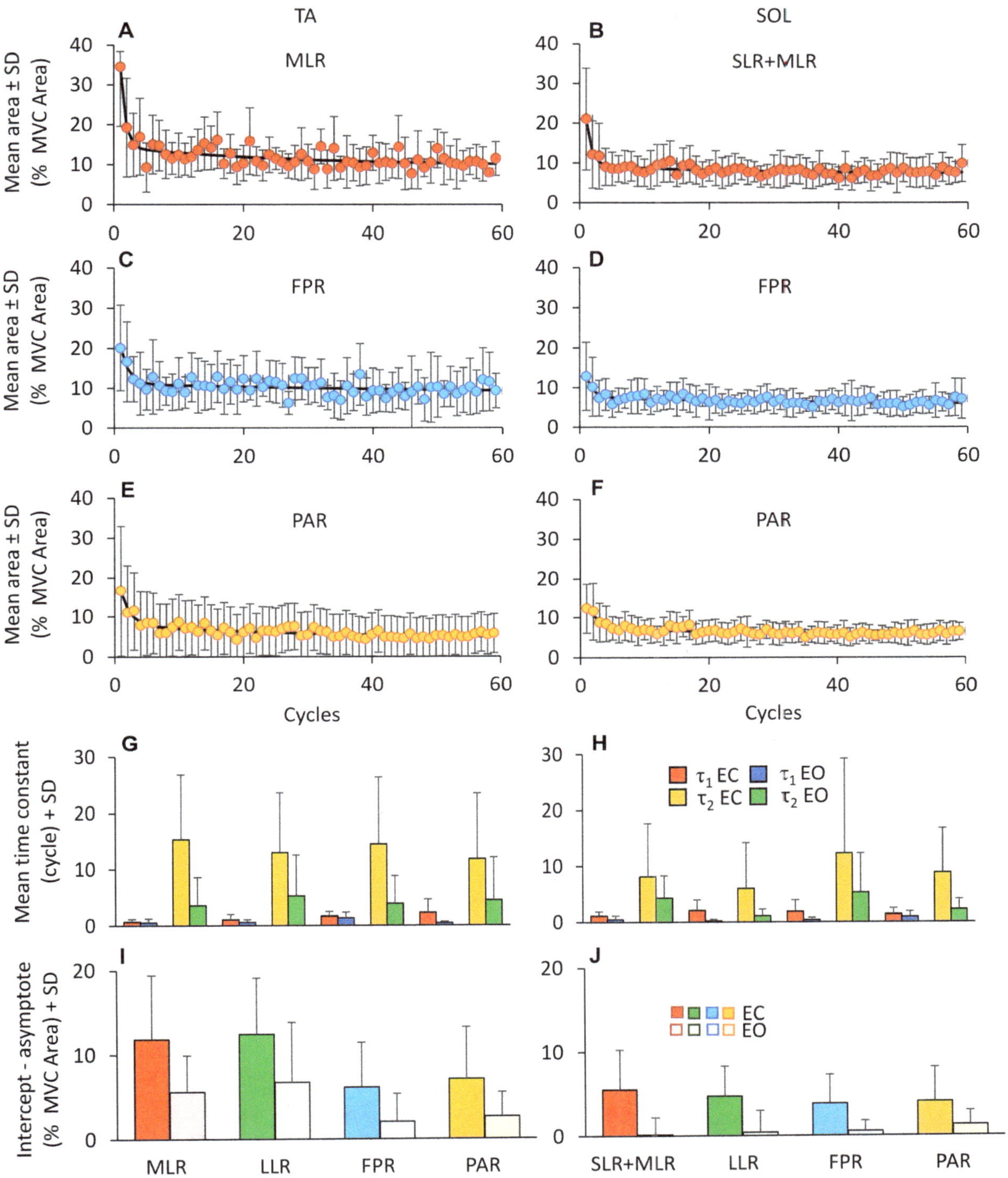

FIGURE 6 | Adaptation of reflex and anticipatory response. (A–F) Shows the adaptation of the different TA (MLR, **A**; FPR, **C**; PAR, **E**) and Sol responses (SLR + MLR, **B**; FPR, **D**; PAR, **F**). For TA, the exponential functions fitting the mean burst area are $y = 9.7 + 20.3e^{-t/0.8} + 4.5e^{-t/26.8}$ for MLR, $y = 8.3 + 9.4e^{-t/1.3} + 2.8e^{-t/62.6}$ for FPR and $y = 4.3 + 8.5e^{-t/1.5} + 3.6e^{-t/32.1}$ for PAR. For Sol, the exponential functions are $y = 7.46 + 11.5e^{-t/0.8} + 2e^{-t/17.1}$ for SLR + MLR, $y = 5.7 + 5.4e^{-t/1.0} + 1.9e^{-t/29.8}$ for FPR and $y = 5.5 + 5.2e^{-t/1.8} + 2e^{-t/22.4}$ for PAR. **(G,H)** show the mean time constants obtained by fitting with a double exponential function the TA **(G)** and Sol **(H)** responses EC (τ_1, red bars; τ_2, yellow bars) and EO (τ_1, blue bars; τ_2, green bars). The time constants differ between EC and EO and between TA and Sol. The extent of adaptation in the amplitude of the response bursts **(I,J)** is higher for TA than Sol, higher with EO than EC and different between reflex and anticipatory responses.

On average, the oscillation indexes of head and CoM were not different with EO (*post hoc*, $p = 0.05$), while closing the eyes induced a larger oscillation for head than CoM (*post hoc*, $p < 0.001$).

The CoM A-P positions with respect to malleolus are critical to balance, since any translation of the CoM behind the malleolus increases the risk of falling backwards. There was no difference in the CoM position between EC and EO condition ($F_{(1,9)} = 0.12$, $p = 0.7$), both at the beginning (the intercept value of the exponential fit, *post hoc*, $p = 0.34$) and end of the perturbation cycles (the asymptotic value of the fit, *post hoc*, $p = 0.75$; **Figures 7A,B**). The CoM mean positions **(A,B)** exhibited a moderate shift forwards of about 1 cm with respect to its position in the first cycle, with a time-constant of 3.4 ± 2.9 cycles (EC) and 2.0 ± 1.9 cycles (EO). There was no difference in the time-constant between EC and EO (*t*-test, $p = 0.2$), but a difference in the CoM position between the first cycle and the final cycles ($F_{(1,9)} = 20.45$, $p < 0.05$), both for EC and EO (*post hoc*, $p < 0.05$). After the initial forward shift, the CoM position remained remarkably constant throughout the following cycles with both EC and EO, indicating an overall similar inclination of the body with respect to the ankle joint. The bottom panels show that, on collapsing all trials and subjects, CoM **(C)** and head **(D)** backward-most positions infrequently (EC) and never (EO) bypassed the position of the malleolus. The graphs also show the limited scatter of CoM compared with the larger head data scatter (EC) across subjects and trials. Overall, the control of the CoM position relative to the base of support (critical for preventing backward fall) proved to be effective from the beginning to the end of the perturbation cycles regardless of the major attenuation of the EMG bursts.

The anterior displacement of the CoM was accompanied by an increase in the height of the malleolus marker, as a sign of deformation of the foot arch. The direct relationship between CoM advancement and malleolus height in a representative subjects during EC condition is shown in **Figure 7E**. Across subjects, the average slope of the line best fitting that relationship **(F)** was 0.019 ± 0.012 (EC) and 0.018 ± 0.016 (EO) (*t*-test, $p = 0.95$), indicating that the malleolus height increased by about 0.2 mm for 1 cm of CoM advancement, both under EC and EO condition.

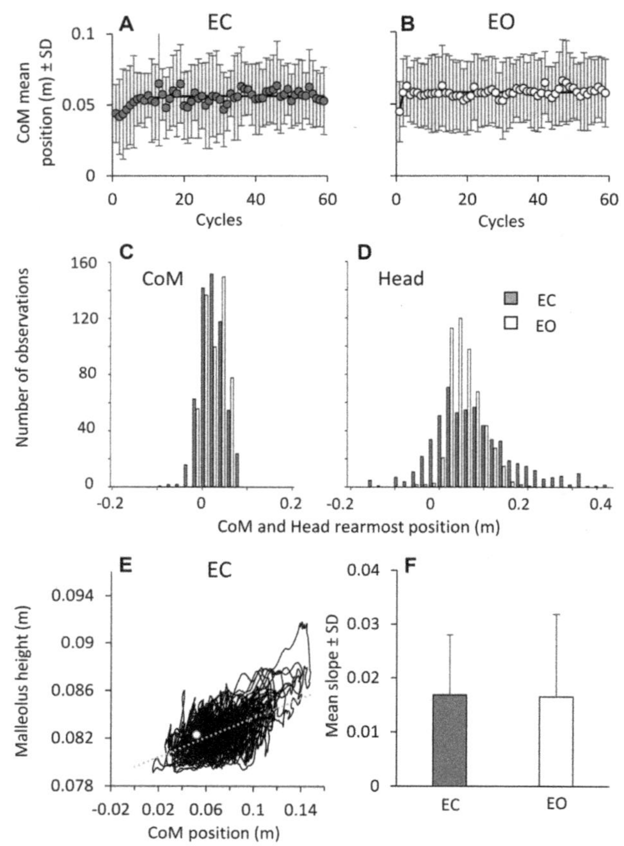

FIGURE 7 | Changes in CoM positions over time. During the perturbation cycles, the CoM mean positions with respect to malleolus **(A,B)** exhibited a minor shift forwards, both EC (left) and EO (right). The exponential functions fitted to the mean positions of CoM are $y = 0.056 - 0.015e^{-t/4.4}$ in EC and $y = 0.058 - 0.013e^{-t/0.1}$ in EO. **(C,D)** show CoM and head backward-most position (all trials and all subjects collapsed). These only infrequently EC (gray bars) and never EO (white bars) bypass the position of the malleolus (backwards negative in the abscissa). **(E)** shows the direct relationship ($y = 0.04x + 0.08$; $r^2 = 0.3$; $p < 0.001$) between CoM position with respect to malleolus and the height of the marker placed on malleolus in a representative subject under EC condition. The white dot indicates the values of CoM position and malleolus height during quite stance. The mean slope across subjects of the regression line indicating the relationship between CoM position and malleolus height is reported in **(F)** for EC (gray bar) and EO (white bar).

Changes in the Temporal Relationship of the CoM Position With Respect to the Moving Base of Support

Figures 8A–C show the progressive time-shift of the CoM with respect to the support base in a representative subject (EC). For all subjects, the CC coefficient between the traces of CoM and platform (**Figure 8D**) was high from the beginning ($R = 0.77 \pm 0.2$, the average of the first cycle across subjects) and tended to increase and level off over time. The mean R of the last 5 cycles was 0.84 ± 0.07. The mean time-constant of this change in R over time was 11.9 ± 11.5 cycles. With EO (**Figure 8E**), the CC coefficient was high at the first cycle ($R = 0.84 \pm 0.11$) and increased slightly during the successive perturbation cycles ($R = 0.89 \pm 0.06$) with a mean time-constant across subjects of 4.8 ± 3.0 cycles. The time-constant of the changes in CC over time was not strongly affected by vision (EC and EO, paired *t*-test, $p = 0.08$).

Figures 8F,G show the average values over time of the CoM-platform time lags, under EC and EO conditions. At the beginning, the displacement of CoM trailed the platform displacement by about 0.16 s with EC and 0.1 s with EO (paired *t*-test, $p = 0.15$). The mean time-lag diminished with cycle repetition to about 0.1 s with EC and 0.07 s with EO (paired *t*-test, $p = 0.06$) with a mean time-constant **(F)** of

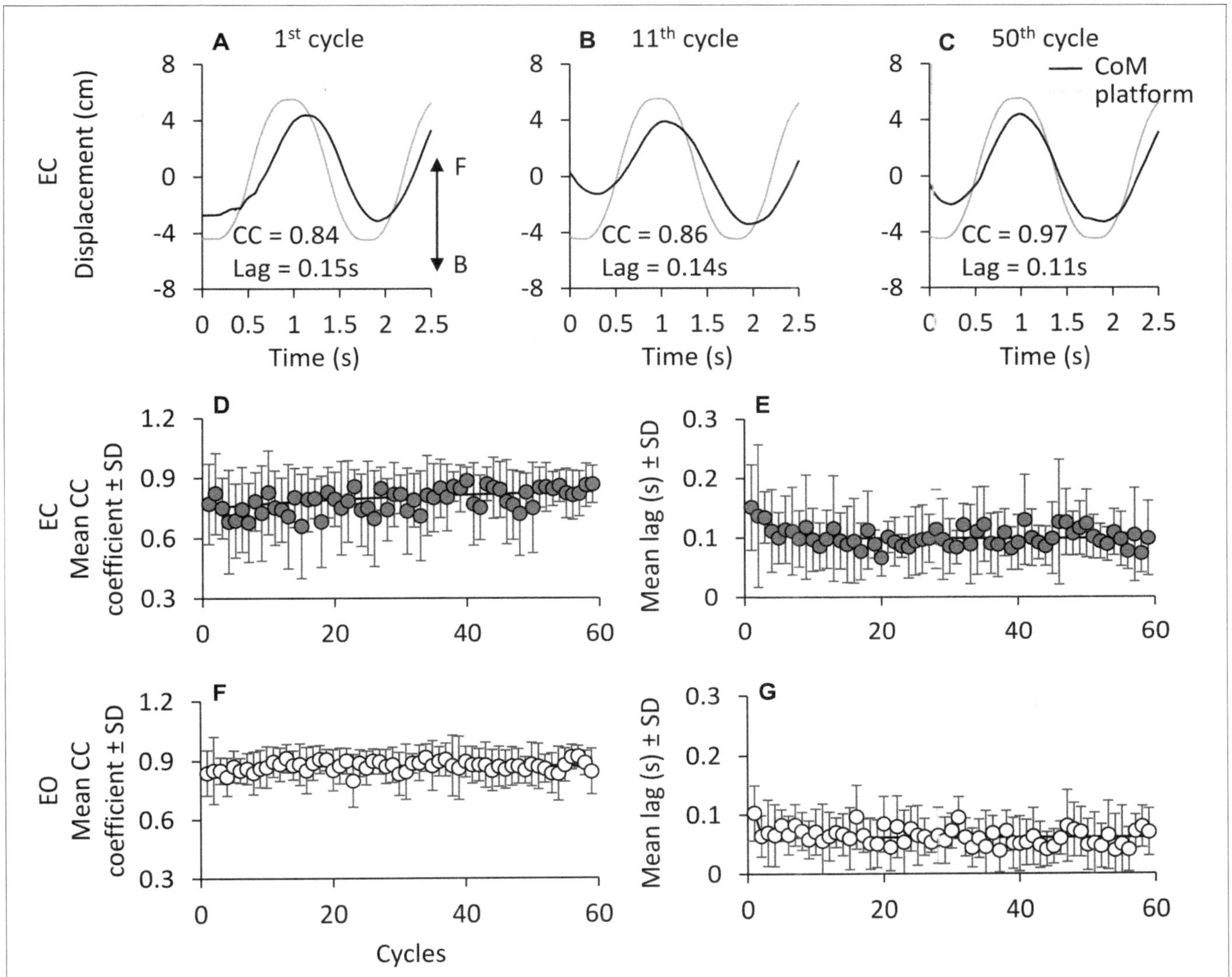

FIGURE 8 | Cross correlation (CC) between CoM and platform displacement. (A–C) show CoM (black line) and platform displacement (gray line; both referred to the laboratory space) during three non-consecutive cycles in one subject EC (F, forward; B, backward). **(D,E)** show the grand mean of the CC coefficient at time lag = 0 between CoM and platform displacement traces. CC values slightly increase with cycle repetition under both EC **(D)** and EO **(E)** condition. The exponential functions fitted to the mean CC coefficient data points are $y = 0.83 - 0.15e^{-t/36.3}$ in EC and $y = 0.87 - 0.04e^{-t/4.7}$ in EO. At the beginning of the oscillation cycles, CoM follows the platform with a lag of about 0.16 s EC, and 0.1 s EO. The time lag between CoM and platform diminishes with cycle **(F,G)** both EC and EO. The exponential function is $y = 0.10 + 0.05e^{-t/2.7}$ in EC and $y = 0.06 + 0.04e^{-t/0.5}$ in EO.

7.8 ± 9.7 cycles with EC, and of 4.6 ± 2.9 cycles with EO (paired t-test, $p = 0.33$). These lags were small, but significantly different from zero in most perturbation cycles of all subjects (EC, 83%; EO, 80%). Overall, the delay of the CoM with respect to the platform back-and-forth displacement was very limited, as a sign of effective synchrony of body to platform movements, but tended to become in-phase with the platform translation.

The regularity of the CoM cyclic displacement was at the expense of a presumably complex control. When the CoM back-and-forth displacement with respect to malleolus was plotted against ankle angle for each successive cycle (**Figure 9**), the coefficient of determination of the linear regression (r^2) was initially very low, and improved with time. Then, the "easy" balancing synergy (CoM moving forward when the ankle angle decreased and vice versa), featuring a coefficient of determination approaching unity, was reached with a time-constant of about 10 cycles (**J**). When the mean time course of r^2 was calculated for all subjects, this finding was replicated. This time-course proved to be much shorter with EO than EC (*post hoc*, $p < 0.001$), as shown in the bottom panel *(K)* of **Figure 9**, indicating a strong coupling between CoM displacement and ankle angular change with EO from the very beginning.

We note that both the time-constants of the coefficient of determination (r^2) and the time-constant of the co-contraction

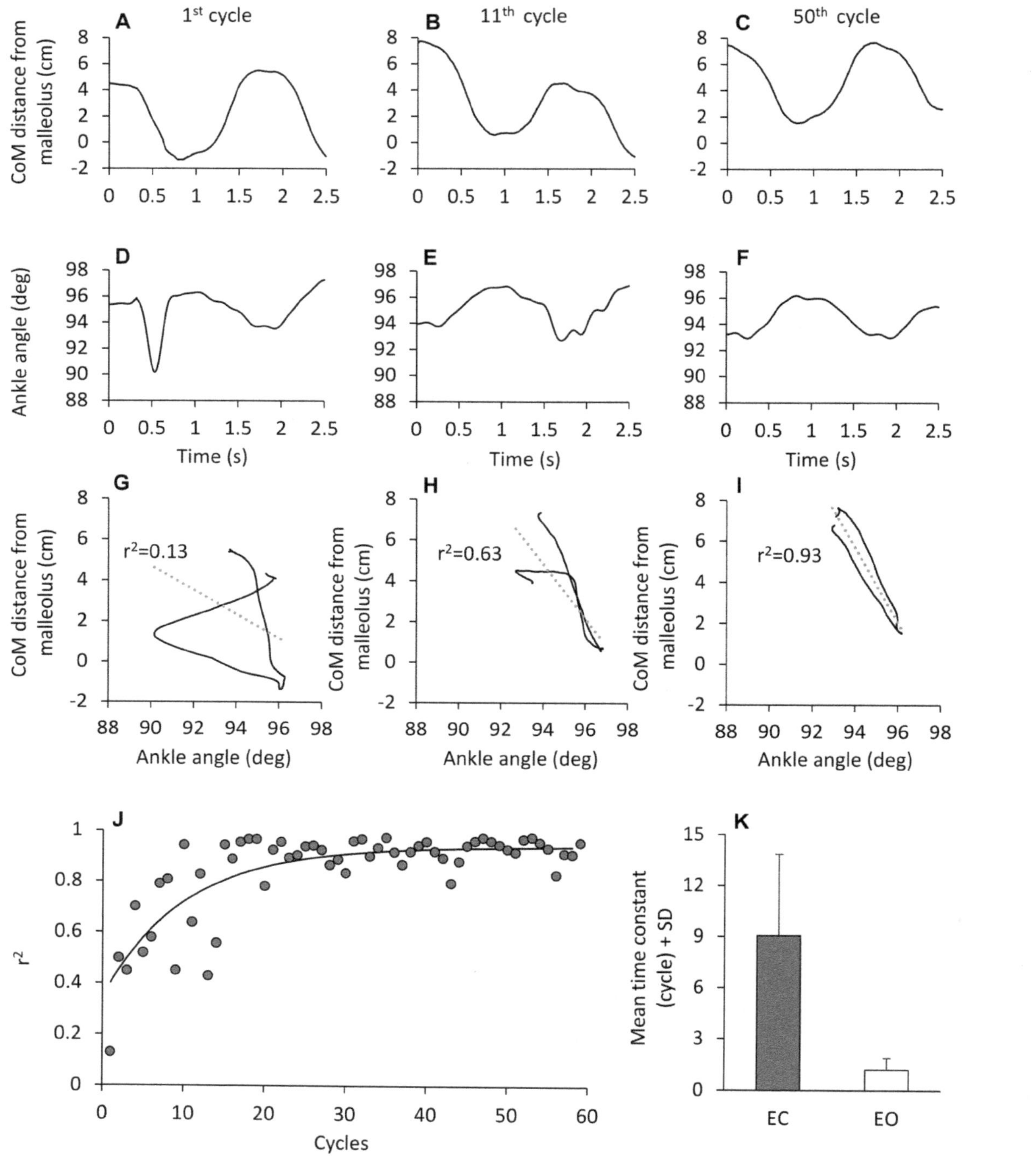

FIGURE 9 | Time-dependence of the correlation between CoM displacement and ankle angle variation. (A–F) CoM horizontal distance from malleolus **(A–C)** and ankle angle variation **(D–F)** in one subject during three different cycles of perturbation EC. When the CoM distance from malleolus is plotted against ankle angle **(G–I)**, the association between the two traces improves with cycle number. **(J)** show the value of the determination coefficient (r^2) calculated for each cycle EC. The r^2 values increase with cycle repetition with a time-constant of 10.1 cycles ($y = 0.93 + 0.6e^{-t/10.1}$). **(K)** show the mean time-constant across subjects, EC (gray bar) and EO (white bar).

index (**k**) (**Figure 3**) were not significantly different ($F_{(1,9)} = 4.19$, $p = 0.07$), suggesting a parallel time-course of both parameters. There was an effect of vision ($F_{(1,9)} = 28.52$, $p < 0.001$), since the time-course was much more rapid for EO than EC. There was no interaction between visual conditions and time-constants ($F_{(1,9)} = 3.44$, $p = 0.09$).

DISCUSSION

Progressive Decrease in Leg Muscle EMG Activity

Healthy young subjects underwent repeated and predictable perturbations of stance, featuring continuous A-P translations of the support base calling into action feedback responses and proactive postural adjustments related to the repetitive rhythmic platform displacements (Milner and Franklin, 2005; Franklin et al., 2008). Our aim was to confirm that: (a) leg muscle EMG activity decreases over the perturbation cycles (Schmid et al., 2011) and to assess whether; (b) adaptation is differently modulated for the reflex and anticipatory responses elicited in the leg postural muscles; (c) adaptation implies changes in both amplitude and latency of the response bursts; (d) a relationship exists between EMG response adaptation and critical kinematic variables; in addition, we addressed; and (e) the role of vision on adaptation. We will first discuss the no-vision data (EC), to later consider the effect of vision (EO) on the balancing behavior.

The TA muscle showed in all subjects a progressive decrease in activity, common to both legs (Vieira et al., 2014). The time-constant of this decrease with EC was such that the activity tended to level off to about 30% of its initial value after 15–20 cycles. The time course and the steady-state level of this decrease were not exactly the same in all the subjects, though, as indicated by the variance of the mean data. This could be connected with cycle-to-cycle differences in the balancing behavior, whereby some subjects kept their body straight, trying to counteract the platform displacement, while others allowed a moderate bending of their body by hip and ankle angle changes. In addition, since the stimulation pattern implied a fixed-support strategy and precluded the option of grasping (Maki and McIlroy, 1997), four subjects initially made a short step that was soon corrected. In other subjects, there was a transient phase wherein, after the initial smooth adaptation (Adi-Japha et al., 2008), the balancing performance was possibly disturbed by a gradual forward or backward body lean that required a corrective intervention by modulating the amplitude of the leg muscle bursts.

The Sol muscle also showed a progressive decrease in amplitude, with a time-constant just as like that of the TA, showing a contribution of the Sol to the general process of adaptation. However, contrary to TA, the steady-state EMG level remained elevated in the Sol (about 60% of the initial value). This is likely connected with the need to continuously counteract gravity, since in all subjects and cycles the CoM lay always in front of the malleolus, requiring a continuous plantar-flexor activity. The limited reduction of Sol activity could be also connected to the forward displacement of the CoM (about 1 cm) occurring during the first few initial cycles and persisting until the last cycles (Keshner et al., 1987), which would have increased the gravity torque (Schieppati et al., 1994). In addition, in the course of adaptation, TA activity progressively diminished. Overall, while CoM advancement requires a larger Sol activity to keep the body from falling, the diminishing TA force requires less counter-action by Sol so that, in the end, Sol activity may remain approximately constant.

The Timing of the Bursts Within Cycles, and the "First-Trial" Effect

Averaging the EMG traces across subjects and perturbation cycles gave a clear-cut profile of the time-varying muscle activity within a cycle. This presented a series of bursts that could be easily encompassed by distinct time-windows. The large TA bursts occurring during the first few cycles had the same latency as the corresponding smaller-amplitude bursts recorded during the following cycles. Hence, the latency of the bursts was independent from the process leading to the attenuation of burst amplitude over time. This was not necessarily predicted, since latency changes *can* occur under a continuous perturbation protocol similar to ours, as after deliberately produced fatigue of TA (Kennedy et al., 2012). One might argue that, in the latter case, the changes in latency take into account the smaller capacity of muscle force production, compelling the neural command to change its timing since changes in force recruitment would be less effective. Without fatigue, the strategy of reducing amplitude but not timing of activation would be adequate.

The latency of the first large TA burst is not different from that of the corresponding bursts of the following cycles. This reduces the probability that the first large burst is a startle reaction (Oude Nijhuis et al., 2010; Campbell et al., 2013), and suggests it to be a true stretch-induced balance-correcting response. McIlroy and Maki (1993) had already emphasized that a response to an unexpected perturbation can contain a compensatory reaction. The fact that subjects wore soundproof earphones also renders unlikely that they reacted with a startle reaction to the noise produced by the platform. The extent to which any "startling" effect of proprioceptive or vestibular origin (Bisdorff et al., 1994; Álvarez-Blanco et al., 2009; Sanders et al., 2015) might have contributed to the large amplitude of the first TA MLR and LLR bursts cannot be settled based on the present data. However, we would note that the body position was closer to the vertical at the time of the first perturbation cycle, as shown by the large ankle angle and the short distance between CoM and malleolus. The greater length of the TA at this time with respect to the subsequent cycles would favor a larger reflex response to the rapid TA stretch induced by the platform forward displacement. As to the bursts following the initial TA reflex responses, namely the so-called FPR and PAR, it seems even less likely that any startle reaction *per se* could have extended its effect to the muscle activity occurring later.

Adaptation of Reflex and Anticipatory Responses

For almost all cycles of the sequence, the TA burst occurring at the beginning of each platform forward translation had similar latency, in turn similar to the latency of the response to the very first perturbation. This occurred in spite of the burst being triggered by "dynamic" consecutive perturbations, while the first perturbation started from the "neutral" static postural configuration. The amplitude of these TA bursts were always related to the velocity of the increase in ankle angle. These bursts were considered medium- and long-latency stretch reflexes (MLR and LLR), since the angular velocity is a variable appropriate for estimating the velocity of change in muscle length. The latter is the adequate stimulus for triggering the stretch reflex, given the velocity-dependence of the sensitivity of the muscle spindle receptors. The responses occurring at about the anterior platform turn-around points and during the backward translation periods bore instead no relation to the ankle angular velocity. For this reason, these were considered proactive activities and were named FPR and anticipatory PAR, respectively. In this connection, we would point out that continuous sinusoidal rather than single support surface perturbations were employed in this study, and that only leg muscle stretch was considered. Input from other muscles synchronous with some phase of the perturbation displacement might have produced phasic responses in the leg muscles triggered by changes in body segment movements that we have not examined. However, the similarity in the responses' latencies between EC and EO, two conditions producing different displacements of the body parts, would not readily favor that possibility. Of note, since the ankle angle *decreases* during the period where the PAR occurred (and the TA shortens accordingly), that burst might include the so-called "shortening reaction" (Katz and Rondot, 1978; Bathien et al., 1981; Berardelli and Hallett, 1984), the amplitude of which is known to depend on the central set (Miscio et al., 2001). This would be in keeping with the notion that, during adaptation, PAR can be modulated at cortical level, since the cortex is certainly involved in controlling critical postures (Taube et al., 2006; Maki and McIlroy, 2007; Nardone et al., 2008; Petersen et al., 2009; Tokuno et al., 2009; Bolton et al., 2011; Zwergal et al., 2012; Obata et al., 2014; Fujiwara et al., 2016). It has been recently suggested that the motor cortex confers sophisticated feedback to these responses, thereby potentially participating in their calibration (Pruszynski et al., 2011; Pruszynski and Scott, 2012).

The absolute decrease in amplitude of burst area from the second cycle (in order to exclude the "first-trial effect" from the computation) to steady state was larger for the reflex than for the anticipatory responses. Consequently, the weight of the anticipatory responses *relatively* increased over the series of perturbations. Hence, it can be inferred that adaptation does not prioritize reflex responses, but appropriately weights feedback and feed-forward control. This inference is not in contrast with the conclusion of previous studies (Cenciarini and Peterka, 2006) asserting that, during continuous perturbations, subject's reliance on information from the stimulus decreases, whereas a sensory reweighting mechanism ensues, tending to favor information that encode body orientation relative to vertical. A difference in the time course of the decrease in burst amplitude between reflex and PARs might potentially reside in muscle mechanical factors (Proske et al., 1993), such as thixotropy. This is dependent on the history of the changes in length and activation of muscle's extra- and intrafusal fibers. While we would not deny a contribution of these factors to the early adaptation phase, in particular for the ample decrease in amplitude of the reflex response at the 2nd cycle, we would note that the relatively low amplitude and high frequency of the changes in muscle length would not favor a history-dependent change in muscle fiber stiffness in active muscle (Gurfinkel et al., 1997; Altman et al., 2015, in rabbit in Ca^{++}-activated single fiber), which might contribute to the overall adaptation process. Further, the latency of the reflex responses did not change over time, whereas thixotropy would be expected to affect latency (Hagbarth et al., 1995). Besides, in our hands, similar changes in leg muscle length occurred during EC and EO perturbations, but the adaptation time course was very different.

Fast and Slow Adaptation

At first sight, both reflex and anticipatory TA responses decreased over successive cycles almost in parallel, as an indication of progressive general attenuation of the responsiveness of the TA motor pool to all converging excitatory inputs. However, their time-course (both reflex and anticipatory) was fitted by an equation with two exponential terms, in order to comply with the initial rapid decrease (τ_1) followed by a slower decrease (τ_2), and to better address possible differences in adaptation between bursts. The time-constant of the initial rapid decay was the shortest (albeit not significantly so) for the MLR, shaped by the vanishing of the "first-trial effect" (Oude Nijhuis et al., 2010) discussed above. The time-course of the other bursts was also best fitted by two time-constants. A difference was present between τ_1 and τ_2, since all bursts exhibited a rapid decrease during the initial few cycles and all slowly decreased with a similar time-course, until a steady state was reached after 20–30 cycles. We would argue that the first rapid adaptation produces a coarse adjustment of the corrective torques to promptly counteract the risk of falling (Peterka and Loughlin, 2004), while the second slow process would progressively fine tune muscle activity to the new sensory references (Assländer and Peterka, 2014). It is becoming clear that distinct processes can contribute to sensorimotor adaptation (Huberdeau et al., 2015). In a visuomotor adaptation paradigm requiring to overcome perturbation while reaching, one process learns rapidly and depends on an explicit component, the other learns slowly and in an implicit mode (Taylor et al., 2014). It would not be surprising if these processes also applied to balancing, whereby the early rapid and the later slow adaptation would be expression of an explicit and implicit process, respectively.

Parallel analysis of the Sol bursts allowed to identify stretch responses and anticipatory responses as well. As expected, the pattern of Sol EMG activity profile, as obtained by the same averaging procedure as for TA, showed a half-cycle delay with respect to that of TA. This was in keeping with the TA and Sol similar involvement in counteracting oppositely directed platform translations (the Sol reflex burst appeared at the beginning of the backward displacement of the platform, in response to the rapid Sol muscle stretch, and so on for the other response bursts). For Sol, both reflex and anticipatory responses showed a rapid small reduction (τ_1) followed by a further slower reduction (τ_2). The decrease in amplitude from the second cycle to steady state was also similar for the feedback and PARs, but much less pronounced than for TA. It might be suggested that all Sol responses serve the main task of counteracting gravity by being less susceptible to *selective* adaptation. Also in a different context, task- and context-related changes were more clearly present in the TA than in the Sol muscle (Schieppati and Nardone, 1995).

Relationship Between Muscle Activity and Kinematics During Adaptation

The constant latencies of the response bursts matched the substantial invariance of the CoM, which is kept within safe margins from the beginning. Possibly, this consistency would be guided by the need to keep stable the CoM that is the important variable for balance control (Safavynia and Ting, 2013; Welch and Ting, 2014). The progressive decrease in muscle activity (particularly so in the case of TA) would not alter the critical time-relationships between biomechanical body parameters and instantaneous position of the continuously translating support base.

At the beginning of the perturbation cycles, the coordination between CoM and ankle joint angle was very poor, and gradually achieved larger determination coefficients. Other body muscles (not recorded here) must therefore be recruited to help keep CoM stable at the earliest cycles, compensating for the poorly controlled ankle angle. Cappa et al. (2008) attributed to the upper limbs (free to move) an anticipatory role in counteracting perturbations similar to ours. In our case, subjects' arms were deliberately kept crossed so that only small not-monitored motions would have minimally affected the CoM displacement (Assländer and Peterka, 2014). Maki and McIlroy (1997) have reviewed the role of limb movements in maintaining upright stance, and suggested that they are substantially finalized in spite of their apparently chaotic production (Corbeil et al., 2013). In a sense, our protocol "forced" the leg muscles to compensate for absence of assistance of the upper limb motion.

Co-contraction around the ankle joint occurs during tasks such as standing on one leg, balancing on an unstable platform or reacting to rotation of a support surface, or walking on a narrow beam (Diener et al., 1983; Keshner et al., 1987; Nielsen and Kagamihara, 1992; Geertsen et al., 2013) or after fatigue (Kennedy et al., 2012). However, co-contraction is not a rule under different critical postures (Sozzi et al., 2013). In our protocol, TA-Sol co-contraction was present during the initial few cycles, and then gradually vanished. Interestingly, the changes over time of the coefficient of determination of CoM displacement vs. ankle angle increased exponentially toward $r^2 \cong 1$ with a time-constant almost equal to that of the TA-Sol co-contraction index, suggesting that co-activation can be a major disturbing factor. This feature, whereby higher co-contraction is associated with poor performances, and lower co-contraction with good performances, seems to be a general phenomenon in motor adaptation (Thoroughman and Shadmehr, 1999; Osu et al., 2002; Cordo and Gurfinkel, 2004). Following Osu et al. (2002), we would suggest that increased stiffness is a sign of inaccurate knowledge of the task, and that this subsides as learning builds up. At steady state, co-contraction is almost absent, and riding the platform becomes smoother and more coordinated while stability of the CoM is maintained.

The slight surge in height of the malleolus (about 0.2 mm per cm of CoM advancement) gives evidence of a significant deformation of the foot arch as the CoM of the body moves forward. As shown by Wright et al. (2012), such deformation would contribute to a change in ankle joint angle ($<1°$) that accompanies CoM advancement. Regrettably, we are not in the position of dissecting out the role in this event of the change in torque over the ankle joint or of any potential activation of plantar foot muscles or toe-extensor muscle (Schieppati et al., 1994), since no electrodes were fixed to the foot plantar surface or dorsum as in Schieppati et al. (1995). On the one hand, we can only argue that plantar foot muscle activity likely occurred when the CoM moved ahead of the malleolus, and that its activity would parallel that of Sol given that these two muscles are agonist and co-active during backward platform translations (Schieppati et al., 1995). On the other hand, the strong similarity of the slopes of the lines best fitting malleolus height and CoM position with EC and EO (two conditions exhibiting large difference in TA activity) would point to a role for the mechanical constraint rather than for the TA EMG adaptation.

The Effect of Vision on the Adaptation of the Balancing Behavior

When the same perturbation protocol was administered with EO, clear-cut differences and invariances were observed with respect to EC. As a preliminary note, we would remind here that the EC and EO tests were not performed in a randomized order. The fact that subjects under EO condition were familiar with the protocol, having previously performed the same protocol with EC, might have influenced the adaptation pattern (Pai and Bhatt, 2007; Patel and Bhatt, 2015). However, in *ad hoc* experiments performed in a different group of matched subjects, EO administered first produced a very rapid adaptation, equivalent to that observed in the main subject group. For this reason, we are confident that the very rapid adaptation with EO did not depend critically on the earlier EC trial.

The time-constant τ_1 of the profile of the TA bursts with EO was very short and not significantly different from EC. This suggests that the proprioceptive control predominates for the responses to the first perturbation cycle also when vision is available. The time-constant τ_2 was also short with EO (significantly shorter than EC). In some subjects and bursts (especially in the case of the FPR response), the fitting algorithm did not even converge to an exponential curve, since the EMG activity was low from the very beginning. Therefore, we would put forward the notion that the effect of vision does not only consist in speeding up the adaptation process. It would also consist in a generalized down-modulation of the excitability of the motor neurons of the postural muscles, which are the final common pathway for both reflex and proactive activation (Schieppati et al., 2002; De Nunzio et al., 2005; Schmid et al., 2011).

The time-constant τ_1 (EO) was about one cycle. Hence, with vision, experience of one single cycle is enough to reprogram the balancing behavior in the successive cycles. With EO, the adaptation rate may almost be the sole consequence of the vanishing of the "first-trial effect" (Allum et al., 2011). In a different study from this laboratory, an equally similar rapid adaptation in the balancing strategy and EMG activity was observed when passing from EC to EO condition *during* a series of perturbations similar to that used here (De Nunzio and Schieppati, 2007), generalizing the effect of vision beyond the first-trial effect. Also the stabilization of a standing posture (as measured by the reduction of body sway) on adding vision or haptic information is fast (Sozzi et al., 2011; Blouin et al., 2014). This suggests that addition of vision can very rapidly entrain a low-motion, low-activity balancing pattern.

The prediction that, with adaptation, the final level of TA activity with EC at steady state could have reached the level of activity observed with EO, signifying the attainment of a more energy-efficient mode of balancing, was not verified. The absolute level of TA activity at steady state was in fact substantially larger EC than EO. Therefore, even if TA activity *can* decrease to very low levels, absence of vision precludes what would seem an easily attainable task. On the contrary, Sol activity at steady state with EO remained almost similar to that recorded for EC, indicating major differences in the functional outcomes of adaptation according to muscles having different purposes, as mentioned above. With EO, the TA-Sol co-activation index was also low from the beginning and rapidly diminished further in the following cycles. Also, the coordination between CoM and ankle angle under EO promptly reached a high value. Moreover, the time lag between CoM and back-and-forth movement of the platform, which was just smaller for EO than EC, reached steady state very soon. Conversely, the mean position and the extent of back-and-forth displacement of the CoM were similar across cycles between EC and EO, both in amplitude and rapidity to attain a steady state. Therefore, vision does not confer any particular stability to the body' CoM. In contrast, the back-and-forth displacement of the head was remarkably reduced by vision, in keeping with previous findings (Buchanan and Horak, 1999; Corna et al., 1999; Schieppati et al., 2002; De Nunzio and Schieppati, 2007; Schmid et al., 2007). Therefore, we would interpret the head stabilization in space with EO as the direct consequence of vision, an input that critically helps defining the reference frame for balance control by conferring the nervous system information about the environment (Dokka et al., 2009; Isableu et al., 2010; Joseph Jilk et al., 2014). Since it is the head that bears the eyes, the rapid head stabilization in space with EO and minimization of its peak-to-peak displacement would mainly contribute to minimizing the changes in visual flow connected with the platform displacement (Schmid et al., 2008; Dokka et al., 2009; Kiemel et al., 2011). In the absence of the possibility of exploiting vision, our brain accepts some extra activity in the postural muscles.

Perhaps, minimization in the metabolic cost has a neural *computational* cost. While the process of adaptation put in action under EC seems to be insufficient for completing this minimization, the neural computation would be easily afforded with vision. Moreover, with clear perception of environment and body movement in space (Gresty and Bronstein, 1992), the brain need not previously experience repeated cyclic events, but uses sort of a "default" strategy as a substitute of a costly adaptation process. It is tempting to assume that the brain without vision undergoes a complex trial-and-error course, whereby balancing improvements are gained from repeated practice by processing down-up information, whereas vision allows an almost immediate shift from a down-up to a top-down control strategy. Admittedly, the possibility of generalizing these inferences is limited by the absence of concurrent recording of the EMG activity of other muscles, potentially relevant in the process of the bodily adaptation to the continuous perturbations. Further studies are needed for detailing the contribution of (rapid or slow) adaptation of other muscle groups in this task.

CONCLUDING REMARKS

Taken together, the findings show that adaptation occurs when a subject's balance is challenged by repeated perturbations. Under these circumstances, the underlying sensorimotor adaptive processes would include the initial collection of information about the task to handle (among others, from the moving support surface and the position of the CoM), determine how to improve the performance (e.g., reducing redundant muscle activity), to then implement these changes as enhanced motor control performance by repeated trial and error procedure. Contrary to what happens with a self-paced movement, under this balance task condition, the initiator of the process is the initial exposure to an external stimulus (the onset of the series of platform oscillation cycles). This implies reflexive stability-enhancing countermeasures at the same time as it produces an important volley of afferent information about the bodily events. Progressive improvements in balancing behavior, underscored by reduced postural muscle activity and better intersegmental coordination, supervenes from repeated practice.

The ensuing adaptation process selectively affects different neural circuits, since TA activity shows a rapid followed by a slow reduction, while Sol shows a rapid minor adaptation followed by no-reduction in activity (prioritizing antigravity action). Both feedback and feed-forward controls are gradually tuned: yet, the smallest reduction is observed for anticipatory responses (featuring a partial shift from feedback to feed-forward control). Further, any initial TA-Sol co-contraction subsides with the repetition of successive cycles passing from a stiffening strategy to antagonist muscles reciprocal activation. With vision, almost no adaptation is observed after the first few cycles, and the head reduces its motion already at the 2nd perturbation cycle regardless of the persistent CoM back-and-forth displacement.

We therefore suggest that adaptation serves the purpose of: (a) reducing muscle activity and co-contraction while allowing continuous CoM back-and-forth displacement in compliance with the platform translations (*"effort-reducing" adaptation*); (b) improving body segment coordination, reducing over time the number of unnecessary movements (*"entropy-reducing" adaptation*); (c) diminishing head back-and-forth displacement when eyes are open, allowing stable vision (*"visual-field stabilizing" adaptation*). We would also note that standing and balancing on the continuously translating platform shares several features of voluntary control: subjects are aware of the critical stance condition particularly in the absence of visual input, clearly perceive the body displacements accompanying platform displacements, and produce anticipatory adjustments or react to it with correcting counter-movements (Ouchi et al., 1999). Hence, the role of the sensory input in maintaining equilibrium may not be different from the role sensory input plays in directing and correcting voluntary movements of the upper limb (Patla et al., 2002; Soto et al., 2006; Crevecoeur et al., 2012; Hemami and Moussavi, 2014). This ultimately suggests that the cerebral cortex may be the site of the sensorimotor integration and reweighting processes underlying balance control (Taube et al., 2007; Sumner and Husain, 2008; Honeine et al., 2015) and suggests that a similar repertoire of basic mechanisms lies behind skill acquisition in voluntary and postural tasks (Elion et al., 2015).

Postural adaptations occurring from day to day have been reported (Tjernström et al., 2010b; Nardone et al., 2015) and suggested to underpin the rehabilitation effects of repeated perturbations. Predictable balance perturbations by sinusoidal translations have been successfully employed for rehabilitation of balance in selected patient groups (Nardone et al., 2010, 2014) including vestibular patients (Corna et al., 2003), who may badly behave on the platform when not compensated (Buchanan and Horak, 2001–2002). Interestingly, the complex processes of adaptive behavior in a balancing task are able to produce true learning, the uniqueness of which would be to prepare the body to counteract more general features of platform motion (Van Ooteghem et al., 2008; Kanekar and Aruin, 2015). The analytical approach described here could be easily applied to patients with balance problems of different nature, as for instance patients with Parkinson's disease, who may well show adaptation problems contributing to their balance dysfunction (Schieppati and Nardone, 1991; De Nunzio and Schieppati, 2007; Weissblueth et al., 2008; Nanhoe-Mahabier et al., 2012; Paul et al., 2013; Schoneburg et al., 2013), and patients with stroke (Kitago and Krakauer, 2013) or spinal cord injury, in which co-activation of TA and Sol contribute to impaired balance and walking ability (Beauparlant et al., 2013; Manella et al., 2013).

AUTHOR CONTRIBUTIONS

MS and AN conceptualized the study and designed the experiments. SS performed the experiments. SS and MS performed the data analysis. All the authors made contributions in drafting the manuscript and have approved the final version.

FUNDING

Supported in part by "Ricerca Finalizzata" grants (RF-2010-2312497, RF-2011-02352379) from the Italian Ministry of Health to AN and MS, and by "PRIN" grants (2009JMMYFZ and 2010MEFNF7) from the Italian Ministry of University to MS.

REFERENCES

Adi-Japha, E., Karni, A., Parnes, A., Loewenschuss, I., and Vakil, E. (2008). A shift in task routines during the learning of a motor skill: group-averaged data may mask critical phases in the individuals' acquisition of skilled performance. *J. Exp. Psychol. Learn Mem. Cogn.* 34, 1544–1551. doi: 10.1037/a0013217

Allum, J. H., Tang, K. S., Carpenter, M. G., Oude Nijhuis, L. B., and Bloem, B. R. (2011). Review of first trial responses in balance control: influence of vestibular loss and Parkinson's disease. *Hum. Mov. Sci.* 30, 279–295. doi: 10.1016/j.humov.2010.11.009

Altman, D., Minozzo, F. C., and Rassier, D. E. (2015). Thixotropy and rheopexy of muscle fibers probed using sinusoidal oscillations. *PLoS One* 10:e0121726. doi: 10.1371/journal.pone.0121726

Álvarez-Blanco, S., Leon, L., and Valls-Solé, J. (2009). The startle reaction to somatosensory inputs: different response pattern to stimuli of upper and lower limbs. *Exp. Brain Res.* 195, 285–292. doi: 10.1007/s00221-009-1784-7

Aruin, A. S., Forrest, W. R., and Latash, M. L. (1998). Anticipatory postural adjustments in conditions of postural instability. *Electroencephalogr. Clin. Neurophysiol.* 109, 350–359. doi: 10.1016/s0924-980x(98)00029-0

Aruin, A. S., Kanekar, N., and Lee, Y. J. (2015). Anticipatory and compensatory postural adjustments in individuals with multiple sclerosis in response to external perturbations. *Neurosci. Lett.* 591, 182–186. doi: 10.1016/j.neulet.2015.02.050

Assländer, L., and Peterka, R. J. (2014). Sensory reweighting dynamics in human postural control. *J. Neurophysiol.* 111, 1852–1864. doi: 10.1152/jn.00669.2013

Bathien, N., Toma, S., and Rondot, P. (1981). Shortening reaction in man in various neurological disorders. *Electroencephalogr. Clin. Neurophysiol.* 51, 156–164. doi: 10.1016/0013-4694(81)90004-3

Beauparlant, J., van den Brand, R., Barraud, Q., Friedli, L., Musienko, P., Dietz, V., et al. (2013). Undirected compensatory plasticity contributes to neuronal dysfunction after severe spinal cord injury. *Brain.* 136, 3347–3361. doi: 10.1093/brain/awt204

Berardelli, A., and Hallett, M. (1984). Shortening reaction of human tibialis anterior. *Neurology* 34, 242–245. doi: 10.1212/wnl.34.2.242

Berger, W., Discher, M., Trippel, M., Ibrahim, I. K., and Dietz, V. (1992). Developmental aspects of stance regulation, compensation and adaptation. *Exp. Brain Res.* 90, 610–619. doi: 10.1007/bf00230945

Bisdorff, A. R., Bronstein, A. M., and Gresty, M. A. (1994). Responses in neck and facial muscles to sudden free fall and a startling auditory stimulus. *Electroencephalogr. Clin. Neurophysiol.* 93, 409–416. doi: 10.1016/0013-4694(94)00232-a

Blouin, J., Saradjian, A. H., Lebar, N., Guillaume, A., and Mouchnino, L. (2014). Opposed optimal strategies of weighting somatosensory inputs for planning reaching movements toward visual and proprioceptive targets. *J. Neurophysiol.* 112, 2290–2301. doi: 10.1152/jn.00857.2013

Bolton, D. A., Patel, R., Staines, W. R., and McIlroy, W. E. (2011). Transient inhibition of primary motor cortex suppresses hand muscle responses during a reactive reach to grasp. *Neurosci. Lett.* 504, 83–87. doi: 10.1016/j.neulet.2011.09.001

Bouisset, S., and Do, M. C. (2008). Posture, dynamic stability and voluntary movement. *Neurophysiol. Clin.* 38, 345–362. doi: 10.1016/j.neucli.2008.10.001

Buchanan, J. J., and Horak, F. B. (1999). Emergence of postural patterns as a function of vision and translation frequency. *J. Neurophysiol.* 81, 2325–2339.

Buchanan, J. J., and Horak, F. B. (2001–2002). Vestibular loss disrupts control of head and trunk on a sinusoidally moving platform. *J. Vestib. Res.* 11, 371–389.

Campbell, A. D., Squair, J. W., Chua, R., Inglis, J. T., and Carpenter, M. G. (2013). First trial and Start React effects induced by balance perturbations to upright stance. *J. Neurophysiol.* 110, 2236–2245. doi: 10.1152/jn.00766.2012

Cappa, P., Patanè, F., Rossi, S., Petrarca, M., Castelli, E., and Berthoz, A. (2008). Effect of changing visual condition and frequency of horizontal oscillations on postural balance of standing healthy subjects. *Gait Posture* 28, 615–626. doi: 10.1016/j.gaitpost.2008.04.013

Cenciarini, M., and Peterka, R. J. (2006). Stimulus-dependent changes in the vestibular contribution to human postural control. *J. Neurophysiol.* 95, 2733–2750. doi: 10.1152/jn.00856.2004

Corbeil, P., Bloem, B. R., van Meel, M., and Maki, B. E. (2013). Arm reactions evoked by the initial exposure to a small balance perturbation: a pilot study. *Gait Posture* 37, 300–303. doi: 10 1016/j.gaitpost.2012.07.017

Cordo, P. J., and Gurfinkel, V. S. (2004). Motor coordination can be fully understood only by studying complex movements. *Prog. Brain Res.* 143, 29–38. doi: 10.1016/s0079-6123(03)43003-3

Corna, S., Nardone, A., Prestinari, A., Galante, M., Grasso, M., and Schieppati, M. (2003). Comparison of Cawthorne-Cooksey exercises and sinusoidal support surface translations to improve balance in patients with unilateral vestibular deficit. *Arch. Phys. Med. Rehabil.* 84, 1173–1184. doi: 10.1016/s0003-9993(03)00130-8

Corna, S., Tarantola, J., Nardone, A., Giordano, A., and Schieppati, M. (1999). Standing on a continuously moving platform: is body inertia counteracted or exploited? *Exp. Brain Res.* 124, 331–341. doi: 10.1007/s002210050630

Crevecoeur, F., Kurtzer, I., and Scott, S. H. (2012). Fast corrective responses are evoked by perturbations approaching the natural variability of posture and movement tasks. *J. Neurophysiol.* 107, 2821–2832. doi: 10.1152/jn.00849.2011

De Nunzio, A. M., Nardone, A., Picco, D., Nilsson, J., and Schieppati, M. (2008). Alternate trains of postural muscle vibration promote cyclic body displacement in standing parkinsonian patients. *Mov. Disord.* 23, 2186–2193. doi: 10.1002/mds.22201

De Nunzio, A. M., Nardone, A., and Schieppati, M. (2005). Head stabilization on a continuously oscillating platform: the effect of a proprioceptive disturbance on the balancing strategy. *Exp. Brain Res.* 165, 261–272. doi: 10.1007/s00221-005-2297-7

De Nunzio, A. M., and Schieppati, M. (2007). Time to reconfigure balancing behaviour in man: changing visual condition while riding a continuously moving platform. *Exp. Brain Res.* 178, 18–36. doi: 10.1007/s00221-006-0708-z

Diener, H. C., Bootz, F., Dichgans, J., and Bruzek, W. (1983). Variability of postural "reflexes" in humans. *Exp. Brain Res.* 52, 423–428. doi: 10.1007/bf00238035

Dietz, V., Trippel, M., Ibrahim, I. K., and Berger, W. (1993). Human stance on a sinusoidally translating platform: balance control by feedforward and feedback mechanisms. *Exp. Brain Res.* 93, 352–362. doi: 10.1007/bf00228405

Dokka, K., Kenyon, R. V., and Keshner, E. A. (2009). Influence of visual scene velocity on segmental kinematics during stance. *Gait Posture* 30, 211–216. doi: 10.1016/j.gaitpost.2009.05.001

Elion, O., Sela, I., Bahat, Y., Siev-Ner, I., Weiss, P. L., and Karni, A. (2015). Balance maintenance as an acquired motor skill: delayed gains and robust retention after a single session of training in a virtual environment. *Brain Res.* 1609, 54–62. doi: 10.1016/j.brainres.2015.03.020

Franklin, D. W., Burdet, E., Tee, K. P., Osu, R., Chew, C. M., Milner, T. E., et al. (2008). CNS learns stable, accurate and efficient movements using a simple algorithm. *J. Neurosci.* 28, 11165–11173. doi: 10.1523/JNEUROSCI.3099-08.2008

Fransson, P. A., Hjerpe, M., and Johansson, R. (2007). Adaptation of multi-segmented body movements during vibratory proprioceptive and galvanic vestibular stimulation. *J. Vestib. Res.* 17, 47–62.

Fujiwara, K., Irei, M., Kiyota, N., Yaguchi, C., and Maeda, K. (2016). Event-related brain potential and postural muscle activity during standing on an oscillating table while the knee, hip and trunk are fixed. *J. Physiol. Anthropol.* 35:6. doi: 10.1186/s40101-016-0088-4

Fujiwara, K., Kiyota, T., Maeda, K., and Horak, F. B. (2007). Postural control adaptability to floor oscillation in the elderly. *J. Physiol. Anthropol.* 26, 485–493. doi: 10.2114/jpa2.26.485

Fujiwara, K., Maeda, K., Irei, M., Mammadova, A., and Kiyota, N. (2012). Changes in event-related potentials associated with postural adaptation during floor oscillation. *Neuroscience* 213, 122–132. doi: 10.1016/j.neuroscience.2012.03.027

Fujiwara, K., Toyama, H., Kiyota, T., and Maeda, K. (2006). Postural muscle activity patterns during standing at rest and on an oscillating floor. *J. Electromyogr. Kinesiol.* 16, 448–457. doi: 10.1016/j.jelekin.2005.08.008

Geertsen, S. S., Kjær, M., Pedersen, K. K., Petersen, T. H., Perez, M. A., and Nielsen, J. B. (2013). Central common drive to antagonistic ankle muscles in relation to short-term cocontraction training in nondancers and professional ballet dancers. *J. Appl. Physiol. (1985)* 115, 1075–1081. doi: 10.1152/japplphysiol.00707.2012

Gresty, M. A., and Bronstein, A. M. (1992). Visually controlled spatial stabilisation of the human head: compensation for the eye's limited ability to roll. *Neurosci. Lett.* 140, 63–66. doi: 10.1016/0304-3940(92)90682-w

Gurfinkel, V. S., Ivanenko, Y. P., and Levik, Y. S. (1997). Muscle resistance to slow ramp weakly depends on activation level. *Neuroscience* 80, 299–306. doi: 10.1016/s0306-4522(97)00130-9

Hagbarth, K. E.,, Nordin, M., and Bongiovanni, L. G. (1995). After-effects on stiffness and stretch reflexes of human finger flexor muscles attributed to muscle thixotropy. *J. Physiol.* 482, 215–223. doi: 10.1113/jphysiol.1995.sp020511

Hemami, H., and Moussavi, Z. (2014). A model of the basal ganglia in voluntary movement and postural reactions. *Comput. Methods Biomech. Biomed. Engin.* 17, 1432–1446. doi: 10.1080/10255842.2012.751983

Honeine, J. L., Crisafulli, O., Sozzi, S., and Schieppati, M. (2015). Processing time of addition or withdrawal of single or combined balance-stabilizing haptic and visual information. *J. Neurophysiol.* 114, 3097–3110. doi: 10.1152/jn.00618.2015

Horak, F. B., Diener, H. C., and Nashner, L. M. (1989). Influence of central set on human postural responses. *J. Neurophysiol.* 62, 841–853.

Horak, F. B., and Nashner, L. M. (1986). Central programming of postural movements: adaptation to altered support surface configurations. *J. Neurophysiol.* 55, 1369–1381.

Huberdeau, D. M., Krakauer, J. W., and Haith, A. M. (2015). Dual-process decomposition in human sensorimotor adaptation. *Curr. Opin. Neurobiol.* 33, 71–77. doi: 10.1016/j.conb.2015.03.003

Isableu, B., Ohlmann, T., Cremieux, J., Vuillerme, N., Amblard, B., and Gresty, M. A. (2010). Individual differences in the ability to identify, select and use appropriate frames of reference for perceptuo-motor control. *Neuroscience* 169, 1199–1215. doi: 10.1016/j.neuroscience.2010.05.072

Jacobs, J. V., and Horak, F. B. (2007). External postural perturbations induce multiple anticipatory postural adjustments when subjects cannot pre-select their stepping foot. *Exp. Brain Res.* 179, 29–42. doi: 10.1007/s00221-006-0763-5

Joseph Jilk, D., Safavynia, S. A., and Ting, L. H. (2014). Contribution of vision to postural behaviors during continuous support-surface translations. *Exp. Brain Res.* 232, 169–180. doi: 10.1007/s00221-013-3729-4

Kanekar, N., and Aruin, A. S. (2015). Improvement of anticipatory postural adjustments for balance control: effect of a single training session. *J. Electromyogr. Kinesiol.* 25, 400–405. doi: 10.1016/j.jelekin.2014.11.002

Katz, R., and Rondot, P. (1978). Muscle reaction to passive shortening in normal man. *Electroencephalogr. Clin. Neurophysiol.* 45, 90–99. doi: 10.1016/0013-4694(78)90345-0

Kennedy, A., Guevel, A., and Sveistrup, H. (2012). Impact of ankle muscle fatigue and recovery on the anticipatory postural adjustments to externally initiated perturbations in dynamic postural control. *Exp. Brain Res.* 223, 553–562. doi: 10.1007/s00221-012-3282-6

Keshner, E. A., Allum, J. H., and Pfaltz, C. R. (1987). Postural coactivation and adaptation in the sway stabilizing responses of normals and patients with bilateral vestibular deficit. *Exp. Brain Res.* 69, 77–92. doi: 10.1007/bf00247031

Kiemel, T., Zhang, Y., and Jeka, J. J. (2011). Identification of neural feedback for upright stance in humans: stabilization rather than sway minimization. *J. Neurosci.* 31, 15144–15153. doi: 10.1523/JNEUROSCI.1013-11.2011

Kitago, T., and Krakauer, J. W. (2013). Motor learning principles for neurorehabilitation. *Handb. Clin. Neurol.* 110, 93–103. doi: 10.1016/B978-0-444-52901-5.00008-3

Laessoe, U., and Voigt, M. (2008). Anticipatory postural control strategies related to predictive perturbations. *Gait Posture* 28, 62–68. doi: 10.1016/j.gaitpost.2007.10.001

Li, L., and Caldwell, G. E. (1999). Coefficient of cross correlation and the time domain correspondence. *J. Electromyogr. Kinesiol.* 9, 385–389. doi: 10.1016/s1050-6411(99)00012-7

Lison, L. (1960). *Statistique Appliquée à La Biologie Expérimentale. La Planification De L'éxperience Et l'analyse Des Résultats.* France: Gauthier-Villars.

Lotze, M., Braun, C., Birbaumer, N., Anders, S., and Cohen, L. G. (2003). Motor learning elicited by voluntary drive. *Brain* 126, 866–872. doi: 10.1093/brain/awg079

Maki, B. E., and McIlroy, W. E. (1997). The role of limb movements in maintaining upright stance: the "change-in-support" strategy. *Phys. Ther.* 77, 488–507.

Maki, B. E., and McIlroy, W. E. (2007). Cognitive demands and cortical control of human balance-recovery reactions. *J. Neural Transm. (Vienna)* 114, 1279–1296. doi: 10.1007/s00702-007-0764-y

Manella, K. J., Roach, K. E., and Field-Fote, E. C. (2013). Operant conditioning to increase ankle control or decrease reflex excitability improves reflex modulation and walking function in chronic spinal cord injury. *J. Neurophysiol.* 109, 2666–2679. doi: 10.1152/jn.01039.2011

Massion, J. (1992). Movement, posture and equilibrium: interaction and coordination. *Prog. Neurobiol.* 38, 35–56. doi: 10.1016/0301-0082(92)90034-c

McIlroy, W. E., and Maki, B. E. (1993). Do anticipatory postural adjustments precede compensatory stepping reactions evoked by perturbation? *Neurosci. Lett.* 164, 199–202. doi: 10.1016/0304-3940(93)90891-n

Mierau, A., Hülsdünker, T., and Strüder, H. K. (2015). Changes in cortical activity associated with adaptive behavior during repeated balance perturbation of unpredictable timing. *Front. Behav. Neurosci.* 9:272. doi: 10.3389/fnbeh.2015.00272

Milner, T. E., and Franklin, D. W. (2005). Impedance control and internal model use during the initial stage of adaptation to novel dynamics in humans. *J. Physiol.* 567, 651–664. doi: 10.1113/jphysiol.2005.090449

Miscio, G., Pisano, F., Del Conte, C., Pianca, D., Colombo, R., and Schieppati, M. (2001). The shortening reaction of forearm muscles: the influence of central set. *Clin. Neurophysiol.* 112, 884–894. doi: 10.1016/s1388-2457(01)00468-0

Nanhoe-Mahabier, W., Allum, J. H., Overeem, S., Borm, G. F., Oude Nijhuis, L. B., and Bloem, B. R. (2012). First trial reactions and habituation rates over successive balance perturbations in Parkinson's disease. *Neuroscience* 217, 123–129. doi: 10.1016/j.neuroscience.2012.03.064

Nardone, A., Galante, M., Grasso, M., and Schieppati, M. (2008). Stance ataxia and delayed leg muscle responses to postural perturbations in cervical spondylotic myelopathy. *J. Rehabil. Med.* 40, 539–547. doi: 10.2340/16501977-0214

Nardone, A., Galante, M., Pareyson, D., and Schieppati, M. (2007). Balance control in sensory neuron disease. *Clin. Neurophysiol.* 118, 538–550. doi: 10.1016/j.clinph.2006.11.012

Nardone, A., Giordano, A., Corrà, T., and Schieppati, M. (1990). Responses of leg muscles in humans displaced while standing. *Brain* 113, 65–84. doi: 10.1093/brain/113.1.65

Nardone, A., Godi, M., Artuso, A., and Schieppati, M. (2010). Balance rehabilitation by moving platform and exercises in patients with neuropathy or vestibular deficit. *Arch. Phys. Med. Rehabil.* 91, 1869–1877. doi: 10.1016/j.apmr.2010.09.011

Nardone, A., Grasso, M., and Schieppati, M. (2006). Balance control in peripheral neuropathy: are patients equally unstable under static and dynamic conditions? *Gait Posture* 23, 364–373. doi: 10.1016/j.gaitpost.2005.04.002

Nardone, A., Grasso, M., Tarantola, J., Corna, S., and Schieppati, M. (2000). Postural coordination in elderly subjects standing on a periodically moving platform. *Arch. Phys. Med. Rehabil.* 81, 1217–1223. doi: 10.1053/apmr.2000.6286

Nardone, A., and Schieppati, M. (1998). Medium-latency response to muscle stretch in human lower limb: estimation of conduction velocity of group II fibres and central delay. *Neurosci. Lett.* 249, 29–32. doi: 10.1016/s0304-3940(98)00383-8

Nardone, A., and Schieppati, M. (2006). Balance in Parkinson's disease under static and dynamic conditions. *Mov. Disord.* 21, 1515–1520. doi: 10.1002/mds.21015

Nardone, A., Schieppati, M., Arcolin, M., Godi, M., Grasso, M., Guglielmetti, S., et al. (2015). "Continuous and predictable perturbation of balance in Parkinson's disease: a way of testing reflex and anticipatory responses of leg muscles and of training balance," in *Proceedings of the Congress Neurorehabilitation and Neural Repair* (Maastricht), 27.

Nardone, A., Turcato, A. M., and Schieppati, M. (2014). Effects of balance and gait rehabilitation in cerebellar disease of vascular or degenerative origin. *Restor. Neurol. Neurosci.* 32, 233–245. doi: 10.3233/RNN-130315

Nashner, L. M. (1976). Adapting reflexes controlling the human posture. *Exp. Brain Res.* 26, 59–72. doi: 10.1007/bf00235249

Nielsen, J., and Kagamihara, Y. (1992). The regulation of disynaptic reciprocal Ia inhibition during co-contraction of antagonistic muscles in man. *J. Physiol.* 456, 373–391. doi: 10.1113/jphysiol.1992.sp019341

Nonnekes, J., Carpenter, M. G., Inglis, J. T., Duysens, J., and Weerdesteyn, V. (2015). What startles tell us about control of posture and gait. *Neurosci. Biobehav. Rev.* 53, 131–138. doi: 10.1016/j.neubiorev.2015.04.002

Obata, H., Sekiguchi, H., Ohtsuki, T., and Nakazawa, K. (2014). Posture-related modulation of cortical excitability in the tibialis anterior muscle in humans. *Brain Res.* 1577, 29–35. doi: 10.1016/j.brainres.2014.06.027

Osu, R., Franklin, D. W., Kato, H., Gomi, H., Domen, K., Yoshioka, T., et al. (2002). Short- and long-term changes in joint cocontraction associated with motor learning as revealed from surface EMG. *J. Neurophysiol.* 88, 991–1004.

Ouchi, Y., Okada, H., Yoshikawa, E., Nobezawa, S., and Futatsubashi, M. (1999). Brain activation during maintenance of standing postures in humans. *Brain* 122, 329–338. doi: 10.1093/brain/122.2.329

Oude Nijhuis, L. B., Allum, J. H., Borm, G. F., Honegger, F., Overeem, S., and Bloem, B. R. (2009). Directional sensitivity of "first trial" reactions in human balance control. *J. Neurophysiol.* 101, 2802–2814. doi: 10.1152/jn.90945.2008

Oude Nijhuis, L. B., Allum, J. H., Valls-Solé, J., Overeem, S., and Bloem, B. R. (2010). First trial postural reactions to unexpected balance disturbances: a comparison with the acoustic startle reaction. *J. Neurophysiol.* 104, 2704–2712. doi: 10.1152/jn.01080.2009

Pai, Y. C., and Bhatt, T. S. (2007). Repeated-slip training: an emerging paradigm for prevention of slip-related falls among older adults. *Phys. Ther.* 87, 1478–1491. doi: 10.2522/ptj.20060326

Patel, P., and Bhatt, T. (2015). Adaptation to large-magnitude treadmill-based perturbations: improvements in reactive balance response. *Physiol. Rep.* 3:12247. doi: 10.14814/phy2.12247

Patla, A. E., Ishac, M. G., and Winter, D. A. (2002). Anticipatory control of center of mass and joint stability during voluntary arm movement from a standing posture: interplay between active and passive control. *Exp. Brain Res.* 143, 318–327. doi: 10.1007/s00221-001-0968-6

Paul, S. S., Sherrington, C., Fung, V. S., and Canning, C. G. (2013). Motor and cognitive impairments in Parkinson disease: relationships with specific balance and mobility tasks. *Neurorehabil. Neural Repair* 27, 63–71. doi: 10.1177/1545968312446754

Peterka, R. J., and Loughlin, P. J. (2004). Dynamic regulation of sensorimotor integration in human postural control. *J. Neurophysiol.* 91, 410–423. doi: 10.1152/jn.00516.2003

Petersen, T. H., Rosenberg, K., Petersen, N. C., and Nielsen, J. B. (2009). Cortical involvement in anticipatory postural reactions in man. *Exp. Brain Res.* 193, 161–171. doi: 10.1007/s00221-008-1603-6

Prokop, T., Berger, W., Zijlstra, W., and Dietz, V. (1995). Adaptational and learning processes during human split-belt locomotion: interaction between central mechanisms and afferent input. *Exp. Brain Res.* 106, 449–456. doi: 10.1007/bf00231067

Proske, U., Morgan, D. L., and Gregory, J. E. (1993). Thixotropy in skeletal muscle and in muscle spindles: a review. *Prog. Neurobiol.* 41, 705–721. doi: 10.1016/0301-0082(93)90032-n

Pruszynski, J. A., Kurtzer, I., and Scott, S. H. (2011). The long-latency reflex is composed of at least two functionally independent processes. *J. Neurophysiol.* 106, 449–459. doi: 10.1152/jn.01052.2010

Pruszynski, J. A., and Scott, S. H. (2012). Optimal feedback control and the long-latency stretch response. *Exp. Brain Res.* 218, 341–359. doi: 10.1007/s00221-012-3041-8

Rogers, M. W., Hedman, L. D., Johnson, M. E., Martinez, K. M., and Mille, M. L. (2003). Triggering of protective stepping for the control of human balance: age and contextual dependence. *Brain Res. Cogn. Brain Res.* 16, 192–198. doi: 10.1016/s0926-6410(02)00273-2

Safavynia, S. A., and Ting, L. H. (2013). Sensorimotor feedback based on task-relevant error robustly predicts temporal recruitment and multidirectional tuning of muscle synergies. *J. Neurophysiol.* 109, 31–45. doi: 10.1152/jn.00684.2012

Saling, L. L., and Phillips, J. G. (2007). Automatic behaviour: efficient not mindless. *Brain Res. Bull.* 73, 1–20. doi: 10.1016/j.brainresbull.2007.02.009

Sanders, O. P., Savin, D. N., Creath, R. A., and Rogers, M. W. (2015). Protective balance and startle responses to sudden freefall in standing humans. *Neurosci. Lett.* 586, 8–12. doi: 10.1016/j.neulet.2014.11.034

Schieppati, M., Giordano, A., and Nardone, A. (2002). Variability in a dynamic postural task attests ample flexibility in balance control mechanisms. *Exp. Brain Res.* 144, 200–210. doi: 10.1007/s00221-002-1028-6

Schieppati, M., Hugon, M., Grasso, M., Nardone, A., and Galante, M. (1994). The limits of equilibrium in young and elderly normal subjects and in parkinsonians. *Electroencephalogr. Clin. Neurophysiol.* 93, 286–298. doi: 10.1016/0013-4694(94)00036-k

Schieppati, M., and Nardone, A. (1991). Free and supported stance in Parkinson's disease. The effect of posture and 'postural set' on leg muscle responses to perturbation, and its relation to the severity of the disease. *Brain* 114, 1227–1244. doi: 10.1093/brain/114.3.1227

Schieppati, M., and Nardone, A. (1995). Time course of 'set'-related changes in muscle responses to stance perturbation in humans. *J. Physiol.* 487, 787–796. doi: 10.1113/jphysiol.1995.sp020918

Schieppati, M., Nardone, A., Siliotto, R., and Grasso, M. (1995). Early and late stretch responses of human foot muscles induced by perturbation of stance. *Exp. Brain Res.* 105, 411–422.

Schmid, M., Bottaro, A., Sozzi, S., and Schieppati, M. (2011). Adaptation to continuous perturbation of balance: progressive reduction of postural muscle activity with invariant or increasing oscillations of the center of mass depending on perturbation frequency and vision conditions. *Hum. Mov. Sci.* 30, 262–278. doi: 10.1016/j.humov.2011.02.002

Schmid, M., Casabianca, L., Bottaro, A., and Schieppati, M. (2008). Graded changes in balancing behavior as a function of visual acuity. *Neuroscience* 153, 1079–1091. doi: 10.1016/j.neuroscience.2008.03.024

Schmid, M., Nardone, A., De Nunzio, A. M., Schmid, M., and Schieppati, M. (2007). Equilibrium during static and dynamic tasks in blind subjects: no evidence of cross-modal plasticity. *Brain* 130, 2097–2107. doi: 10.1093/brain/awm157

Schoneburg, B., Mancini, M., Horak, F., and Nutt, J. G. (2013). Framework for understanding balance dysfunction in Parkinson's disease. *Mov. Disord.* 28, 1474–1482. doi: 10.1002/mds.25613

Shadmehr, R., Smith, M. A., and Krakauer, J. W. (2010). Error correction, sensory prediction and adaptation in motor control. *Annu. Rev. Neurosci.* 33, 89–108. doi: 10.1146/annurev-neuro-060909-153135

Siegmund, G. P., Blouin, J. S., and Inglis, J. T. (2008). Does startle explain the exaggerated first response to a transient perturbation? *Exerc. Sport Sci. Rev.* 36, 76–82. doi: 10.1097/JES.0b013e318168f1ce

Solopova, I. A., Selionov, V. A., Kazennikov, O. V., and Ivanenko, Y. P. (2014). Effects of transcranial magnetic stimulation during voluntary and non-voluntary stepping movements in humans. *Neurosci. Lett.* 579, 64–69. doi: 10.1016/j.neulet.2014.07.015

Soto, O., Valls-Solé, J., Shanahan, P., and Rothwell, J. (2006). Reduction of intracortical inhibition in soleus muscle during postural activity. *J. Neurophysiol.* 96, 1711–1717. doi: 10.1152/jn.00133.2006

Sozzi, S., Honeine, J. L., Do, M. C., and Schieppati, M. (2013). Leg muscle activity during tandem stance and the control of body balance in the frontal plane. *Clin. Neurophysiol.* 124, 1175–1186. doi: 10.1016/j.clinph.2012.12.001

Sozzi, S., Monti, A., De Nunzio, A. M., Do, M. C., and Schieppati, M. (2011). Sensori-motor integration during stance: time adaptation of control mechanisms on adding or removing vision. *Hum. Mov. Sci.* 30, 172–189. doi: 10.1016/j.humov.2010.06.002

Sumner, P., and Husain, M. (2008). At the edge of consciousness: automatic motor activation and voluntary control. *Neuroscientist* 14, 474–486. doi: 10.1177/1073858408314435

Tang, K. S., Honegger, F., and Allum, J. H. (2012). Movement patterns underlying first trial responses in human balance corrections. *Neuroscience* 225, 140–151. doi: 10.1016/j.neuroscience.2012.09.004

Taube, W., Gruber, M., Beck, S., Faist, M., Gollhofer, A., and Schubert, M. (2007). Cortical and spinal adaptations induced by balance training: correlation between stance stability and corticospinal activation. *Acta Physiol. (Oxf)* 189, 347–358. doi: 10.1111/j.1748-1716.2007.01665.x

Taube, W., Schubert, M., Gruber, M., Beck, S., Faist, M., and Gollhofer, A. (2006). Direct corticospinal pathways contribute to neuromuscular control of perturbed stance. *J. Appl. Physiol. (1985)* 101, 420–429. doi: 10.1152/japplphysiol.01447.2005

Taylor, J. A., Krakauer, J. W., and Ivry, R. B. (2014). Explicit and implicit contributions to learning in a sensorimotor adaptation task. *J. Neurosci.* 34, 3023–3032. doi: 10.1523/JNEUROSCI.3619-13.2014

Thoroughman, K. A., and Shadmehr, R. (1999). Electromyographic correlates of learning internal models of reaching movements. *J. Neurosci.* 19, 8573–8588.

Tjernström, F., Bagher, A., Fransson, P. A., and Magnusson, M. (2010a). Short and long-term postural learning to withstand galvanic vestibular perturbations. *J. Vestib. Res.* 20, 407–417. doi: 10.3233/VES-2010-0391

Tjernström, F., Fransson, P. A., Patel, M., and Magnusson, M. (2010b). Postural control and adaptation are influenced by preceding postural challenges. *Exp. Brain Res.* 202, 613–621. doi: 10.1007/s00221-010-2166-x

Tokuno, C. D., Taube, W., and Cresswell, A. G. (2009). An enhanced level of motor cortical excitability during the control of human standing. *Acta Physiol. (Oxf)* 195, 385–395. doi: 10.1111/j.1748-1716.2008.01898.x

Van Ooteghem, K., Frank, J. S., Allard, F., Buchanan, J. J., Oates, A. R., and Horak, F. B. (2008). Compensatory postural adaptations during continuous, variable amplitude perturbations reveal generalized rather than sequence-specific learning. *Exp. Brain Res.* 187, 603–611. doi: 10.1007/s00221-008-1329-5

Vieira, O. Jr., Coelho, D. B., and Teixeira, L. A. (2014). Asymmetric balance control between legs for quiet but not for perturbed stance. *Exp. Brain Res.* 232, 3269–3276. doi: 10.1007/s00221-014-4018-6

Weissblueth, E., Schwartz, M., and Hocherman, S. (2008). Adaptation to cyclic stance perturbations in Parkinson's disease depends on postural demands. *Parkinsonism Relat. Disord.* 14, 489–494. doi: 10.1016/j.parkreldis.2007.12.002

Welch, T. D., and Ting, L. H. (2014). Mechanisms of motor adaptation in reactive balance control. *PLoS One* 9:e96440. doi: 10.1371/journal.pone.0096440

Winter, D. A. (2009). *Biomechanics and Motor Control of Human Movement.* 4th Edn. New York, NY: John Wiley & Sons.

Wright, W. G., Ivanenko, Y. P., and Gurfinkel, V. S. (2012). Foot anatomy specialization for postural sensation and control. *J. Neurophysiol.* 107, 1513–1521. doi: 10.1152/jn.00256.2011

Zwergal, A., Linn, J., Xiong, G., Brandt, T., Strupp, M., and Jahn, K. (2012). Aging of human supraspinal locomotor and postural control in fMRI. *Neurobiol. Aging* 33, 1073–1084. doi: 10.1016/j.neurobiolaging.2010.09.022

8

The Throw-and-Catch Model of Human Gait: Evidence from Coupling of Pre-Step Postural Activity and Step Location

*Matthew J. Bancroft and Brian L. Day**

Sobell Department of Motor Neuroscience and Movement Disorders, UCL Institute of Neurology, University College London, London, UK

***Correspondence:**
Brian L. Day
brian.day@ucl.ac.uk

Postural activity normally precedes the lift of a foot from the ground when taking a step, but its function is unclear. The throw-and-catch hypothesis of human gait proposes that the pre-step activity is organized to generate momentum for the body to fall ballistically along a specific trajectory during the step. The trajectory is appropriate for the stepping foot to land at its intended location while at the same time being optimally placed to catch the body and regain balance. The hypothesis therefore predicts a strong coupling between the pre-step activity and step location. Here we examine this coupling when stepping to visually-presented targets at different locations. Ten healthy, young subjects were instructed to step as accurately as possible onto targets placed in five locations that required either different step directions or different step lengths. In 75% of trials, the target location remained constant throughout the step. In the remaining 25% of trials, the intended step location was changed by making the target jump to a new location 96 ms ± 43 ms after initiation of the pre-step activity, long before foot lift. As predicted by the throw-and-catch hypothesis, when the target location remained constant, the pre-step activity led to body momentum at foot lift that was coupled to the intended step location. When the target location jumped, the pre-step activity was adjusted (median latency 223 ms) and prolonged (on average by 69 ms), which altered the body's momentum at foot lift according to where the target had moved. We conclude that whenever possible the coupling between the pre-step activity and the step location is maintained. This provides further support for the throw-and-catch hypothesis of human gait.

Keywords: postural balance, gait initiation, motor activity, humans, gait, biomechanical phenomena, locomotion, walking

INTRODUCTION

When taking a step, postural activity usually precedes the lift of the stepping foot by around half a second. It modulates the force between the feet and ground to accelerate the body sideways and forwards, and is observed during single steps as well as during locomotion (Carlsöö, 1966; Mann et al., 1979; Crenna and Frigo, 1991; Jian et al., 1993; MacKinnon and Winter, 1993). What is the function of this pre-step activity? One possibility is that its job is to move the body mass directly over the upcoming stance foot, allowing the stepping foot to be lifted freely without compromising balance. However, this is not what is usually observed during single steps or locomotion. At the instant the stepping foot is lifted, the vertical projection of the body's center of mass (CoM) commonly lies outside and medial to the base of support formed by the stance foot (Jian et al., 1993; MacKinnon and Winter, 1993; Lyon and Day, 1997, 2005). This means that the body is not balanced, but is falling sideways under gravity during a step.

An alternative function of the pre-step activity has been proposed by the throw-and-catch model of human gait (Lyon and Day, 1997). This hypothesis states that the pre-step activity represents a "throw", which gives the body a specific position and momentum at the time of foot lift. At this point, the body enters a ballistic phase during the step where it falls under gravity along a trajectory determined by the pre-step activity, just as a ball would after being thrown. The direction and magnitude of the throw is finely tuned to take into account the initial state of the body and the intended final position of the stepping foot. Thus, during the step, the stepping foot swings towards its intended target while at the same time being optimally placed when it lands to "catch" the body and regain balance.

The throw-and-catch model predicts that the pre-step activity depends on both the body's initial conditions and the intended step location. In support of this are the findings that the resulting position and velocity of the body's CoM at the point of foot lift depend on both the initial stance width (Lyon and Day, 1997) and whether the step is to a forward or diagonal location (Lyon and Day, 1997, 2005), but are not influenced by the final position of the trailing foot (Lyon and Day, 2005). However, the predicted coupling between the pre-step activity and the intended step location has been shown to be breakable under certain circumstances. If the intended step location changes after the stepping foot leaves the ground, for example by shifting the position of a target, it is possible for the foot to land at a location different to that originally planned (Reynolds and Day, 2005, 2007; Kim and Brunt, 2009, 2013; Tseng et al., 2009; Nonnekes et al., 2010). This ability to de-couple the pre-step activity from the step location represents a challenge to the throw-and-catch hypothesis.

Here we investigate the strength of coupling between the pre-step activity and the step location under conditions previously unexplored. First, we study stepping onto five (for each foot) possible target locations, either demanding different step directions with the same step length, or demanding different step lengths with the same direction. The throw-and-catch hypothesis predicts that the pre-step activity will differ and be unique for each target location. Second, we occasionally make the central target jump to another location just after the pre-step activity has been initiated, but before the stepping foot has been lifted. This timing of target jump potentially allows the pre-step activity to be adjusted should it be advantageous to do so. The crucial question, therefore, is whether the pre-step activity is adjusted to take account of the new target location, or is unchanged such that all necessary adjustments are made later during the step, similar to that observed with later target jumps. Support for the throw-and-catch hypothesis would be obtained if: (1) the pre-step activity were modulated by the target jump; and (2) the modulation were dependent on the final location of the target.

MATERIALS AND METHODS

Ten human subjects (7 male; 24 ± 2 years; 64 ± 7 kg; mean ± standard deviation (SD)) gave written informed consent to participate in the experiment and reported no known neurological, sensory, muscular or orthopedic disorders. The experiment was approved by the UCL Research Ethics Committee and conformed to the *Declaration of Helsinki*. Participants were provided a written information sheet detailing the experimental procedures. Further to this, the experimental procedures were explained verbally. All subjects were naïve to the purpose of the study.

Protocol

Subjects performed a step onto a floor-bound target. Prior to the step, subjects stood barefoot and still with both feet parallel. The medial borders of the feet were separated by 15 cm. This starting position was chalk-marked to ensure a consistent starting location for all steps. The positions of the targets required a forwards movement, with five targets located on each of the left and right sides (**Figure 1**). Subjects were instructed to step as accurately as possible to the target, and bring the trailing foot alongside. An accurate step to each target was self-defined by all participants prior to the experiment. To achieve this, participants placed the appropriate foot over each of the 10 targets without time constraints in a manner they deemed accurate. For these accuracy trials, subjects were allowed to adjust their foot's position until they felt it represented an accurate step to a target. The step was redone if the subject or experimenter felt it necessary. Subjects were instructed to land their foot in this way for all subsequent steps and the position of their foot when it landed was compared to this ideal position. By instructing subjects to step accurately to the targets, rather than as quickly as possible, we sought to minimize variability in the placement of the stepping foot and thereby minimize variability in the step location.

The final position of the stepping foot was emphasized as being paramount and non-adjustable following foot landing. After the stepping foot landed subjects were required to step with the trailing foot and bring it alongside their stepping foot. The final position of the trailing foot does not affect the performance of the initial step (Lyon and Day, 2005) so no specific instruction was given as to where to place the trailing foot. However, subjects were encouraged to finish the step in a balanced state, similar to which they started. When a target illuminated to the left, a left-foot leading step was required and when a target illuminated to the right, a right-foot leading step was required. Multiple targets on both left and right sides were used to prevent prediction of target jump location or stepping side, thereby ensuring unbiased conditions at the time of target presentation and target jump.

A trial began with an audible beep, which was followed by a random delay and illumination of a step target. Illumination of the target acted as a cue for the subject to initiate a step

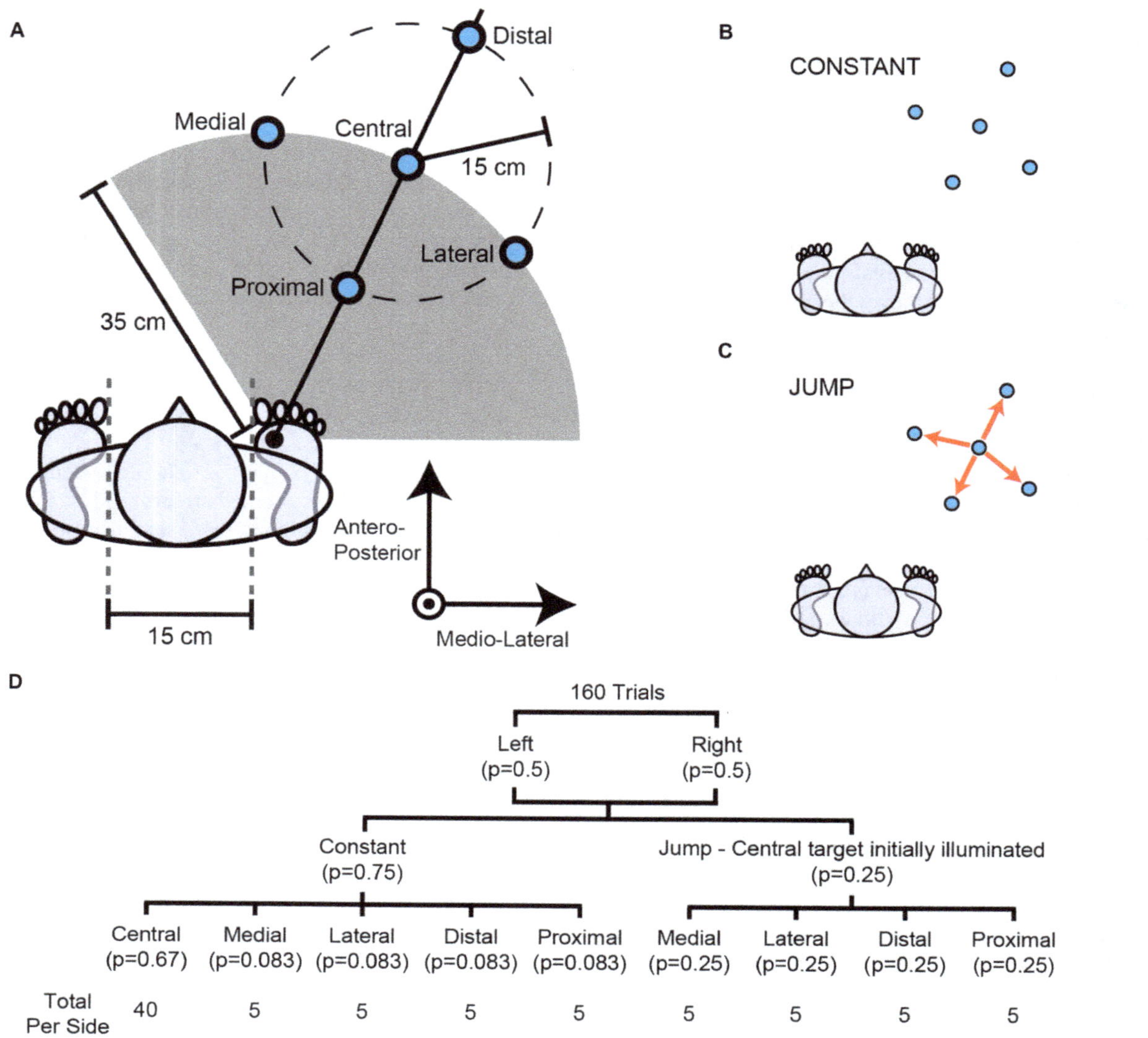

FIGURE 1 | Experimental set-up. (A) Right-sided targets are depicted; an identical configuration was present on the left side. The vertical axis protrudes directly out of the page. Subjects were instructed to step to a visually-presented target (blue circles). In most trials a target illuminated on either the left or right side and its location did not change **(B)**. In some trials the target jumped 15 cm from the central target to one of four peripheral targets (medial, lateral, distal or proximal) shortly after initiation of the pre-step activity **(C)**. **(D)** Probability tree outlining the number of trials and probability per condition. A target jump occurred with a probability of 0.33 after illumination of the central target.

to its location in their own time. The stepping targets were oriented so that step length and direction could be independently manipulated (**Figure 1A**). That is, for medial, central and lateral targets, step length was constant (35 cm) but step direction was different (0°, 25°, 50° forward of the stepping foot respectively). Equally, for proximal, central and distal targets, step direction was constant (25° forward of the stepping foot) but step length was different (20 cm, 35 cm, 50 cm respectively).

Experimental Conditions

In 75% of trials, one of the five targets on either the left or right side was selected pseudo-randomly and illuminated for the duration of the step (constant condition; **Figure 1B**). The central target was selected most frequently (probability = 0.67), whereas the peripheral targets were selected less often but each with equal frequency (probability = 0.083).

In 25% of trials, the central target was illuminated on either the left or right side and was made to unpredictably jump to one of its four peripheral targets selected pseudo-randomly (jump condition; **Figure 1C**). The peripheral targets were selected with equal frequency when a target jumped to a new location (probability = 0.25). After illumination of the central target, the probability of it jumping was 0.33.

The target jump was achieved by simultaneously extinguishing the central target and illuminating one of the four peripheral targets. Target jumps were triggered when the difference in vertical force between the stepping and trailing foot sides exceeded 80 N. This related to a mean (SD) of 7.8 (0.9)% (range: 5.7%–8.8%) of total body weight. Due to inherent electrical transmission delays, the new target would emit light 16.5 ms after the trigger signal. This delay is accounted for in all reported data. The new target appeared shortly after the initiation of the pre-step activity (mean (SD) latency: 96 (43) ms), long before the stepping foot lifted. The locations of the new targets meant that the required magnitude of foot adjustment remained constant (15 cm) but either step direction (medial- or lateral-jump) or length (distal- or proximal-jump) required modification.

A total of 160 trials were completed and performed in 10 blocks of 16 steps. The number of trials and its probability for each condition is summarized in **Figure 1D**.

Apparatus

Targets were circular (2.5 cm diameter) and illuminated via electroluminescent paper (Light Tape UK Limited, Barnsley, Yorkshire, UK) within a low-profile display on the floor in front of the subject. Ambient light conditions were dim (<0.1 Lux; Isotech 1332A Digital Illuminance Meter, Southport, Merseyside, UK) to eliminate potential distractors and ensure that the target light was compelling. Three infrared-emitting diode markers were placed at the base of the first metatarsal and head of the first (hallux) and fifth metatarsals of each foot. Marker positions were tracked at 200 Hz by two motion capture units comprising six "cameras" (Codamotion cx-1, Charnwood Dynamics, Leicestershire, UK). At the start of a trial, subjects stood with each foot over separate force platforms (9281C1, Kistler, Winterthur, Switzerland) which were embedded in the floor. Force was acquired at 1000 Hz.

Data Analysis

Both marker position and force data were digitally low-pass filtered using a zero-lag, second order Butterworth filter with 15 Hz and 30 Hz cut-off frequencies respectively. An anti-aliasing analog filter was used on force data prior to this.

The two force platforms were summed to evaluate the net force acting on the body in three-dimensions. From Newton's Second Law of Motion, the acceleration of the body's CoM was calculated by dividing net force by a subject's mass. The net acceleration of the body's CoM while the subject stood still (from the beginning of a trial until target illumination) was assumed to be zero and used as a baseline for the remainder of the trial. CoM velocity at foot lift, which has previously been shown to be an important variable in stepping (Lyon and Day, 1997, 2005), was then estimated by numerical integration of the CoM acceleration during the pre-step activity (trapezoidal method).

Typically, the center of pressure initially moves laterally towards the stepping side heel during the pre-step activity (Mann et al., 1979; Breniere et al., 1987). Therefore, the pre-step activity's initiation was calculated as the first point after target illumination that the medio-lateral (ML) center-of-pressure velocity towards the stepping foot exceeded 5 $cm.s^{-1}$ for at least 50 ms. Stepping foot lift was the first point that the stepping side's vertical force went below 1% of total body weight. Pre-step activity duration was the time from its initiation to stepping foot lift. The time the stepping foot landed was the first point after foot lift that the ML, antero-posterior (AP) and vertical speed of the stepping foot hallux marker went below 2 $cm.s^{-1}$. Speed was calculated as the absolute value of the first derivative of marker position. The final position of the stepping foot was the mean position of the three foot markers upon landing.

To investigate whether the pre-step activity was modulated when the intended step location changed, the body's horizontal (AP and ML) motion in jump trials was compared to constant-central (the initial target in a jump trial) steps over time after alignment. All trials were aligned to the initiation of the pre-step activity and CoM acceleration was differentiated to calculate jerk. Two-dimensional 95% confidence intervals (confidence ellipses) were then generated at each time point for the constant-central condition. **Figure 2** shows an example of this for one subject. The latency of any modulation was defined as the first time, at least 100 ms after a target jump, that a jump trial diverged from the constant-central confidence interval. The delay of 100 ms after a target jump was chosen as this relates to the shortest reported latencies to adjust lower limb trajectory or modulate ground reaction forces in visuomotor tasks (Reynolds and Day, 2005, 2007; Leonard et al., 2011). Modulation latency was measured for each jump condition and subject.

Sixteen jump trials (1% of total trials, 4% of jump trials) were excluded from the analysis due to the target jump being triggered

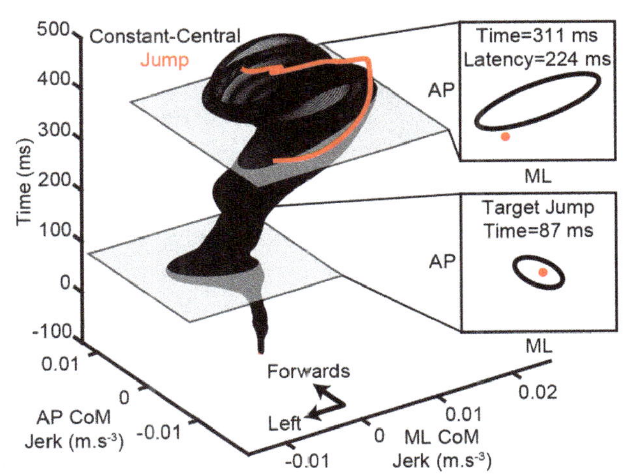

FIGURE 2 | Calculation of modulation latency. An example is shown for one subject's step to the right-side lateral target after the target jumped (red). Medio-lateral (ML) and antero-posterior (AP) center-of-mass (CoM) jerk traces were aligned to the initiation of the pre-step activity (time = 0) and 95% confidence ellipses were calculated at each time point for the constant-central steps (black). A modulation was detected when a jump trial diverged from the confidence ellipse. In this example the modulation occurred 224 ms after the target jumped and before the stepping foot lifted (time = 488).

either before the initiation of the pre-step activity or shortly before the stepping foot lifted.

Statistical Analysis

No bias was found between the left and right sides or dominant and non-dominant legs in the latency of the target jump from the pre-step activity's initiation, final position of the stepping foot, CoM velocity at foot lift, or duration of the pre-step activity (all $P > 0.05$). Therefore left-sided steps were reflected about the laboratory AP axis and combined with right-sided steps. All steps are reported as if they were right-sided.

Foot placement and CoM velocity at foot lift contained both ML and AP components and as such are multidimensional variables requiring analysis by multidimensional statistical methods. Ideally, a repeated-measures ANOVA capable of analyzing differences in multidimensional variables would be used to test whether the foot landed accurately or whether CoM velocity differed with target location. However, to the best of our knowledge, no such test exists. Therefore, paired *t*-tests for multidimensional variables (one-sample Hotelling's tests; Batschelet, 1981; Zar, 2010) were used to distinguish differences between conditions. Using multidimensional statistical methods, rather than examining the data in two dimensions separately, is advantageous as power is increased (Batschelet, 1981) and no *a priori* assumptions are required about which dimension of the data an effect is expected. CoM velocity at foot lift was paired within-subject by subtracting the mean of the constant-central condition from all other stepping conditions.

Unidimensional temporal variables (pre-step activity duration and modulation latency) were submitted to repeated-measures ANOVA with the within-subject factor of step location. ANOVAs were performed using SPSS statistical software (IBM Corporation, New York, NY, USA). Hotelling's tests and all other analyses were performed using custom written Matlab scripts (The Mathworks Inc., Natick, MA, USA). Statistical significance was set at an alpha level of 0.05 after Bonferroni correction for multiple comparisons. Greenhouse Geisser correction was used in ANOVAs when the assumption of sphericity was violated. Normality of data analyzed by Hotelling's tests was confirmed by Mardia's test of skewness and kurtosis (Mardia, 1970).

RESULTS

Steps When the Target Location Remained Constant

All subjects were able to land the stepping foot on or near the target when its location remained constant. On average, the final position of the foot was not different to each subject's self-defined ideal step, which was the case when stepping to all target locations (**Figure 3**, black symbols; all $T^2_{(2,8)} < 5.3, P > 0.7$). This indicated that a successful step was taken to all targets.

In order to land the foot in this position, all subjects produced pre-step activity that accelerated the body sideways, away from the stepping foot, and forwards. The mean (SD) time from the pre-step activity's initiation until foot lift was

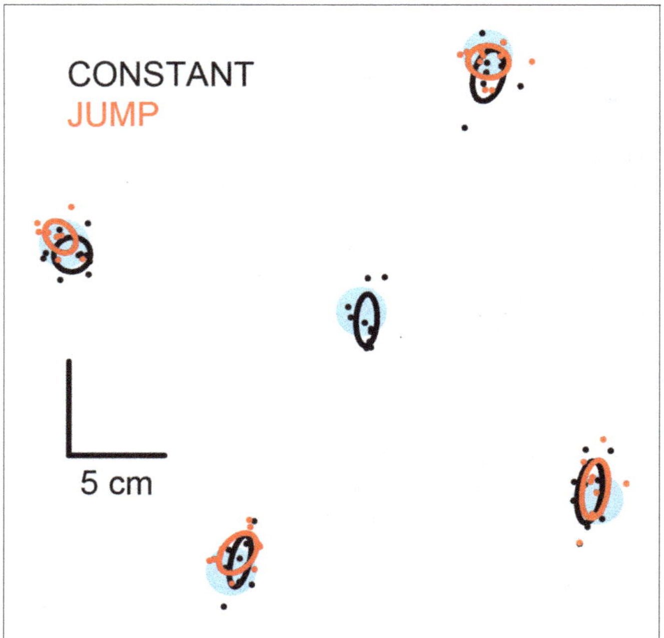

FIGURE 3 | Mean final position of the stepping foot. Filled blue circles are the stepping targets. Filled black and red circles are each subject's mean final position of the stepping foot for the constant and jump conditions respectively. Ellipses are Hotelling's 95% confidence ellipses of the group mean. The size and spacing of the stepping targets is to scale.

561 (89) ms and was not consistently affected by the step location ($F_{(4,36)} = 0.8$, $P = 0.520$). However, the pre-step activity that accelerated the CoM differed with target location (**Figure 4**). **Figures 4A,C** depict the mean CoM acceleration for one subject and shows activity before the lift of the stepping foot. **Figures 4B,D** show that for this subject the pre-step acceleration resulted in the body gaining velocity that was specific for each intended step location. For the group analysis, each subject's mean CoM velocity at foot lift for steps to the central target was subtracted from the mean value for steps to each peripheral target. The resulting two-dimensional (AP and ML) representation of relative CoM velocity at foot lift showed a target-specific organization that resembled the relative positions of the targets in Cartesian coordinates (**Figure 4E**). The confidence ellipses of CoM velocity at foot lift for steps to medial, lateral, distal and proximal locations were all significantly different from each other (all $T^2_{(2,8)} > 82.5$, $P < 0.001$), indicating that the pre-step activity was coupled to the planned step location.

Steps When the Target Location Changed

All subjects adjusted their step when the target jumped to a new position shortly after initiation of the pre-step activity. This was demonstrated by the final position of the foot being different to that originally planned (constant-central steps) for steps to all target-jump locations (**Figure 3**, red symbols; all $T^2_{(2,8)} > 1900$, $P < 0.001$). Furthermore, the mean final position of the foot was not different to each subject's self-defined ideal step for any target jump location (all $T^2_{(2,8)} < 8.0$, $P > 0.3$), indicating

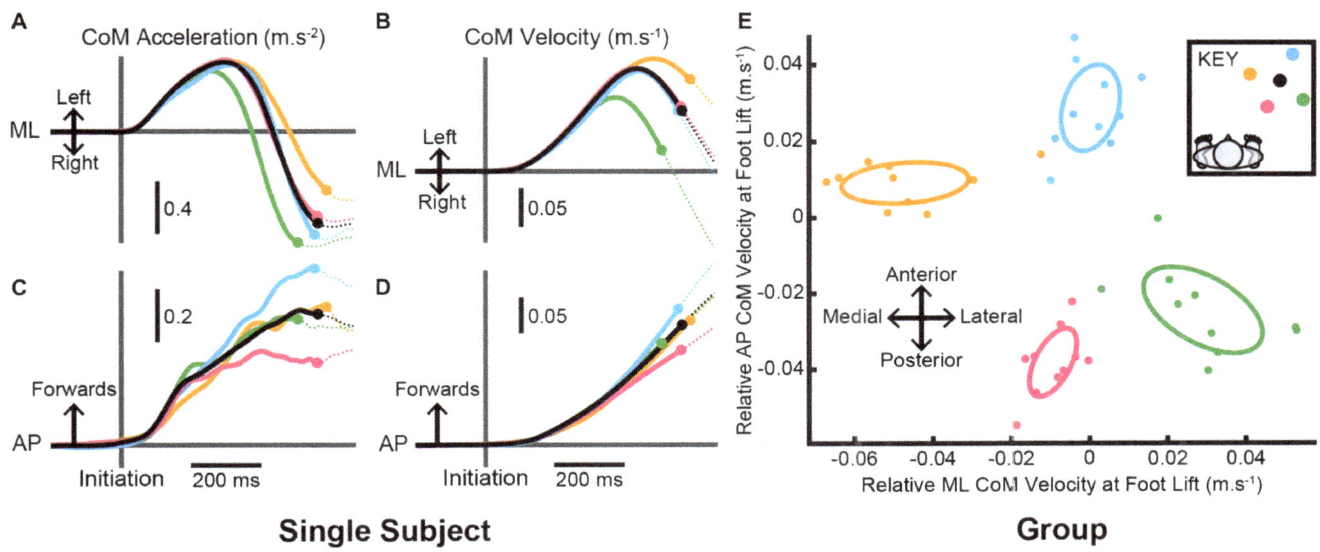

FIGURE 4 | Centre-of-mass (CoM) motion when the target location remained constant. (A–D) Mean estimated CoM acceleration **(A,C)** and velocity **(B,D)** over time from an individual subject in the ML **(A,B)** and AP **(C,D)** dimensions. Trials were aligned to the time of pre-step activity initiation. Filled circles denote the mean time the stepping foot lifted in steps to each target and the traces are dotted thereafter. **(E)** Estimated CoM velocity at foot lift for the group after within-subject pairing by subtracting the constant-central mean. Filled circles are each subject's mean estimated CoM velocity at foot lift for each target. Ellipses are Hotelling's 95% confidence ellipses of the group mean. As per the key, black= central; yellow= medial; green= lateral; blue= distal; magenta= proximal.

that the step adjustments were successful and accurate. The final position of the foot after a target jump was mostly the same as when stepping without a target jump (lateral, distal and proximal all $T^2_{(2,8)} < 10.5$, $P > 0.18$), however medial steps were modestly but significantly different from each other (mean vector distance = 1.1 cm; $T^2_{(2,8)} = 49.2$, $P = 0.002$).

To determine whether the pre-step activity was modulated in response to a change in step location, the CoM motion when subjects stepped to the constant-central target was compared with that when the target jumped (see **Figure 2** for details). An initial modulation could be reliably detected in 94% of all jump trials, with 6% of trials being excluded because their jerk trace lay outside the constant-central ellipse at the time of target jump. The first detectable modulation occurred before the foot lifted from the ground in the vast majority (93%) of the remaining trials, with a modulation after foot lift in 7% of trials (**Figure 5**). The median modulation latency was 223 ms (interquartile range = 158) and was not affected by the new target's location ($F_{(3,27)} = 1.0$, $P = 0.41$). Subjects would also delay the lift of the stepping foot to elongate the pre-step activity in response to the change of target location. When compared with steps to the constant-central target, foot lift was significantly delayed by 69 (55) ms in jump trials ($P = 0.003$), but did not depend on target-jump location ($F_{(3,27)} = 1.8$, $P = 0.178$). The stepping foot was also lifted later in jump trials than in steps to the same location without a target jump ($F_{(1,9)} = 10.9$, $P = 0.009$). The mean (SD) pre-step activity duration of steps with a target jump was 629 (129) ms.

Typically, the initial response to a change in target location acted to reduce the forward acceleration of the body, as shown for a single subject in **Figure 6C**. This "braking" effect was apparent for all target jump locations even if an increase in

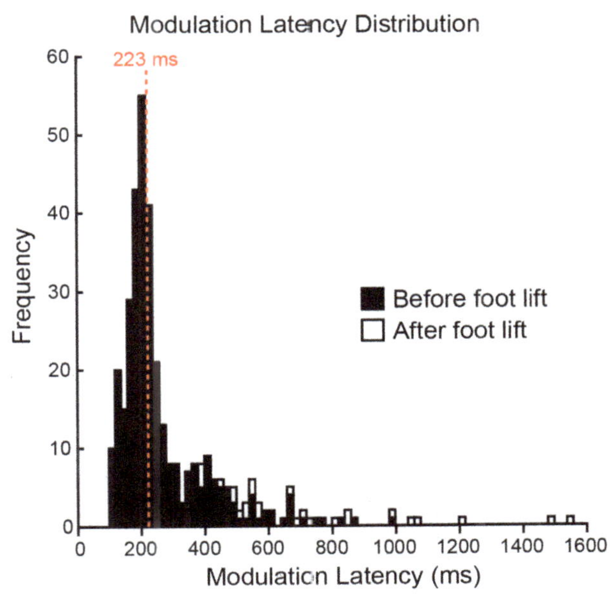

FIGURE 5 | Distribution of modulation latencies. A histogram of all jump trials for all subjects is depicted. The distribution was skewed and the average modulation latency was determined by the median (223 ms, red dashed line). Filled bars represent modulations occurring before the lift of the stepping foot and open bars represent modulations occurring after the lift of the stepping foot. Each bin is 20 ms.

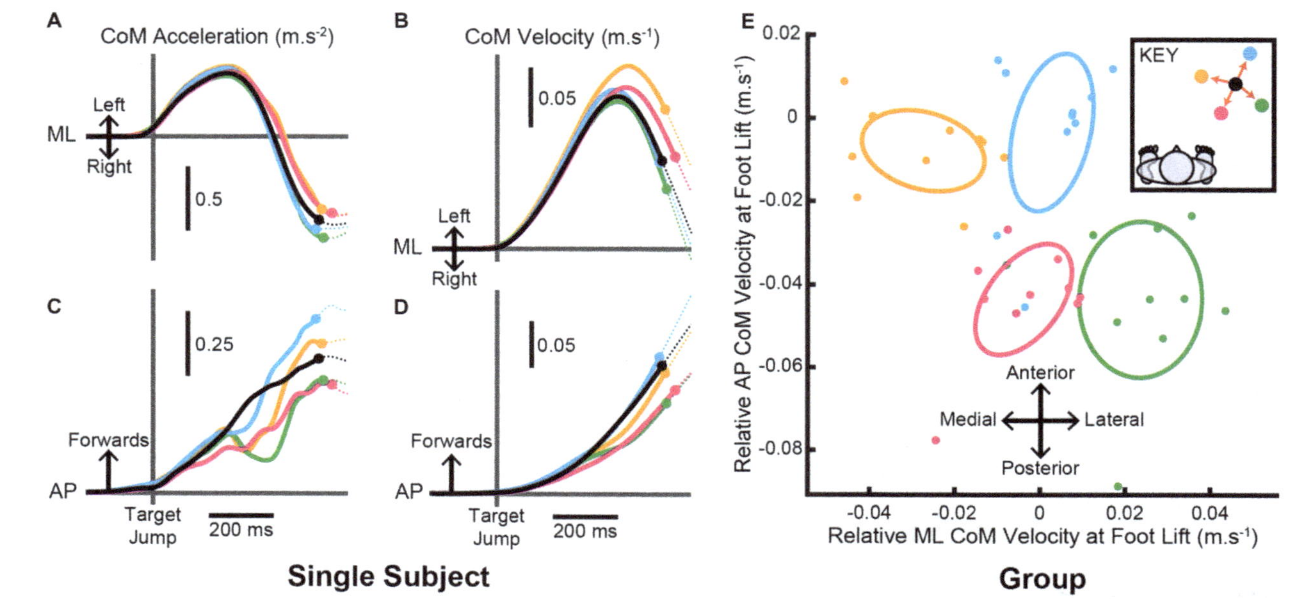

FIGURE 6 | Centre-of-mass (CoM) motion when the target location changed. (A–D) Mean estimated CoM acceleration **(A,C)** and velocity **(B,D)** over time from an individual subject in the ML **(A,B)** and AP **(C,D)** dimensions. Trials were aligned to the time a target jumped. Filled circles denote the mean time the stepping foot lifted in steps to each target and the traces are dotted thereafter. **(E)** Estimated CoM velocity at foot lift for the group after within-subject pairing by subtracting the constant-central mean. Filled circles are each subject's mean estimated CoM velocity at foot lift for each target. Ellipses are Hotelling's 95% confidence ellipses of the group mean. As per the key, black = constant-central; yellow = medial; green = lateral; blue = distal; magenta = proximal.

forward acceleration seemed more appropriate, for example during a jump that required an increased step length. The initial non-specific response was rapidly followed by a target-specific acceleration of the CoM (**Figures 6A,C**) leading to different CoM velocities at the point of foot lift (**Figures 6B,D**). For the group, the confidence ellipses of the change in CoM velocity at foot lift for steps with a medial, lateral, distal and proximal target jump were all significantly different from each other (**Figure 6E**; all $T^2_{(2,8)} > 83.9, P < 0.001$) demonstrating that the pre-step activity modulation was target-specific. The modulated CoM velocity at foot lift reflected the positions of the new stepping target, similar to that observed when the target position remained constant, suggesting that an attempt was made to re-couple the pre-step activity and step location.

DISCUSSION

The experiments were designed to test the throw-and-catch hypothesis of human gait. This was achieved by measuring the coupling between the pre-step activity (the throw) and the final stepping-foot position (the catch). The hypothesis states that the two actions are intimately coupled such that the pre-step activity differs with the planned step location. This was verified in the experiment where the final location was known to the subject throughout the movement. For the experiment in which the final location changed just after the throw was initiated, which effectively de-coupled the two actions, the throw was found to be adjusted so that it was re-coupled to the new step location. Together these results provide support for the throw-and-catch hypothesis of human gait.

Steps When the Target Location Remained Constant

The throw-and-catch model predicts that the pre-step activity depends on the intended step location. This is because the direction and magnitude of the body throw would need to be tuned differently in order for the body to fall towards its target during steps to different locations. Previous research identified a coupling between the pre-step activity and step location for forwards and diagonal steps (Lyon and Day, 1997, 2005). We sought to investigate whether this finding, and the throw-and-catch model, generalized to steps of different lengths and directions. The resulting data therefore required that both ML and AP body motion was analyzed together using multidimensional statistics (Hotelling's tests and confidence ellipses). The results confirmed that the pre-step activity systematically differed with target location in steps of both different lengths and directions (**Figure 4**). The net result of these changes was such that when the stepping foot lifted from the ground, the body had gained velocity, and therefore momentum, that was specific to the intended step location. Lyon and Day (1997) demonstrated that the body's momentum at the point of foot lift is a key factor that predicts the body's trajectory during the step. The coupling between the body's momentum and step location in the present results suggests that this ballistic model generalizes and the throw is fine-tuned for steps of different lengths and directions.

In order to test the throw-and-catch model's generality, steps were initiated from an imposed initial posture which allowed both step length and direction to be precisely controlled. Although the initial posture may not have been a natural stance width or foot angle for all subjects, it is unlikely to have affected their behavior significantly. The step was otherwise natural for each subject as the initiation and duration of the step was unconstrained. This lack of temporal constraint is unlikely to have affected the use of a ballistic strategy, as it has been demonstrated both for temporally unconstrained steps (Lyon and Day, 1997, 2005) and when initiating gait as quickly as possible (Yiou et al., 2016). It is possible that differences in step duration may have influenced the throws to different targets (Zettel et al., 2002a,b; Yiou et al., 2016). However, this is unlikely to explain our data because although step duration changed with step length, it did not change with step direction (data not shown). In exploring the throw-and-catch in steps of different lengths and directions, subjects would often step beyond the force platforms. Subsequently, CoM position was unable to be reliably estimated (for a discussion of CoM position estimation from force data see Lyon and Day, 1997). The position from which the body initiates its fall is an important aspect of the throw (Lyon and Day, 1997, 2005) but, by demonstrating a step location-specific change in CoM velocity, the present results show that the pre-step activity is tuned to the future foot position.

The between-subject variability of the throw in this experiment (**Figure 4E**) and in Lyon and Day (1997) shows that there is no "one-size-fits-all" throw to achieve a successful step. Even for the same subject, different throws could successfully be caught by identical foot-landing positions. This likely reflects both the ability to make mid-step adjustments (Reynolds and Day, 2005, 2007; Kim and Brunt, 2009, 2013; Tseng et al., 2009; Nonnekes et al., 2010) and the numerous solutions that exist to catch the body without losing balance (Koolen et al., 2012). However, the present results show that there is pressure to maintain the throw within limits which differ for different step locations. This suggests there is some advantage in coupling the pre-step activity and step location.

Steps When the Target Location Changed

The pre-step activity and the step location can be uncoupled, for example by changing the location of a target. In this scenario the body throw and step location become uncoupled if the pre-step activity remains unchanged while the foot position changes. Previous work has shown that if the target is made to jump after the foot leaves the ground, so that the pre-step activity cannot be changed, the final position of the stepping foot can still be altered, albeit with varying degrees of success depending on the extent and direction of the target jump (Reynolds and Day, 2005, 2007; Kim and Brunt, 2009, 2013; Tseng et al., 2009; Nonnekes et al., 2010). This de-coupling does not necessarily disprove the throw-and-catch hypothesis, but may be interpreted as there being some flexibility in the coupling which can be exploited under certain circumstances. A better test of the hypothesis is to measure whether there is an attempt to re-couple the pre-step activity with the new step location under conditions when the pre-step activity has an opportunity to be adjusted. Here we made the target change location during the pre-step activity, long before the stepping foot left the ground, thus allowing time for a re-coupling of the pre-step activity with the new target location. The target jump was unpredictable, as more often than not the target location did not change and could be to any one of four locations when it did. This procedure resulted in substantial uncertainty and rendered attempts at anticipating the target jump unlikely to be of value to the subject. We argue that an attempt to re-couple the pre-step activity with the new step location would provide support for the throw-and-catch hypothesis given that an adjustment could be initiated after the foot leaves the ground.

Previous research is conflicted on whether the pre-step activity can be modulated. Experiments that unpredictably perturbed the trajectory of the body during the pre-step activity via mechanical pulls have returned mixed results, with muscle activity being altered to correct the body's trajectory in response to resistive (Mouchnino et al., 2012; Mille et al., 2014) but not assistive perturbations (Mouchnino et al., 2012). Additionally, stimulation of proprioceptive (Ruget et al., 2008) and vestibular (Bent et al., 2002) afferents were found not to affect the pre-step activity, suggesting it may be immutable once it has been initiated. This was not found to be the case in the present experiment, since the pre-step activity was modulated in the vast majority of trials when prompted by a visual cue. Furthermore, the precise modulation of the pre-step activity depended on the new target location. This suggests that an attempt was made to re-couple the pre-step activity to the new target location and provides causal evidence that the pre-step activity is fine-tuned to take the final position of the foot into account. According to the throw-and-catch hypothesis, re-coupling the pre-step activity to the new target location would have promoted a more appropriate fall of the body towards its intended target after the lift of the stepping foot. This does not rule out the possibility that further adjustments were made during the step.

Although the net adjustment of the pre-step activity was different depending on where the target jumped, a non-specific initial response to the perturbation was evident that reduced the forward acceleration of the body. Similar "braking" responses to visual cues have been reported after the lift of the stepping foot during both single steps and locomotion (Kim and Brunt, 2013; Potocanac et al., 2016). In the present experiment, this braking was used irrespective of where the target moved. Although the braking could have been expected when the step length required shortening, it was surprising that it was also used when a longer step was required. This is because greater forward acceleration was observed for longer steps when the target did not move (**Figure 4**). The braking may have enabled a pause whilst the necessary actions for a successful step were reconsidered (Potocanac et al., 2016), which would explain the increase in pre-step duration that was observed when a target jumped. Mille et al. (2014) also report a similar delay in stepping after a mechanical pull to the body prior to a step. Presumably, in the current experiments, the extra time was needed to re-program and adjust the body throw so that it was re-coupled to the new final foot location.

What Advantage Does the Throw-and-Catch Coupling Offer?

Stepping can be considered a ballistic action if, as we suggest, gravity drives the fall of the body during the step with its trajectory being controlled by the pre-step activity. The ballistic nature of stepping is sometimes misinterpreted as sensory information not being attended to or usable during the step. This interpretation is clearly false given that adjustments to the step are possible both before the lift of the stepping foot, as shown in this paper, and after foot lift when suitable sensory cues are provided (Reynolds and Day, 2005, 2007; Kim and Brunt, 2009, 2013; Tseng et al., 2009; Nonnekes et al., 2010). However, the magnitude and direction of mid-step adjustments are limited by the fall of the body and the subsequent balance constraints. For example, the size of medially-directed foot adjustments cannot be made as large as laterally-directed adjustments (Reynolds and Day, 2005). This limitation may underlie the incentive to maintain the coupling between the pre-step activity and final foot location demonstrated in the present experiment. At the same time, the ability to rapidly alter the intended foot position mid-step offers a degree of flexibility in the coupling, which would be essential for responding to an unexpected environmental threat or maintaining foot landing accuracy in the presence of error in the initial throw.

CONCLUSION

We find that there is a close coupling between pre-step activity and final foot position during unperturbed steps of different lengths and directions. Furthermore, there is pressure to maintain this coupling when the demanded step location unpredictably changes shortly after initiation of the pre-step activity. We conclude that these results support the throw-and-catch hypothesis of human stepping.

AUTHOR CONTRIBUTIONS

MJB and BLD conceptualized and designed the experiment, analyzed the data, drafted and revised the manuscript and approved its final version. MJB acquired the data.

FUNDING

This work was funded by a University College London (UCL) Grand Challenge studentship.

ACKNOWLEDGMENTS

We would like to thank Mr. Dan Voyce for technical assistance.

REFERENCES

Batschelet, E. (1981). *Circular Statistics in Biology*. London: Academic Press.

Bent, L. R., Inglis, J. T., and McFadyen, B. J. (2002). Vestibular contributions across the execution of a voluntary forward step. *Exp. Brain Res.* 143, 100–105. doi: 10.1007/s00221-001-0967-7

Breniere, Y., Do, M. C., and Bouisset, S. (1987). Are dynamic phenomena prior to stepping essential to walking? *J. Mot. Behav.* 19, 62–76. doi: 10.1080/00222895.1987.10735400

Carlsöö, S. (1966). The initiation of walking. *Acta. Anat.* 65, 1–9. doi: 10.1159/000142864

Crenna, P., and Frigo, C. (1991). A motor programme for the initiation of forward-oriented movements in humans. *J. Physiol. Lond.* 437, 635–653. doi: 10.1113/jphysiol.1991.sp018616

Jian, Y., Winter, D. A., Ishac, M. G., and Gilchrist, L. (1993). Trajectory of the body COG and COP during initiation and termination of gait. *Gait Posture* 1, 9–22. doi: 10.1016/0966-6362(93)90038-3

Kim, H.-D., and Brunt, D. (2009). The effect of a sensory perturbation on step direction or length while crossing an obstacle from quiet stance. *Gait Posture* 30, 1–4. doi: 10.1016/j.gaitpost.2009.02.016

Kim, H.-D., and Brunt, D. (2013). Effect of a change in step direction from a forward to a lateral target in response to a sensory perturbation. *J. Electromyogr. Kinesiol.* 23, 851–857. doi: 10.1016/j.jelekin.2013.03.001

Koolen, T., de Boer, T., Rebula, J., Goswami, A., and Pratt, J. (2012). Capturability-based analysis and control of legged locomotion, Part 1: Theory and application to three simple gait models. *Int. J. Robot. Res.* 31, 1094–1113. doi: 10.1177/0278364912452673

Leonard, J. A., Gritsenko, V., Ouckama, R., and Stapley, P. J. (2011). Postural adjustments for online corrections of arm movements in standing humans. *J. Neurophysiol.* 105, 2375–2388. doi: 10.1152/jn.00944.2010

Lyon, I. N., and Day, B. L. (1997). Control of frontal plane body motion in human stepping. *Exp. Brain Res.* 115, 345–356. doi: 10.1007/pl00005703

Lyon, I. N., and Day, B. L. (2005). Predictive control of body mass trajectory in a two-step sequence. *Exp. Brain Res.* 161, 193–200. doi: 10.1007/s00221-004-2058-z

MacKinnon, C. D., and Winter, D. A. (1993). Control of whole body balance in the frontal plane during human walking. *J. Biomech.* 26, 633–644. doi: 10.1016/0021-9290(93)90027-c

Mann, R. A., Hagy, J. L., White, V., and Liddell, D. (1979). The initiation of gait. *J. Bone Joint Surg. Am.* 61, 232–239.

Mardia, K. V. (1970). Measures of multivariate skewness and kurtosis with applications. *Biometrika* 57, 519–530. doi: 10.2307/2334770

Mille, M. L., Simoneau, M., and Rogers, M. W. (2014). Postural dependence of human locomotion during gait initiation. *J. Neurophysiol.* 112, 3095–3103. doi: 10.1152/jn.00436.2014

Mouchnino, L., Robert, G., Ruget, H., Blouin, J., and Simoneau, M. (2012). Online control of anticipated postural adjustments in step initiation: evidence from behavioral and computational approaches. *Gait Posture* 35, 616–620. doi: 10.1016/j.gaitpost.2011.12.009

Nonnekes, J. H., Talelli, P., de Niet, M., Reynolds, R. F., Weerdesteyn, V., and Day, B. L. (2010). Deficits underlying impaired visually triggered step adjustments in mildly affected stroke patients. *Neurorehab. Neural Repair* 24, 393–400. doi: 10.1177/1545968309348317

Potocanac, Z., Pijnappels, M., Verschueren, S. M., van Dieën, J. H., and Duysens, J. (2016). Two stage muscle activity responses in decisions about leg movement adjustments during trip recovery. *J. Neurophysiol.* 115, 143–156. doi: 10.1152/jn.00263.2015

Reynolds, R. F., and Day, B. L. (2005). Rapid visuo-motor processes drive the leg regardless of balance constraints. *Curr. Biol.* 15, R48–R49. doi: 10.1016/j.cub.2004.12.051

Reynolds, R. F., and Day, B. L. (2007). Fast visuomotor processing made faster by sound. *J. Physiol.* 583, 1107–1115. doi: 10.1113/jphysiol.2007.136192

Ruget, H., Blouin, J., Teasdale, N., and Mouchnino, L. (2008). Can prepared anticipatory postural adjustments be updated by proprioception? *Neuroscience* 155, 640–648. doi: 10.1016/j.neuroscience.2008.06.021

Tseng, S.-C., Stanhope, S. J., and Morton, S. M. (2009). Impaired reactive stepping adjustments in older adults. *J. Gerontol. A Biol. Sci. Med. Sci.*, 807–815. doi: 10.1093/gerona/glp027

Yiou, E., Artico, R., Teyssedre, C. A., Labaune, O., and Fourcade, P. (2016). Anticipatory postural control of stability during gait initiation over obstacles of different height and distance made under reaction-time and self-initiated instructions. *Front. Hum. Neurosci.* 10:449. doi: 10.3389/fnhum.2016.00449

Zar, J. H. (2010). *Biostatistical Analysis.* Upper Saddle River, NJ: Prentice Hall.

Zettel, J. L., McIlroy, W. E., and Maki, B. E. (2002a). Can stabilizing features of rapid triggered stepping reactions be modulated to meet environmental constraints? *Exp. Brain Res.* 145, 297–308. doi: 10.1007/s00221-002-1083-z

Zettel, J. L., McIlroy, W. E., and Maki, B. E. (2002b). Environmental constraints on foot trajectory reveal the capacity for modulation of anticipatory postural adjustments during rapid triggered stepping reactions. *Exp. Brain Res.* 146, 38–47. doi: 10.1007/s00221-002-1150-5

9

Multi-Trial Gait Adaptation of Healthy Individuals during Visual Kinematic Perturbations

*Trieu Phat Luu *, Yongtian He, Sho Nakagome, Kevin Nathan, Samuel Brown, Jeffrey Gorges and Jose L. Contreras-Vidal*

Noninvasive Brain-Machine Interface System Laboratory, Department of Electrical and Computer Engineering, University of Houston, Houston, TX, United States

***Correspondence:**
Trieu Phat Luu
ptluu2@central.uh.edu

Optimizing rehabilitation strategies requires understanding the effects of contextual cues on adaptation learning. Prior studies have examined these effects on the specificity of split-belt walking adaptation, showing that contextual visual cues can be manipulated to modulate the magnitude, transfer, and washout of split-belt-induced learning in humans. Specifically, manipulating the availability of vision during training or testing phases of learning resulted in differences in adaptive mechanisms for temporal and spatial features of walking. However, multi-trial locomotor training has been rarely explored when using visual kinematic gait perturbations. In this study, we investigated multi-trial locomotor adaptation in ten healthy individuals while applying visual kinematic perturbations. Subjects were instructed to control a moving cursor, which represented the position of their heel, to follow a prescribed heel path profile displayed on a monitor. The perturbations were introduced by scaling all of the lower limb joint angles by a factor of 0.7 (i.e., a gain change), resulting in visual feedback errors between subjects' heel trajectories and the prescribed path profiles. Our findings suggest that, with practice, the subjects learned, albeit with different strategies, to reduce the tracking errors and showed faster response time in later trials. Moreover, the gait symmetry indices, in both the spatial and temporal domains, changed significantly during gait adaptation ($P < 0.001$). After-effects were present in the temporal gait symmetry index whens the visual perturbations were removed in the post-exposure period ($P < 0.001$), suggesting adaptation learning. These findings may have implications for developing novel gait rehabilitation interventions.

Keywords: locomotor adaptation, visuo-motor adaptation, gait symmetry, human locomotion, motor adaptation

NEW AND NOTEWORTHY

This study deployed a novel gait adaptation paradigm in which healthy subjects learned to move their lower limbs to control a cursor in response to visuo-motor perturbations (i.e., gain change). Our findings suggest that, with practice, the subjects learned, albeit with different strategies, to reduce the tracking errors and showed faster response time in later trials. Moreover, we observed differential effects of adaptation to the kinematic perturbation on the temporal and spatial symmetry (i.e., after-effects were only observed in the temporal domain of gait symmetry, indicating its adaptation). Overall, these findings may have implications for the development of novel gait interventions for people with lower-limb disabilities.

INTRODUCTION

Motor adaptation can be defined as an error-driven process that allows humans to adjust sensorimotor mappings of well-learned movements to adapt to new, predictable demands (Bastian, 2008; Malone et al., 2011). Thus, motor adaptation mechanisms are generally engaged in response to changing intrinsic (e.g., muscle fatigue, aging, and neurological disease) and/or extrinsic (e.g., visual kinematic or dynamic perturbations) conditions. Motor adaptation to extrinsic perturbations has been investigated in the context of gait rehabilitation for people with walking disabilities (Torres-Oviedo et al., 2011). Both visual and dynamic disturbances induce sensorimotor errors, which initiate motor adaptation. Indeed, experimental studies of motor adaptation have been performed by applying extrinsic perturbations including introducing abnormal visual feedback (Contreras-Vidal and Kerick, 2004; Krakauer et al., 2005; Cheng and Sabes, 2007; Wei and Kording, 2009; Izawa and Shadmehr, 2011; Luu et al., 2015, 2016), manipulating physical dynamics (split-belt treadmill; Scheidt et al., 2001; Choi and Bastian, 2007; Emken et al., 2007; Izawa et al., 2008; Malone et al., 2012), or both (Kim et al., 2010).

Helm and Reisman have reviewed the split-belt walking paradigm, which has been widely used to explore motor learning and spatiotemporal asymmetry for post-stroke conditions (Helm and Reisman, 2015). The locomotor adaptation to split-belt treadmill training can improve walking symmetry in post-stroke patients (Reisman et al., 2007), and the persistence of improved gait symmetry on a treadmill partially transfers to over-ground walking (Reisman et al., 2009). Moreover, the temporal and spatial control for symmetric gait can be adapted separately, which suggests we could potentially develop interventions targeting either temporal or spatial domain of gait deficits (Malone et al., 2012). However, split-belt treadmill is not the only way to disrupt normal gait patterns. In some cases, this purpose can also be achieved by altering the visual-motor representation of locomotion.

Prior studies have examined the effect of altering visual feedback in walking adaptation. Torres-Oviedo and Bastian showed that removing vision via blindfolds improved the transfer of split-belt treadmill adaptation to natural walking (Torres-Oviedo and Bastian, 2010). This agreed with a prior study that reported the transferring of motor learning occurs in the intrinsic coordinates (Imamizu et al., 1998; Malfait et al., 2002). Prisms are used in many studies to distort vision and interrupt the visuo-motor neural pathway (Morton and Bastian, 2004; Alexander et al., 2013; Nemanich and Earhart, 2015). On the other hand, visual cues can be provided and manipulated in rehabilitation. Kim et al. used a cursor on a screen to represent the sagittal position of a subject's foot when walking with a robotic system (Kim et al., 2010). They suggested that combining both dynamics (interaction force between subjects and robot) and visual perturbations to the gait pattern retained the gait adaptation for longer than training with either dynamics or visual perturbation alone. Statton et al. used bars on a screen to show subjects the amount of their knee flexion (Statton et al., 2016). By manipulating the height of the bars, they created illusions in subjects that they had to over-correct their gait. Long et al. showed the position of steps on a screen so that the subjects would know where their feet landed (Long et al., 2016). Although the effect induced in the gait pattern from these studies vary greatly, they can usually be labeled as either spatial (Long et al., 2016; Statton et al., 2016) or temporal (Hussain et al., 2013; Finley et al., 2014) gait patterns but not both, partially limited by the paradigm of interruption to the visual-motor system.

In this study, we proposed a novel method to explore multi-day gait adaptation of human treadmill walking under visual kinematic perturbations. Participants were instructed to control a moving cursor, representing the heel position in the sagittal plane, to follow a specific trajectory displayed on a screen. Visual kinematic perturbations were introduced by scaling the lower limb joint angles (factor of 0.7) therefore distorting the mapping of the actual heel position on the screen, resulting in mismatch between the moving cursor and the prescribed heel path. Participants adapted their locomotor patterns to visual perturbations as demonstrated by a reduction of tracking errors across trials. After-effects were present when the visual perturbations were removed in the post-exposure period suggesting adaptation learning had taken place. We also found that individual subjects are idiosyncratic in which joints they use to control the heel positions during the adaptation. The modifications in the spatial and temporal symmetry of gait induced by the visual kinematic perturbations were also investigated. These findings have implications for developing novel effective gait rehabilitation interventions.

METHODS

Experimental Setup and Procedure

Ten healthy individuals (six males, four females; aged from 22 to 30) with no history of neurological disease or lower limb pathology participated in this study. All participants provided written and informed consent as approved by the Institutional Review Board at the University of Houston. Each subject participated in two sessions (two consecutive days, two trials per session). There were two phases in each day at trial 1 and trial 3 (**Table 1**). In the first phase, the subjects were instructed to walk normally and consistently for 3 min on a treadmill at a fixed speed of 1 mile per hour (mph), or 0.45 meter per second (m/s). A 52-inch TV monitor was placed in front of the treadmill at eye level and it showed a black screen in this phase. The subjects were also instructed to look at the screen during the entire protocol. Heel path profiles of their normal walking were computed for each session from the goniometer data using Matlab 2016a (The MathWorks, Inc.). Details of the calculation are provided in Section Forward Kinematic Model. In the second phase, the subjects first stood still (rest) on the treadmill for 2 min, then started walking at 1 mph without visual feedback on the screen for 5 min, following by a walking period with visual feedback. The subjects stood still for another 2 min at the end of each trial The walking period without the

TABLE 1 | The experimental procedure for 4 trials in 2 consecutive days.

		Phase 1	Phase 2					
		Template generation	**Rest**	**Without visual feedback**	**With visual feedback**			**Rest**
					Pre-	**Exposure**	**Post-**	
Day 1	Trial 1	3	2	5	8	8	–	2
	Trial 2	–	2	5	–	8	–	2
Day 2	Trial 3	3	2	5	–	8	–	2
	Trial 4	–	2	5	–	8	5	2

Heel path profiles (template generation) were generated in Phase 1. In Phase 2, subjects stood for 2 min in the beginning and the end (rest) and walked in periods without and with visual feedback. Small dash "–" represents periods that were excluded in a trial. All values are in minutes.

visual feedback serves as a baseline to normalize gait symmetry indices. The visual feedback to the subjects included a moving cursor, which was linked to their right heel position in the sagittal plane, and a desired heel path. During the entire visual feedback period, the subjects were instructed to control a moving cursor to follow prescribed right heel path profiles displayed on the screen. The tracking task was mainly spatial because the subjects performed the task without considering the time to reach a specific point. In the pre-exposure phase (8 min) in Trial 1, the moving cursor was driven by the goniometer data (right hip, knee, and ankle). In the exposure period (8 min), a visual kinematic perturbation was introduced by scaling the goniometer data of the right leg by 0.7 and the moving cursor departed from the prescribed heel profiles. The subjects controlled the moving cursor to follow the prescribed heel profiles by adapting their gait patterns. A gain of 0.7 was chosen because the visual perturbation is detectable with this gain and the physical demand to compete the task at this gain is not so high. In the post-exposure period (5 min), the perturbations were removed and the moving cursor was driven by the goniometer data again. We defined early- and late- exposure phases in each trial as the first and the last 30 gait cycles (~1 min), respectively. Similarly, early post-exposure phase was defined as the first 30 gait cycles in the post-exposure period. For safety purposes, all subjects were instructed to hold onto a front handle bar while walking on the treadmill.

Data Collection

Lower limb joint angles (hip, knee, and ankle) in the sagittal plane were recorded by goniometers (SG150 & SG110/A Gonio electrodes, Biometrics Ltd., UK) at 100 Hz using our customized C++ program. We visually estimated the joint locations and placed six sensors on both legs. To improve the consistency of sensor placement across days, we used the same sensor for each joint, 3D-printed a tool to hold the two pieces of a goniometer in place, and recorded the distance (from the ground) of each goniometer after the sensors were attached. Details for the goniometer sensor setup are provided in the Supplementary Material. Three wireless inertial motion sensors (OPAL, APDM Inc., Portland, OR) were mounted on the head, left heel, and right heel of the subject. Each sensor included accelerometer, gyroscope, and magnetometer sampled at 128 Hz. Electroencephalography (EEG) signals were also collected but will be reported elsewhere. **Figure 1** shows raster plot of these signals and illustrates the movements of the right leg in a full gait cycle during pre- and early-exposure phases.

Data Analysis

Data analysis and statistical analysis were performed using custom software written in Matlab R2016a (The MathWorks, Inc.). Joint angle data were low-pass filtered at 6 Hz by using a second order Butterworth filter. Because subjects walked at a slow speed (1 mph), the 0–6 Hz band covers most power of joint angle signals (Antonsson and Mann, 1985; Luu et al., 2014). Heel position in sagittal plane was calculated using a forward kinematic model (Section Forward Kinematic Model).

Forward Kinematic Model

The forward kinematic model of human treadmill walking (in sagittal plane) and the definitions of lower limb joint angles are shown in **Figure 2**. In this model, the hip joint position is assumed to be fixed. The prescribed heelpaths and trajectories of moving circle displayed on a screen during experiment were calculated by using the following equations:

$$\begin{aligned} z_{heel} &= l_1 \sin(\theta_h) + l_2 \sin(\theta_h + \theta_k) + l_3 \sin(\theta_h + \theta_k + \theta_a) \\ &\quad + l_4 \cos(\theta_h + \theta_k + \theta_a) \\ y_{heel} &= -l_1 \cos(\theta_h) - l_2 \cos(\theta_h + \theta_k) - l_3 \cos(\theta_h + \theta_k \\ &\quad + \theta_a) + l_4 \sin(\theta_h + \theta_k + \theta_a) \end{aligned} \tag{1}$$

where z_{heel} and y_{heel} are horizontal and vertical heel position in sagittal plane, respectively; θ_h, θ_k, θ_a are hip, knee, and ankle joint angles, respectively; l_1 is the length from the greater trochanter to the lateral epicondyle of the femur, l_2 is the length from the lateral epicondyle of the femur to the lateral malleolus of the fibula, l_3 is the perpendicular distance from the lateral malleolus of the fibula to the plantar surface of the foot, and l_4 is the distance from the posterior aspect of the calcaneus (heel) to the projection of ankle onto the foot.

To assess the rate of change of y_{heel} with respect to the changes of each lower limb joint angle, the gradient of y_{heel} was also

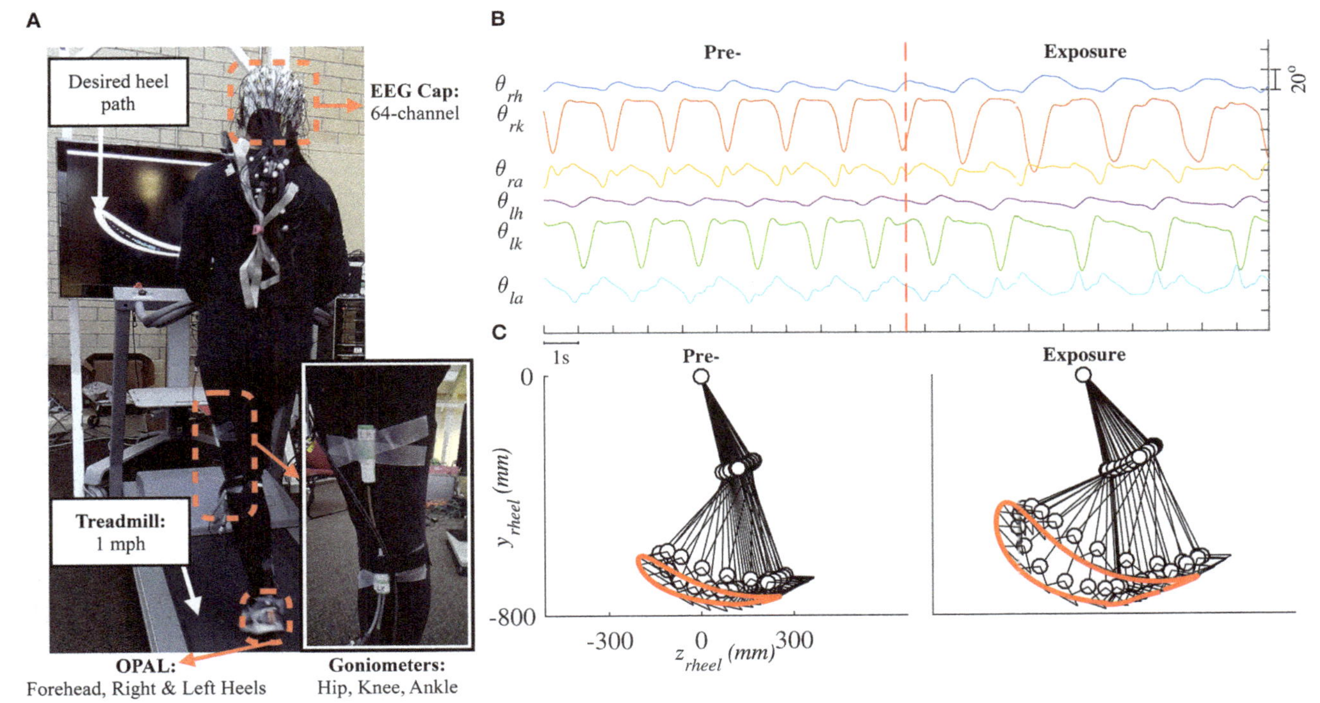

FIGURE 1 | (A) Experimental setup in this study. Each subject was instructed to walk on a treadmill while controlling a moving cursor to follow prescribed heel path profiles. Lower limb joint angles (θ_h, θ_k, θ_a) were recorded using six goniometers. **(B)** Example of joint angles in 20 s, vertical rec line represents the time when the perturbation was introduced. **(C)** Illustration of the right leg in a full gait cycle during pre- and early-exposure.

derived as:

$$\nabla y_{heel} = \begin{bmatrix} \dfrac{\partial y_{heel}}{\partial \theta_h} \\ \dfrac{\partial y_{heel}}{\partial \theta_k} \\ \dfrac{\partial y_{heel}}{\partial \theta_a} \end{bmatrix} = \begin{bmatrix} l_1 \sin(\theta_h) + l_2 \sin(\theta_h + \theta_k) + l_3 \sin(\theta_h + \theta_k + \theta_a) \\ \quad + l_4 \cos(\theta_h + \theta_k + \theta_a) \\ l_2 \sin(\theta_h + \theta_k) + l_3 \sin(\theta_h + \theta_k + \theta_a) \\ \quad + l_4 \cos(\theta_h + \theta_k + \theta_a) \\ l_3 \sin(\theta_h + \theta_k + \theta_a) + l_4 \cos(\theta_h + \theta_k + \theta_a) \end{bmatrix} \quad (2)$$

Gait Segmentation and Temporal Gait Parameters

Kinematic data were segmented into gait cycles. Data from each trial were first divided into non-overlapping windows (window size of 10 s). Heel-strike and toe-off events for right and left legs were determined by using heel velocity profiles in the sagittal plane. Toe-off events in each window were defined by local maximum peaks of the heel velocity profile in the vertical direction (v_{yheel}) (Winter, 1992). The minimum distance between two consecutive peaks is 80% of signal period which was computed by using auto-correlation method. Subsequently, heel-strike was determined by the first local minimum peak of heel velocity profile in the horizontal direction (v_{zheel}) between two consecutive toe-offs. **Figure 3** illustrates the alignment of gait events with lower limb joint angles and heel velocity profiles. Definitions of temporal gait parameters are also depicted. *ST* is stance time period from heel-strike (*HS*) to toe-off (*TO*) for the same leg. Double support time *DS* in a walking gait cycle is the time when both feet are in contact with the floor. Right double support, DS_r, was defined as the time from left heel-strike to right toe-off, and vice versa for left double support, DS_l. Interlimb heel-strike duration (t) is defined as the time between the heel-strike of one leg to the subsequent heel-strike of the other.

Assessment of Subjects' Performance during Visual Kinematic Perturbations

In order to evaluate the performance of participants in adapting to the visual kinematic perturbations, we defined tracking error and response time as performance measurements. Tracking error for each gait cycle was defined as the difference between the moving cursor path and the prescribed heel path (average of gait templates across gait cycles). A value closed to zero would signify that the moving cursor which represents the subjects' heel position followed the prescribed heel path profile correctly. We first converted the desired heel path and the moving cursor's path into regions and placed them on an image of 1,000 × 1,000 pixels. The tracking error was then computed by subtracting the area inside the moving cursor to the area inside the desired heel path (in pixels). Positive tracking error was defined when the

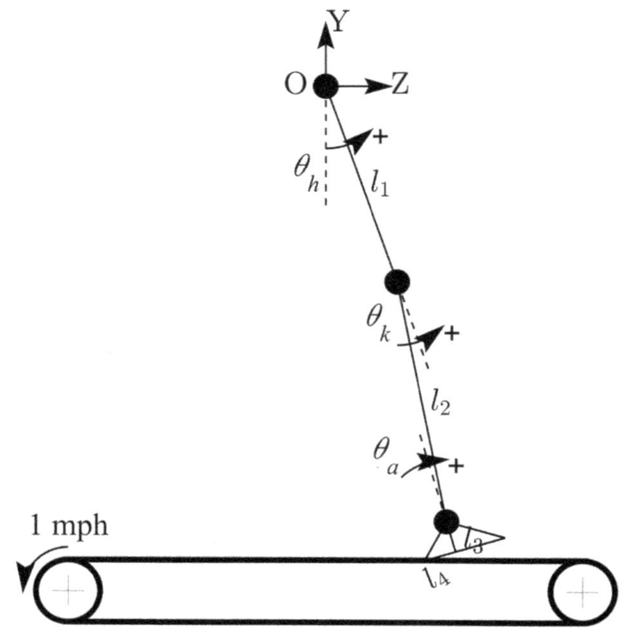

FIGURE 2 | Forward kinematic model of human walking in sagittal plane. Coordinate OZY was placed at hip position and hip joint position is assumed to be fixed. Hip joint angle was defined to increase during flexion, knee joint angle increased during extension, and ankle joint angle increased during plantar-flexion.

area of the moving cursor was larger than the area of the desired heel path and vice versa. **Figure 4** illustrates the computation of tracking error in one gait cycle.

We defined response time to measure how fast a subject responded to the visual perturbations. **Figure 5** illustrates the computation for the response time. First, the initial tracking error was computed as the average of tracking errors in the first 10 gait cycles before the subjects started responding to the perturbations, and the final tracking error was obtained by averaging tracking errors in the late exposure. We then applied cumulative sum (cusum) to track the deviations of each sample away from the initial tracking error. Cusum chart is especially useful in detecting if a signal has drifted beyond a pre-defined deviation above and below a target value. We identified the response time T_s by applying cusum with target value is the initial tracking error and the pre-defined deviation is the difference between the final and the initial tracking errors. The response time T_s was computed in the number of gait cycles.

Assessment of the Adaptations of Lower Limb Joint Angles across Subjects

To analyze the adaptation of lower limb joint angles under the presence of the visual perturbations, we computed the ratio between the range of movement (ROM) in late-exposure (Trial 4) and the ROM in normal walking (without visual feedback). The ROM ratios were computed for all joints (hip, knee, and ankle) of the right leg.

Assessment of Gait Symmetry during Visual Kinematic Perturbations

The changes of gait symmetry under constraint of visual kinematic perturbations were measured in both temporal and spatial domains. Previous studies on locomotion adaptation using split-belt treadmill have demonstrated that the motor system may generate temporal motor outputs to minimize the difference in double support times when the subjects were walking under perturbations (Reisman et al., 2005; Malone et al., 2012). These studies also suggested that the temporal motor outputs from motor system approach a desired value defined as the normalized stance time difference. In this study, the gait symmetry index in the temporal domain is defined as follows:

$$S_{temporal} = \frac{ST_l - ST_r}{t_r + t_l} \tag{3}$$

where t_r and t_l are right and left step times; ST_r and ST_l are stance times of right and left legs, respectively.

In the spatial domain, the differences between lower limb joint angles of the right and left legs were defined to characterize spatial asymmetry. The gait symmetry index in the spatial domain were defined as the difference between the range of motion (ROM) of the right and the left legs normalized by their sum:

$$S_{spatial} = \frac{ROM_{r\gamma} - ROM_{l\gamma}}{ROM_{r\gamma} + ROM_{l\gamma}} \tag{4}$$

where γ is the angle between the vertical line (to the ground) and the line that connects right hip (greater trochanter) and heel (the posterior aspect of the calcaneus) positions.

Gait symmetry indices in both temporal and spatial domains were normalized by subtracting the mean of these values in the period when the subjects walked without the visual feedback on the screen. Gait symmetry values closed to zero indicate that a subject's gait pattern was highly symmetrical.

Statistical Analysis

Statistical analyses were performed to analyze the changes of tracking errors, which had non-normal distributions, across different phases in the 4 training trials: pre-exposure, exposure (from trial 1 to trial 4), and post-exposure. Kruskal-Wallis non-parametric statistical tests with Tukey-Kramer correction for *post-hoc* multiple comparison was applied to assess the changes of tracking errors and response time across all trials. This model was also applied to test the adaptation of the spatial and temporal gait symmetry across all trials. To compare the adaptation of lower limb joint angles, which had normal distributions, under the presence of perturbations, we used a within subject, repeated-measures one-way ANOVA test.

RESULTS

Subjects Adapted Their Gait in Response to Visual Kinematic Perturbations

We observed changes in both tracking errors and response time across training trials. **Figure 6A** shows the group means

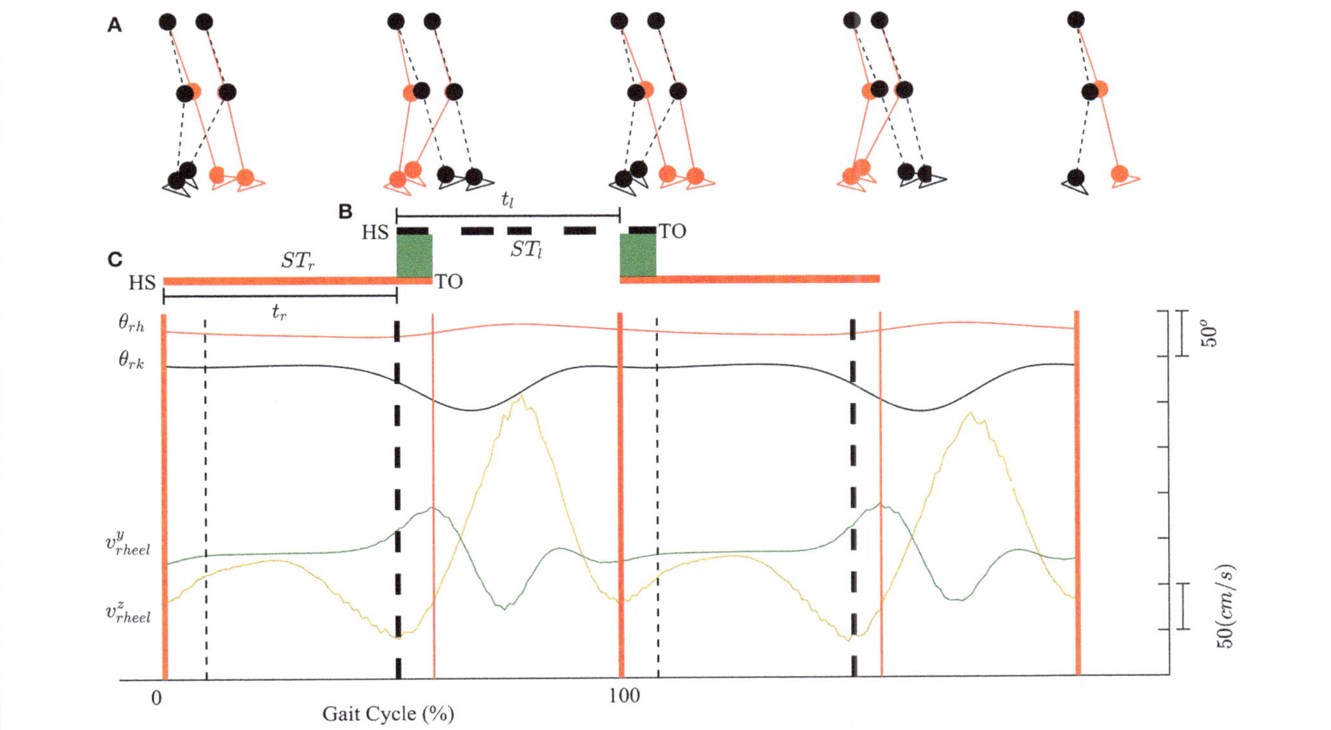

FIGURE 3 | (A) Diagram for human walking at different gait events, walking speed 1 mph. **(B)** Definitions of temporal parameters of human locomotion. HS, heel strike; TO, toe-off. Solid and dashed horizontal lines represent stance time period (*ST*) for the right (ST_r) and left (ST_l) legs, respectively. Shaded areas indicate double support periods when both feet are on the ground; DS_r and DS_l are the right and left double support periods, respectively. Step times (interlimb heel-strike durations) of the right and left legs (t_r and t_l) are defined as the time between consecutive heel-strikes. **(C)** θ_{rh}, and θ_{rk} are hip and knee joint angles of the right leg, respectively. v_{yheel}, and v_{zheel} are velocity profiles of heel in y and z directions. Thick solid and dashed vertical lines represent gait events for the right and left legs, respectively.

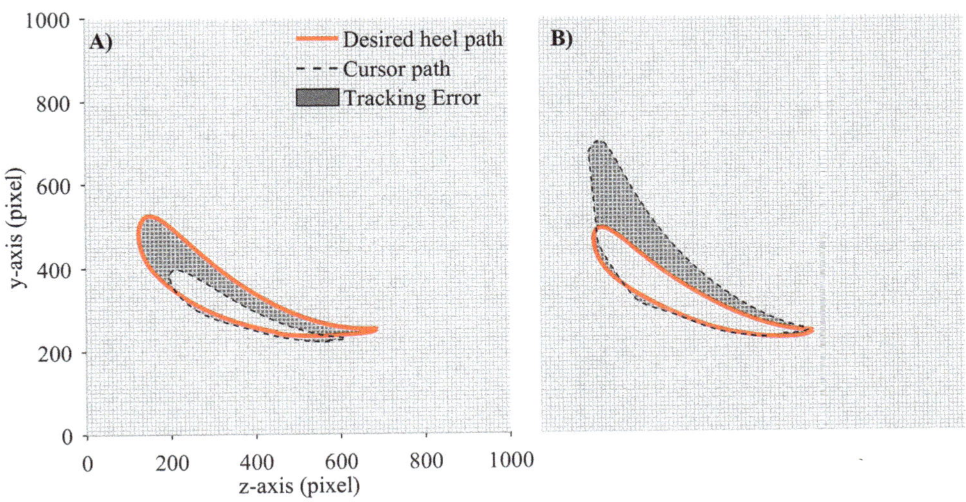

FIGURE 4 | Computation of tracking error in each gait cycle. Desired heel path (solid red line) and cursor path (dashed black line) were placed on a 1,000 × 1,000 pixel image. Tracking error was defined as the number of pixels in gray area. Each small square block in the grid contains 100 pixels. **(A)** Tracking error is negative and **(B)** Tracking error is positive.

of tracking errors in different phase of training: pre-, exposure, and post-. During pre-exposure, subjects walked normally on treadmill and the moving cursor was closed to the prescribed heel path. When visual kinematic perturbations were introduced (lower limb joint angles were scaled down by 0.7), the moving cursor departed from the prescribed heel path and subjects

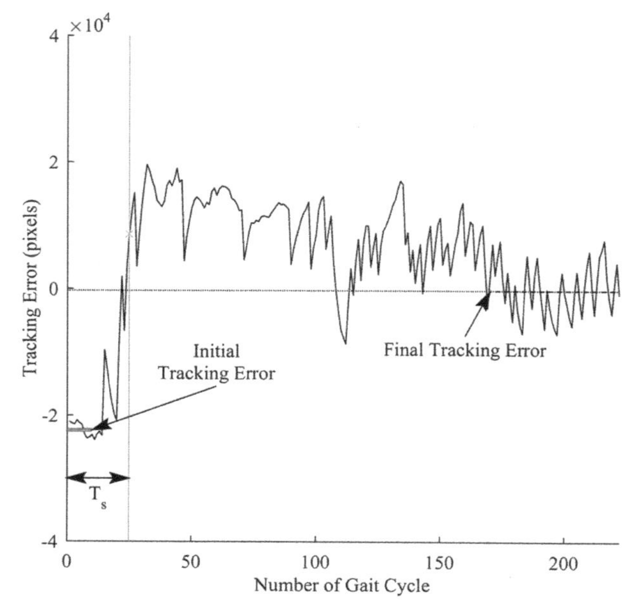

FIGURE 5 | Illustration of response time definition for each trial. Thick red line represents the initial tracking error (at the beginning of perturbation), and dashed line represents final tracking error (at late exposure). T_S is the response time computed in the number of gait cycles. Vertical green line is time when a subject responded to the visual perturbations.

started adapting their gait to the perturbation. The tracking errors in the early exposures gradually decreased across trials (from Trial 1 to Trial 4) as subjects were adapting to the visual perturbation. When subjects resolved the perturbation problem, the moving cursor were closed the prescribed heel path profiles again. In the post-exposure phase, the visual kinematic perturbation was removed. In this phase, the moving cursor departed from the prescribed heel path profiles again but in the opposite direction (positive tracking errors), reflecting after-effects of gait adaptation. By the end of this trial, the tracking errors returned to pre-exposure levels.

Figure 6B shows the results of statistical analysis for tracking errors. Significant increases in tracking errors [block means ($\times 10^4$ pixels): pre $= -0.47 \pm 1.21$; early exposure (the first 30 gait cycles in Trial 1) $= -2.07 \pm 1.25$, $P < 0.001$] were found immediately after the introduction of visual kinematic perturbations. As expected, the tracking errors gradually decreased with practice from Trial 1 to Trial 3 and reached a plateau in Trial 4 [block means for early-exposure ($\times 10^4$ pixels): Trial 1 $= -2.07 \pm 1.25$; Trial 2 $= -0.54 \pm 1.57$; Trial 3 $= -0.28 \pm 1.26$, and Trial 4 $= -0.29 \pm 0.97$]. There were significant after-effects for tracking errors in the early post-exposure phase (the first 1 min) when the visual perturbation was removed [group means ($\times 10^4$ pixels): pre $= -0.47 \pm 1.21$; early post $= 0.68 \pm 1.54$, $P < 0.001$]. **Figure 6C** shows the results of response time during exposure periods across 4 trials. When the visual perturbation was introduced in the first trial, the mean and one standard deviation of the response time across all subjects was 148.5 ± 69.1 gait cycles. These value substantially decreased in later trials except for Trial 4 (Trial 2: 56.2 ± 36.0; Trial 3: 19.3 ± 20.7; Trial 4: 35.7 ± 36.7). Although the response time in the trial 4 is higher than in the trial 3, the difference is non-significant (p-value > 0.05).

Strategies of Gait Adaptation Varied across Subjects

Figure 7 depicts the changes in lower limb joint angles during late-exposure (Trial 4) when subjects adapted to the visual kinematic perturbations. Results from *post-hoc* analysis show that subjects varied joint angles differently when adapting to the perturbation. For example, SG01 had more changes in ankle joint angles (Hip: 1.35 ± 0.14; Knee: 1.57 ± 0.10; Ankle: 3.11 ± 0.34, $P < 0.001$), while SG02 had more changes in knee joint angles (Hip: 1.09 ± 0.15; Knee: 1.61 ± 0.09; Ankle: 1.02 ± 0.06, $P < 0.001$). **Figure 7A** shows that different strategies of gait adaptation affect tracking errors in the late-exposure. Specifically, the tracking errors of subjects SG01: 12.61 ± 6.95, SG06: 11.06 ± 6.25, and SG08: 10.46 ± 2.80 were significantly higher than the other subjects: 8.67 ± 4.45 (these values are in $\times 10^3$ pixels). **Figure 7B** reveals that SG01, SG06, and SG08 adapted more on the ankle joint angles instead of the hip and knee joints. This gait adaptation strategy resulted in larger tracking errors because the changes in the ankle joint angles have lesser effect on the variations of heel position as compared to the changes in the hip and knee joint angles (Equation 2).

Gait Symmetry in the Spatial and Temporal Domains during Visual Kinematic Perturbations

Figure 8 illustrates the changes of gait symmetry in the temporal domain to visual kinematic perturbations. Theoretically, the right and left double support limb periods are equal during normal walking conditions (pre-exposure). When visual kinematic perturbations were introduced and subjects started adapting their gait to the perturbation, the double support periods are different and the gait asymmetry in temporal domain increase. In the post-exposure phase, visual kinematic perturbations were removed and double support periods gradually return to symmetric step times.

We observed that $S_{spatial}$ and $S_{temporal}$ can characterize the adaptation of gait symmetry in the spatial and temporal domains, respectively. For example, results from **Figure 9** show that $S_{spatial}$ and $S_{temporal}$ significantly increased between the early (Trial 1) and late exposure phase (Trial 4), indicating the adaptation of motor outputs for gait symmetry ($S_{spatial}$ − Trial 1: 0.09 ± 0.09, Trial 4: 0.19 ± 0.06, $P < 0.001$; $S_{temporal}$ − Trial 1: 0.05 ± 0.07, Trial 4: 0.08 ± 0.08, $P < 0.001$). Moreover, there was significant difference between pre- and post-exposure ($S_{temporal}$ − Pre: 0.02 ± 0.07, Post-Exposure: 0.06 ± 0.09, $P < 0.001$), indicating that there were significant storages of new gait symmetry indices in the temporal domains.

Figure 9 also illustrates that the gait symmetry in the temporal domain is less sensitive to the visual kinematic perturbations and its after-effects are larger than those in the spatial domain. For example, when the perturbations were introduced, $S_{spatial}$

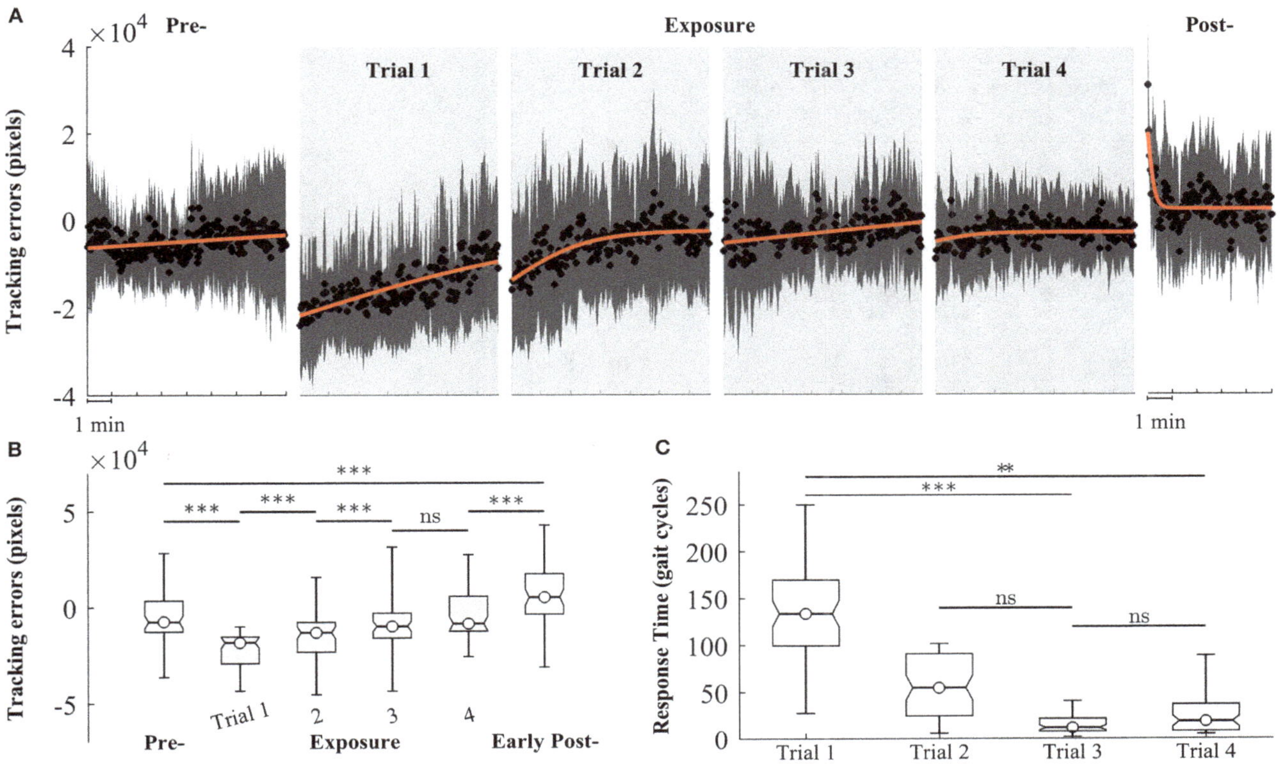

FIGURE 6 | Group averages of tracking errors across 4 trials of training, gray areas represent early exposure period. **(A)** Black circles represent mean of tracking errors across subjects, and shaded areas indicate one standard deviation. Solid lines are fitting curves using a sigmoidal model. **(B,C)** Statistical analysis of tracking errors and response time using multiple comparison test with Tukey-Kramer adjustment, respectively. $^{**}P < 0.01$ and $^{***}P < 0.001$. ns, non-significant.

increased from -0.002 ± 0.07 (Pre-) to 0.12 ± 0.14 (Exposure, trial 1) while $S_{temporal}$ increased from 0.02 ± 0.07 to 0.05 ± 0.07. When the perturbations were removed, $S_{spatial}$ decreased from 0.18 ± 0.08 (Exposure, trial 4) to 0.006 ± 0.09 (Post-) while $S_{temporal}$ decreased from 0.08 ± 0.08 to 0.06 ± 0.09. Moreover, gait symmetry index in the spatial domain approached a new-steady state faster than in the temporal domain. For example, $S_{spatial}$ reached a new steady state on Trial 2 ($S_{spatial}$ was not significantly different from Trial 2 to Trial 4) while $S_{temporal}$ reached a new steady-state on Trial 4. The perturbation resulted in a stronger after-effect in the temporal domain as compared to the spatial domain. The temporal gait symmetry was significantly different between the pre- and post-exposure phase ($P < 0.001$) and it lasted for more than 5 min. However, there is no significant difference in the spatial gait symmetry index between pre- and post-exposure phase. When the perturbation was removed, the spatial gait symmetry index returned to the pre-exposure condition in <1 min.

DISCUSSION

This study investigated gait adaptation of healthy individual in the presences of visual kinematic perturbation (i.e., a gain change) of gait during treadmill walking across several trials. The visual kinematic perturbations, which caused a mismatch between actual and prescribed heel path trajectories displayed on a screen, were introduced to investigate visual-motor adaptation of human locomotion. We observed that, with practice, the subjects could reduce the errors induced by the visual kinematic perturbations and showed faster response time in later trials (Trial 1 to Trial 3). Thus, by late exposure, subjects have found a solution for the visual kinematic perturbations problem and acquired, at least partially, the internal model of the visuomotor transformation. Moreover, the strategies of gait adaptation varied across subjects and affected steady-state tracking errors in late-exposure. Our results also showed that the temporal gait symmetry in the post-exposure phase was significantly different from the pre-exposure phase. This after-effect suggested that there were significant storages of new temporal gait symmetry index.

Introduction of the kinematic gait perturbation showed an initial rise of tracking errors in early-exposure, the reduction of tracking errors in exposure, and the after-effect in post-exposure (**Figure 6**). The presence of after-effects is an indication that motor adaptation has occurred (Shadmehr and Mussa-Ivaldi, 1994; Kagerer et al., 1997; Buch et al., 2003; Krakauer et al., 2005; Scheidt et al., 2005; Choi and Bastian, 2007; Reisman et al., 2009; Kim et al., 2010). Although the experimental setup in this study is simple, the results reflect the decreases of tracking errors

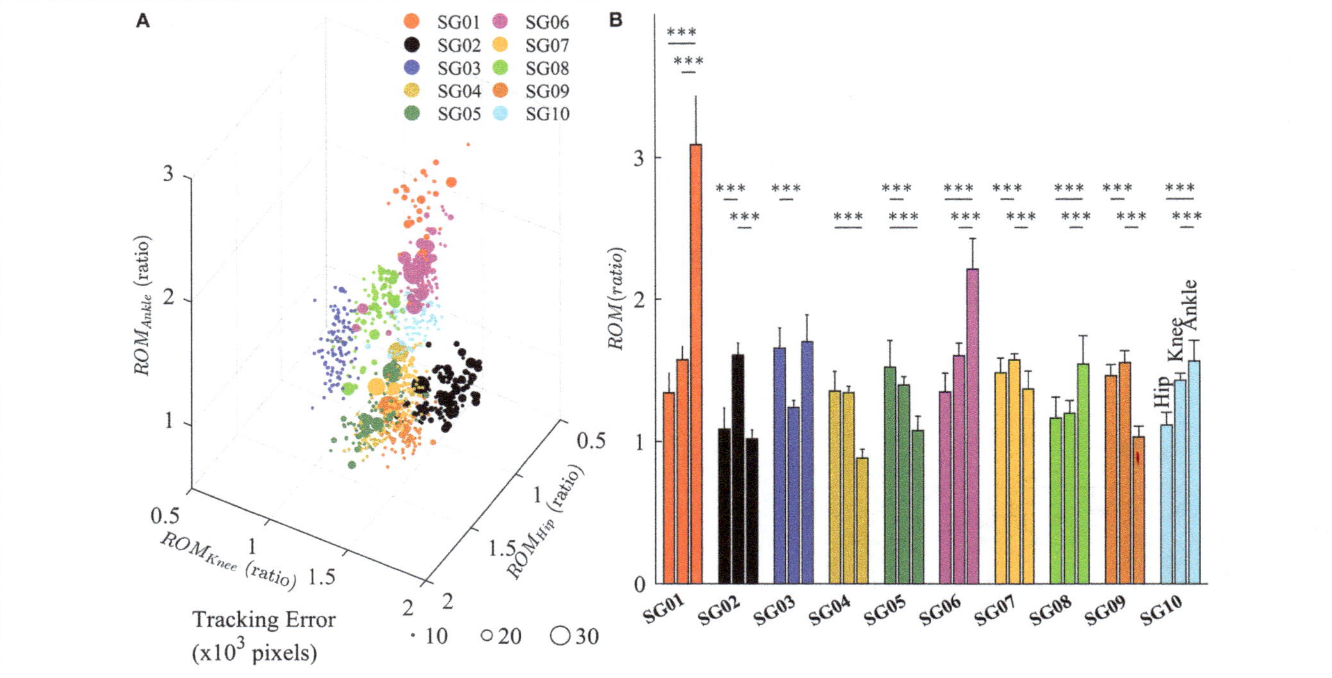

FIGURE 7 | (A) Variations of lower limb joint angles (hip, knee, and ankle) in the right leg for 10 subjects in late-exposure (Trial 4). The size of the symbols represents the tracking error. **(B)** ROM ratio is the proportion of range of motion in late-exposure compared to pre-exposure. *Post-hoc* analyses using multiple comparison with Tukey-Kramer adjustment. ***$P < 0.001$.

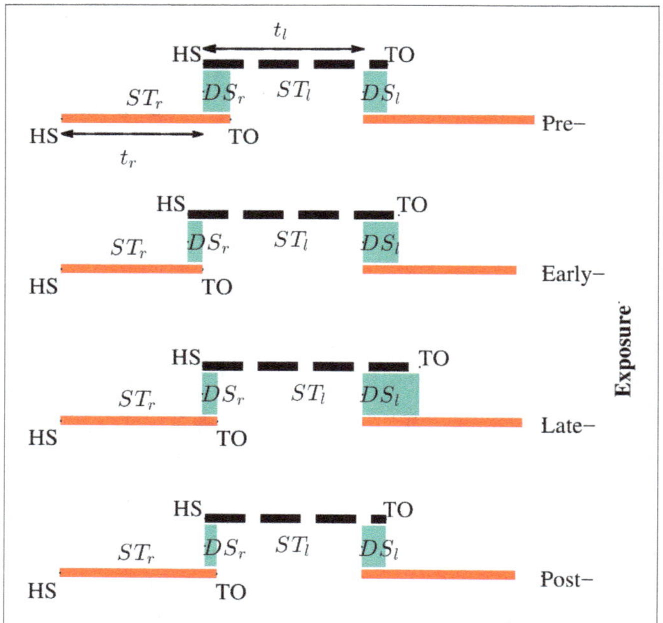

FIGURE 8 | Adaptation of temporal parameters during visual kinematic perturbations for subject SG04. The solid red line and dashed black line represent stance periods of the right and left leg, respectively. Double support periods are represented by the shaded sea green area. During the pre-exposure phase, the subject walked normally and the right and left double support times were equal. Temporal asymmetry increased in the exposure phases and sustained in post-exposure.

across trials and the after-effects that characterize the motor adaptation process. We hypothesize that the training method used in this study could be a feasible intervention to potentially improve asymmetries in post-stroke gait rehabilitation. Previous studies have shown that after-effects of locomotor or visuomotor adaptation improve task performance in individuals post-stroke (Rossetti et al., 1998; Patton et al., 2006). Moreover, Reisman et al. demonstrated that the improvements of task performance following split-belt treadmill adaptation could transfer to real world tasks such as overground walking (Reisman et al., 2009).

Gait asymmetry is an important gait characteristic that may have a role in guiding the clinician's treatment decisions (Patterson et al., 2008, 2010). Gait asymmetry may be associated with negative effects on human locomotion such as decreases in gait efficiency, balance control, and gait speed (Jorgensen et al., 2000). For example, asymmetric step length results in decreased walking speed, and both decreased propulsive force and increased severity of the paretic limb (Bowden et al., 2006; Balasubramanian et al., 2007; Jonkers et al., 2009). Asymmetric double support time is related to decreased gait speed (Olney et al., 1994). Asymmetric walking gait patterns are commonly found in individuals post-stroke. However, some individuals post-stroke have asymmetry in only one domain. For example, they only have either step length asymmetry (spatial) or double support time asymmetry (temporal). Therefore, it could be more efficient to target therapeutic rehabilitation to only the domain (spatial or temporal) of gait symmetry in which the post-stroke persons experience difficulty. Separate control of the

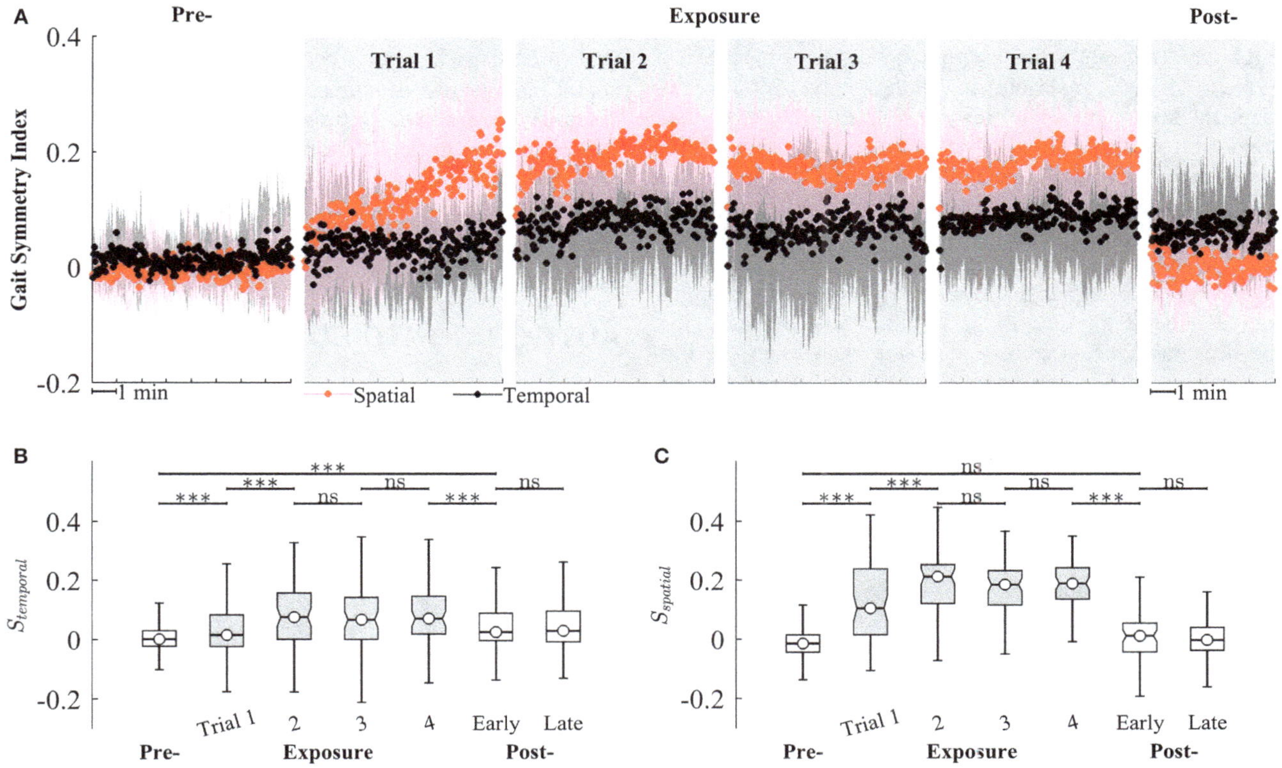

FIGURE 9 | (A) Group averages of gait symmetry indices across 4 trials of training. Black and red circles represent mean values of temporal and spatial gait symmetry indices, respectively. Shaded areas indicate one standard deviation. **(B,C)** Statistical analysis for gait symmetry index in the temporal ($S_{temporal}$), and spatial ($S_{spatial}$) domain using multiple comparison with Tukey-Kramer adjustment. ***P < 0.001, *ns*, non-significant. Box plots in gray represent exposure period.

temporal and spatial control of human locomotion has been demonstrated in studies of locomotor adaptation to split-belt treadmill training (Reisman et al., 2009; Malone et al., 2012). However, interventions that target only one domain of gait asymmetry have not been fully developed. In this study, multi-trial locomotor training using visual kinematic perturbations was implemented and the subjects adapted to the perturbations by modifying their gait patterns. Once adapted, the subjects could not retrieve their normal gait pattern immediately when the perturbations were removed. Instead, they had to "de-adapt" their gait patterns back to original state. This after-effect was a strong clue that motor adaptation has occurred and a new representation of visuomotor mapping has been learned. Results in **Figure 9** show the after-effects of gait symmetry indices in the temporal domains in early post-exposure phase, indicating that there were significant storages of new temporal gait symmetry index. However, after-effects were not observed for the spatial gait symmetry index. These findings have implications for a possible intervention to improve gait symmetry in the temporal domain for individuals post-stroke and the setup in this study could be beneficial to gait rehabilitation.

Our results suggest differential temporal and spatial symmetry effects to the kinematic perturbations. For example, we observed after-effects of the temporal gait symmetry index after the presence of kinematic perturbations, indicating its adaptation. However, the after-effect or adaptation of the spatial gait symmetry was missing. These results support previous findings suggesting that the adaptation of spatial and temporal gait symmetry is dissociable (Malone et al., 2012). The tracking task in this study was mainly spatial because the subjects followed the desired heel path without considering the time to reach a specific point. Interestingly, the adaptation occurred nevertheless in the temporal gait symmetry. This could have the implication that the subjects unconsciously adapted temporal gait symmetry under the visual kinematic perturbations. This findings are aligned with previous studies suggesting that subjects may not be able to consciously prevent adapting temporal motor output under split-belt conditions (Malone et al., 2012), and that temporal gait symmetry is harder to influence with conscious efforts (Malone and Bastian, 2010). Additionally, our findings support the hypothesis that the temporal control of human gait is more automatic and depends more heavily on subcortical circuits. Vasudevan et al. (2011) also showed that temporal adaptation was found to be fully developed earlier than spatial adaptation (by 3 year old and until adolescence, respectively).

The feasibility of this intervention to improve gait asymmetry might also be extended to target only specific joints that may be affected more than others. Our results demonstrated that subjects use multiple solutions, i.e., multiple ways for subjects to alter their joint movements, to adapt to the visual kinematic perturbations (**Figure 7**). For example, while the subject SG01 preferred to adapt the ankle joint angles, the subject SG02 favored to adapt the knee joint angles instead. **Figure 7** illustrates that different strategies of gait adaptation affect tracking errors in late-exposure. Moreover, **Figure 7B** reveals that subjects who adapted more on the ankle joint angle instead of the hip and knee joints (SG01, SG06, and SG08) showed larger steady-state tracking errors in the late-exposure phase. This gait adaptation strategy resulted in higher tracking errors because the changes in the ankle joint angles have lesser effect on the variations of the heel positions as compared to the changes in the hip and knee joint angles (Equation 2). Overall, these findings are supported by the motor equivalence problem (Bernstein, 1967), which characterizes the kinematic redundancy of motor control systems: in this case, using three degrees of freedom (hip, knee, and ankle joints) to control the heel position in a two-dimensional space. Therefore, even though there are multiple solutions (due to redundant degrees of freedom) to accomplish a motor task, we can indirectly influence the motor system to favor one solution by controlling the rules that generate visual kinematic perturbations (i.e., using different scaling factors for each joint angle), which can allow for personalized gait therapy based on the current state of the patient.

Findings of this study are currently limited to healthy individuals. Future investigations should consider implementing the framework of visual kinematic perturbations for gait rehabilitation in individuals post-stroke. In this regard, the motor task is expected to be more challenging for persons post-stroke. The number of trials required to achieve significant performance improvement may also increase. It will also be important to examine the changes in the representations of gait at cortical level during the visual kinematic perturbations. The understanding of neural mechanisms of human gait adaptation is important for designing an effective training paradigm of gait rehabilitation in a top-down approach. Noninvasive electroencephalography (EEG) studies could be designed to investigate the underlying patterns of neural activity during the visual kinematic perturbations.

AUTHOR CONTRIBUTIONS

TPL contributed to task design, developing software for data collection, acquisition of the data, interpretation for the work, and manuscript draft. YH contributed to developing software for data collection, acquisition of the data, and literature review. SN, KN, and JG contributed to experimental design, data acquisition, and revising the draft. SB contributed in developing software for data collection and manuscript review. JC conceived the experiment, edited the manuscript and approved the final version of the paper.

ACKNOWLEDGMENTS

This research was supported by award R01NS075889 from the National Institute of Neurological Disorders And Stroke (NINDS). The content is solely the responsibility of the authors and does not necessarily represent the official views of the NINDS or the National Institutes of Health (NIH).

REFERENCES

Alexander, M. S., Flodin, B. W., and Marigold, D. S. (2013). Changes in task parameters during walking prism adaptation influence the subsequent generalization pattern. *J. Neurophysiol.* 109, 2495–2504. doi: 10.1152/jn.00810.2012

Antonsson, E. K., and Mann, R. W. (1985). The frequency content of gait. *J. Biomech.* 18, 39–47. doi: 10.1016/0021-9290(85)90043-0

Balasubramanian, C. K., Bowden, M. G., Neptune, R. R., and Kautz, S. A. (2007). Relationship between step length asymmetry and walking performance in subjects with chronic hemiparesis. *Arch. Phys. Med. Rehabil.* 88, 43–49. doi: 10.1016/j.apmr.2006.10.004

Bastian, A. J. (2008). Understanding sensorimotor adaptation and learning for rehabilitation. *Curr. Opin. Neurol.* 21:628. doi: 10.1097/WCO.0b013e328315a293

Bernstein, N. A. (1967). *The Co-ordination and Regulation of Movements.* Oxford: Pergamon Press.

Bowden, M. G., Balasubramanian, C. K., Neptune, R. R., and Kautz, S. A. (2006). Anterior-posterior ground reaction forces as a measure of paretic leg contribution in hemiparetic walking *Stroke* 37, 872–876. doi: 10.1161/01.STR.0000204063.75779.8d

Buch, E. R., Young, S., and Contreras-Vidal, J. L. (2003). Visuomotor adaptation in normal aging. *Learn. Mem.* 10, 55–63. doi: 10.1101/lm.50303

Cheng, S., and Sabes, P. N. (2007). Calibration of visually guided reaching is driven by error-corrective learning and internal dynamics. *J. Neurophysiol.* 97, 3057–3069. doi: 10.1152/jn.00897.2006

Choi, J. T., and Bastian, A. J. (2007). Adaptation reveals independent control networks for human walking. *Nat. Neurosci.* 10, 1055–1062. doi: 10.1038/nn1930

Contreras-Vidal, J. L., and Kerick, S. E. (2004). Independent component analysis of dynamic brain responses during visuomotor adaptation *Neuroimage* 21, 936–945. doi: 10.1016/j.neuroimage.2003.10.037

Emken, J. L., Benitez, R., Sideris, A., Bobrow, J. E., and Reinkensmeyer, D. J. (2007). Motor adaptation as a greedy optimization of error and effort. *J. Neurophysiol.* 97, 3997–4006. doi: 10.1152/jn.01095.2006

Finley, J. M., Statton, M. A., and Bastian, A. J. (2014). A novel optic flow pattern speeds split-belt locomotor adaptation *J. Neurophysiol.* 111, 969–976. doi: 10.1152/jn.00513.2013

Helm, E. E., and Reisman, D. S. (2015). The split-belt walking paradigm: exploring motor learning and spatiotemporal asymmetry poststroke. *Phys. Med. Rehabil. Clin. N. Am.* 26, 703–713. doi: 10.1016/j.pmr.2015.06.010

Hussain, S. J., Hanson, A. S., Tseng, S. C., and Morton, S. M. (2013). A locomotor adaptation including explicit knowledge and removal of postadaptation errors induces complete 24-hour retention. *J. Neurophysiol.* 110, 916–925. doi: 10.1152/jn.00770.2012

Imamizu, H., Uno, Y., and Kawato, M. (1998). Adaptive internal model of intrinsic kinematics involved in learning an aiming task. *J. Exp. Psychol. Hum. Percept. Perform.* 24:812. doi: 10.1037/0096-1523.24.3.812

Izawa, J., Rane, T., Donchin, O., and Shadmehr, R. (2008). Motor adaptation as a process of reoptimization. *J. Neurosci.* 28, 2883–2891. doi: 10.1523/JNEUROSCI.5359-07.2008

Izawa, J., and Shadmehr, R. (2011). Learning from sensory and reward prediction errors during motor adaptation. *PLoS Comput. Biol.* 7:e1002012. doi: 10.1371/journal.pcbi.1002012

Jonkers, I., Delp, S., and Patten, C. (2009). Capacity to increase walking speed is limited by impaired hip and ankle power generation in lower functioning persons post-stroke. *Gait Posture* 29, 129–137. doi: 10.1016/j.gaitpost.2008.07.010

Jorgensen, L., Crabtree, N., Reeve, J., and Jacobsen, B. (2000). Ambulatory level and asymmetrical weight bearing after stroke affects bone loss in the upper and lower part of the femoral neck differently: bone adaptation after decreased mechanical loading. *Bone* 27, 701–707. doi: 10.1016/S8756-3282(00)00374-4

Kagerer, F. A., Contreras-Vidal, J. L., and Stelmach, G. E. (1997). Adaptation to gradual as compared with sudden visuo-motor distortions. *Exp. Brain Res.* 115, 557–561. doi: 10.1007/PL00005727

Kim, S. H., Banala, S. K., Brackbill, E. A., Agrawal, S. K., Krishnamoorthy, V., and Scholz, J. P. (2010). Robot-assisted modifications of gait in healthy individuals. *Exp. Brain Res.* 202, 809–824. doi: 10.1007/s00221-010-2187-5

Krakauer, J. W., Ghez, C., and Ghilardi, M. F. (2005). Adaptation to visuomotor transformations: consolidation, interference, and forgetting. *J. Neurosci.* 25, 473–478. doi: 10.1523/JNEUROSCI.4218-04.2005

Long, A. W., Roemmich, R. T., and Bastian, A. J. (2016). Blocking trial-by-trial error correction does not interfere with motor learning in human walking. *J. Neurophysiol.* 115, 2341–2348. doi: 10.1152/jn.00941.2015

Luu, T. P., He, Y., Brown, S., Nakagame, S., and Contreras-Vidal, J. L. (2016). Gait adaptation to visual kinematic perturbations using a real-time closed-loop brain–computer interface to a virtual reality avatar. *J. Neural Eng.* 13:036006. doi: 10.1088/1741-2560/13/3/036006

Luu, T. P., He, Y., Brown, S., Nakagome, S., and Contreras-Vidal, J. L. (2015). "A closed-loop brain computer interface to a virtual reality avatar: gait adaptation to visual kinematic perturbations," in *Virtual Rehabilitation Proceedings (ICVR), 2015 International Conference on* (Valencia), 30–37.

Luu, T. P., Low, K. H., Qu, X., Lim, H. B., and Hoon, K. H. (2014). An individual-specific gait pattern prediction model based on generalized regression neural networks. *Gait Posture* 39, 443–448. doi: 10.1016/j.gaitpost.2013.08.028

Malfait, N., Shiller, D. M., and Ostry, D. J. (2002). Transfer of motor learning across arm configurations. *J. Neurosci.* 22, 9656–9660. Available online at: http://www.jneurosci.org/content/22/22/9656.long

Malone, L. A., and Bastian, A. J. (2010). Thinking about walking: effects of conscious correction versus distraction on locomotor adaptation. *J. Neurophysiol.* 103, 1954–1962. doi: 10.1152/jn.00832.2009

Malone, L. A., Bastian, A. J., and Torres-Oviedo, G. (2012). How does the motor system correct for errors in time and space during locomotor adaptation? *J. Neurophysiol.* 108, 672–683. doi: 10.1152/jn.00391.2011

Malone, L. A., Vasudevan, E. V., and Bastian, A. J. (2011). Motor adaptation training for faster relearning. *J. Neurosci.* 31, 15136–15143. doi: 10.1523/JNEUROSCI.1367-11.2011

Morton, S. M., and Bastian, A. J. (2004). Prism adaptation during walking generalizes to reaching and requires the cerebellum. *J. Neurophysiol.* 92, 2497–2509. doi: 10.1152/jn.00129.2004

Nemanich, S. T., and Earhart, G. M. (2015). Prism adaptation in Parkinson disease: comparing reaching to walking and freezers to non-freezers. *Exp. Brain Res.* 233, 2301–2310. doi: 10.1007/s00221-015-4299-4

Olney, S. J., Griffin, M. P., and McBride, I. D. (1994). Temporal, kinematic, and kinetic variables related to gait speed in subjects with hemiplegia: a regression approach. *Phys. Ther.* 74, 872–885. doi: 10.1093/ptj/74.9.872

Patterson, K. K., Parafianowicz, I., Danells, C. J., Closson, V., Verrier, M. C., Staines, W. R., et al. (2008). Gait asymmetry in community-ambulating stroke survivors. *Arch. Phys. Med. Rehabil.* 89, 304–310. doi: 10.1016/j.apmr.2007.08.142

Patterson, K. K., Gage, W. H., Brooks, D., Black, S. E., and McIlroy, W. E. (2010). Evaluation of gait symmetry after stroke: a comparison of current methods and recommendations for standardization. *Gait Posture* 31, 241–246. doi: 10.1016/j.gaitpost.2009.10.014

Patton, J. L., Stoykov, M. E., Kovic, M., and Mussa-Ivaldi, F. A. (2006). Evaluation of robotic training forces that either enhance or reduce error in chronic hemiparetic stroke survivors. *Exp. Brain Res.* 168, 368–383. doi: 10.1007/s00221-005-0097-8

Reisman, D. S., Block, H. J., and Bastian, A. J. (2005). Interlimb coordination during locomotion: what can be adapted and stored? *J. Neurophysiol.* 94, 2403–2415. doi: 10.1152/jn.00089.2005

Reisman, D. S., Wityk, R., Silver, K., and Bastian, A. J. (2007). Locomotor adaptation on a split-belt treadmill can improve walking symmetry post-stroke. *Brain* 130, 1861–1872. doi: 10.1093/brain/awm035

Reisman, D. S., Wityk, R., Silver, K., and Bastian, A. J. (2009). Split-belt treadmill adaptation transfers to overground walking in persons poststroke. *Neurorehabil. Neural Repair* 23, 735–744. doi: 10.1177/1545968309332880

Rossetti, Y., Rode, G., Pisella, L., Farné, A., Li, L., Boisson, D., et al. (1998). Prism adaptation to a rightward optical deviation rehabilitates left hemispatial neglect *Nature* 395, 166–169. doi: 10.1038/25988

Scheidt, R. A., Conditt, M. A., Secco, E. L., and Mussa-Ivaldi, F. A. (2005). Interaction of visual and proprioceptive feedback during adaptation of human reaching movements. *J. Neurophysiol.* 93, 3200–3213. doi: 10.1152/jn.00947.2004

Scheidt, R. A., Dingwell, J. B., and Mussa-Ivaldi, F. A. (2001). Learning to move amid uncertainty. *J. Neurophysiol.* 86, 971–985. Available online at: http://jn.physiology.org/content/86/2/971.short

Shadmehr, R., and Mussa-Ivaldi, F. A. (1994). Adaptive representation of dynamics during learning of a motor task. *J. Neurosci.* 14, 3208–3224.

Statton, M. A., Toliver, A., and Bastian, A. J. (2016). A dual-learning paradigm can simultaneously train multiple characteristics of walking. *J. Neurophysiol.* 115, 2692–2700. doi: 10.1152/jn.00090.2016

Torres-Oviedo, G., and Bastian, A. J. (2010). Seeing is believing: effects of visual contextual cues on learning and transfer of locomotor adaptation. *J. Neurosci.* 30, 17015–17022. doi: 10.1523/JNEUROSCI.4205-10.2010

Torres-Oviedo, G., Vasudevan, E., Malone, L., and Bastian, A. J. (2011). Locomotor adaptation. *Prog. Brain Res.* 191, 65–74. doi: 10.1016/B978-0-444-53752-2.00013-8

Vasudevan, E. V., Torres-Oviedo, G., Morton, S. M., Yang, J. F., and Bastian, A. J. (2011). Younger is not always better: development of locomotor adaptation from childhood to adulthood. *J. Neurosci.* 31, 3055–3065. doi: 10.1523/JNEUROSCI.5781-10.2011

Wei, K., and Kording, K. (2009). Relevance of error: what drives motor adaptation? *J. Neurophysiol.* 101, 655–664. doi: 10.1152/jn.90545.2008

Winter, D. A. (1992). Foot trajectory in human gait: a precise and multifactorial motor control task. *Phys. Ther.* 72, 45–53. doi: 10.1093/ptj/72.1.45

10

Recovery from Multiple APAs Delays Gait Initiation in Parkinson's Disease

Rajal G. Cohen[1], John G. Nutt[2] and Fay B. Horak[2,3]*

[1] *Department of Psychology and Communication Studies, University of Idaho, Moscow, ID, USA,* [2] *Department of Neurology, Oregon Health and Science University, Portland, OR, USA,* [3] *Research Department, Veterans Affairs Portland Health Care System, Portland, OR, USA*

Correspondence:
Rajal G. Cohen
rcohen@uidaho.edu

Background: Freezing of gait in Parkinson's disease (PD) has been linked with deficits in inhibitory control, but causal mechanisms are not established. Freezing at gait initiation (start hesitation) is often accompanied by multiple anticipatory postural adjustments (APAs). If inhibition deficits contribute to freezing by interfering with ability to inhibit initial weight shifts in the wrong direction, then PD subjects should experience more episodes of multiple APAs than healthy controls (HCs) do. If inhibition deficits contribute to freezing by interfering with ability to release a previously inhibited step following multiple APAs, then step onset following multiple APAs should be delayed more in people with PD than in HCs.

Methods: Older adults with PD and HC subjects rapidly initiated stepping in response to a light cue in blocks of simple (SRT) and choice (CRT) conditions. We recorded kinematics and ground reaction forces, and we administered the Stroop task to assess inhibitory control.

Results: Multiple APAs were more common in CRT than SRT conditions but were equally common in HC and PD subjects. Step onsets were delayed in both conditions and further delayed in trials with multiple APAs, except for HC subjects in SRT trials. Poor Stroop performance correlated with many multiple APAs, late step onset, and rearward position of center of mass (COM) at cue presentation. Forward motion of the COM during the APA was higher in trials with multiple APAs than in trials with single APAs, especially in CRT trials and in PD subjects *without* self-reported freezing.

Conclusion: Start hesitation is not caused by multiple APAs *per se*, but may be associated with difficulty recovering from multiple APAs, due to difficulty releasing a previously inhibited step.

Keywords: Parkinson's disease, anticipatory postural adjustment, freezing of gait, start hesitation, inhibition, inhibitory control, gait initiation, voluntary stepping

INTRODUCTION

People with Parkinson's disease (PD) commonly experience a gait problem known as *start hesitation*, a brief episode of freezing of gait in which step initiation is involuntarily delayed (Nutt et al., 2011). While the precise causes of start hesitation (and the wider category of gait freezing) are not yet known, several intriguing clues exist. For instance, start hesitation is often accompanied by trembling of the knees and multiple lateral weight shifts, termed anticipatory postural adjustments, or *APAs* (Jacobs et al., 2009). The dissociation between APA onset and step onset in these cases led to the proposal that freezing may be caused by decoupling between the postural preparation and the step (Jacobs et al., 2009). Freezing of gait has also been associated with cognitive deficits in the domain of executive function, especially inhibitory control (Amboni et al., 2008; Vandenbossche et al., 2011; Cohen et al., 2014). We postulate that posture-step decoupling and inhibitory deficits may play a joint role in the etiology of start hesitation.

Previous work investigating start hesitation in PD demonstrated multiple APAs in protective stepping but did not elicit substantial numbers of multiple APAs in voluntary stepping (Jacobs et al., 2009). In everyday life, however, start hesitation is particularly problematic during voluntary stepping; the accepted definition of freezing, "brief, episodic absence or marked reduction of forward progression of the feet despite the intention to walk" (Nutt et al., 2011), implies the thwarting of a voluntary act. Therefore, the present study makes use of a protocol known to elicit multiple APAs in voluntary stepping in healthy adults (Cohen et al., 2011).

To initiate a step, it is necessary to select a stepping leg and shift the weight off the stepping leg onto the stance leg. Shifting the weight off of the intended stepping leg is achieved by first briefly *increasing* vertical ground reaction force under the stepping foot, in order to push off (Brenière et al., 1987). Because the needed initial weight shift is toward the stepping foot (in the opposite direction from the goal), inhibition may be required to avoid shifting the weight in the wrong direction when attempting to step. Therefore, inhibitory control may be challenged experimentally by forcing subjects to make rapid choices about which foot to step with. In a previous study, we asked healthy older subjects to perform a stepping task in a choice reaction time (CRT) condition, which presented a foot selection challenge, as well as a simple reaction time (SRT) condition, in which the stepping foot was known in advance (Cohen et al., 2011). We found that in the CRT condition only, healthy older adults made initial weight shift errors, leading to multiple APAs in 25% of trials. The presence of multiple APAs resulted in statistically significant step onset delays of about 130 ms. Furthermore, the proportion of trials with weight shift errors was strongly correlated with the time to complete the conflict condition of the Stroop task, a typical measure of inhibitory control. Thus, a possible mechanism by which inhibitory deficits could contribute to freezing of gait is by making foot selection more difficult, leading to multiple APAs and start hesitation. However, questions remain as to whether and how the multiple APAs elicited by CRT stepping in healthy older adults are related to start hesitation in subjects with PD.

Parkinson's disease impairs frontostriatal circuitry, which is important for selection and inhibition of actions (Mostofsky and Simmonds, 2008). Individuals with PD who freeze have significantly reduced structural and functional connectivity in the right hemisphere inhibitory circuit between the SMA and STN compared to individuals with PD who do not freeze (Fling et al., 2013, 2014). Furthermore, freezing of gait is specifically associated with deficits in cognitive inhibitory control and conflict resolution (Amboni et al., 2008; Vandenbossche et al., 2011; Cohen et al., 2014) and especially with difficulty releasing inhibition (Cohen et al., 2014). We investigated two (non-exclusive) ways that deficits in inhibitory control could interact with multiple APAs and lead to posture-step decoupling and start hesitation. One possible way that inhibitory deficits could contribute to start hesitation is if individuals with PD who experience freezing of gait are particularly *predisposed* to multiple APAs, due to problems selecting the correct stepping leg initially. Another possibility is that individuals with PD who freeze might have a particularly difficult time *recovering* from multiple APAs, due to difficulty releasing inhibition.

The primary purpose of the present study was to examine the prevalence and influence of multiple APAs on step onset in adults with PD who did and did not report freezing, compared with healthy older adults, and to relate these findings to differences in inhibitory control. A secondary purpose of the study was to examine the kinematics of step onset associated with multiple APAs. Freezing of gait is strongly associated with fall risk (e.g., Bloem et al., 2004; Delval et al., 2014b). If, during a delayed step onset, the center of mass (COM) continues to move forward in adults with PD, this could predispose these individuals to falls.

Subjects performed a cued step initiation task in which trials were presented with (SRT) or without (CRT) foreknowledge of the stepping foot. To assess start hesitation, we measured kinematics and forces under subjects' feet; we then identified trials with multiple APAs and looked at onset times of weight shifts and first steps, as well as body position. Our hypotheses were as follows: (1) If inhibition is important for step initiation, we predicted that poor performance on the Stroop task would correlate with high prevalence of multiple APAs and delayed step onset. (2) If difficulty selecting the stepping leg (and inhibiting shifting weight in the wrong direction) contributes to start hesitation, we predicted that PD subjects who freeze would demonstrate a larger proportion of multiple APAs (especially in the CRT condition) relative to subjects who do not freeze. (3) If difficulty recovering from a multiple APA (and releasing inhibition of the step) contributes to start hesitation, we predicted that multiple APAs would lead to a larger step onset delay in PD subjects (especially those who freeze) than in subjects without PD. (4) We also predicted that the COM would travel forward farther during multiple APAs in subjects with PD (especially in those who tend to freeze) than in subjects without PD.

MATERIALS AND METHODS

Subjects

Twenty-five adults with idiopathic PD in a practical (14-h) OFF state participated in the study. Twelve self-identified as experiencing freezing of gait, and 13 did not. These subjects were compared with 12 previously studied healthy comparison (HC) subjects without PD (Cohen et al., 2011). None of the subjects had orthopedic problems or identified neurological disorders other than PD. All had normal or corrected-to-normal vision and hearing. See **Table 1** for details. The experiment was conducted in accordance with the Declaration of Helsinki and its later amendments. All procedures were carried out with adequate understanding and written consent by the subjects involved and

TABLE 1 | Demographic attributes of participants in healthy control (HC), non-freezing Parkinson's (NF), and Parkinson's with freezing (FR) groups; mean (SD); UPDRS, Unified Parkinson's Disease Rating Scale (Fahn and Elton, 1987).

	HC	*NF*	*FR*
Age	66.9 (6.6)	66.6 (5.9)	67.7 (8.9)
Number Men/Women	11/2	10/3	10/2
UPDRS III total	–	32.2 (7.7)	43.0 (14.0)
UPDRS: bradykinesia	–	15.0 (5.4)	19.9 (5.4)
UPDRS: PIGD	–	2.6 (2.2)	5.2 (3.4)
UPDRS: rigidity	–	8.0 (5.2)	8.9 (3.7)
Disease duration (Years)	–	6.2 (3.6)	10.0 (9.0)
H&Y (Hoehn and Yahr, 1967)	–	2.2 (0.4)	3.0 (0.8)

with the ethical approval of the institutional review board at Oregon Health and Science University.

Design and Protocol

The task was to initiate walking as quickly as possible in response to a cue, taking three steps before stopping. Subjects completed 2 blocks of 20 trials in a counterbalanced repeated measures design, with and without foreknowledge of stepping foot. Subjects began each trial looking straight ahead, with their body weight evenly balanced across two separate force platforms. Their feet were placed at a self-chosen comfortable width for walking, marked with tape so that every trial would begin from the same foot position. Before each trial, the experimenter monitored the force on each force plate on a computer screen and, when necessary, instructed the subject to shift to the left or right to achieve a balanced weight distribution (with no more than 51% of weight on either foot). An eight-camera motion-capture system (Motion Analysis System, Santa Rosa, CA, USA) gathered position data from passive reflective markers on each subject's trunk, head, and limbs, sampled at 60 Hz. Markers were placed bilaterally on the calcaneus, fifth metatarsal, lateral malleolus, lateral condyle, trochanter, acromial extremity of the clavicle, proximal and distal ends of the ulna, tragus, and supraorbital foramen of the subject, and on the force plate for reference.

The "go" cue was a point of light that appeared on a low wall about 4 m in front of the subjects, approximately 30 cm either to the left or right of the subject's midline. A vertical line of tape halfway between the locations of the target lights ensured that subjects could distinguish which side the light was on **Figure 1** shows the setup. Subjects were instructed to initiate stepping with whichever foot was indicated by the light, to respond quickly, and to take three steps before stopping. The light cue appeared 2200 ms after the start of the trial and remained on for 600 ms. Data collection lasted 4000 ms. In the block with foreknowledge of the stepping foot (SRT trials), subjects were informed in advance that the light cue would always appear on the same side as their dominant foot. In the block without foreknowledge (CRT trials), subjects were informed that the cue could appear on either side. In half of these trials the cue appeared on the left, and in half it appeared on the right, in pseudo-random order.

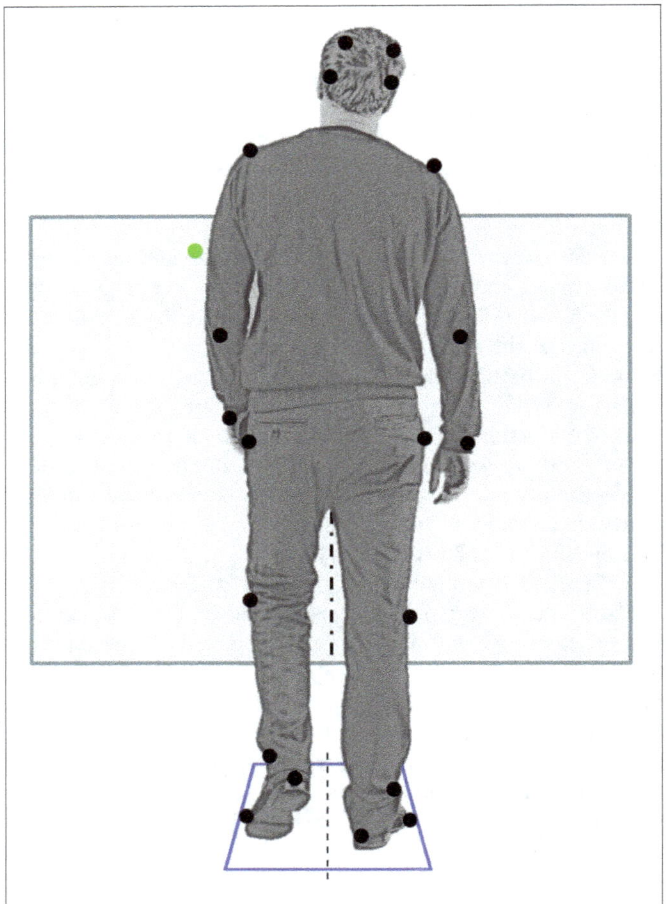

FIGURE 1 | Setup: rear view of a subject beginning to step. The subject's feet are on two separate force plates. Black dots show the placement of reflective markers on bony landmarks and force platform (top two markers are actually above eyebrows). The subject faces a low wall 4 m away. A green laser pointer light appears either on the left (shown) or on the right. The subject steps with the foot on the same side as the light. Figure modified from an image by Konstantin Kamenetskiy © 1234RF.com.

Data Analysis

Our main dependent measures were the onset times of the first APA and the first step as a function of group (HC, PD without freezing, PD with freezing), trial type (SRT, CRT), and presence or absence of multiple APAs. The first APA onset was defined as the time when the difference in vertical force under the two feet increased by 5% of body weight. The step onset was defined as the time when vertical force under either foot decreased to zero. Post-processing was performed in Matlab (R2014a, The Mathworks Inc, Natick, MA, USA). We also examined APA duration, defined as (time of step onset – time of APA onset).

Variables of secondary interest were the relative location of the COM in the anteroposterior (A/P) axis at cue and step onset, the peak velocity of stepping foot, and the first step length. To determine whole body COM, we computed the weighted average of the position of each body segment (Vaughan et al., 1992) based on measurements of the length, width, and circumference of 26 body segments, and self-reported heights and weights for each subject (Chandler et al., 1975). Peak velocity and step length were computed from a reflective marker on the foot. Finally, we looked at correlations between APA/step measures and score on the Stroop task. **Figure 2** shows the vertical force under the stepping foot and the A/P position of the COM for three exemplar trials from a single PD subject with freezing: a normal step with a single weight shift, a trial with two weight shifts, and a trial with more than two weight shifts.

To assess inhibitory function, we had subjects complete the Stroop color-word task (Stroop, 1935). This task measures how well subjects can inhibit a well-learned response to a common stimulus (reading words) in order to respond to another aspect of the stimulus (color names). The task includes three conditions: color naming, reading, and conflict. The conditions are tested in blocks, in fixed order. For each condition, subjects viewed a page containing 100 stimuli (4 columns of 25 items). Words were written in 20-point Times New Roman font, and the page was placed at a comfortable reading distance in front of the subject. Subjects were to respond verbally to each stimulus in order, pointing to each item as they responded to it, to facilitate the experimenter's monitoring of errors. For the color naming condition, the stimuli were blocks of black, red, blue, purple, and green, arranged in random order. For the reading condition, the stimuli were words naming the colors previously presented, printed in black ink and arranged in random order. For the conflict condition, stimuli were the same words as those in the second condition, printed in the same colors as those in the first condition, with words and colors randomly paired. For this condition, subjects were required to ignore the words and name the ink colors. Before every condition, a few practice trials were conducted to assure that subjects understood the task and were able to correctly read the words and name the colors. The Stroop interference score was computed as (time + errors in conflict condition – time in reading condition).

Before analyzing the data, we removed trials in which subjects (1) drifted laterally so that one side had >52.5% of the weight during the baseline period, (2) initiated an APA before the light cue, (3) stepped with the wrong foot, or (4) did not step within the 6 s window of data collection, as well as (5) trials during which the equipment did not properly record. Statistics were computed with R (R Development Core Team, 2014), with an alpha of 0.05 for all tests. We first conducted 2 × 3 ANOVAs on each dependent variable, with foreknowledge of stepping foot (SRT vs. CRT) and group (HC vs. PD with freezing vs. PD without freezing) as the factors. Because we were comparing three groups, we followed significant ANOVA results on the group factor with Tukey *post hoc* comparisons.

For a more in-depth analysis, we then further divided the trials by presence or absence of multiple APAs and performed three-way ANOVAs. Because these included the effect of multiple APAs as a factor, we did not have equal numbers of trials in each cell. Therefore, we used a linear mixed model approach in which data from each trial were entered individually into each model using subject as a random effect. This approach accounts for different numbers of trials in different cells (Stroup, 2012). *Post hoc* comparisons were computed using the "phia" (*post hoc* interaction analysis) package in R, with Bonferroni corrections applied to the *p*-values. Finally, we computed the correlations between Stroop score and step characteristics.

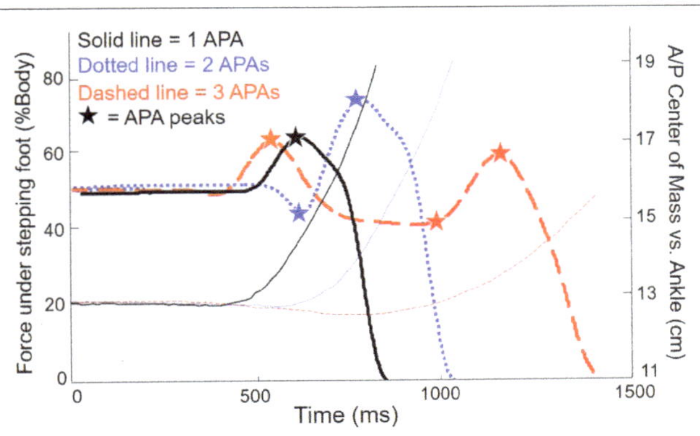

FIGURE 2 | Force and anteroposterior (A/P) center of mass (COM) for three exemplary trials from one subject with PD. Thick lines: vertical force under stepping foot. Thin lines: COM with respect to ankles (baseline shifted to emphasize forward motion of COM). Solid lines: single APA. Dotted lines: two APAs. Dashed lines: three APAs.

RESULTS

Two-Way ANOVAs

After cleaning the data as described above, we were left with 1205 trials for analyses (an average of 32.6 per subject). **Figure 3** shows the proportion of trials with multiple APAs, as a function of group and condition. Multiple APAs were four times more prevalent in the CRT condition (~20%) than in the SRT condition (~5%),

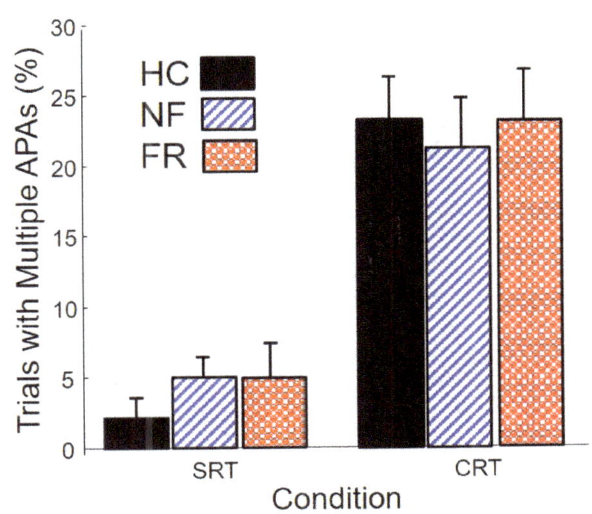

FIGURE 3 | Percentage of trials with multiple APAs in healthy control subjects (HC), PD subjects without freezing (NF), and PD subjects with freezing (FR), in simple reaction time (SRT) and choice reaction time (CRT) stepping.

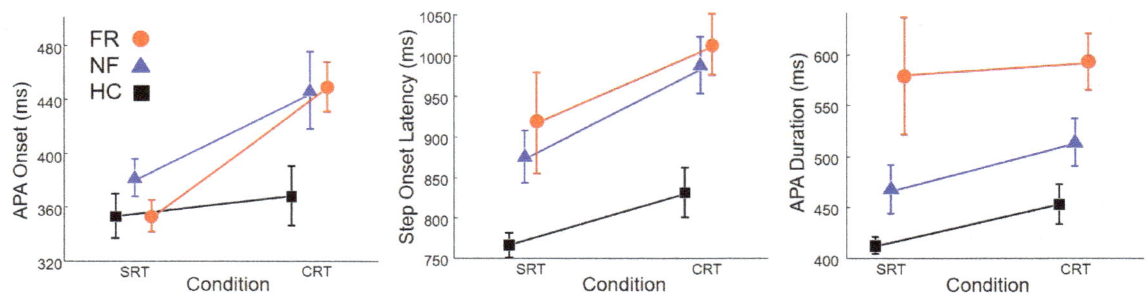

FIGURE 4 | Onset of anticipatory postural adjustment (APA; Left), step onset (Middle), and APA duration (Right) in healthy control subjects (HC, Squares), PD subjects without freezing (NF, Triangles), and PD subjects with freezing (FR, Circles), in SRT and CRT stepping. Note that the scale on the *y*-axis is different in each sub-figure.

$F(1,68) = 45.2, p < 0.0001$. Surprisingly, there were no differences in prevalence of multiple APAs among the groups.

Onset times of the first APA and first step, as well as APA duration, are shown in **Figure 4**. APA onset was 88 ms earlier in SRT trials than in CRT trials (left plot), $F(1,68) = 12.8, p < 0.0001$. There was also a significant effect of group, $F(2,68) = 3.9$, $p = 0.02$. *Post hoc* comparison indicated that PD subjects without freezing initiated APAs later than HC subjects.

In addition, step onset (middle plot) was 91 ms earlier in SRT trials than in CRT trials, $F(1,68) = 7.6$, $p = 0.008$, and was also affected by group, $F(2,68) = 11.5$, $p < 0.0001$. *Post hoc* comparison indicated that HC subjects stepped 155 ms earlier than PD subjects without freezing and 183 ms earlier than PD subjects with freezing.

Anticipatory postural adjustment duration (right plot) was not affected by trial type but was affected by group, $F(2,68) = 10.1$, $p = 0.0001$. APA duration in HC subjects was 101 ms shorter than in PD subjects without freezing and 146 ms shorter than in PD subjects with freezing.

Three-Way Mixed Model ANOVAs

To determine the influence of multiple APAs on step preparation, we analyzed the outcome variables with trials divided according to whether or not there were multiple APAs. The primary results can be seen in **Figure 5**, and the statistics are shown in **Table 2**. The top row shows initial APA onsets. There was a main effect of the presence of multiple APAs, with initial APAs occurring, on average, 70 ms earlier in trials with multiple APAs than in trials with single APAs. There was also an interaction between group and trial type, with *post hoc* tests revealing that trial type had less influence on APA initiation in HC subjects (51 ms) than in PD subjects with freezing (136 ms).

The effect of multiple APAs on step onset time depended on the group and trial type, as seen in the middle row of **Figure 5**. Multiple APAs caused a step onset delay in PD subjects with freezing (134 ms) and in PD subjects without freezing (153 ms) but not in HC subjects. There were also interactions between group and trial type and between trial type and presence of multiple APAs that are best understood by examining the three-way interaction: multiple APAs delayed step onset in both trial types for PD subjects, but only in CRT trials for HC subjects.

Anticipatory postural adjustment durations, shown in the bottom row of **Figure 5**, were longer in PD subjects with freezing (613 ms) and in PD subjects without freezing (604 ms) than in HC subjects (449 ms). Multiple APAs lengthened APA duration an average of 174 ms; the effect was larger in PD subjects with freezing (199 ms) and in PD subjects without freezing (220 ms) than in HC subjects (102 ms). There was also a three-way interaction: the effect of multiple APAs on APA duration was smallest in HC subjects in SRT trials.

Most of the multiple weight shifts we observed were actually *dual* weight shifts, in which the initial weight shift was in the wrong direction and was followed by a single corrective weight shift. Occasionally, subjects exhibited *more than two* APAs before a step. This pattern only occurred in six subjects (one HC, two PD without freezing, and three PD with freezing), so there were not enough trials with more than two APAs to perform a statistical analysis on these trials separately. Instead, we examined their influence by removing them from the data and reanalyzing it (see **Table 3**). The reanalysis did not substantially alter the results.

Kinematic data are presented in **Figure 6**. The left plot shows the length the initial step as a function of group, trial type, and presence or absence of multiple APAs. Only group had an effect, $F(2,34) = 12.4$, $p < 0.0001$: initial steps of PD subjects with freezing were 16 cm shorter than those of PD subjects without freezing and 21 cm shorter than those of HC subjects, but there was no difference between non-freezing PD subjects and healthy controls, and no significant effect of condition or number of APAs. Peak velocity (not pictured) was 0.98 correlated with peak velocity and showed the same effect of group, $F(2,34) = 15.6$, $p < 0.0001$. *Post hoc* tests indicated that PD subjects with freezing stepped at approximately 90 cm/s, which was 52 cm/s more slowly than PD subjects without freezing and 78 cm/s more slowly than HC subjects, but there was no other difference.

At the time of the "go" cue, the anteroposterior location of the COM relative to the ankles averaged 7.7 cm and was not affected by group, trial type, or presence or absence of multiple APAs. The center and right plots of **Figure 6** show the amount of forward motion of the COM between the time of the "go" cue and the step onset. There was an interaction between group and presence/absence of multiple APAs, $F(2,1144) = 8.0$, $p = 0.0004$, with multiple APAs leading to the largest increase in forward

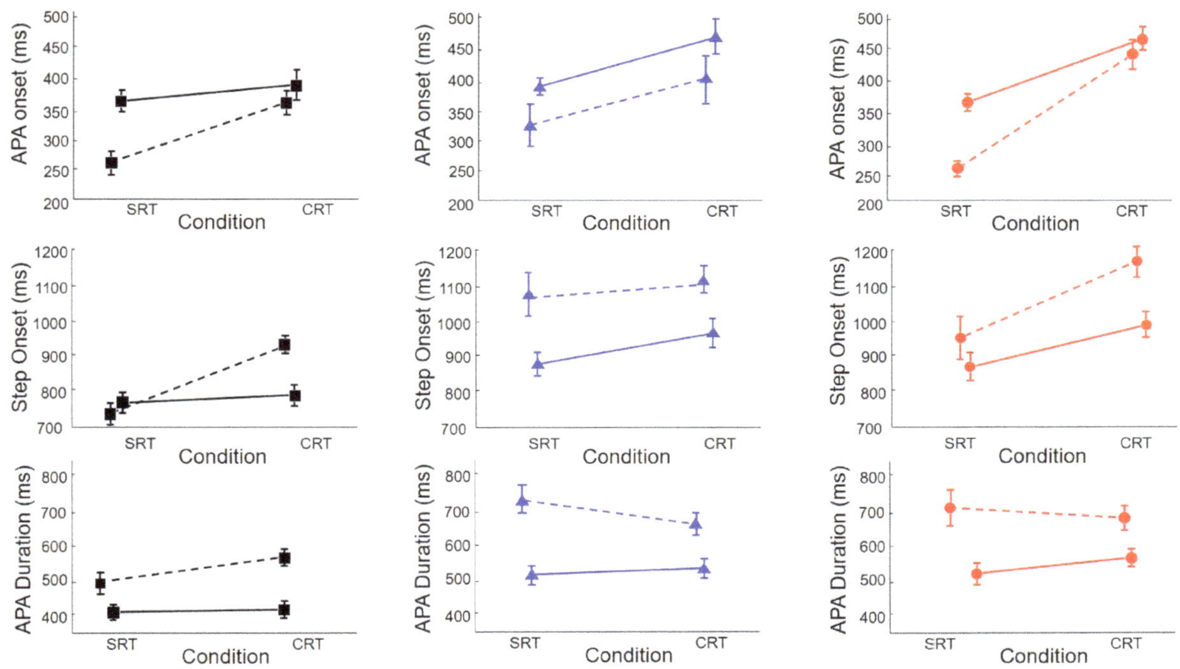

FIGURE 5 | Onset of APA (Top), step onset (Middle), and APA duration (Bottom) in healthy control subjects (HC, Squares, Left), PD subjects without freezing (NF, Triangles, Middle), and PD subjects with freezing (FR, Circles, Right), in SRT and CRT stepping, divided according to whether there was only a single APA (solid lines) or multiple APAs (dashed lines).

TABLE 2 | Anticipatory postural adjustment (APA) and step onset latencies as a function of group, condition, and single vs. multiple APAs; df, degrees of freedom.

	APA onset latency			Step onset latency			APA duration		
	df	F	p	df	F	p	df	F	p
Group	2,34	0.6	0.56	2,34	3.1	0.06	2,34	4.1	**0.03**
Condition	1,1159	2.8	0.09	1,1159	2.8	0.10	1,1159	0.4	0.54
Single vs. Multiple APAs	1,1159	9.9	**0.002**	1,1159	1.0	0.31	1,1159	4.3	**0.04**
Group × Condition	2,1159	9.1	**0.0001**	2,1159	10.0	**0.0001**	2,1159	2.0	0.13
Group × Multiple APAs	2,1159	0.6	0.52	2,1159	7.1	**0.0008**	2,1159	12.6	**<0.0001**
Condition × Multiple APAs	1,1159	2.7	0.10	1,1159	8.4	**0.004**	1,1159	6.5	**0.01**
Group × Condition × Multiple APAs	2,1159	2.1	0.12	2,1159	4.4	**0.01**	2,1159	6.2	**0.002**

Bolded p values are < 0.05.

TABLE 3 | Anticipatory postural adjustment and step onset latencies as a function of group, condition, and single vs. dual APA; df, degrees of freedom.

	APA onset latency			Step Onset Latency			APA Duration		
	df	F	p	df	F	p	df	F	p
Group	2,34	0.6	0.57	2,34	3.2	0.06	2,34	4.3	**0.02**
Condition	1,1151	2.8	0.09	1,1151	3.0	0.08	1,1151	0.4	0.50
Single APA vs. Dual APA	1,1151	9.4	**0.002**	1,1151	2.0	0.16	1,1151	2.6	0.10
Group × Condition	1,1151	9.2	**0.0001**	1,1151	10.9	**<0.0001**	1,1151	2.5	0.08
Group × Dual APA	1,1151	0.8	0.45	1,1151	8.2	**0.0003**	1,1151	16.6	**<0.0001**
Condition × Dual APA	1,1151	2.5	0.12	1,1151	9.7	**0.002**	1,1151	9.4	**0.002**
Group × Condition × Dual APA	1,1151	1.8	0.17	1,1151	5.4	**0.005**	1,1151	10.2	**<0.0001**

Bolded p values are < 0.05.

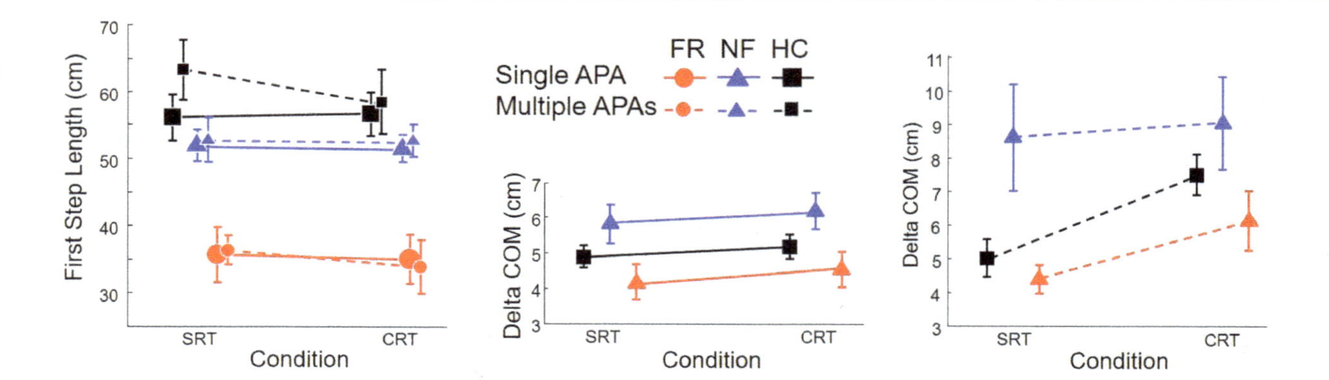

FIGURE 6 | Kinematics for healthy control subjects (HC, Squares), PD subjects without freezing (NF, Triangles), and PD subjects with freezing (FR, Circles), in SRT and CRT stepping. Left: length of first step. Middle and Right: Forward motion of the COM from the time of the "go" cue to the time of step onset. Solid lines: trials with single APAs. Dashed lines: trials with multiple APAs.

motion in PD subjects without freezing (28 mm), to a lesser increase of forward motion in HC subjects (13 mm), and to no significant change in forward motion of COM in PD subjects with freezing. There was also an interaction between trial type and presence/absence of multiple APAs, $F(1{,}1144) = 12.0, p = 0.0005$, with multiple APAs increasing forward motion more in CRT trials (21 mm) than SRT trials (10 mm). A three-way interaction, $F(2{,}1144) = 3.2$, $p = 0.04$, reflected the large forward lean of PD subjects without freezing during SRT trials.

Correlations between Stroop score and APA/step measures are shown in **Figure 7** and **Table 4**. High values for Stroop score indicate poor inhibitory control. There was no overall difference in Stroop score between PD subjects with and without self-reported freezing of gait. Poor Stroop performance correlated with high proportion of trials with multiple APAs, with slow step onset latency and APA duration, and with COM farther back at the time when the cue appeared. Stroop scores were not related to APA onset, step velocity, or forward motion of the COM during

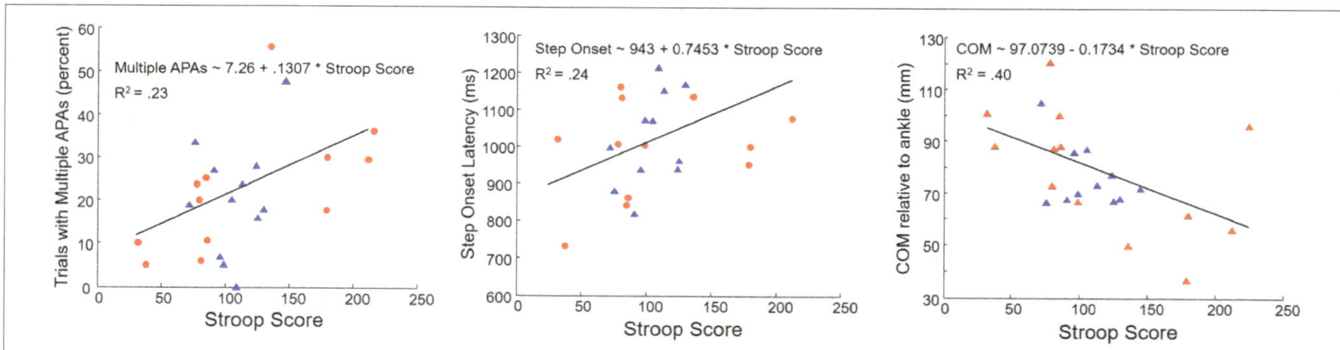

FIGURE 7 | Correlations between Stroop Score and percent trials with multiple APAs (Left), step onset latency (Middle), and COM at cue presentation (Right) in subjects with PD. Triangles: subjects without freezing. Circles: subjects with freezing.

TABLE 4 | Pearson's correlation coefficient (and two-tailed *p*-value) for main outcome variables (PD subjects only).

	Multiple APAs	APA onset latency	Step onset latency	Peak velocity	COM at Cue	Change in COM	UPDRS
Stroop score	**0.48 (0.02)**	0.24 (0.26)	**0.49 (0.02)**	−0.33 (0.12)	**−0.63 (0.001)**	−0.18 (0.40)	0.34 (0.10)
Multiple APAs	–	0.06 (0.76)	0.13 (0.52)	−0.36 (0.08)	−0.33 (0.10)	−0.29 (0.16)	0.01 (0.95)
APA onset	–	–	**0.65 (0.005)**	−0.12 (0.56)	−0.17 (0.45)	−0.16 (0.45)	0.08 (0.71)
Step onset	–	–	–	−0.18 (0.38)	−0.15 (0.48)	0.14 (0.51)	**0.60 (0.001)**
Peak velocity	–	–	–	–	0.26 (0.21)	**0.69 (0.001)**	−0.31 (0.12)
COM at cue	–	–	–	–	–	0.28 (0.18)	−0.01 (0.95)
Change in COM	–	–	–	–	–	–	0.08 (0.68)

Bolded p values are < 0.05.

the APA. The proportion of trials with multiple APAs was not related to any other measured aspect of step initiation.

DISCUSSION

This study investigated the relationships among inhibition, foot selection, multiple APAs, and start hesitation in voluntary stepping. Previous results indicated that when protective steps are evoked by postural perturbations, multiple APAs are more common in PD subjects who tend to freeze than in HC subjects (Jacobs et al., 2009). Previous findings also indicated that challenging foot selection leads to a substantial increase in the prevalence of multiple APAs during voluntary step initiation in healthy older adults (Cohen et al., 2011). The experiment described here built on both of those studies by introducing challenging foot selection during voluntary step initiation in subjects with PD. To manipulate foot selection difficulty, we compared step initiation during SRT and CRT conditions. To assess inhibitory control, we measured performance on a Stroop task.

We found some overall differences among the groups that were consistent with the literature: HC subjects had the earliest APA onsets, and PD subjects had the latest step onsets and the longest APA durations. These differences were in the range of 150 ms. In addition, PD subjects with freezing took the shortest initial steps, with the lowest peak velocity. The step length difference between PD subjects with and without freezing was 16 cm, which is a substantial 30% reduction. The difference in peak velocity of the stepping foot was proportional to the difference in step length. These findings are consistent with previous findings, e.g. (Gantchev et al., 1996).

The CRT manipulation was successful at increasing the prevalence of multiple APAs before stepping: multiple APAs were four times more likely in CRT trials than in SRT trials. CRT trials also led to a small (less than 100 ms) delay in onset of the first APA and the first step, relative to the SRT trials. Trial type did not affect APA duration, peak stepping velocity, or step length. In addition (and contrary to our prediction), multiple APAs were no more likely in PD subjects than in HC subjects, nor in PD subjects with a self-reported freezing tendency than in PD subjects without self-reported freezing. This result suggests that the observed link among inhibition deficits, multiple APAs, and freezing is probably *not* due to a greater tendency in people with freezing to initially shift their weight in the wrong direction before stepping. It also emphasizes the fact that although multiple APAs are linked to start hesitation, they are not one and the same thing.

Multiple APAs were associated with early APA onsets in all subjects; however, they were followed by delayed step onsets only in PD subjects, with APA durations increasing about 140 ms. This result is consistent with the idea that PD leads to a reduced ability to release inhibition of the step when the APA has been initiated (Boulinguez et al., 2009; Cohen et al., 2014). The resulting decoupling between the APA and the step could lead to start hesitation (Jacobs et al., 2009; Delval et al., 2014a; Lin et al., 2016). This line of thinking is supported by recent neuroimaging evidence that freezing episodes are associated with functional decoupling between the cognitive control network and the basal ganglia network (Shine et al., 2013) and is in general agreement with a recent review suggesting that freezing of gait is likely due to a combination of cognitive and decoupling factors (Nieuwboer and Giladi, 2013). However, the power of this argument is weakened by our finding that step onset delays following multiple APAs were not larger in PD subjects with freezing than in PD subjects without freezing. Furthermore, PD subjects were more affected than HC subjects by multiple APAs *only* when the stepping foot was known in advance (SRT condition). This relative deficit for PD subjects in SRT trials could indicate a failure to fully benefit from advance knowledge of the stepping foot, which would make sense given the well-established deficit of subjects with PD in automatic movement preparation (Bloxham et al., 1984; Wu and Hallett, 2005; Cameron et al., 2010).

One motivation for studying start hesitation in PD is its association with fall risk (e.g., Bloem et al., 2004; Delval et al., 2014b). If, during a delayed step onset, the COM continued to move forward, this could pose a threat to balance. For all groups of subjects in the present study, the COM moved farther forward during trials with multiple APAs than during trials with single APAs, especially in CRT trials. However, despite the markedly later step onset latencies in subjects with PD and freezing compared to other groups during multiple-APA trials, and contrary to our prediction, the forward travel of the COM was actually affected *less* by multiple APAs in the self-reported freezing group than in the other subject groups. It may be that people with PD who are aware that they might freeze develop compensatory strategies, such as not leaning forward when initiating gait. It is also possible that difficulty shifting weight forward is a primary element of the dysfunction in people who freeze. In support of the latter alternative, the amount of forward weight shift during step preparation was strongly correlated with the subsequent peak velocity of the step. This explanation is also consistent with (Brenière et al., 1987).

We predicted that subjects who performed poorly in the Stroop task would also show a high prevalence of multiple APAs and delayed step onset; this prediction was supported. This result is consistent with previous findings that inhibitory deficits are associated with self-reported freezing severity (Amboni et al., 2008; Vandenbossche et al., 2011; Cohen et al., 2014) and with clinician-rated severity (Cohen et al., 2014). As described above, we propose that inhibition deficits in PD may also play a *causal* role in start hesitation and freezing, by contributing to the decoupling of the APA and the step.

Interestingly, poor Stroop performance was also associated with a tendency to stand with the COM relatively far back while waiting for the cue to appear. This is not an artifact of severity, as UPDRS was related only with step onset latency and not with Stroop or COM. There is a well-known relationship between attentional control and the steadiness or stability of COM during standing balance, e.g. (Woollacott and Shumway-Cook, 2002).

However, few studies have examined the relationship between cognitive factors and postural alignment or standing position, c.f. (Cohen et al., 2016). This relationship may bear further investigation.

This study had several limitations. First, although we examined voluntary stepping (not protective stepping), subjects were provided with a "go" cue. External cues are thought to assist step preparation in people with PD (Delval et al., 2014a), and the basal ganglia are thought to be more critical for self-initiated, rather than externally triggered, voluntary movements (Boecker et al., 2008; Toyomura et al., 2012). Therefore, future studies of step initiation and freezing should eliminate the external cue. Second, although our interest is in freezing of gait and start hesitation, we didn't actually measure freezing episodes. Instead, our primary outcome was latency of step onset, which might reflect a tendency to freeze but is not the same thing. Finally, it should be noted that the PD subjects with self-reported freezing were, on average, more severely affected by the disease than the PD subjects without freezing; thus, the results that we describe as differences between PD subjects with and without self-reported freezing may also be described as differences between PD subjects with greater or lesser disease severity. However, our main interest here was in understanding the phenomenon of delayed stepping and what is associated with it, rather than with distinguishing a subtype of PD, especially given ongoing questions about whether a freezing subtype of PD even exists (Nieuwboer and Giladi, 2013).

In sum, this study provides evidence that start hesitation in PD is associated not with a greater tendency to produce multiple APAs before stepping, but with difficulty recovering when multiple APAs occur. The results are consistent with the proposal that inhibition deficits – especially difficulty releasing inhibition – play a causal role in start hesitation and freezing in PD, by contributing to the decoupling of the APA from the step.

AUTHOR CONTRIBUTIONS

RC participated in study design, data collection, data analysis, and results interpretation, and wrote the manuscript. JN participated in study design and results interpretation, and gave feedback on the manuscript. FH participated in study design and results interpretation, and gave feedback on the manuscript. All authors approved the final version of the manuscript to be published and agree to be accountable for all aspects of the work in ensuring that questions related to the accuracy or integrity of any part of the work are appropriately investigated and resolved.

FUNDING

This research was supported by a VA Merit Award to FBH (I01 RX001075) and by the National Institutes of Health (AG-006457-31, T32-NS045553, and U54 GM104944).

ACKNOWLEDGMENTS

We thank Triana Nagel and Amanda Chao for help with data collection, and we thank the participants for their crucial time and assistance.

REFERENCES

Amboni, M., Cozzolino, A., Longo, K., Picillo, M., and Barone, P. (2008). Freezing of gait and executive functions in patients with Parkinson's disease. *Mov. Disord.* 23, 395–400. doi: 10.1002/mds.21850

Bloem, B. R., Hausdorff, J. M., Visser, J. E., and Giladi, N. (2004). Falls and freezing of Gait in Parkinson's disease: a review of two interconnected, episodic phenomena. *Mov. Disord.* 19, 871–884. doi: 10.1002/mds.20115

Bloxham, C. A., Mindel, T. A., and Frith, C. D. (1984). Initiation and execution of predictable and unpredictable movements in Parkinson's disease. *Brain* 107, 371–384. doi: 10.1093/brain/107.2.371

Boecker, H., Jankowski, J., Ditter, P., and Scheef, L. (2008). A role of the basal ganglia and midbrain nuclei for initiation of motor sequences. *Neuroimage* 39, 1356–1369. doi: 10.1016/j.neuroimage.2007.09.069

Boulinguez, P., Ballanger, B., Granjon, L., and Benraiss, A. (2009). The paradoxical effect of warning on reaction time: demonstrating proactive response inhibition with event-related potentials. *Clin. Neurophysiol.* 120, 730–737. doi: 10.1016/j.clinph.2009.02.167

Brenière, Y., Cuong Do, M., and Bouisset, S. (1987). Are dynamic phenomena prior to stepping essential to walking? *J. Mot. Behav.* 19, 62–76. doi: 10.1080/00222895.1987.10735400

Cameron, I. G. M., Watanabe, M., Pari, G., and Munoz, D. P. (2010). Executive impairment in Parkinson's disease: response automaticity and task switching. *Neuropsychologia* 48, 1948–1957. doi: 10.1016/j.neuropsychologia.2010.03.015

Chandler, R. F., Clauser, C. E., McConville, J. T., Reynolds, H. M., and Young, J. W. (1975). *Investigation of Inertial Properties of the Human Body*. Report DOT HS-801 430. Washington, DC: Department of Transportation.

Cohen, R. G., Klein, K. A., Nomura, M., Fleming, M., Mancini, M., Giladi, N., et al. (2014). Inhibition, executive function, and freezing of gait. *J. Parkinsons Dis.* 4, 111–122. doi: 10.3233/JPD-130221

Cohen, R. G., Nutt, J. G., and Horak, F. B. (2011). Errors in postural preparation lead to increased choice reaction times for step initiation in older adults. *J. Gerontol. A Biol. Sci. Med. Sci.* 66, 705–713. doi: 10.1093/gerona/glr054

Cohen, R. G., Vasavada, A. N., Wiest, M. M., and Schmitter-Edgecombe, M. (2016). Mobility and upright posture are associated with different aspects of cognition in older adults. *Front. Aging Neurosci.* 8:257. doi: 10.3389/fnagi.2016.00257

Delval, A., Moreau, C., Bleuse, S., Tard, C., Ryckewaert, G., Devos, D., et al. (2014a). Auditory cueing of gait initiation in Parkinson's disease patients with freezing of gait. *Clin. Neurophysiol.* 125, 1675–1681. doi: 10.1016/j.clinph.2013.12.101

Delval, A., Tard, C., and Defebvre, L. (2014b). Why we should study gait initiation in Parkinson's disease. *Neurophysiol. Clin.* 44, 69–76. doi: 10.1016/j.neucli.2013.10.127

Fahn, S., and Elton, R. L. (1987). "Unified Parkinson's Disease Rating Scale," in *Recent Developments in Parkinson's Disease*, Vol. 2, eds S. Fahn, C. Marsden, D. Calne, and M. Goldstein (Florham Park, NJ: Macmillan Health Care Information), 153–163.

Fling, B. W., Cohen, R. G., Mancini, M., Carpenter, S. D., Fair, D. A., Nutt, J. G., et al. (2014). Functional reorganization of the locomotor network in Parkinson patients with freezing of gait. *PLoS ONE* 9:e100291. doi: 10.1371/journal.pone.0100291

Fling, B. W., Cohen, R. G., Mancini, M., Nutt, J. G., Fair, D. A., and Horak, F. B. (2013). Asymmetric pedunculopontine network connectivity in parkinsonian patients with freezing of gait. *Brain* 136, 2405–2418. doi: 10.1093/brain/awt172

Gantchev, N., Viallet, F., Aurenty, R., and Massion, J. (1996). Impairment of posturo-kinetic co-ordination during initiation of forward oriented stepping movements in parkinsonian patients. *Electroencephalogr. Clin. Neurophysiol. Mot. Control* 101, 110–120. doi: 10.1016/0924-980X(95)00253-H

Hoehn, M. M., and Yahr, M. D. (1967). Parkinsonism: onset, progression and mortality. *Neurology* 17, 427–442. doi: 10.1212/WNL.17.5.427

Jacobs, J. V., Nutt, J. G., Carlson-Kuhta, P., Stephens, M., and Horak, F. B. (2009). Knee trembling during freezing of gait represents multiple anticipatory postural adjustments. *Exp. Neurol.* 215, 334–341. doi: 10.1016/j.expneurol.2008.10.019

Lin, C.-C., Creath, R. A., and Rogers, M. W. (2016). Variability of anticipatory postural adjustments during gait initiation in individuals with Parkinson disease. *J. Neurol. Phys. Ther.* 40, 40–46. doi: 10.1097/NPT.0000000000000112

Mostofsky, S. H., and Simmonds, D. J. (2008). Response inhibition and response selection: two sides of the same coin. *J. Cogn. Neurosci.* 20, 751–761. doi: 10.1162/jocn.2008.20500

Nieuwboer, A., and Giladi, N. (2013). Characterizing freezing of gait in Parkinson's disease: models of an episodic phenomenon. *Mov. Disord.* 28, 1509–1519. doi: 10.1002/mds.25683

Nutt, J. G., Bloem, B. R., Giladi, N., Hallett, M., Horak, F. B., and Nieuwboer, A. (2011). Freezing of gait: moving forward on a mysterious clinical phenomenon. *Lancet Neurol.* 10, 734–744. doi: 10.1016/S1474-4422(11)70143-0

R Development Core Team (2014). *R: A Language and Environment for Statistical Computing*. Vienna: R Foundation for Statistical Computing.

Shine, J. M., Matar, E., Ward, P. B., Frank, M. J., Moustafa, A. A., Pearson, M., et al. (2013). Freezing of gait in Parkinson's disease is associated with functional decoupling between the cognitive control network and the basal ganglia. *Brain* 136, 3671–3681. doi: 10.1093/brain/awt272

Stroop, J. R. (1935). Studies of interference in serial verbal reactions. *J. Exp. Psychol.* 18, 643–662. doi: 10.1037/h0054651

Stroup, W. W. (2012). *Generalized Linear Mixed Models: Modern Concepts, Methods and Applications*. Boca Raton, FL: CRC Press.

Toyomura, A., Shibata, M., and Kuriki, S. (2012). Self-paced and externally triggered rhythmical lower limb movements: a functional MRI study. *Neurosci. Lett.* 516, 39–44. doi: 10.1016/j.neulet.2012.03.049

Vandenbossche, J., Deroost, N., Soetens, E., Spildooren, J., Vercruysse, S., Nieuwboer, A., et al. (2011). Freezing of gait in Parkinson disease is associated with impaired conflict resolution. *Neurorehabil. Neural Repair* 25, 765–773. doi: 10.1177/1545968311403493

Vaughan, C. L., Davis, B. L., and O'connor, J. C. (1992). *Dynamics of Human Gait*, 2nd Edn. Champaign, IL: Human Kinetics.

Woollacott, M., and Shumway-Cook, A. (2002). Attention and the control of posture and gait: a review of an emerging area of research. *Gait Posture* 16, 1–14. doi: 10.1016/S0966-6362(01)00156-4

Wu, T., and Hallett, M. (2005). A functional MRI study of automatic movements in patients with Parkinson's disease. *Brain* 128, 2250–2259. doi: 10.1093/brain/awh569

11

Computerized Dual-Task Testing of Gait and Visuospatial Cognitive Functions: Test-Retest Reliability and Validity

Tony J. Szturm [1,2]*, *Vedant S. Sakhalkar* [1,3], *Anuprita Kanitkar* [1,4] *and Mayur Nankar* [1]

[1] *Mobility and Cognition Lab, College of Rehabilitation Sciences, University of Manitoba, Winnipeg, MB, Canada,* [2] *Department of Physical Therapy, University of Manitoba, Winnipeg, MB, Canada,* [3] *School of Medical Rehabilitation, University of Manitoba, Winnipeg, MB, Canada,* [4] *Applied Health Sciences, University of Manitoba, Winnipeg, MB, Canada*

Correspondence:
Tony J. Szturm
tony.szturm@med.umanitoba.ca

The common occurrence of age decline in mobility and cognition does cause a decrease in the level of physical activity and an increased falls risk. Consequently, dual -task (DT) assessment that simultaneously addresses both mobility skills and cognitive functions are important because, continued difficulties and fall injuries will have a sizable impact in this population. The first objective of the present study was to assess test-retest reliability of a computerized DT treadmill walking protocol and concurrent outcome measures of gait and visuospatial executive function in a group of healthy older adults. Secondly, discriminative validity was evaluated by examining the effect of DT conditions (single task vs. dual-task) on; (a) spatiotemporal gait measures (average and coefficient of variation) and (b) visuomotor and visuospatial executive performance measures. Twenty-five community-dwelling individuals median age 65 (range 61–67) were recruited from a Fitness Facility. Participants performed a computerized visuomotor tracking task and a visuospatial executive game task in standing and while treadmill walking. Testing was conducted on two occasions, 1 week apart. Moderate to high test-retest reliability (ICC values of 0.65–0.88) were observed for spatiotemporal gait variables. No significant differences between the group means were observed between test periods in any gait variable. Moderate test-retest reliability (ICC values of 0.6–0.65) was observed for measures of visuomotor and visuospatial executive performance during treadmill walking. Significant DT effects were observed for both spatiotemporal gait variables and visuospatial executive performance measures. This study demonstrates the reliability and reproducibility of the computer-based assessment tool for dual task treadmill walking. The high to moderate ICC values and the lack of systematic errors in the measures indicate that this tool has the ability to repeatedly record reliable data from community-dwelling older adults. The present computerized dual-task protocols broaden the types of standardized visuomotor and visuospatial executive activities for use with DT treadmill walking that has previously been reported.

Keywords: treadmill walking, spatiotemporal gait variables, cognitive performance, Dual-task performance, intra-class correlation coefficient

INTRODUCTION

The frequent occurrence of mobility limitations and falls with age can arise due to singular events (e.g., stroke, peripheral vestibular dysfunction) or can have an insidious onset, with the problem source found in multiple predisposing factors, such as, the gradual decline of musculoskeletal and/or neural fitness (sensory, cognitive, motor; Santos-Eggimann et al., 2008). Walking problems and falls, in particular outdoors, become evident when compensatory strategies have failed, or where certain tasks and environmental conditions cannot be avoided (Shumway-Cook et al., 2007; Santos-Eggimann et al., 2008).

For older adults, community ambulation is strongly associated with the preservation of skills for independent living, community participation, and healthy aging (Simonsick et al., 2005). Safe, independent community walking outdoors requires both mobility skills and cognitive flexibility to address threats to balance while attending to a range of environmental demands and concurrent executive tasks. Mobility limitations and executive impairments common to aging often coexist and are prognostic of adverse health events, including falls (Santos-Eggimann et al., 2008; van Iersel et al., 2008; Herman et al., 2010; Ijmker and Lamoth, 2012). Consequently, dual- task screening and training programs that simultaneously address both mobility and cognition are important to consider in the promotion of healthy aging and in rehabilitation (Pichierri et al., 2011; Diamond, 2015; Gregory et al., 2016).

The application of digital media and computer technologies provides a number of promising approaches for dual task (DT) assessments and training. For example, a Virtual reality (VR) environments viewed during treadmill walking have been used to provide a more ecological and task-oriented approach to mobility training. Preliminary results suggest that mixed, augmented VR environments that incorporate both treadmill walking and executive tasks have the potential as a rehabilitation tool. (Mirelman et al., 2013; Park et al., 2015) The application of computer games has also received considerable interest from researchers and clinicians as a method to challenge and train many different aspects of executive functions (Anguera et al., 2013; Wolinsky et al., 2013; Rebok et al., 2014; Strenziok et al., 2014). These emerging rehabilitation technologies have the potential to improve clinical outcomes by making therapies and exercise more engaging more motivating and more effective. For this purpose, an engaging, Game-Based Rehabilitation Platform (GRP) for dual-task training with embedded assessment was developed (Szturm et al., 2013a,b). The platform provides an integrated approach to decline in balance, mobility, visuomotor and gaze control, and visuospatial executive function. The GRP consists of a standard treadmill instrumented with a pressure mapping system to record center of foot pressure, and an interactive computer game subsystem (Betker et al., 2008; Szturm et al., 2015a). The treadmill is equipped with a standard LED monitor, and thus, a broad range of visuomotor and visual-spatial executive game activities can easily be managed concurrently while treadmill walking. The GRP includes a monitoring application which uses advanced data logging and analysis method to record the client's actions and choices while playing designed rehabilitation assessment games. The game activities involve visual attention, visual search and tracking of moving visual targets, and the ability to select and interact with relevant targets and ignore/avoid distracter objects. Visuospatial processing is an important aspect of cognition to explore as a factor involved in age decline in mobility and increased fall risk (Santos-Eggimann et al., 2008; van Iersel et al., 2008; Nagamatsu et al., 2009; Murray et al., 2010). With this method both gait and visuospatial executive performance can be quantified during steady state walking at a constant velocity and over durations of 1–2 min or more, as tolerated (i.e., 40 to hundreds of consecutive steps).

Many over ground walking studies examine how information processing load affects gait rhythm or stability, (i.e., spatiotemporal gait variables (Al-Yahya et al., 2011). However, gait speed is a confounding variable, as spatiotemporal gait variables are sensitive to changes in gait speed (Kang and Dingwell, 2008; Stoquart et al., 2008; Szturm et al., 2013a; Keene et al., 2016). Most of over ground walking studies use an instrumented walkway, which records only 4–6 consecutive steps. This method may reliably measure gait speed, but is not sufficient for measures of gait variability or periodicity, particularly during dual-task walking (Bruijn et al., 2009; Hollman et al., 2010; Galna et al., 2013).

The purpose of this study is to establish the psychometric properties of the test protocols and the dual-task outcome measures of the GRP during treadmill walking. This is an important initial step before it can be routinely used clinically or in community centers for screening, fall risk assessment, and rehabilitation, as well as for preventative measures. Although, the test-retest reliability of mean values of spatiotemporal gait parameters has been assessed for reliability while walking alone, little is known about the test-retest reliability of gait variability while performing concurrent executive tasks (Brach et al., 2008; Paterson et al., 2008; Beauchet et al., 2011; Faude et al., 2012).

The first objective was to establish test-retest reliability of outcome measures that represent gait performance, visuomotor (VM) performance, and visuospatial executive function when tested during dual-task conditions. The second objective was to examine the discriminative validity of the computerized outcome measures. Specifically to examine the influence that information processing load has on gait function, and vice versa to examine the influence that physical demands of walking have on visuospatial cognition. A better understanding of the interactions between physical demands of walking and visuospatial cognition will be important for identifying high-risk scenarios that people might encounter outside the lab, and for designing effective, personalized exercise programs suitable for community applications.

METHODS

Participants

Twenty-five adults participated, 19 male and 6 female, the median age of 65 years (range 60–67) who attended a Medical Fitness Facility. The participants were able to walk outside without any walking aids and had no self-reported history of falling. Exclusion criteria included histories of neurological or musculoskeletal disorders (e.g., stroke, hip/knee joint surgery). All participants provided written consent. The study was approved by the University of Manitoba research ethics committee. Prior to testing, each participant completed a 6-min walk test on a 300-m track, and the average walking speed was determined over a 25-m distance.

Tests and Instrumentation

Figure 1A presents the components of the treadmill platform. Participants stood on a treadmill at a viewing distance of 100 cm from an 80 cm computer monitor. The following tasks were performed while walking on a treadmill at 0.9 m/s: for 1 min:

a) Walk only (single task condition),
b) Walk while performing a Visuomotor (VM) task,
c) Walk while performing a Visuospatial Executive Game (VEG) task.

As presented in **Figure 1** the treadmill is instrumented with a pressure mat (Vista Medical, Canada) which was used to record vertical foot contact forces and to compute spatiotemporal gait variables (Betker et al., 2008). At a walking speed of 0.9 m/s, and duration of 1 min, then data for 30 consecutive steps were obtained. Before starting the tests participants walked for 5 min to acclimate to treadmill walking. Test 2 was conducted 1 week after test 1.

Visuospatial Executive Tasks

A custom computer application with the following two assessment modules was used for this study: (a) a Visuomotor (head tracking) module and (b) a Visuospatial Executive game (VEG) module (Szturm et al., 2013a, 2015a). An inexpensive, commercial motion sense mouse (Gyrations, SMK-Link, USA) was used to control and interact with the visuospatial executive games. The motion-sense mouse is small with inertial sensors which are used to derive instantaneous angular position. The motion sense mouse allows head angular rotation to be translated and interpreted as a standard USB computer mouse. Velcro secures the wireless motion mouse to a headband, and with this simple method, the head rotation is used as the pointing device

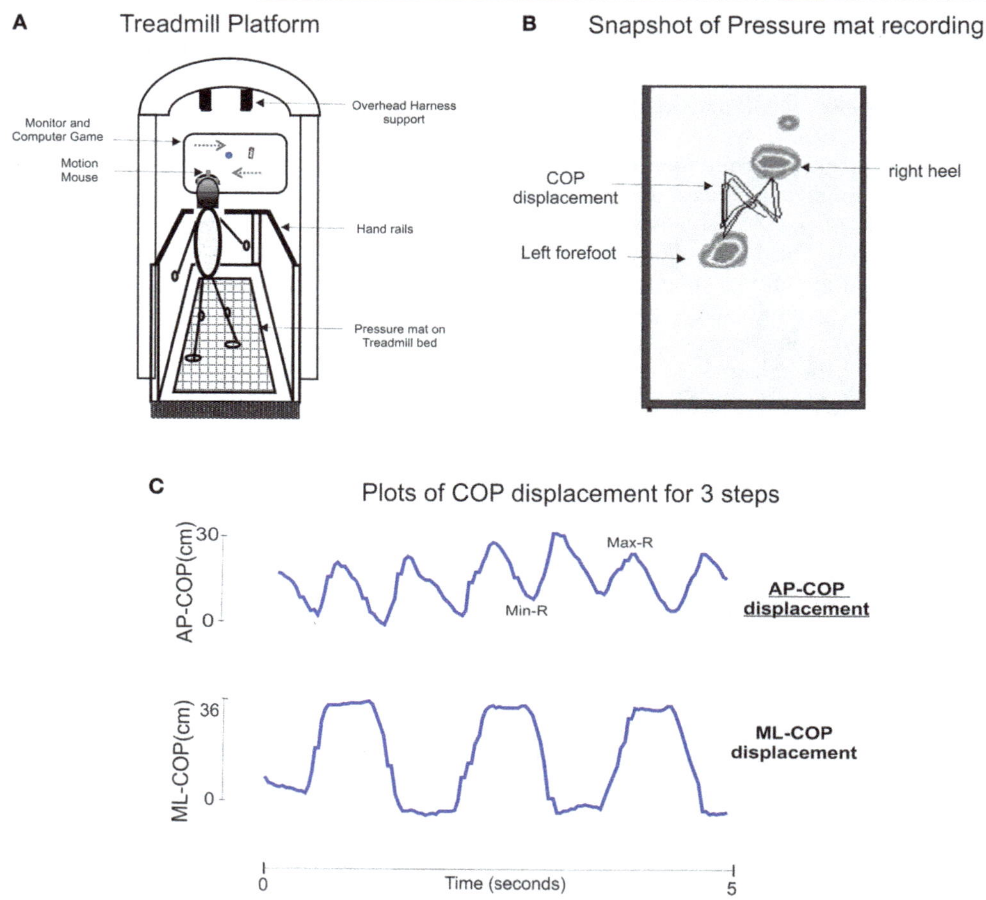

FIGURE 1 | Panel (A) is an illustration of the treadmill platform and experimental set-up. Participant is walking on the instrumented treadmill while viewing a computer monitor. Head rotation (via motion mouse) is used to interact with the visuospatial executive task. Panel **(B)** presents a snapshot of the recorded treadmill pressure mat and the trace of center of foot pressure displacement for a complete gait cycle. Panel **(C)** presents AP and ML COP time-series data for 3 steps. Maxima and minima of COP excursion for right and left steps are quantified, and use to compute swing and step times and step length.

to control the position and motion of the computer game sprite. Therefore, a hands-free computer/game controller to interact with the game activities of the assessment software is introduced. Head pointing movements are among the most natural and can easily be performed with minimal instruction and by most people.

Visuomotor (VM) Task

The goal is to align two moving objects. One object, a bright circular object, is computer controlled and moved horizontally, left and right (cyclic motion) on a computer display for 45 s. Motion frequency was 0.5 Hz and amplitude was 70% of monitor width. The second object, a square, was slaved to head rotation using the head-mounted motion sense mouse (Szturm et al., 2015a). The goal of the task is to maintain an overlap of the two objects for 45 s. The computer application generates a logged data file to record the coordinates of the circle (target) and square (head rotation) at 100 Hz. The data file is processed off-line to quantify visuomotor performance as described below.

Participants were tested in one direction, (a) horizontal motion (left/right).

Visuospatial Executive Game (VEG) Task

The goal was to move a paddle (the game sprite) to interact with moving game objects. Head rotation via the motion sense mouse was used to move the game paddle and catch the target objects while avoiding distractor objects. See **Figure 2A** for illustration of the game function. The target object was a brightly colored circle and the distractor object was an oval shaped object. The target and distractor objects appear at random locations at the top of the monitor and moves to the bottom in a time period of 1.5 s and then disappear. For each game event (target appearance) the participant moves a game paddle along the bottom of the display to catch the target object and avoid any distractor objects. The game was played for 60 s or 45 game events. The software indexes the "times" for the appearance and disappearance of each target game object and logs the position coordinates of the game objects and game paddle (participant's head rotation) at a

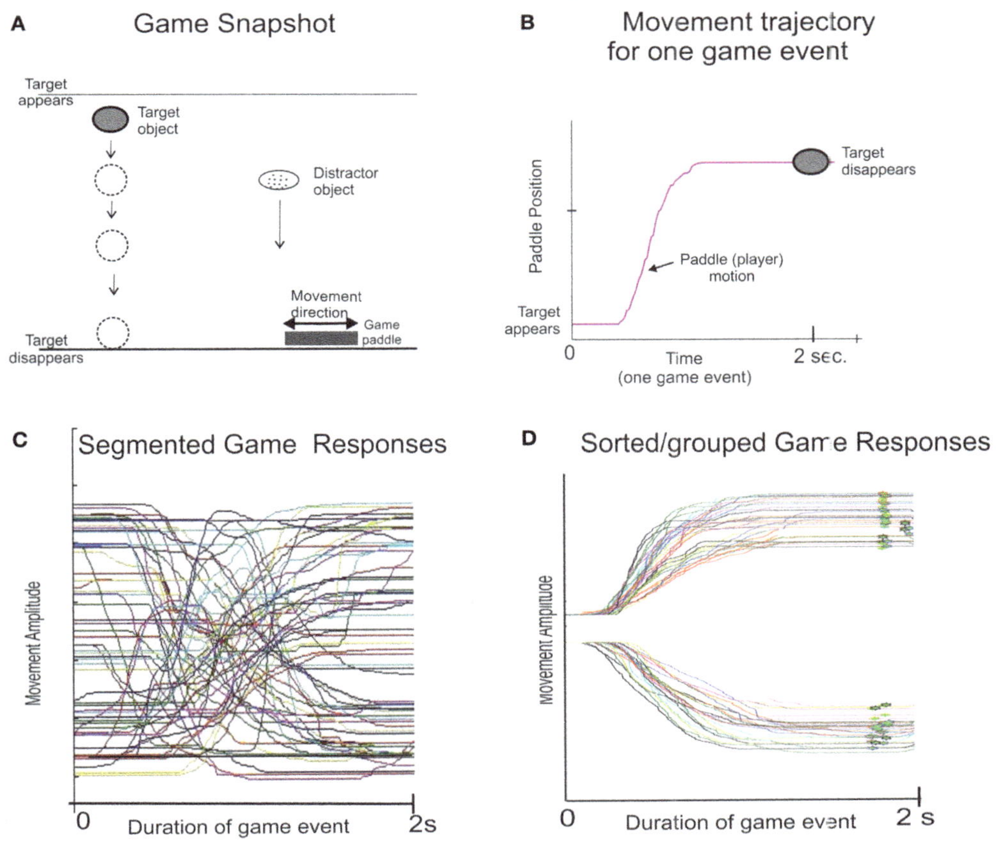

FIGURE 2 | Illustration of the game objects and motions of the visuospatial executive game. Panel **(A)** Screenshot of the VEG game software. The target appears at the top of the screen at a random location and the participant interacts with the target. Panel **(B)** presents the trajectory for one game movement response from target appearance to target disappearance panel **(C)** presents overlay trajectories of all game movement responses (as shown in panel **B**) for one game session of 60 s duration. Some game movements are upward and some downward (i.e., different movement directions), and some game movements are medium and some large amplitudes. Panel **(D)**, the game movement responses of panel **(C)** are sorted and grouped in bins, which in this case represent medium amplitude movement responses for both directions; leftward game movements (upward trajectories), and rightward game movements (downward trajectories).

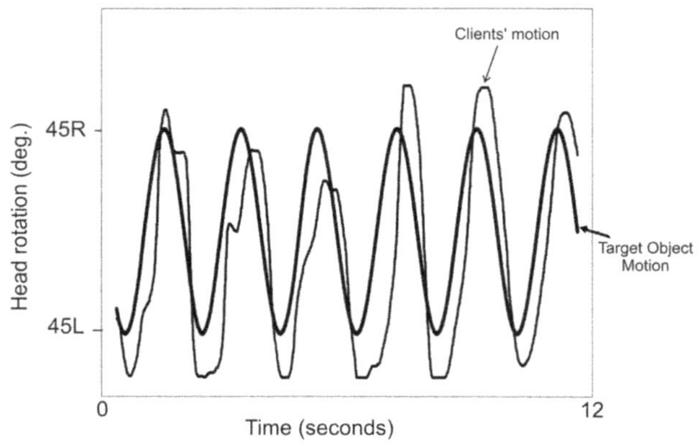

FIGURE 3 | Presents Synchronous plots of the target cursor motion and user movement trajectories (head rotation) for a typical VM tracking task. Maxima are the left most position and minima the right most position.

sampling rate of 100 Hz. The data file is processed off-line to quantify visuospatial executive performance as described below.

The visuomotor and visuospatial executive game tasks were performed in standing (baseline and during treadmill walking (dual-task condition).Prior to testing, the participants were allowed to play the tracking and game tasks while sitting for a few minutes to become familiar with each task.

The treadmill walking tasks were difficult when performing the concurrent game tasks. The treadmill was equipped with safety side rails in easy reach, and participants were fitted with a safety harness secured above to a support system. Also during all test a Physical Therapist stood behind the participants to provide assistance if required.

DATA ANALYSIS

Spatiotemporal Gait Variables

The average and coefficient of variation (COV) over 30 consecutive steps were determined for (a) right step time, (b) right single support times, and (c) right step length. Step time is defined as the time from a right foot off (beginning of left single support) to left foot off. Note analysis was also performed for left steps. Since the statistical analysis showed no significant difference in means of right and left gait variables, only the right gait variables will be presented.

Visuomotor Performance

Figure 3 presents synchronous plots of the target motion (circle) and user head rotation (square) for a typical visuomotor task. A sine-wave function of the reference target cursor waveform was determined, Head rotation trajectories were fit to the sine-wave function, and the coefficient of determination (COD) was computed based on total and the average residual difference between the position (pixel coordinates) of the target and head cursor for all sampled data points. The first two cycles of the tracking tasks were excluded to allow the participants' time to acquire the moving target and begin tracking. MATLAB (The Math Works, Natick, MA, version 2010a) was used to compute the COD.

Visuospatial Executive Performance Measures

Figure 2B presents the trajectory of an individual game movement response. Each game event was 1.5 s in duration from target appearance to target disappearance. **Figure 2C** Presents overlay trajectories of individual game movement responses in one game session. Based on time indices of target appearance and disappearance the software segments all game movement traces for each direction and game movement amplitude. The software then sorts these movement traces by direction and for medium amplitude movements (**Figure 2D**). Thus, the software produces multiple, standardized contextual movement events (Players actions) for each direction. For a detailed description of the game movement indexing and segmentation see (Lockery et al., 2011; Szturm et al., 2015a). The following variables were quantified; (a) success rate determined as the percentage of target objects that were caught, (b) average Response Time: the time from target appearance to the start of the game paddle movement and (c) average Movement Time, the time from start of the game paddle movement to the time it reaches its plateau at the point the target disappears Response Time and Movement Time were averaged over all game movement responses separately for leftward and rightward directions. Statistical analysis (paired t-test) revealed no significant difference in average response time or average movement time between leftward and right game movement responses, and therefore only averages for leftward game movements are presented in the present study.

Statistical Analysis

Relative reliability was assessed using a fixed model intra-class correlation coefficient (ICC) (Weir, 2005). The ICC scores were interpreted as high when equal to or greater than 0.70, as moderate between 0.5 and 0.69, and as low when less than 0.50 (Lexell and Downham, 2005). Absolute reliability was analyzed using standard error of measurement (SEM). Systematic errors between the test periods were evaluated using a paired t-test. Normality of data was assessed using the Shapiro-Wilks test ($n < 50$). This test revealed a normal distribution for all variable ($p > 0.1$).

Discriminative validity was evaluated using a paired t-test to examine the effect of dual-task conditions on; (a) gait performance and (b) visuomotor and visuospatial executive performance. For the VM and VEG performance measures, the single task condition is when performed in standing on a fixed surface and the DT condition is when performed during treadmill walking.

SPSS software for Windows, version 20.0 (SPSS Inc. Chicago) was used for all statistical analysis procedures.

RESULTS

Nineteen females and six males participated. The median age was 65, range 61–68 years. Group average gait speed was 1.1 m/s and a standard deviation (SD) of 0.14, and the average distance walked in 6 min was 532 m and SD of 87. All participants walked outdoors on a regular basis, and none had reported a fall in the last year.

Table 1 presents the results of the test-retest reliability analyses for the temporal and spatial gait variables. With a few exceptions, high ICC values of 0.71–0.85 were observed for both averages and COV. Moderate ICC values were observed for average step length (0.65) during the visuomotor task, and for SL COV (0.65) when performing the executive game task. The standard error of measurement (SEM) as a percentage of the group mean values ranged from 4 to 15% and was less than 10% in the majority of cases. Based on a paired t-test analyses, no systematic errors in the average or COV variables were observed between the two test sessions for either the single or the two DT walk conditions. As presented in **Table 2**, moderate ICC values of 0.6–0.65 were observed for visuomotor and executive game performance measures. The SEM as a percentage of the group mean values for the visuomotor task was 15%, and for the executive game performance measures, it ranged from 5 to 11%. The results of the paired t-tests revealed no significant difference in visuomotor or executive performance measures between the two test periods.

Group means and 95% CI for average and COV of spatiotemporal gait variables obtained during walk only and dual-task walk conditions are presented in **Figures 4, 5** respectively. As presented in **Table 3** all temporal and spatial gait variables did demonstrate a significant change when performing the visuospatial executive tasks (DT condition) as compared to walk alone (single task condition). Average swing time ($p < 0.01$) and average step length ($p < 0.001$) significantly decreased from single to dual-task conditions, whereas average single support time significantly increased ($p < 0.001$) from single to dual-task conditions. Group means and 95% confidence intervals (CI) are presented in **Table 1**. There was a significant increase in COV for all gait variables when performing the visuospatial executive game task as compared to walk alone ($p < 0.01$). As presented in **Table 3** the majority of gait variables did not demonstrate a significant change when performing the visuomotor task. There were two exceptions; a significant decrease in Average step length ($p < 0.001$) and a significant increase in single support time COV ($p < 0.001$) as compared to walk alone.

Figure 6 presents the group means and 95% CI for the visuomotor performance measure obtained during walk only and dual-task walk conditions. As presented in **Table 4** there was a significant decrease in visuomotor performance when tested during treadmill walking as compared to standing; ($p < 0.001$). Group means and 95% confidence intervals (CI) are presented in **Table 2**. When tested in standing visuomotor performance was 0.78 and decreased to 0.65 during walking.

Figure 7 presents the group means and 95% CI for the visuospatial cognitive performance measures obtained during walk only and dual-task walk conditions. As presented in **Table 4** there was a significant decrease in visuospatial executive performance when tested during treadmill walking as compared to standing. There was a significant decrease in success rate ($p < 0.04$), but no significant change in Response time or Movement Time when tested during treadmill walking as compared to standing. Success rate, when tested in standing, was 94%, as compared to 82% during walking.

DISCUSSION

High ICC values (greater than 0.8) have been reported for average gait variables during overground and treadmill walking (Brach et al., 2008; Paterson et al., 2008). In the present study comparable

TABLE 1 | Results of statistical analysis, ICC scores, standard error of measurement (SEM), group means and 95% confidence interval (CI) for the spatial and temporal gait parameters during the three walking conditions.

Task conditions	Test 1 Mean (95%CI)	Test 2 Mean (95%CI)	ICC	SEM
WALK ALONE				
Avg-SsT, ms	376 (359.6–392.4)	386 (369.3–402.7)	0.8	19.1
Avg-SwT, ms	457 (429.6–484.4)	478 (450.6–505.4)	0.7	40.7
Avg-SL, cm	40.4 (38.1–42.7)	41.6 (39.7–43.5)	0.8	2.9
COV-SsT	10.4 (9.48–11.3)	10.7 (9.9–11.5)	0.8	1.1
COV-SwT	12.1 (10.6–13.6)	11.5 (10–13)	0.9	0.5
COV-SL	14.7 (13.1–16.2)	15.3 (13.9–16.8)	0.8	1.6
DT-VM				
Avg-SsT, ms	401 (379.6–422.4)	393 (376.2–409.4)	0.8	30.3
Avg-SwT, ms	437 (409.6–464.4)	421 (393.6–448.4)	0.8	36.1
Avg-SL, cm	32.5 (30.7–34.3)	31.8 (30.3–33.3)	0.7	2.6
COV-SsT	13.2 (12–14.4)	13.7 (12.2–15.2)	0.7	1.5
COV-SwT	12.7 (11.5–13.9)	11.5 (10.3–12.7)	0.7	1.7
COV-SL	16.2 (14.7–17.7)	16.3 (15.2–17.4)	0.9	1.2
DT-VEG				
Avg-SsT, ms	445 (422.2–467.8)	436 (419.7–452.4)	0.7	35.1
Avg-SwT, ms	294 (281.2–306.8)	302 (288.1–315.9)	0.7	18.3
Avg-SL, cm	32.5 (30.7–34.3)	32.5 (30.8–34.2)	0.8	4.1
COV-SsT	16.2 (14.3–18.1)	19.4(17.3–21.5)	0.8	2.1
COV-SwT	19.8 (18.9–20.7)	20.0 (17.7–22.3)	0.7	1.3
COV-SL	23.9 (22.3–25.5)	23.1 (21–25.2)	0.8	2.1

SsT, single support time; SwT, swing time; SL, step length; Avg, Average; COV, coefficient of variation (%).

TABLE 2 | Results of statistical analysis, ICC scores, standard error of measurement (SEM), group means and 95% confidence interval (CI) for visuomotor and Visuospatial Executive Game tasks during treadmill walking.

Outcome measures	Test 1 Mean (95%CI)	Test 2 Mean (95%CI)	ICC	SEM
VISUOMOTOR				
COD	0.6 (0.6–0.7)	0.7 (0.6–0.7	0.7	0.1
VISUOSPATIAL EXECUTIVE GAME				
Success Rate, %	82.5 (79.5–85.5)	84 (83.3–88.7)	0.7	3.6
Avg-Response Time, ms	502 (475.5–528.5)	493 (465.9–508.1)	0.6	41
Avg-Movement Time, ms	526 (505.7–552.3)	514 (482.5–535.5)	0.6	56

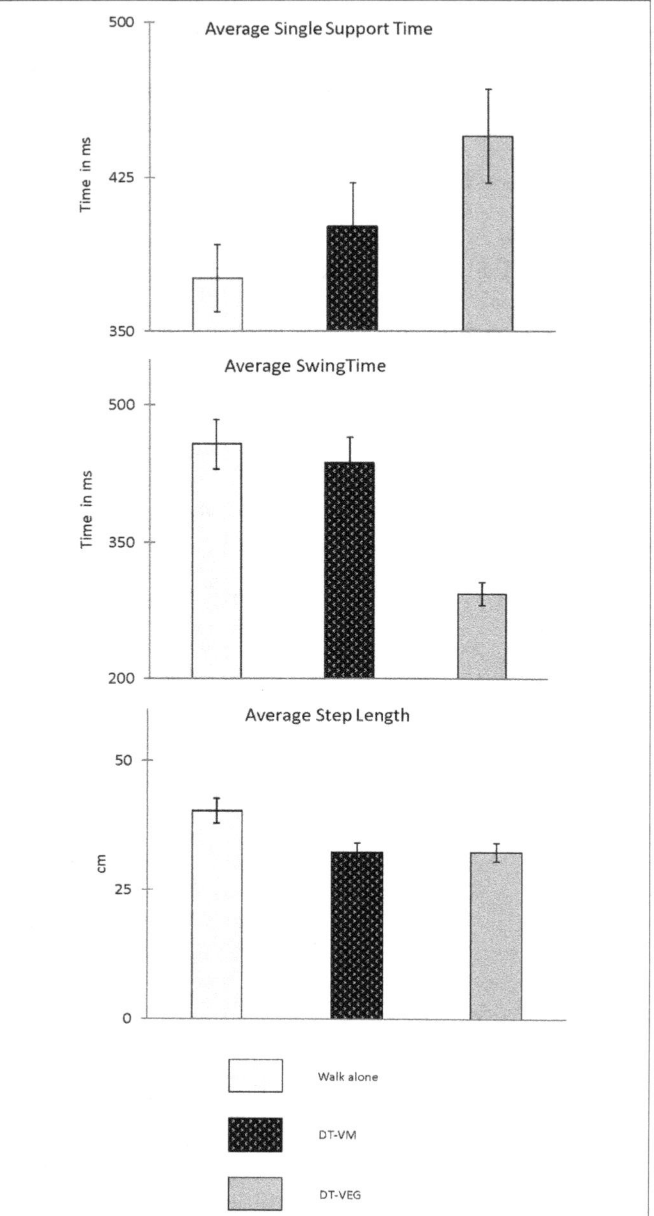

FIGURE 4 | Presented are group means and 95% confidence intervals (CI) for the average spatiotemporal gait variables (SsT, SwT, SL) obtained during walk only and dual-task walk conditions.

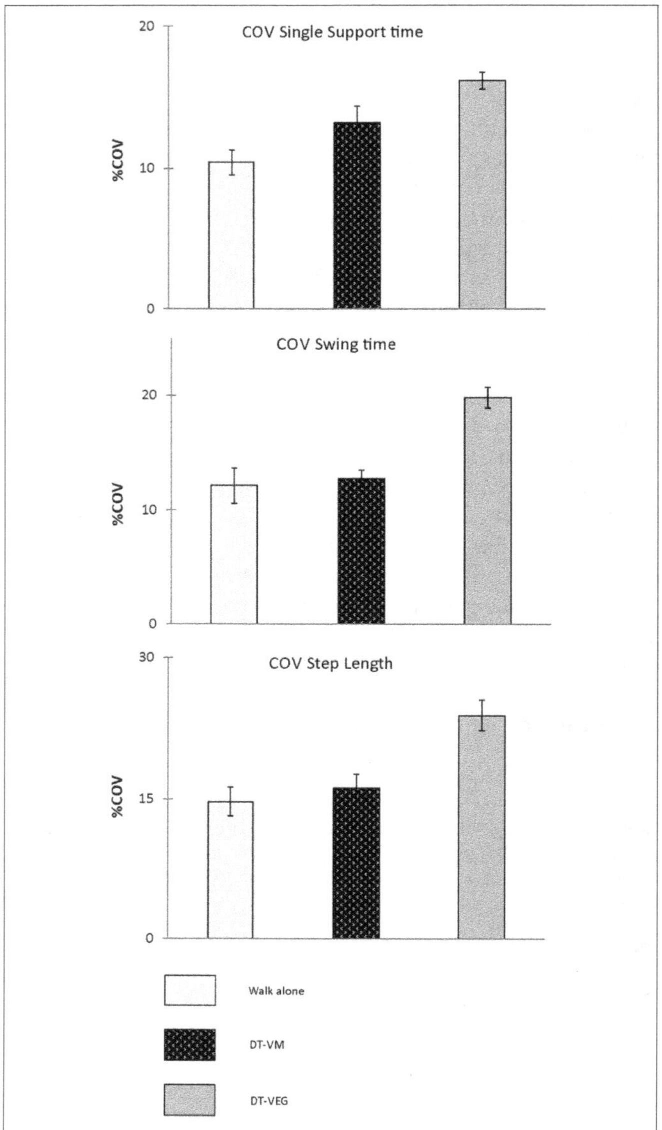

FIGURE 5 | Presented are group means and 95% CI for COV of the spatiotemporal gait variables (SsT, SwT, Sl) obtained during walk only and dual-task walk conditions.

high to moderate ICC values were observed for all average gait variables during walk alone trials. The present results extend reliability analysis to include DT treadmill walking involving computerized visuomotor and visuospatial executive tasks. A number of studies have reported low ICC values (less than 0.4) for measures of gait variation (Brach et al., 2008; Paterson et al., 2008; Faude et al., 2012). Immediate test re-test reliability was examined in older adults (mean age of 75.5 years) during an over ground DT walking test consisting of counting backward (Beauchet et al., 2011). Low ICC values of 0.28 for stride variability were observed. In contrast, the present results show modest to high ICC values for COV of gait variables during DT treadmill walking. There are a few important differences between the present study and the studies using over ground walking. In the present study participants viewed a computer monitor and performed standardized visual-spatial executive tasks for a duration of 60 s. The VEG tasks employed in the present study were executively demanding, requiring timely responses (less than 1 s) to identify a moving object as the target or a distractor, to estimate its final position, and to move the game sprite using head rotation in order to intercept the moving target, i.e., accuracy requirement. Secondly, walking speed was controlled and over 30 consecutive steps were recorded, as opposed to recordings of

TABLE 3 | Effect of dual-tasking on spatiotemporal gait variables (Average and COV).

Gait variables	Walk alone vs. Walk + visuospatial task	Walk alone vs. Walk + visuomotor task
	t-statistics, *p*-value	*t*-statistics, *p*-value
Avg-SsT	4.5, 0.01	1.9, 0.07
Avg-SwT	10.1, 0.01	1.0, 0.3
Avg-SL	8.5, 0.01	6.8, 0.01
COV-SsT	5.4, 0.01	3.7, 0.01
COV-SwT	8.1, 0.01	0.6, 0.5
COV-SL	7.8, 0.01	1.4, 0.18

Degrees of Freedom (df) = 24.

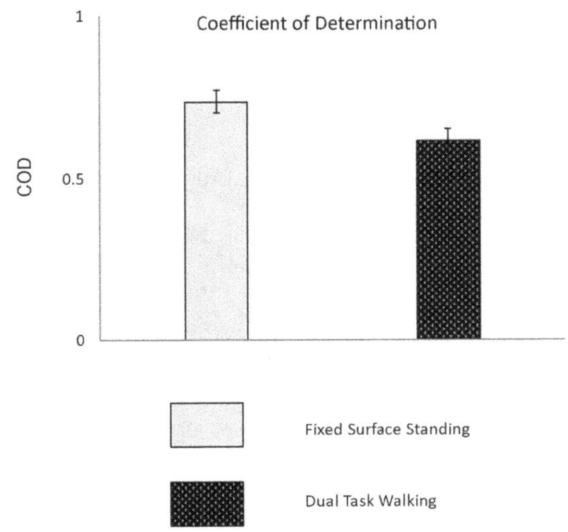

FIGURE 6 | Presented are group means and 95% CI for the visuomotor performance measure obtained during fixed surface standing and dual-task walk conditions.

TABLE 4 | Effect of dual-tasking on Visuomotor and Visuospatial executive game performance measures.

Outcome measures	*t*-statistics, *p*-value
VISUOMOTOR TASK	
Coefficient of Determination (COD)	4.5, 0.01
VISUOSPATIAL EXECUTIVE TASK	
Success Rate, %	2.3, 0.04
Avg-Response Time, ms	0.1, 0.9
Avg-Movement Time, ms	0.9, 0.4

Degrees of Freedom (df) = 24.

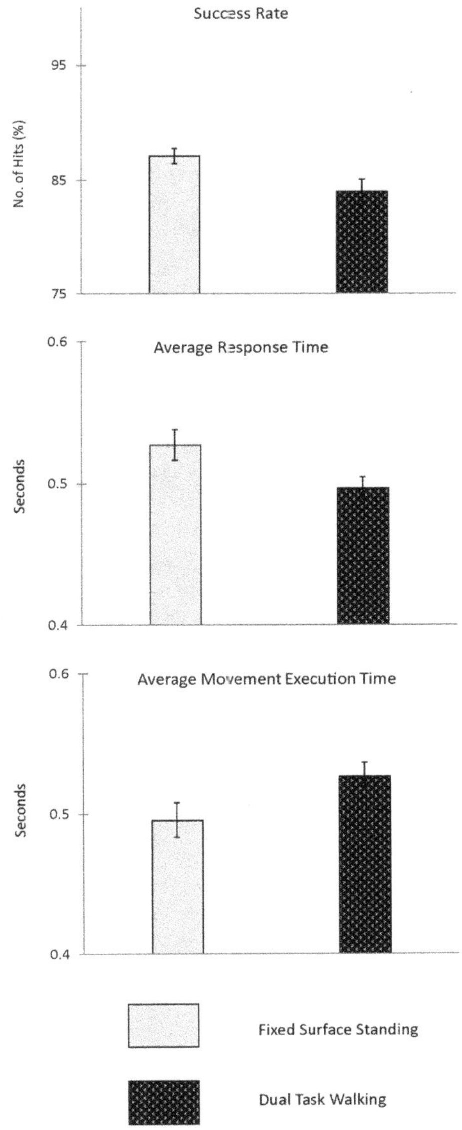

FIGURE 7 | Presented are group means and 95% CI for the visuospatial executive performance measures obtained during fixed surface standing and dual-task walk conditions.

a small number of consecutive steps on a short walkway (i.e., 3–5 m). Many studies have demonstrated that spatiotemporal gait variables are influenced by walking speed (Kang and Dingwell, 2008; Stoquart et al., 2008; Keene et al., 2016). Furthermore, it has been shown that using a continuous walking protocol instead of short intermittent walks, and collecting more than 30 steps improved reliability, in particular for measures of gait variability (Galna et al., 2013). Low between day ICC values (less than 0.4) for gait variation has been reported for active, healthy older adults (mean age of 64 years) when tested on a treadmill (Faude et al., 2012). It is not clear why this large difference (during walk alone condition) is observed between the present study and the results of (Faude et al., 2012). One difference is the walking speed of the two studies; 1.3 vs. 0.9 m/s. A lower speed was used in the present study because the addition of the visuospatial executive activities did make the walking more difficult.

The present results show a small absolute variability; SEM ranged from 4 to 15% of the mean scores and the majority were less than 10%. Taken together the moderate to high ICC values and the small measurement error indicate that this tool has the ability to repeatedly record reliable data from active older adults, and would serve as acceptable outcome measures to examine effects of preventative measures and targeted interventions on dual-task walking performance.

Ability to recover from a sudden loss of balance is only part of the equation that governs the probability of falling; also important is what causes the instability. Besides large physical disturbances, performing a concurrent executive task can lead to a sudden change in locomotor rhythm and even falls. A number of studies have examined the interaction among physical and information processing load as a function of aging using a DT paradigm (Plummer-D'Amato et al., 2012; Xiangde, 2014). In the present study where speed is held constant all gait variables tested (average and COV) except one case were significantly affected when performing the visuospatial executive task as compared to walk alone. Average Single support time did increase when the information processing load was added. These findings for average gait variables would indicate the main effect of visuospatial processing load on locomotor rhythm. There was also a significant increase in COV for all gait variables when the visuospatial load was increased. These results are consistent with other studies which have examined dual-task effects on gait variation during overground walking in healthy young and older adults (Ijmker and Lamoth, 2012; Montero-Odasso et al., 2012). Variation of gait variables has often been used to index gait stability (Baltadjieva et al., 2006; Herman et al., 2010; Lord et al., 2011). Herman et al. (2010) reported swing time variability to be nearly 20% higher in fallers compared to non-fallers. Unlike the dual-task visuospatial trials, there was little change in gait performance during the dual-task visuomotor trials. The VM task has very simple executive demand, overlap two visible objects. This may explain why the dual-task VM trials had little effect on spatiotemporal gait variables.

A significant decrease in the Success Rate of the visuospatial tasks was observed during treadmill walking. However, Response Time and Movement Time were not affected by the increased processing demands of treadmill walking. Motor planning and temporal parameters of precision movements would not be the only factors that contribute to movement accuracy of the visuospatial task. The estimation of the final target position and control requirements of the head rotations would also contribute to movement accuracy. This is an area that will receive further investigation. The performance of the visuomotor task also decreased during treadmill walking as compared to standing. The VM task required continuous visual attention and foveation to determine the relative positions (overlap error) of 2 moving objects, and this spatial feedback would be required to maintain or restore their overlap. The significant decline in VM performance is likely due to the increase in the amount of passive head movement between standing vs. treadmill walking. There is a considerable increase in the magnitude of passive head velocity during walking, as much as 10 times of that seen during standing (Szturm et al., 2015b). Passive head motion will cause increased retinal image slip, and thus affects the ability to stabilize gaze during continuous fixation tasks, such as, tracking and interacting with moving targets (Scherer et al., 2008; Lambert et al., 2010).

Most commonly dual-task studies have utilized executive tasks, like walking while talking, verbal fluency or number subtraction that is typically only assessed qualitatively, do not involve visuospatial processing, and are limited in what individual brain areas are recruited (Al-Yahya et al., 2011).Visual attention, tracking, choice responses and the processing of object locations/trajectories and their spatial relations with respect to other objects are key aspects to consider in locomotor control and are important factors in fall risk (Bagurdes et al., 2008; Nagamatsu et al., 2009; Murray et al., 2010). The present computerized dual-task protocols broaden the types of standardized executive activities for use with treadmill walking that has previously been reported.

Study Limitations

Treadmill walking does constrain gait, for example, by the belt width, and does not reflect all aspects of over ground walking behavior (Hollman et al., 2016). The present visuospatial computer task involves both head rotation and information processing, and at this point we cannot rule out any intersegmental mechanical effect of the head rotation as a cause of the gait changes observed between the walk alone and the DT walk trials. Head rotations during the VEG task were relatively small and slow i.e., the majority of the head rotations for game responses were less than 20° and movement duration was in the order of 500 ms. Therefore, every 2 s the participant produced these small ramp head rotations. The head movements were rotations so the mass center of the head segment would not change relative to body center of mass. Duysens et al. examined COP migration during an open-loop tracking tasks (up to 30° of visual target motion) while treadmill walking (Duysens et al., 2008). Three tasks were performed; tracking with eye movements only (head stationary), tracking by rotating the head in synchrony with the moving visual target (open-loop tracking task), and tracking while rotating the trunk in synchrony with the moving visual target. The results demonstrated no significant deviation of the COP migration when participants performed the tracking task with eye or head rotation, whereas, trunk rotations led to a doubling of ML-COP deviation. The mechanical effect of head rotation on gait rhythm pacing and variation will receive further investigation.

CONCLUSION

This study demonstrates the reliability and reproducibility of the computer-based assessment tool for DT treadmill walking. The high to Moderate ICC values, the small standard errors of measurement and the lack of systematic errors in the measures indicate that this tool has the ability to repeatedly record reliable data from community-dwelling older adults Improved and affordable methods of screening and fall risk assessment in the community particularly are important because continued difficulties and fall injuries will have a sizable impact in this population.

ETHICS STATEMENT

Bannatyne Campus Health Research ethics board at the University of Manitoba (Ethics Reference number H2011:284) approved the study "Computerized Dual-task testing of gait and visuospatial cognitive functions; Test-retest reliability and validity." A written informed consent was acquired from all participants before the screening process by blind assessors. This study was carried out in accordance with the recommendations of "University of Manitoba, Bannatyne campus Health Research Ethics Board" with written informed consent from all subjects. All subjects gave written informed consent in accordance with the Declaration of Helsinki. The protocol was approved by the "University of Manitoba, Bannatyne campus Health Research Ethics Board."

AUTHOR CONTRIBUTIONS

TS and VS: study concept and design; acquisition, analysis, and interpretation of data; preparation of the manuscript. AK: Acquisition, analysis, and interpretation of data; preparation of the manuscript. MN: Analysis, and interpretation of data; preparation of the manuscript.

ACKNOWLEDGMENTS

This study was supported by the Canadian Institute of Health Research (CIHR) grant ITM: 83266. The sponsor had no involvement in any aspect of the research or in the preparation of this manuscript.

REFERENCES

Al-Yahya, E., Dawes, H., Smith, L., Dennis, A., Howells, K., and Cockburn, J. (2011). Cognitive motor interference while walking: a systematic review and meta-analysis. *Neurosci. Biobehav. Rev.* 35, 715–728. doi: 10.1016/j.neubiorev.2010.08.008

Anguera, J. A., Boccanfuso, J., Rintoul, J. L., Al-Hashimi, O., Faraji, F., Janowich, J., et al. (2013). Video game training enhances cognitive control in older adults. *Nature* 501, 97–101. doi: 10.1038/nature12486

Bagurdes, L. A., Mesulam, M. M., Gitelman, D. R., Weintraub, S., and Small, D. M. (2008). Modulation of the spatial attention network by incentives in healthy aging and mild cognitive impairment. *Neuropsychologia* 46, 2943–2948. doi: 10.1016/j.neuropsychologia.2008.06.005

Baltadjieva, R., Giladi, N., Gruendlinger, L., Peretz, C., and Hausdorff, J. M. (2006). Marked alterations in the gait timing and rhythmicity of patients with *de novo* parkinson's disease. *Eur. J. Neurosci.* 24. 1815–1820. doi: 10.1111/j.1460-9568.2006.05033.x

Beauchet, O., Freiberger, E., Annweiler, C., Kressig, R. W., Herrmann, F. R., and Allali, G. (2011). Test-retest reliability of stride time variability while dual tasking in healthy and demented adults with frontotemporal degeneration. *J. Neuroeng. Rehabil.* 8:37. doi: 10.1186/1743-0003-8-37

Betker, A. L., Maharjan, P., Yaduvanshi, C., Szturm., T., and Moussavi, Z. (2008). "Automated quantification and comparison of spatiotemporal GAIT parameters during treadmill and overground walking," in *CCECE 2008. Canadian Conference on, Electrical and Computer Engineering* (Niagara Falls, ON), 165–168.

Brach, J. S., Studenski, S., Perera, S., VanSwearingen, J. M., and Newman, A. B. (2008). Stance time and step width variability have unique contributing impairments in older persons. *Gait Posture* 27, 431–439. doi: 10.1016/j.gaitpost.2007.05.016

Bruijn, S. M., van Dieen, J. H., Meijer, O. G., and Beek, P. J. (2009). Statistical precision and sensitivity of measures of dynamic gait stability. *J. Neurosci. Methods* 178, 327–333. doi: 10.1016/j.jneumeth.2008.12.015

Diamond, A. (2015). Effects of physical exercise on executive functions: Going beyond simply moving to moving with thought. *Ann. Sports Med. Res.* 2, 1011.

Duysens, J., Duysens, J. P., Bastiaanse, C. M., van Sprundel, M., Schubert, M., and Smits-Engelsman, B. C. (2008). How trunk turns affect locomotion when you are not looking where you go. *Hum. Mov. Sci.* 27, 759–770. doi: 10.1016/j.humov.2008.04.004

Faude, O., Donath, L., Roth, R., Fricker, L., and Zahner, L. (2012). Reliability of gait parameters during treadmill walking in community-dwelling healthy seniors. *Gait Posture* 36, 444–448. doi: 10.1016/j.gaitpost.2012.04.003

Galna, B., Lord, S., and Rochester, L. (2013). Is gait variability reliable in older adults and parkinson's disease? towards an optimal testing protocol. *Gait Posture* 37, 580–585. doi: 10.1016/j.gaitpost.2012.09.025

Gregory, M. A., Gill, D. P., Zou, G., Liu-Ambrose, T., Shigematsu, R., Fitzgerald, C., et al. (2016). Group-based exercise combined with dual-task training improves gait but not vascular health in active older adults without dementia. *Arch. Gerontol. Geriatr.* 63, 18–27. doi: 10.1016/j.archger.2015.11.008

Herman, T., Mirelman, A., Giladi, N., Schweiger, A., and Hausdorff, J. M. (2010). Executive control deficits as a prodrome to falls in healthy older adults: a prospective study linking thinking, walking, and falling. *J. Gerontol. Ser. A, Biol. Sci. Med. Sci.* 65, 1086–1092. doi: 10.1093/gerona/glq077

Hollman, J. H., Childs, K. B., McNeil, M. L., Mueller, A. C., Quilter, C. M., and Youdas, J. W. (2010). Number of strides required for reliable measurements of pace, rhythm and variability parameters of gait during normal and dual task walking in older individuals. *Gait Posture* 32, 23–28. doi: 10.1016/j.gaitpost.2010.02.017

Hollman, J. H., Watkins, M. K., Imhoff, A. C., Braun, C. E., Akervik, K. A., and Ness, D. K. (2016). A comparison of variability in spatiotemporal gait parameters between treadmill and overground walking conditions. *Gait Posture* 43, 204–209. doi: 10.1016/j.gaitpost.2015.09.024

Ijmker, T., and Lamoth, C. J. (2012). Gait and cognition: the relationship between gait stability and variability with executive function in persons with and without dementia. *Gait Posture* 35, 126–130. doi: 10.1016/j.gaitpost.2011.08.022

Kang, H. G., and Dingwell, J. B. (2008). Separating the effects of age and walking speed on gait variability. *Gait Posture* 27, 572–577. doi: 10.1016/j.gaitpost.2007.07.009

Keene, D. J., Moe-Nilssen, R., and Lamb, S. E. (2016). The application of multilevel modelling to account for the influence of walking speed in gait analysis. *Gait Posture* 43, 216–219. doi: 10.1016/j.gaitpost.2015.09.026

Lambert, S., Sigrist, A., Delaspre, O., Pelizzone, M., and Guyot, J. P. (2010). Measurement of dynamic visual acuity in patients with vestibular areflexia. *Acta Otolaryngol.* 130, 820–823. doi: 10.3109/00016480903426592

Lexell, J. E., and Downham, D. Y. (2005). How to assess the reliability of measurements in rehabilitation. *Am. J. Phys. Med. Rehabil.* 84, 719–723. doi: 10.1097/01.phm.0000176452.17771.20

Lockery, D., Peters, J. F., Ramanna, S., Shay, B. L., and Szturm, T. (2011). Store-and-feedforward adaptive gaming system for hand-finger motion tracking in telerehabilitation. *IEEE Trans. Inf. Technol. Biomed.* 15, 467–473. doi: 10.1109/TITB.2011.2125976

Lord, S., Howe, T., Greenland, J., Simpson, L., and Rochester, L. (2011). Gait variability in older adults: a structured review of testing protocol and clinimetric properties. *Gait Posture* 34, 443–450. doi: 10.1016/j.gaitpost.2011.07.010

Mirelman, A., Rochester, L., Reelick, M., Nieuwhof, F., Pelosin, E., Abbruzzese, G., et al. (2013). V-TIME: a treadmill training program augmented by virtual reality to decrease fall risk in older adults: study design of a randomized controlled trial. *BMC Neurol.* 13:15. doi: 10.1186/1471-2377-13-15

Montero-Odasso, M., Muir, S. W., and Speechley, M. (2012). Dual-task complexity affects gait in people with mild cognitive impairment: the interplay between gait variability, dual tasking, and risk of falls. *Arch. Phys. Med. Rehabil.* 93, 293–299. doi: 10.1016/j.apmr.2011.08.026

Murray, M. E., Senjem, M. L., Petersen, R. C., Hollman, J. H., Preboske, G. M., Weigand, S. D., et al. (2010). Functional impact of white matter hyperintensities in cognitively normal elderly subjects. *Arch. Neurol.* 67, 1379–1385. doi: 10.1001/archneurol.2010.280

Nagamatsu, L. S., Liu-Ambrose, T. Y., Carolan, P., and Handy, T. C. (2009). Are impairments in visual-spatial attention a critical factor for increased falls risk in seniors? an event-related potential study. *Neuropsychologia* 47, 2749–2755. doi: 10.1016/j.neuropsychologia.2009.05.022

Park, E. C., Kim, S. G., and Lee, C. W. (2015). The effects of virtual reality game exercise on balance and gait of the elderly. *J. Phys. Ther. Sci.* 27, 1157–1159. doi: 10.1589/jpts.27.1157

Paterson, K. L., Hill, K. D., Lythgo, N. D., and Maschette, W. (2008). The reliability of spatiotemporal gait data for young and older women during continuous overground walking. *Arch. Phys. Med. Rehabil.* 89, 2360–2365. doi: 10.1016/j.apmr.2008.06.018

Pichierri, G., Wolf, P., Murer, K., and de Bruin, E. D. (2011). Cognitive and cognitive-motor interventions affecting physical functioning: a systematic review. *BMC Geriatr.* 11:29. doi: 10.1186/1471-2318-11-29

Plummer-D'Amato, P., Brancato, B., Dantowitz, M., Birken, S., Bonke, C., and Furey, E. (2012). Effects of gait and cognitive task difficulty on cognitive-motor interference in aging. *J. Aging Res.* 2012:583894. doi: 10.1155/2012/583894

Rebok, G. W., Ball, K., Guey, L. T., Jones, R. N., Kim, H. Y., King, J. W., et al. (2014). Ten-year effects of the advanced cognitive training for independent and vital elderly cognitive training trial on cognition and everyday functioning in older adults. *J. Am. Geriatr. Soc.* 62, 16–24. doi: 10.1111/jgs.12607

Santos-Eggimann, B., Karmaniola, A., Seematter-Bagnoud, L., Spagnoli, J., Bula, C., Cornuz, J., et al. (2008). The lausanne cohort Lc65+: a population-based prospective study of the manifestations, determinants and outcomes of frailty. *BMC Geriatr.* 8:20. doi: 10.1186/1471-2318-8-20

Scherer, M., Migliaccio, A. A., and Schubert, M. C. (2008). Effect of vestibular rehabilitation on passive dynamic visual acuity. *J. Vestib. Res.* 18, 147–157.

Shumway-Cook, A., Guralnik, J. M., Phillips, C. L., Coppin, A. K., Ciol, M. A., Bandinelli, S., et al. (2007). Age-associated declines in complex walking task performance: the walking InCHIANTI toolkit. *J. Am. Geriatr. Soc.* 55, 58–65. doi: 10.1111/j.1532-5415.2006.00962.x

Simonsick, E. M., Guralnik, J. M., Volpato, S., Balfour, J., and Fried, L. P. (2005). Just get out the door! importance of walking outside the home for maintaining mobility: findings from the women's health and aging study. *J. Am. Geriatr. Soc.* 53, 198–203. doi: 10.1111/j.1532-5415.2005.53103.x

Stoquart, G., Detrembleur, C., and Lejeune, T. (2008). Effect of speed on kinematic, kinetic, electromyographic and energetic reference values during treadmill walking. *Neurophysiol. Clin.* 38, 105–116. doi: 10.1016/j.neucli.2008.02.002

Strenziok, M., Parasuraman, R., Clarke, E., Cisler, D. S., Thompson, J. C., and Greenwood, P. M. (2014). Neurocognitive enhancement in older adults: comparison of three cognitive training tasks to test a hypothesis of training transfer in brain connectivity. *Neuroimage* 85, 1027–1039. doi: 10.1016/j.neuroimage.2013.07.069

Szturm, T., Maharjan, P., Marotta, J. J., Shay, B., Shrestha, S., and Sakhalkar, V. (2013a). The interacting effect of cognitive and motor task demands on performance of gait, balance and cognition in young adults. *Gait Posture* 38, 596–602. doi: 10.1016/j.gaitpost.2013.02.004

Szturm, T., Marotta, J., Wu, C., and nayak, A. (2013b). Technology-assisted and motivational programme for a blended approach to prevent and manage balance, gaze, mobility and cognitive decline with age. *OA Evid. Based Med.* 11:4.

Szturm, T., Reimer, K. M., and Hochman, J. (2015b). Home-based computer gaming in vestibular rehabilitation of gaze and balance impairment. *Games Health J.* 4, 211–220. doi: 10.1089/g4h.2014.0093

Szturm, T., Sakhalkar, V., Boreskie, S., Marotta, J. J., Wu, C., and Kanitkar, A. (2015a). Integrated testing of standing balance and cognition: test-retest reliability and construct validity. *Gait Posture* 41, 146–152. doi: 10.1016/j.gaitpost.2014.09.023

van Iersel, M. B., Kessels, R. P., Bloem, B. R., Verbeek, A. L., and Olde Rikkert, M. G. (2008). Executive functions are associated with gait and balance in community-living elderly people. *J. Gerontol. Ser. A Biol. Sci. Med. Sci.* 63, 1344–1349. doi: 10.1093/gerona/63.12.1344

Weir, J. P. (2005). Quantifying test-retest reliability using the intraclass correlation coefficient and the SEM. *J. Strength Cond. Res.* 19, 231–240. doi: 10.1519/15184.1

Wolinsky, F. D., Vander Weg, M. W., Howren, M. B., Jones, M. P., and Dotson, M. M. (2013). A randomized controlled trial of cognitive training using a visual speed of processing intervention in middle aged and older adults. *PLoS ONE* 8:e61624. doi: 10.1371/journal.pone.0061624

Xiangde, Q. (2014). Age-related cognitive task effects on gait characteristics: do different working memory components make a difference? *J. NeuroEng. Rehabil.* 11:149. doi: 1186/1743-0003-11-149

12

Effects of Changing Body Weight Distribution on Mediolateral Stability Control during Gait Initiation

Teddy Caderby[1], Eric Yiou[2,3], Nicolas Peyrot[1], Xavier de Viviés[1], Bruno Bonazzi[1] and Georges Dalleau[1]*

[1]Laboratoire IRISSE, UFR des Sciences de l'Homme et de l'Environnement, Université de la Réunion, Ile de la Réunion, France, [2]Laboratoire CIAMS, Université Paris Sud, Université Paris-Saclay, Orsay, France, [3]Laboratoire CIAMS, Université d'Orléans, Orléans, France

***Correspondence:**
Eric Yiou
eric.yiou@u-psud.fr

During gait initiation, anticipatory postural adjustments (APA) precede the execution of the first step. It is generally acknowledged that these APA contribute to forward progression but also serve to stabilize the whole body in the mediolateral direction during step execution. Although previous studies have shown that changes in the distribution of body weight between both legs influence motor performance during gait initiation, it is not known whether and how such changes affect a person's postural stability during this task. The aim of this study was to investigate the effects of changing initial body weight distribution between legs on mediolateral postural stability during gait initiation. Changes in body weight distribution were induced under experimental conditions by modifying the frontal plane distribution of an external load located at the participants' waists. Fifteen healthy adults performed a gait initiation series at a similar speed under three conditions: with the overload evenly distributed over both legs; with the overload strictly distributed over the swing-limb side; and with the overload strictly distributed over the stance-leg side. Our results showed that the mediolateral location of center-of-mass (CoM) during the initial upright posture differed between the experimental conditions, indicating modifications in the initial distribution of body weight between the legs according to the load distribution. While the parameters related to the forward progression remained unchanged, the alterations in body weight distribution elicited adaptive changes in the amplitude of APA in the mediolateral direction (i.e., maximal mediolateral shift of the center of pressure (CoP)), without variation in their duration. Specifically, it was observed that the amplitude of APA was modulated in such a way that mediolateral dynamic stability at swing foot-contact, quantified by the margin of stability (i.e., the distance between the base of support boundary and the extrapolated CoM position), did not vary between the conditions. These findings suggest that APA seem to be scaled as a function of the initial body weight distribution between both legs so as to maintain optimal conditions of stability during gait initiation.

Keywords: anticipatory postural adjustments, postural stability, gait initiation, external load, weight bearing asymmetry, margin of stability, balance

INTRODUCTION

Gait initiation, which corresponds to the transition from an upright stance to walking, is a locomotor task that is frequently executed in daily life. This task can be decomposed into two successive phases: a "postural phase", which precedes the swing heel-off time, followed by a "step execution phase" (Brenière et al., 1987; Brunt et al., 1999). During the postural phase, dynamic phenomena known as "anticipatory postural adjustments" (APA) are developed along the progression (or anteroposterior) axis (Brenière et al., 1987; Crenna and Frigo, 1991). These APA are manifested by a backwards shift in the center of pressure (CoP), which acts to propel the center of mass (CoM) forwards. It is acknowledged that these anticipatory dynamic phenomena create the conditions that are needed to reach the intended gait speed at the end of the first step (Brenière et al., 1987; Lepers and Brenière, 1995; Michel and Do, 2002).

APA are also described along the mediolateral axis. They are characterized by a CoP shift towards the swing-leg side, which propels the CoM towards the stance-leg side prior to swing foot-off (Jian et al., 1993; Elble et al., 1994). These postural dynamics are known to be crucial for stabilizing the whole body during step execution (McIlroy and Maki, 1999; Rogers et al., 2001; Yiou et al., 2012a). Indeed, the act of lifting the swing foot may create a mediolateral "gap" between the CoM and the CoP, which is then located in a new position beneath the stance foot. This gap may be responsible for a disequilibrium torque, which accelerates the CoM towards the swing-leg side and can potentially lead to a sideways fall. During gait initiation, this disequilibrium torque is invariably attenuated by the CoM displacement towards the stance leg-side during APA. Mediolateral APA are thus generally considered a feed-forward mechanism; one that is responsible for controlling mediolateral stability during gait initiation (McIlroy and Maki, 1999; Mille et al., 2014). Nevertheless, it is noteworthy that the mediolateral swing-foot placement (i.e., step width) may also be modulated in order to control mediolateral stability during gait initiation (Zettel et al., 2002a,b; Caderby et al., 2014). Modulating the swing-foot placement allows the CoM to be repositioned inside the base of support, thus ensuring postural stability.

The question of whether and how the initial body weight distribution between both legs may influence the gait initiation process in able-bodied subjects has been addressed in recent studies (Patchay and Gahéry, 2003; Azuma et al., 2007). In these studies, weight distribution between both legs were experimentally modified by asking subjects to shift their weight either onto the stance leg-side or swing leg-side prior to gait initiation, thus yielding an asymmetrical body weight distribution between the legs. Overall, these studies reported that an increase in the weight distribution over the swing leg-side induced APA of a longer duration, a shorter duration of step execution, and faster forward progression velocity compared with gait initiation performed with a posture with symmetrical body weight distribution over both legs. This effect was reversed when subjects shifted their weight over the stance leg-side. Despite the efforts made by the aforementioned authors, there is still an overall lack of understanding of how initial body weight distribution between the legs influences mediolateral postural stability during gait initiation. Such knowledge would be particularly significant for the prevention of falls, because mediolateral instability is known to be responsible for sideways falls and serious hip fractures (Nevitt and Cummings, 1993; Kannus et al., 2006).

When body weight is positioned closer to the stance leg-side in the initial upright posture, the amplitude of the mediolateral postural dynamics generated during APA needs to be scaled down (when compared with posture with symmetrical body weight distribution) to maintain postural stability during step execution. If it is not, the CoM may be propelled beyond the base of support with the risk of an imbalance towards the stance leg-side. Conversely, when body weight is positioned closer towards the swing leg-side in the initial posture, the amplitude of the mediolateral postural dynamics during APA needs to be scaled up to maintain postural stability during step execution. If it is not, the tendency of the CoM to fall towards the swing leg-side during step execution will be exacerbated, with a potential risk of imbalance. A strategy of increasing step width may then be required to maintain balance. Thus, body weight distribution between both legs can influence mediolateral stability during gait initiation, according to the loaded limb side. Nevertheless, recent results have suggested that the central nervous system is able to modulate the stabilizing features of gait initiation, i.e., mediolateral APA and swing-foot placement, so as to maintain an invariant mediolateral stability in situations with a postural constraint, e.g., induced by a lateral arm motion (Yiou and Do, 2011), an obstacle to clear (Yiou et al., 2016b) or a faster gait speed (Caderby et al., 2014). Therefore, the question arises as to whether such adaptations occur when gait initiation is performed and body weight distribution between both legs is modified.

It should be noted that, in contrast with some specific cases of pathological patients (e.g., patients that have suffered a stroke Marigold and Eng, 2006; Tessem et al., 2007), healthy adults evenly distribute their body weight between both legs during quiet standing (Bouisset and Maton, 1995; Hill and Vandervoort, 1996). In able-bodied subjects, natural posture with asymmetrical body weight distribution between the legs can be found in ecological situations, typically when one side of the body is loaded with an additional mass (e.g., carrying an object with a single hand or a backpack on one shoulder, etc.). Some authors have reported that, under such conditions, CoM location during quiet stance is shifted towards the overloaded limb side (Wu and MacLeod, 2001; Haddad et al., 2011). To our knowledge, although recent studies have investigated the effect of changes in body weight distribution induced by load carriage and by overweight on postural control during various motor tasks (e.g., Li and Aruin, 2007, 2009; Robert et al., 2007; Cau et al., 2014; Chen et al., 2015), no study has sought to examine the effect of changes in body weight distribution between the legs induced by load carriage on postural stability during gait initiation.

Thus, the aim of this study was to investigate the effect of changes in body weight distribution between both legs induced by an external load on mediolateral stability control during gait initiation. Based on previous findings from the literature (Yiou and Do, 2011; Caderby et al., 2014; Yiou et al., 2016b), we hypothesized that healthy young adults would modulate the stabilizing features of gait initiation (i.e., mediolateral APA and/or step width) as a function of initial body weight distribution so that the mediolateral stability remains unchanged.

MATERIALS AND METHODS

Subjects

Fifteen healthy subjects (13 males, 2 females; mean age: 21 ± 2 years, height: 176 ± 9 cm, weight: 70 ± 10 kg) participated in this experiment. All gave written consent after being fully informed of the test procedure, which was approved by the Institutional Review Board for the Protection of Human Research of the University of La Réunion and conducted in accordance with the Declaration of Helsinki.

Experimental Set-Up and Procedure

Gait initiation was performed from a first force-plate located at the beginning of a 5-m walkway. A second force-plate was located immediately in front of this initial force-plate so that the first step naturally landed on it. The two force-plates (40 × 60 cm, AMTI, Watertown, MA, USA), embedded in the walkway, recorded the ground reaction forces and moments at 1000 Hz. Beforehand, a foot switch sensor (25 mm, Biometrics, France) was secured to the first force-plate, under the heel of the subject's swing leg. Force-plate and foot switch signals were synchronized and transmitted to an acquisition system.

Initially, subjects were instructed to stand barefoot in a comfortable and natural upright posture with their arms alongside their trunk. They were asked to stand as still as possible and to fixate their gaze on a target placed at eye level, at a distance of 6 m. After receiving a verbal "all set" signal, subjects initiated gait on their own initiative and continued walking straight ahead to the end of the walkway. The swing leg was selected by the subject and was maintained throughout the experiment. After each trial, the subjects repositioned themselves in the standardized foot position (see McIlroy and Maki, 1997) previously marked on the first force-plate. The experimenter triggered the data acquisition when the subjects were motionless and at least 1 s before the "all set" signal.

Each subject performed a gait initiation series under three experimental conditions (**Figure 1**): with a load symmetrically distributed around the waist (Symmetrical condition), with an asymmetrical load strictly placed over the stance-limb side (Stance condition), and with an asymmetrical load strictly placed over the swing-limb side (Swing condition). The overload consisted of a belt positioned at a height that was close to the subject's body CoM, which in this study corresponded to 57% of the subject's height (Winter, 1990). Weights were attached to this belt ventrally and dorsally in order to reach the desired load. The chosen mass was 10% of the subject's body mass, because this was shown to be sufficient to modify the CoM location in quiet standing (Wu and MacLeod, 2001). In all conditions, the weights were placed symmetrically with respect to the sagittal plane so as avoid modifying the anteroposterior CoM location during the upright posture (Caderby et al., 2013a).

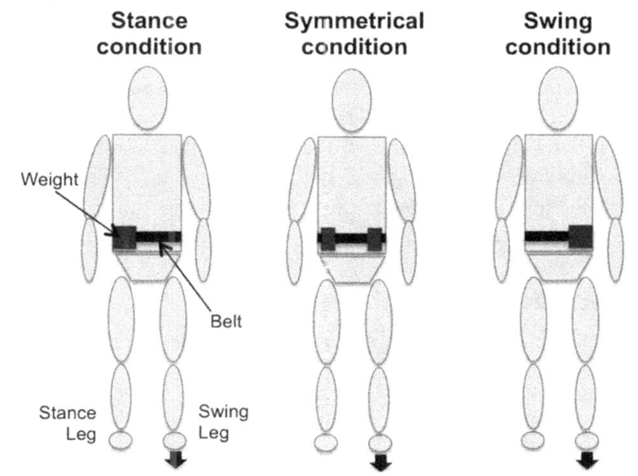

FIGURE 1 | Schematic representation of the various experimental conditions (Stance, Symmetrical and Swing). Note that the weights were ventrally and dorsally added.

To enable a comparison to be made between the various experimental conditions, the subjects were instructed to maintain a similar self-selected gait speed in all conditions. The order of the experimental conditions was randomized across subjects. In each condition, the subjects performed two familiarization trials, followed by eight trials from which data were collected. The subjects rested for 3 min between each condition.

Data Analysis

Before analysis, the force-plate signals were filtered using a low-pass Butterworth filter with a 10 Hz cut-off frequency. The anteroposterior and mediolateral CoP coordinates were calculated from force-plate data in accordance with the manufacturer's instructions (AMTI Manual). The anteroposterior (x"CoM) and mediolateral (y"CoM) accelerations of the CoM were determined from ground reaction forces according to Newton's second law. The anteroposterior and mediolateral CoM velocities and displacements were computed by successive numerical integrations of the corresponding acceleration using the trapezoidal rule. Calculations were performed with integration constant null, i.e., initial velocity and displacement equal to zero (Brenière et al., 1987). By convention, the CoM displacement and velocity and the CoP displacement were considered positive when directed forwards and towards the swing leg-side.

Several temporal events were determined to calculate our various dependent variables. The APA onset was detected when y"CoM deviated 2.5 standard deviations from its baseline value (Yiou et al., 2012b). Time of heel-off was detected from the foot switch sensor (Caderby et al., 2013b). The instant of swing foot-contact was determined when the vertical force signal of the second force-plate exceeded 10 N. The instant of swing foot-off was identified from the mediolateral CoP displacement (Melzer et al., 2007; Uemura et al., 2011), at the precise point when the slope of the CoP shift toward the stance leg suddenly changed (absolute CoP slope <100 mm/s, 2 samples in a row). The instant of stance foot-off was determined when the vertical force signal of the first force-plate dropped below 5 N.

Dependent Variables

The main dependent variables are illustrated in **Figure 2**. Initial anteroposterior and mediolateral CoM locations were estimated by averaging respectively the anteroposterior and mediolateral CoP positions during the 250 ms period preceding the "all set" signal (McIlroy and Maki, 1999). These initial locations also served as initial constants for computing the CoM position from its displacement during the time course of the gait initiation movement.

APA duration corresponded to the delay between APA onset and the heel-off of the swing leg. Step execution duration corresponded to the time between the swing heel-off and the swing foot-contact. Anteroposterior and mediolateral APA amplitudes were characterized respectively by the maximal backwards CoP shift and the maximal mediolateral CoP shift towards the swing leg during APA. The anteroposterior and mediolateral CoM velocities to time of heel-off and foot-contact were analyzed. Both the peak of mediolateral CoM displacement towards the stance leg during gait initiation and the mediolateral distance between the CoM and the CoP at this instant were calculated. Progression velocity was quantified at the peak of the anteroposterior CoM velocity reached at the end of the first step (Brenière et al., 1987). Step length was calculated as the anteroposterior distance between the CoP position at the swing foot-off time and the stance foot-off time (Gélat et al., 2006).

The concept of "margin of stability" (MoS) introduced by Hof et al. (2005) was used to quantify mediolateral dynamic stability in the present study. The MoS corresponded to the difference between the mediolateral boundary of the base of support (BoS_{ymax}) and the mediolateral position of the "extrapolated CoM" at foot-contact ($YcoM_{FC}$), i.e., $MoS = BoS_{ymax} - YcoM_{FC}$. As in Hof et al. (2005), BoS_{ymax} was determined from CoP data. Specifically, BoS_{ymax} was defined as the mediolateral CoP position at the time of stance foot-off, which at this point was located beneath the swing-foot (Hof et al., 2005). The mediolateral distance between the CoP position at this time (i.e., stance foot-off) and the mean CoP position over the single stance period of the leg stance represented the step width, and was representative of the size of the mediolateral base of support.

Based on the study of Hof et al. (2005), the mediolateral position of the extrapolated CoM at foot-contact ($YcoM_{FC}$) was calculated as follows:

$$YcoM_{FC} = yCoM_{FC} + \frac{y'CoM_{FC}}{\omega_0},$$

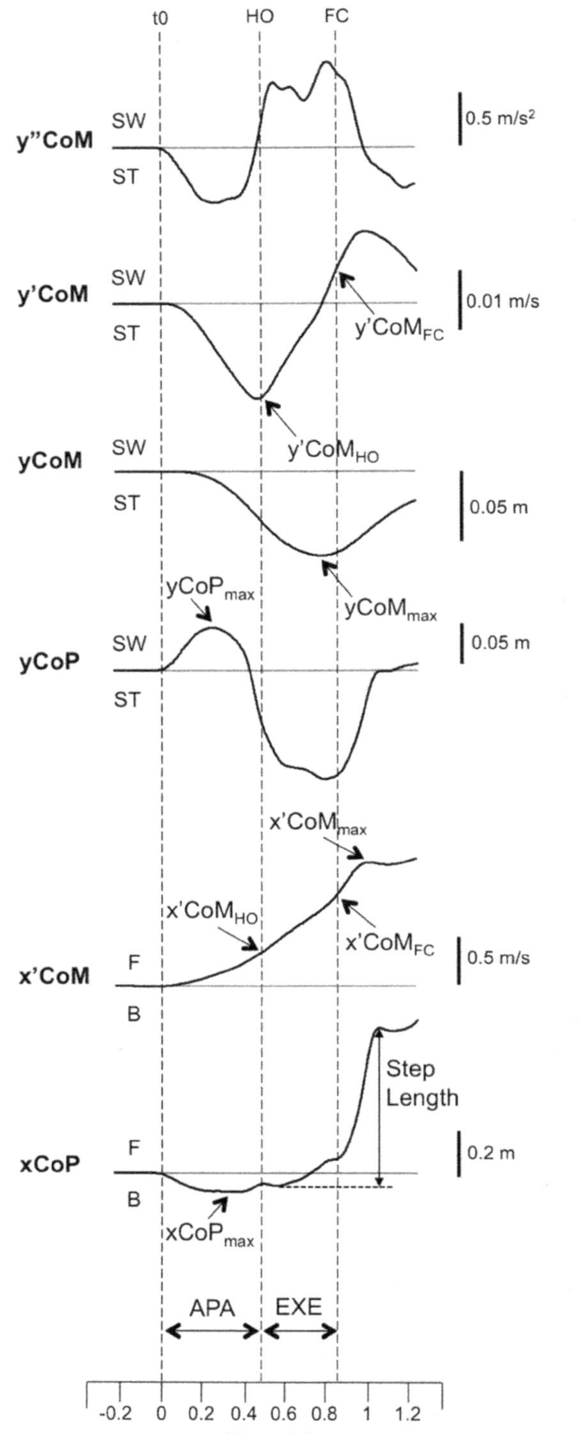

FIGURE 2 | Example of the main biomechanical traces obtained for one subject during gait initiation gait (one trial) under the Symmetrical condition. y"CoM, y'CoM, yCOM, yCoP: mediolateral center-of-mass (CoM) acceleration, velocity and displacement, mediolateral center-of-pressure (CoP) displacement, respectively. x'COM, xCoP: anteroposterior CoM velocity and *(Continued)*

FIGURE 2 | Continued
anteroposterior CoP displacement, respectively. T0 indicates the onset variation of the y"CoM trace from the baseline. HO and FC: swing heel-off and swing foot-contact, respectively. F and B indicate forward and backward movement, respectively. ST and SW indicate stance limb and swing limb, respectively. $x'CoM_{HO}$, $x'CoM_{FC}$, $x'CoM_{max}$, $xCoP_{max}$: anteroposterior CoM velocity at heel-off, at foot-contact, at the end of the first step and maximal backwards CoP shift, respectively. $y'CoM_{HO}$, $y'CoM_{FC}$, $yCoM_{max}$, $yCoP_{max}$: mediolateral CoM velocities at heel-off, at foot-contact, maximal mediolateral CoM displacement towards the stance leg and maximal mediolateral CoP displacement towards the swing leg during anticipatory postural adjustments (APA). APA and EXE: time windows for APA and step execution.

where $yCoM_{FC}$ and $y'CoM_{FC}$ are respectively the mediolateral CoM position and velocity at foot-contact, and ω_0 is the eigenfrequency of the body modeled as an inverted pendulum, calculated as:

$$\omega_0 = \sqrt{\frac{g}{l}},$$

where $g = 9.81$ m/s^2 is the gravitational acceleration and l is the length of the inverted pendulum, which in this study corresponded to 57.5% of the body height (Winter, 1990).

Mediolateral dynamic stability at foot-contact is ensured on condition that $YcoM_{HC}$ is within BoS_{ymax}, which corresponds to a positive MoS. A negative MoS indicates mediolateral instability and implies that a corrective action (e.g., in the form of an additional lateral step) has to be undertaken to maintain balance.

Statistical Analysis

Mean and standard deviation values for each dependent variable were calculated over the eight trials performed in each experimental condition. Repeated measures ANOVA with the load distribution condition (Stance, Symmetrical and Swing) as within-subject factors were conducted on each of these variables in turn. For each ANOVA, partial eta-squared value (η_p^2) was presented as a measure of effect size. When a significant statistical difference was found, *post hoc* comparisons were performed using pairwise comparisons with a Holm-Bonferroni correction (Holm, 1979). The level of significance was set at $\alpha = 0.05$.

RESULTS

Description of the Biomechanical Traces

Gait initiation movement globally followed a similar pattern under the various load distribution conditions. This pattern is illustrated in **Figure 2**. The heel-off of the swing leg was systematically preceded by postural dynamics that corresponded to APA. During APA, CoP shifted backwards and laterally towards the swing leg. In the mediolateral direction, CoP displacement reached a peak value towards the swing leg, while CoM displacement and velocity were directed towards the stance leg. The mediolateral CoM velocity trace reached the first peak value towards the stance-leg side at around heel-off. This trace then dropped towards the swing-leg side. The second peak value towards this side was reached a few milliseconds after foot-contact. The CoM displacement reached a peak value towards the stance-leg side during the execution phase. The CoM then fell towards the swing-leg side. In the anteroposterior direction, the CoM velocity increased progressively until it reached a peak value a few milliseconds after foot-contact.

Initial Posture

Load distribution significantly affected the initial CoM location in the mediolateral direction $F_{(1,14)} = 73.34$, $P < 0.001$, $\eta_p^2 = 0.84$), but not along the anteroposterior direction ($P > 0.05$, $\eta_p^2 = 0.02$). *Post hoc* analysis revealed that the initial mediolateral CoM location differed significantly between the three experimental conditions ($P < 0.001$). In the Symmetrical condition, the initial mediolateral CoM location was 0.1 ± 0.7 cm on the swing-leg side with respect to the midline between both feet. This initial mediolateral CoM position (with respect to the midline between both feet) was significantly closer to the swing leg in the Swing condition (0.8 ± 0.7 cm at the swing-leg side), and significantly closer to the stance leg in the Stance condition (0.8 ± 0.8 cm at the stance-leg side) compared with the Symmetrical condition.

Anticipatory Postural Adjustments

No effect of the load distribution was found on APA duration ($P > 0.05$, $\eta_p^2 = 0.17$, **Figure 3**). Similarly, statistical analysis indicated that the load distribution did not affect the maximal backward CoP shift ($P > 0.05$, $\eta_p^2 = 0.02$, **Figure 4**) and the anteroposterior CoM velocity at heel-off ($P > 0.05$, $\eta_p^2 = 0.05$, **Figure 4**), indicating that the anticipatory postural dynamics in the anteroposterior direction were not modified by changes in body weight distribution. In contrast, with regard to the mediolateral postural dynamics, a significant effect of the load distribution was found for the peak of the mediolateral CoP shift during APA ($F_{(1,14)} = 13.46$, $P < 0.001$, $\eta_p^2 = 0.49$) and the mediolateral CoM velocity at heel-off ($F_{(1,14)} = 20.42$, $P < 0.001$, $\eta_p^2 = 0.59$). *Post hoc* analysis indicated that these parameters differed significantly between all of the conditions (**Figure 3**). More specifically, when compared with the Symmetrical condition, these parameters were significantly higher in the Swing condition, and lower in the Stance condition.

Mediolateral Stability

A significant effect of the load distribution was found for the maximal mediolateral CoM displacement towards the stance leg during step execution ($F_{(1,14)} = 22.53$, $P < 0.001$, $\eta_p^2 = 0.62$). Compared with the Symmetrical condition, this parameter was significantly higher in the Swing condition, and significantly lower in the Stance condition (**Figure 5**). Despite these variations, both the mediolateral CoP position ($P > 0.05$, $\eta_p^2 = 0.10$) and the mediolateral gap between the CoP and CoM at the time of maximal mediolateral CoM displacement were unchanged in all of the conditions ($P > 0.05$, $\eta_p^2 = 0.13$, **Figure 5**). A significant effect of the load distribution was also found for the mediolateral CoM velocity at foot-contact ($F_{(1,14)} = 4.65$, $P < 0.05$, $\eta_p^2 = 0.25$). Specifically, the mediolateral CoM velocity was significantly higher in the Stance condition

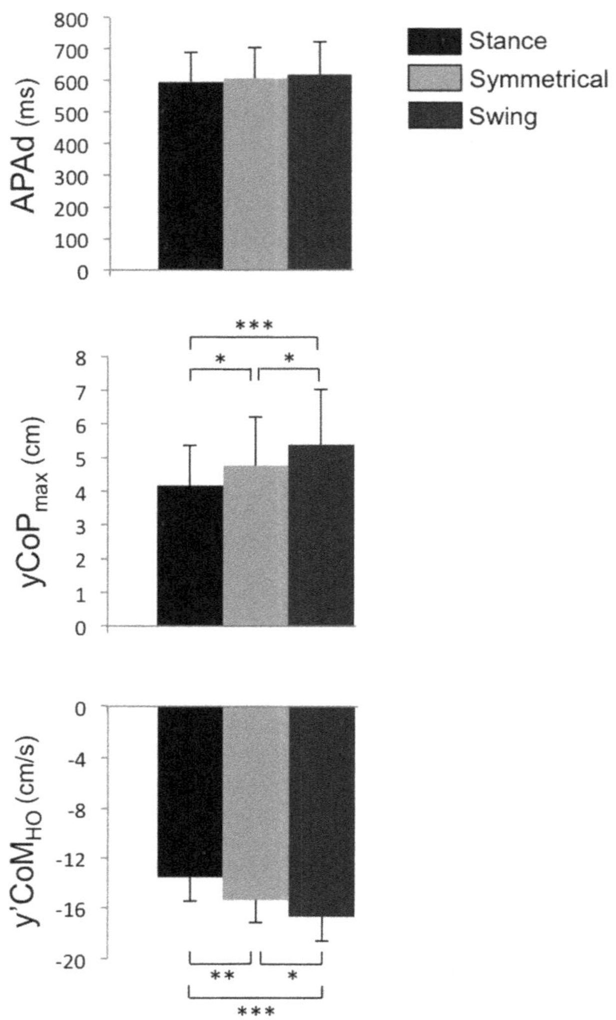

FIGURE 3 | Mean of temporo-spatial features of APA under the Stance, Symmetrical and Swing conditions. APAd: APA duration; yCoP$_{max}$: peak of mediolateral CoP shift towards the swing leg during APA. y'CoM$_{HO}$: mediolateral CoM velocity at heel-off. Negative values indicate a displacement or velocity directed towards the stance leg. *,**,***Significant difference with $P < 0.05$, $P < 0.01$ and $P < 0.001$, respectively.

than in the Swing condition (**Figure 5**), whilst the *post hoc* analysis revealed no other difference. Finally, there was no effect of load distribution on the mediolateral CoM position at foot-contact ($P > 0.05$, $\eta_p^2 = 0.06$, **Figure 5**), the mediolateral position of the extrapolated CoM at foot-contact ($P > 0.05$, $\eta_p^2 = 0.07$, **Figure 5**), the margin of stability ($P > 0.05$, $\eta_p^2 = 0.14$, **Figure 5**), and step width ($P > 0.05$, $\eta_p^2 = 0.03$, **Figure 5**).

Motor Performance

Our results showed that the load distribution had no effect on the parameters related to forward progression (**Figure 4**): the anteroposterior CoM velocity at foot-contact ($P > 0.05$, $\eta_p^2 = 0.17$), the peak of the anteroposterior CoM velocity at the end of the first step ($P > 0.05$, $\eta_p^2 = 0.08$), the duration of step execution ($P > 0.05$, $\eta_p^2 = 0.15$), and the step length ($P > 0.05$, $\eta_p^2 = 0.13$).

DISCUSSION

The aim of this study was to investigate the effects of changing the initial body weight distribution between both legs on the control of mediolateral dynamic stability during gait initiation. Changes in body weight distribution were experimentally induced by modifying the distribution along the frontal plane of an external load located at the participants' waists.

External Load Induced Changes in Body Weight Distribution between Both Legs

The changes in body weight distribution induced by the external load were attested by the significant differences observed in the initial mediolateral CoM location between the various experimental conditions. In the Symmetrical condition, the CoM was almost located at the midline between both feet (0.1 cm from the swing leg), reflecting a quasi-symmetrical body weight distribution between both legs. In the asymmetrical loading conditions (Stance and Swing conditions), we observed that the initial CoM location was significantly shifted towards the overloaded leg side, which is in accordance with previous studies on quiet standing (Wu and MacLeod, 2001; Haddad et al., 2011). This indicates an increase in the body weight distribution over the overloaded leg side. To be precise, the CoM was displaced by ~0.8 cm on the overloaded side (stance or swing leg) compared with the Symmetrical condition. This finding is in accordance with the deviations observed in the study by Wu and MacLeod (2001) for an asymmetrical load of 10% of body weight (≈1 cm in this previous study). The initial anteroposterior CoM location, in contrast, was not affected by changes in the external load distribution. This suggests that, in the present study, the distribution of body weight along the sagittal plane did not change between the various experimental conditions.

Effects of the Changes in Body Weight Distribution on Mediolateral Dynamic Stability Control

In accordance with our hypothesis, our results showed that the mediolateral dynamic stability at swing foot-contact, quantified by the margin of stability, was unaffected by the changes in the initial body weight distribution. This finding suggests that the subjects developed adaptive postural strategies in order to reach an equivalent mediolateral stability when the initial body weight distribution was modified. It has been shown that mediolateral stability during gait initiation is mainly regulated by the mediolateral APA and the mediolateral swing foot-placement, i.e., the step width (McIlroy and Maki, 1999; Caderby et al., 2014; Yiou et al., 2016a). In the present study, the step width was not

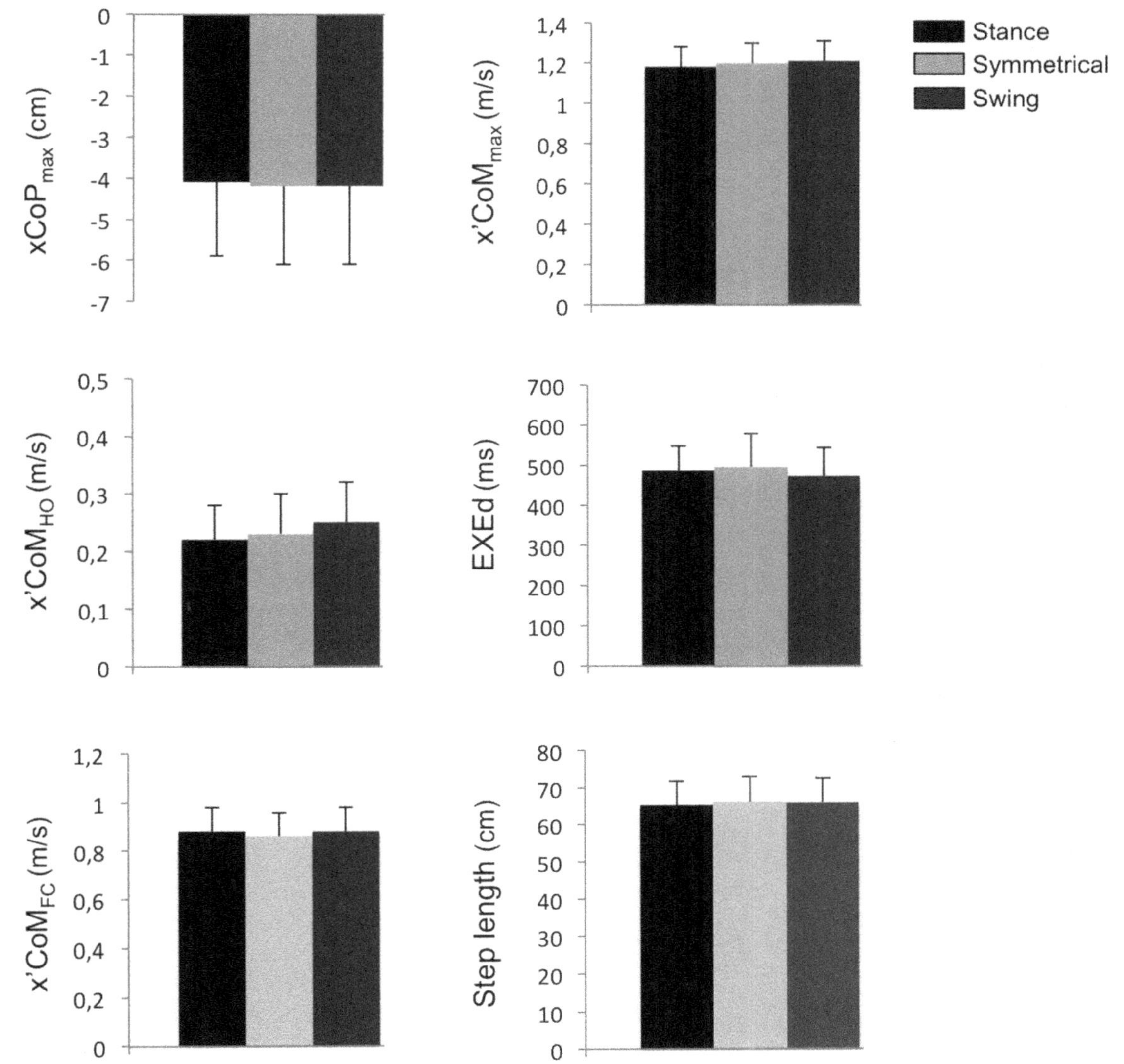

FIGURE 4 | Mean of parameters related to the forward progression under the Stance, Symmetrical and Swing conditions. $xCoP_{max}$: maximal backward shift of the CoP during APA. $x'CoM_{HO}$: anteroposterior velocity of the CoM at heel-off. $x'CoM_{FC}$: anteroposterior CoM velocity at foot-contact. $x'CoM_{max}$: peak of the anteroposterior CoM velocity at the end of the first step. EXEd: duration of step execution. Negative values indicate a displacement or velocity directed backwards.

modified between the various experimental conditions. This implies that other forms of postural adaptations occurred in order to maintain an invariant mediolateral dynamic stability when the body weight distribution between the legs was modified.

It is well known that mediolateral APA, often considered as a lateral thrust exerted on the ground (Mouchnino and Blouin, 2013), serve to propel the CoM towards the stance foot prior to swing foot-off. Although the CoM is never repositioned over the stance foot, mediolateral APA help to minimize the extent to which the body subsequently falls towards the swing-leg side during step execution, i.e., mediolateral instability (Jian et al., 1993; Winter, 1995; Lyon and Day, 1997; McIlroy and Maki, 1999; Rogers et al., 2001; Yiou et al., 2016a). In the present study, the results showed that APA duration, i.e., the time allocated to propel the CoM toward the stance foot, did not differ between the various conditions. In contrast, the amplitude of mediolateral APA, characterized by the peak of mediolateral CoP shift towards the swing leg during APA, varied as a function of the body weight distribution over both legs. Specifically, when compared with the Symmetrical condition, mediolateral APA amplitude increased when body weight was further distributed onto the swing leg (in the Swing condition), and

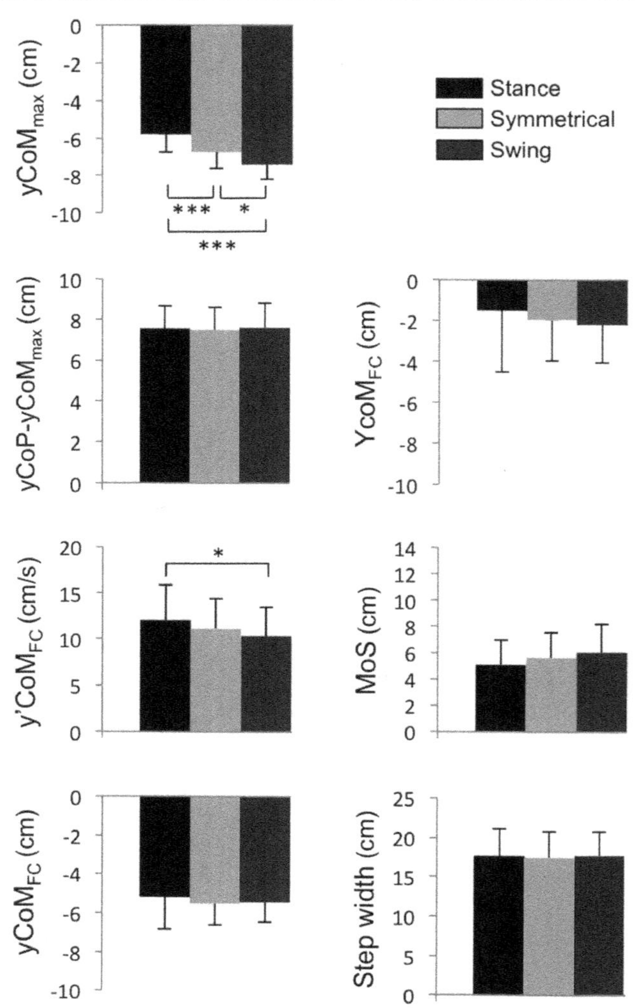

FIGURE 5 | Mean of parameters related to the mediolateral stability under the Stance, Symmetrical and Swing conditions. yCoM$_{max}$: maximal CoM displacement towards the stance leg. yCoP-yCoM$_{max}$: mediolateral distance between CoP and CoM at the instant when the CoM reaches its maximal displacement towards the stance leg. y'CoM$_{FC}$: mediolateral CoM velocity at foot-contact. yCoM$_{FC}$: mediolateral CoM position at the time of foot-contact. YcoM$_{FC}$: mediolateral extrapolated CoM position at the time of foot-contact. Margin of stability (MoS). Negative values indicate a displacement or velocity directed towards the stance leg. *,***Significant difference with $P < 0.05$ and $P < 0.001$, respectively.

decreased when body weight was further distributed onto the stance leg (Stance condition). It has been shown that this anticipatory CoP shift towards the swing leg generates the propulsive forces responsible for accelerating the CoM in the opposite direction, i.e., towards the stance leg (Brenière et al., 1987; Jian et al., 1993; Winter, 1995). Consequently, these modulations in the mediolateral amplitude of APA influenced the propulsion of the CoM towards the stance foot, as attested by the differences in mediolateral CoM velocity at heel-off and the peak of mediolateral CoM displacement towards the stance foot during step execution. To be precise, compared with the Symmetrical condition, both the displacement and velocity of the CoM directed towards the stance leg increased in the Swing condition, and decreased in the Stance condition. Similar findings were observed in previous studies that investigated the effect of body weight distribution between both legs on the gait initiation process (Patchay and Gahéry, 2003; Azuma et al., 2007). However, none of these existing studies established the link between these postural adaptations and mediolateral dynamic stability during gait initiation.

Our results suggest that mediolateral APA changes in the present study aimed to compensate for the differences in the initial CoM location during the upright posture. By modulating the mediolateral APA amplitude, the subjects were able to adapt the propulsive forces so that the CoM reached a similar position relative to the stance foot during the step execution phase. Indeed, we observed that the gap between the CoP and CoM at the time of the maximal mediolateral CoM displacement towards the stance foot during step execution did not vary. This indicates that the CoM was propelled at a similar distance from the stance foot during step execution. As a consequence, the extent that the body fell laterally towards the swing leg, reflected by the mediolateral CoM position at the time of foot-contact, did not change between the various conditions. Thus, we were able to achieve an equivalent extrapolated CoM position at foot-contact in the various conditions, although the mediolateral CoM velocity at foot-contact was slightly higher in the Stance condition than in the Swing condition. In short, these adaptive changes in the mediolateral APA avoided the eventual modulation of the step width to maintain the extrapolated CoM inside the base-of-support. In addition, they helped to maintain the mediolateral stability invariant in the various conditions. These results are in line with findings from previous studies, which have shown that healthy subjects are able to modulate the features of APA in order to maintain an unchanged mediolateral stability when confronted with postural perturbation (Yiou et al., 2012a, 2016b; Caderby et al., 2014). Furthermore, these results reinforce the hypothesis that the extrapolated CoM could be a robust parameter for human balance control (Hasson et al., 2008; Yiou et al., 2012a; Caderby et al., 2014).

Our findings, which show that APA are scaled as a function of body weight distribution between the legs, are congruent with findings from the existing literature on gait initiation (Patchay and Gahéry, 2003; Azuma et al., 2007) for a task that combines stepping and pointing (Robert et al., 2007), and on a leg flexion task (Mille and Mouchnino, 1998). Recent data has provided evidence that cutaneous mechanoreceptors in the sole of the foot may be involved in the setting of APA associated with gait initiation (Mouchnino and Blouin, 2013). These receptors are sensitive to changes in pressure plantar distribution (Kavounoudias et al., 1998), which may be induced by modifications in the body weight distribution between both legs. Thus, it may be assumed that the adaptive APA changes observed in our study were associated with the integrity of these receptors in our healthy young subjects. Further investigations are required to determine whether the present results are applicable in populations that suffer from a decline in the sensitivity of these plantar receptors, such as elderly people (Wells et al., 2003; Perry, 2006). Specifically, future studies should investigate whether, like young healthy adults, the elderly are able to adapt the APA to changes in body weight distribution between the legs so as to maintain unchanged the mediolateral stability during gait initiation. Such studies may allow to identify abnormalities in the generation of APA under conditions requiring postural adaptation and may thus offer a better understanding of the causes of the frequent falls that occur among the elderly during gait initiation (Robinovitch et al., 2013).

Effects of the Changes in Body Weight Distribution on Motor Performance

Our results indicate that changes in body weight distribution between both legs did not influence the temporal (i.e., duration of APA and step execution) and spatial (i.e., amplitude of anteroposterior APA, step length and anteroposterior CoM velocities at the various selected events) variables related to forward progression. These results are in marked contrast with those from previous studies (Patchay and Gahéry, 2003; Azuma et al., 2007; Dalton et al., 2011), which noted changes in these variables as a function of body weight distribution between both legs. This discrepancy may be explained by the fact that, contrary to these previous studies, the participants of the present study were instructed to maintain a similar progression velocity under the various experimental conditions, as attested by the absence of change in the peak of anteroposterior CoM velocity at the end of the first step. Thus, in our study, it may be assumed that the subjects scaled the temporo-spatial features of gait initiation in such way that forward progression velocity remained equivalent across all conditions. These results support the hypothesis that young healthy adults are able to independently create the conditions for both forward progression and mediolateral stability during gait initiation (Caderby et al., 2014). Interestingly, a recent study has shown that modifications in the body weight distribution over the legs along the anteroposterior direction led to scaling of the amplitude of anteroposterior APA without consistent changes in the amplitude of mediolateral APA (Hansen et al., 2016). These findings suggest that changes in the body weight distribution along the anteroposterior direction might affect the biomechanical organization of gait initiation in that direction, but not in the mediolateral direction. Further investigation is however required to confirm this hypothesis.

Conclusion

The results of the present study highlight that young healthy adults are able to modulate mediolateral APA so as to maintain optimal conditions of dynamic stability during gait initiation with the modification of the initial body weight distribution between both legs. Bearing in mind the fact that elderly people's falls frequently occur during gait initiation, the present findings may provide a basis for future studies that aim to better understand the mechanisms of falls in this population.

AUTHOR CONTRIBUTIONS

TC, EY and GD designed the study. TC, GD and BB collected the data. TC, EY, NP, XV, BB and GD analyzed and interpreted the data, drafted the manuscript and gave final approval.

FUNDING

This work was supported by a grant from the University of La Reunion. The present study was funded by the French government.

ACKNOWLEDGMENTS

The authors thank Mr. Grath Erdki for his technical assistance.

REFERENCES

Azuma, T., Ito, T., and Yamashita, N. (2007). Effects of changing the initial horizontal location of the center of mass on the anticipatory postural adjustments and task performance associated with step initiation. *Gait Posture* 26, 526–531. doi: 10.1016/j.gaitpost.2006.11.203

Bouisset, S., and Maton, B. (1995). *Muscles, Posture et Mouvement: Bases et Applications de la Méthode Électromyographique.* Paris: Hermann.

Brenière, Y., Do, M. C., and Bouisset, S. (1987). Are dynamic phenomena prior to stepping essential to walking. *J. Mot. Behav.* 19, 62–76. doi: 10.1080/00222895.1987.10735400

Brunt, D., Liu, S.-M., Trimble, M., Bauer, J., and Short, M. (1999). Principles underlying the organization of movement initiation from quiet stance. *Gait Posture* 10, 121–128. doi: 10.1016/s0966-6362(99)00020-x

Caderby, T., Dalleau, G., Leroyer, P., Bonazzi, B., Chane-Teng, D., and Do, M. C. (2013a). Does an additional load modify the anticipatory postural adjustments in gait initiation? *Gait Posture* 37, 144–146. doi: 10.1016/j.gaitpost.2012.06.012

Caderby, T., Yiou, E., Peyrot, N., Bonazzi, B., and Dalleau, G. (2013b). Detection of swing heel-off event in gait initiation using force-plate data. *Gait Posture* 37, 463–466. doi: 10.1016/j.gaitpost.2012.08.011

Caderby, T., Yiou, E., Peyrot, N., Begon, M., and Dalleau, G. (2014). Influence of gait speed on the control of mediolateral dynamic stability during gait initiation. *J. Biomech.* 47, 417–423. doi: 10.1016/j.jbiomech.2013.11.011

Cau, N., Cimolin, V., Galli, M., Precilios, H., Tacchini, E., Santovito, C., et al. (2014). Center of pressure displacements during gait initiation in individuals with obesity. *J. Neuroeng. Rehabil.* 11:82. doi: 10.1186/1743-0003-11-82

Chen, B., Lee, Y. J., and Aruin, A. S. (2015). Anticipatory and compensatory postural adjustments in conditions of body asymmetry induced by holding an object. *Exp. Brain Res.* 233, 3087–3096. doi: 10.1007/s00221-015-4377-7

Crenna, P., and Frigo, C. (1991). A motor programme for the initiation of forward-oriented movements in humans. *J. Physiol.* 437, 635–653. doi: 10.1113/jphysiol.1991.sp018616

Dalton, E., Bishop, M., Tillman, M. D., and Hass, C. J. (2011). Simple change in initial standing position enhances the initiation of gait. *Med. Sci. Sports Exerc.* 43, 2352–2358. doi: 10.1249/MSS.0b013e318222bc82

Elble, R. J., Moody, C., Leffler, K., and Sinha, R. (1994). The initiation of normal walking. *Mov. Disord.* 9, 139–146. doi: 10.1002/mds.870090203

Gélat, T., Pellec, A. L., and Brenière, Y. (2006). Evidence for a common process in gait initiation and stepping on to a new level to reach gait velocity. *Exp. Brain Res.* 170, 336–344. doi: 10.1007/s00221-005-0214-8

Haddad, J. M., Rietdyk, S., Ryu, J. H., Seaman, J. M., Silver, T. A., Kalish, J. A., et al. (2011). Postural asymmetries in response to holding evenly and unevenly distributed loads during self-selected stance. *J. Mot. Behav.* 43, 345–355. doi: 10.1080/00222895.2011.596169

Hansen, C., LaRue, J., Do, M. C., and Latash, M. L. (2016). Postural preparation to stepping: coupled center of pressure shifts in the anterior-posterior and medio-lateral directions. *J. Hum. Kinet.* 54, 5–14. doi: 10.1515/hukin-2016-0030

Hasson, C. J., Van Emmerik, R. E., and Caldwell, G. E. (2008). Predicting dynamic postural instability using center of mass time-to-contact information. *J. Biomech.* 41, 2121–2129. doi: 10.1016/j.jbiomech.2008.04.031

Hill, K. M., and Vandervoort, A. A. (1996). "Posture and gait in healthy elderly individuals and survivors of stroke," in *Changes in Sensory Motor Behavior in Aging*, eds A. M. Ferrandez and N. Teasdale (New York, NY: Elsevier), 163–199.

Hof, A. L., Gazendam, M. G., and Sinke, W. E. (2005). The condition for dynamic stability. *J. Biomech.* 38, 1–8. doi: 10.1016/j.jbiomech.2004.03.025

Holm, S. (1979). A simple sequential rejective method procedure. *Scand. J. Stat.* 6, 65–70.

Jian, Y., Winter, D. A., Ishac, M. G., and Gilchrist, L. (1993). Trajectory of the body COG and COP during initiation and termination of gait. *Gait Posture* 1, 9–22. doi: 10.1016/0966-6362(93)90038-3

Kannus, P., Leiponen, P., Parkkari, J., Palvanen, M., and Järvinen, M. (2006). A sideways fall and hip fracture. *Bone* 39, 383–384. doi: 10.1016/j.bone.2006.01.148

Kavounoudias, A., Roll, R., and Roll, J. (1998). The plantar sole is a 'dynamometric map' for human balance control. *Neuroreport* 9, 3247–3252. doi: 10.1097/00001756-199810050-00021

Lepers, R., and Brenière, Y. (1995). The role of anticipatory postural adjustments and gravity in gait initiation. *Exp. Brain Res.* 107, 118–124. doi: 10.1007/bf00228023

Li, X., and Aruin, A. S. (2007). The effect of short-term changes in the body mass on anticipatory postural adjustments. *Exp. Brain Res.* 181, 333–346. doi: 10.1007/s00221-007-0931-2

Li, X., and Aruin, A. S. (2009). The effect of short-term changes in body mass distribution on feed-forward postural control. *J. Electromyogr. Kinesiol.* 19, 931–941. doi: 10.1016/j.jelekin.2008.05.003

Lyon, I. N., and Day, B. L. (1997). Control of frontal plane body motion in human stepping. *Exp. Brain Res.* 115, 345–356. doi: 10.1007/pl00005703

Marigold, D. S., and Eng, J. J. (2006). The relationship of asymmetric weight-bearing with postural sway and visual reliance in stroke. *Gait Posture* 23, 249–255. doi: 10.1016/j.gaitpost.2005.03.001

McIlroy, W. E., and Maki, B. E. (1997). Preferred placement of the feet during quiet stance: development of a standardized foot placement for balance testing. *Clin. Biomech. (Bristol Avon)* 12, 66–70. doi: 10.1016/s0268-0033(96)00040-x

McIlroy, W. E., and Maki, B. E. (1999). The control of lateral stability during rapid stepping reactions evoked by antero-posterior perturbation: does anticipatory control play a role? *Gait Posture* 9, 190–198. doi: 10.1016/s0966-6362(99)00013-2

Melzer, I., Kurz, I., Shahar, D., Levi, M., and Oddsson, L. (2007). Application of the voluntary step execution test to identify elderly fallers. *Age Ageing* 36, 532–537. doi: 10.1093/ageing/afm068

Michel, V., and Do, M. C. (2002). Are stance ankle plantar flexor muscles necessary to generate propulsive force during human gait initiation? *Neurosci. Lett.* 325, 139–143. doi: 10.1016/s0304-3940(02)00255-0

Mille, M.-L., and Mouchnino, L. (1998). Are human anticipatory postural adjustments affected by a modification of the initial position of the center of gravity? *Neurosci. Lett.* 242, 61–64. doi: 10.1016/s0304-3940(98)00047-0

Mille, M. L., Simoneau, M., and Rogers, M. W. (2014). Postural dependence of human locomotion during gait initiation. *J. Neurophysiol.* 112, 3095–3103. doi: 10.1152/jn.00436.2014

Mouchnino, L., and Blouin, J. (2013). When standing on a moving support, cutaneous inputs provide sufficient information to plan the anticipatory postural adjustments for gait initiation. *PLoS One* 8:e55081. doi: 10.1371/journal.pone.0055081

Nevitt, M. C., and Cummings, S. R. (1993). Type of fall and risk of hip and wrist fractures: the study of osteoporotic fractures. The study of osteoporotic fractures research group. *J. Am. Geriatr. Soc.* 41, 1226–1234. doi: 10.1111/j.1532-5415.1993.tb07307.x

Patchay, S., and Gahéry, Y. (2003). Effect of asymmetrical limb loading on early postural adjustments associated with gait initiation in young healthy adults. *Gait Posture* 18, 85–94. doi: 10.1016/s0966-6362(02)00167-4

Perry, S. D. (2006). Evaluation of age-related plantar-surface insensitivity and onset age of advanced insensitivity in older adults using vibratory and touch sensation tests. *Neurosci. Lett.* 392, 62–67. doi: 10.1016/j.neulet.2005.08.060

Robert, G., Blouin, J., Ruget, H., and Mouchnino, L. (2007). Coordination between postural and movement controls: effect of changes in body mass distribution on postural and focal component characteristics. *Exp. Brain Res.* 181, 159–171. doi: 10.1007/s00221-007-0916-1

Robinovitch, S. N., Feldman, F., Yang, Y., Schonnop, R., Leung, P. M., Sarraf, T., et al. (2013). Video capture of the circumstances of falls in elderly people residing in long-term care: an observational study. *Lancet* 381, 47–54. doi: 10.1016/S0140-6736(12)61263-X

Rogers, M. W., Hedman, L. D., Johnson, M. E., Cain, T. D., and Hanke, T. A. (2001). Lateral stability during forward-induced stepping for dynamic balance recovery in young and older adults. *J. Gerontol. A Biol. Sci. Med. Sci.* 56, M589–M594. doi: 10.1093/gerona/56.9.m589

Tessem, S., Hagstrøm, N., and Fallang, B. (2007). Weight distribution in standing and sitting positions and weight transfer during reaching tasks, in seated stroke subjects and healthy subjects. *Physiother. Res. Int.* 12, 82–94. doi: 10.1002/pri.362

Uemura, K., Yamada, M., Nagai, K., and Ichihashi, N. (2011). Older adults at high risk of falling need more time for anticipatory postural adjustment in the precrossing phase of obstacle negotiation. *J. Gerontol. A Biol. Sci. Med. Sci.* 66, 904–909. doi: 10.1093/gerona/glr081

Wells, C., Ward, L. M., Chua, R., and Inglis, J. T. (2003). Regional variation and changes with ageing in vibrotactile sensitivity in the human footsole. *J. Gerontol. A Biol. Sci. Med. Sci.* 58, 680–686. doi: 10.1093/gerona/58.8.b680

Winter, D. A. (1990). *Biomechanics and Motor Control of Human Movement.* New York, NY: Wiley.

Winter, D. A. (1995). *A.B.C (Anatomy, Biomechanics and Control) of Balance During Standing and Walking.* Waterloo: Waterloo biomechanics.

Wu, G., and MacLeod, M. (2001). The control of body orientation and center of mass location under asymmetrical loading. *Gait Posture* 13, 95–101. doi: 10.1016/s0966-6362(00)00102-8

Yiou, E., Artico, R., Teyssedre, C. A., Labaune, O., and Fourcade, P. (2016a). Anticipatory postural control of stability during gait initiation over obstacles of different height and distance made under reaction-time and self-initiated instructions. *Front. Hum. Neurosci.* 10:449. doi: 10.3389/fnhum.2016.00449

Yiou, E., Fourcade, P., Artico, R., and Caderby, T. (2016b). Influence of temporal pressure constraint on the biomechanical organization of gait initiation made with or without an obstacle to clear. *Exp. Brain Res.* 234, 1363–1375. doi: 10.1007/s00221-015-4319-4

Yiou, E., Caderby, T., and Hussein, T. (2012a). Adaptability of anticipatory postural adjustments associated with voluntary movement. *World J. Orthop.* 3, 75–86. doi: 10.5312/wjo.v3.i6.75

Yiou, E., Hussein, T., and Larue, J. (2012b). Influence of temporal pressure on anticipatory postural control of medio-lateral stability during rapid leg flexion. *Gait Posture* 35, 494–499. doi: 10.1016/j.gaitpost.2011.11.015

Yiou, E., and Do, M. C. (2011). Effects of medio-lateral postural perturbation induced by voluntary arm raising on the biomechanical organization of rapid step initiation. *Motor Control* 15, 507–524. doi: 10.1123/mcj.15.4.507

Zettel, J. L., McIlroy, W. E., and Maki, B. E. (2002a). Can stabilizing features of rapid triggered stepping reactions be modulated to meet environmental constraints? *Exp. Brain Res.* 145, 297–308. doi: 10.1007/s00221-002-1083-z

Zettel, J. L., McIlroy, W. E., and Maki, B. E. (2002b). Environmental constraints on foot trajectory reveal the capacity for modulation of anticipatory postural adjustments during rapid triggered stepping reactions. *Exp. Brain Res.* 146, 38–47. doi: 10.1007/s00221-002-1150-5

13

Anodal Transcranial Direct Current Stimulation does not Facilitate Dynamic Balance Task Learning in Healthy Old Adults

*Elisabeth Kaminski [1], Maike Hoff [1], Viola Rjosk [1], Christopher J. Steele [1,2], Christopher Gundlach [1,3], Bernhard Sehm [1], Arno Villringer [1,4] and Patrick Ragert [1,5]**

[1] Department of Neurology, Max Planck Institute for Human Cognitive and Brain Sciences, Leipzig, Germany, [2] Department of Psychiatry, Cerebral Imaging Centre, Douglas Mental Health Institute, McGill University, Montreal, QC, Canada, [3] Faculty of Psychology, Department of Experimental Psychology and Methods, University of Leipzig, Leipzig, Germany, [4] Mind and Brain Institute, Charité and Humboldt University, Berlin, Germany, [5] Faculty of Sport Science, Institute for General Kinesiology and Exercise Science, University of Leipzig, Leipzig, Germany

Correspondence:
Patrick Ragert
patrick.ragert@uni-leipzig.de

Older adults frequently experience a decrease in balance control that leads to increased numbers of falls, injuries and hospitalization. Therefore, evaluating older adults' ability to maintain balance and examining new approaches to counteract age-related decline in balance control is of great importance for fall prevention and healthy aging. Non-invasive brain stimulation techniques such as transcranial direct current stimulation (tDCS) have been shown to beneficially influence motor behavior and motor learning. In the present study, we investigated the influence of tDCS applied over the leg area of the primary motor cortex (M1) on balance task learning of healthy elderly in a dynamic balance task (DBT). In total, 30 older adults were enrolled in a cross-sectional, randomized design including two consecutive DBT training sessions. Only during the first DBT session, either 20 min of anodal tDCS (a-tDCS) or sham tDCS (s-tDCS) were applied and learning improvement was compared between the two groups. Our data showed that both groups successfully learned to perform the DBT on both training sessions. Interestingly, between-group analyses revealed no difference between the a-tDCS and the s-tDCS group regarding their level of task learning. These results indicate that the concurrent application of tDCS over M1 leg area did not elicit DBT learning enhancement in our study cohort. However, a regression analysis revealed that DBT performance can be predicted by the kinematic profile of the movement, a finding that may provide new insights for individualized approaches of treating balance and gait disorders.

Keywords: dynamic balance task, balance learning, healthy aging, non-invasive brain stimulation, kinematics, transcranial direct current stimulation

---

Abbreviations: a-tDCS, anodal transcranial direct current stimulation; DBT, dynamic balance task; M1, primary motor cortex; s-tDCS, sham transcranial direct current stimulation; tDCS, transcranial direct current stimulation; TD, Training Day; TiB, Time in Balance; ZC, number of zero crossings.

INTRODUCTION

Due to the demographic change, the older population is constantly increasing. Therefore, understanding the mechanisms of aging processes and examining strategies to decelerate age-related decline is of great importance. One significant problem of the aging process is impaired motor ability (Smith et al., 1999; Krampe, 2002) which is the result of a complex interaction of peripheral and central processes involving losses in muscle strength/power (Frontera et al., 1991; McNeil et al., 2007) and alterations in the central nervous system (CNS; Burke and Barnes, 2006). Age-related decline in muscle strength most severely affects the dorsiflexor and extensor muscles of the lower extremities (Frontera et al., 1991; McNeil et al., 2007), which is why older adults often show increased postural sway (Baloh et al., 1994; Liaw et al., 2009). On the other hand, older adults, compared with younger adults, show a reduced amount of structural and functional brain plasticity (Burke and Barnes, 2006) and also learning-dependent plasticity decreases with age (Sawaki et al., 2003). All these factors contribute to an age-related decrease of postural stability, which is an important risk factor for falls (Granacher et al., 2008; Panel on Prevention of Falls in Older Persons, American Geriatrics Society and British Geriatrics Society, 2011). According to the Clinical Practice Guidelines for Prevention of Falls in Older Persons from 2011, exercise in the form of strength, balance, gait, and coordination training was shown to be effective in reducing falls in older adults (Panel on Prevention of Falls in Older Persons, American Geriatrics Society and British Geriatrics Society, 2011). Besides reducing the number of falls (Gardner et al., 2000), balance training also had a positive effect on gait and reduced the fear of falling (Wolf et al., 1996; Liu-Ambrose et al., 2004) and therefore is considered an effective intervention for treating age-related mobility losses. One study revealed that balance training is also capable of inducing neuroplastic changes in elderly but also in patients suffering from Parkinson's disease (Sehm et al., 2014). Interestingly, these neuroplastic changes were correlated with the learning performance (Sehm et al., 2014) and therefore seem to be an important prerequisite for balance learning. Techniques of non-invasive brain stimulation have also been shown to induce neuroplastic changes and thereby also successfully facilitate task performance (Nitsche and Paulus, 2000; Madhavan and Shah, 2012). Transcranial direct current stimulation (tDCS) can facilitate motor performance by up-regulating neural activity in the underlying brain tissue (Nitsche and Paulus, 2000). Following on training studies attempting to enhance postural stability, recent studies have successfully targeted the leg area of the primary motor cortex (M1) by means of anodal tDCS (a-tDCS) to improve static balance (Dutta et al., 2014) and locomotion (Kaski et al., 2012) in young adults. A study in hemiplegic stroke patients showed that single-session tDCS can improve patients' balance ability and increases the isometric strength of the affected lower extremity (Sohn et al., 2013). Therefore, combining the assessment of older adults balance ability with concurrent use of lower limb tDCS seems reasonable to evaluate the effect of brain stimulation on balance learning. In our previous study, the effect of tDCS on balance learning ability was investigated in healthy young subjects using a dynamic balance task (DBT; Kaminski et al., 2016). Our results showed that tDCS over M1 leg area is capable of enhancing balance performance in the DBT as participants showed higher task performance and lower error rates during and after tDCS compared to a control group. To follow up on these findings, in the present study we wanted to examine the feasibility of using the DBT as a balance learning task in elderly participants. Our main objective was to evaluate the effect of a-tDCS on DBT learning in older adults. Additionally, we analyzed the kinematic profile of DBT learning performance in our aged cohort as kinematic variables have been shown to be sensitive markers of postural stability (Yu et al., 2008; Bisson et al., 2014). In specific, we aimed to identify whether kinematic variables velocity, acceleration, jerk and postural sway frequency can predict balance performance in healthy elderly. In our previous study, we found that kinematic variables can well predict DBT performance in younger adults (Kaminski et al., 2013). Additionally, our results showed that performance improvements were mediated by tDCS-induced changes in movement velocity. According to this previous study, we hypothesized that (A) a-tDCS over M1 leg area during DBT learning facilitates learning performance compared with a group receiving s-tDCS in an older age cohort. Additionally, we expected that (B) the kinematic profile assessed during DBT learning predicts the DBT performance level of elderly with a special impact of velocity on performance improvement.

MATERIALS AND METHODS

Participants

Thirty healthy elderly participants (17 females, mean age = 67.7 ± 6 years) were enrolled in this study. All participants gave written informed consent and the study procedures were approved by the local ethics committee of the University of Leipzig and conducted in accordance with the Declaration of Helsinki and only healthy participants were included. To exclude the presence of any neurological disease and/or contraindications, all participants underwent a detailed neurological examination prior to the testing phase. All participants were free of any medication affecting the CNS and were task naïve. All participants were right-handed as assessed by the Edinburgh Handedness Inventory (mean score 90.03; range 55–100; Oldfield, 1971) and did not show any signs of cognitive impairment, measured by the Mini Mental State Examination (MMSE, mean score: 29.23, range: 27–30; Folstein et al., 1975). Furthermore, we assessed participants standing balance ability before the experimental procedure using the Fullerton Advanced Balance (FAB) Scale (Rose et al., 2006), a multidimensional balance scale specifically designed to evaluate balance ability of functionally independent older adults. We also assessed participants' level of physical activity with the long version of the International Physical Activity Questionnaire (IPAQ; Craig et al., 2003).

Study Design

The study was comprised of two consecutive training sessions that were separated by 24 h. On the first training day (TD1), participants performed 15 trials of DBT training while 20 min of tDCS were applied over the leg motor cortex (M1 leg area). Participants were randomly assigned to either the experimental condition, where they received 20 min of a-tDCS, or the sham-control condition, where s-tDCS was applied. On the second training day (TD2), another 15 trials of DBT training were performed without tDCS. This was done to examine the effects of a-tDCS on consolidation of the newly acquired motor skill and to capture longer lasting a-tDCS effects on a consecutive training session. During each session, the platform position of each subject in each trial was continuously recorded using the Spike2 (Cambridge Electronic Design Ltd., Cambridge, UK) software.

Whole-Body Dynamic Balancing Task (DBT)

The DBT was performed on a stability platform (model 16030, LaFayette Instruments, Lafayette, IN, USA) with a maximal deviation of 26° to each side. A detailed description of the procedure is provided elsewhere (Taubert et al., 2010; Kaminski et al., 2013). In brief, subjects were instructed to stand on the movable platform and to keep it in a horizontal position as long as possible during a trial length of 30 s. On each training day, 15 trials were performed with between-trial rest intervals of 90 s to avoid muscle fatigue. Hence, each training session lasted approximately 29 min, including breaks. To prevent falls, participants were secured with a safety harness during training. The primary performance measure was the total time participants were able to keep the platform in a horizontal position within a range of ±3° to each side, henceforth referred as Time in Balance (TiB). After each trial, participants were provided with their TiB value as verbal feedback but besides that, no strategy on how to best perform the task was provided (discovery learning approach; Wulf et al., 2003; Orrell et al., 2006).

Transcranial Direct Current Stimulation (tDCS)

For tDCS, a weak direct current of 1 mA was delivered for 20 min using a battery driven stimulator (neuroConn GmbH, Ilmenau, Germany). On TD1, either a-tDCS or s-tDCS was applied to the bilateral M1 leg area during the first 10 trials of DBT performance. While the anode (5 cm × 5 cm) was placed over the M1 leg area target region, the cathode (reference electrode) was placed over the right frontal orbit (10 cm × 5 cm). The anatomical landmark for M1 leg area was chosen according to the 10–20 system and the anode was placed 1 cm behind the vertex on the mid-sagittal line (Madhavan and Stinear, 2010; Laczó et al., 2014). TDCS was applied using a highly conductive electrode paste (Ten20 CONDUCTIVE Neurodiagnostic Electrode Paste, Weaver and Company) and flexible elastic straps were used to fixate the electrodes on the head. Current was ramped up for 30 s in the beginning of tDCS eliciting a transient tingling sensation on the scalp that faded over seconds (Nitsche et al., 2003; Gandiga et al., 2006) and also ramped down for 30 s. During s-tDCS, the current was increased, maintained and decreased for 30 s each. Before and after tDCS, participants rated their level of attention (1 = not attentive, 10 = very attentive), fatigue (1 = very tired, 10 = not tired at all) and discomfort (1 = no discomfort, 10 = strong discomfort) on a visual analog scale (VAS).

Data Analysis

For detailed data analysis, we recorded the platform position of each subject in each trial. This was done by transforming voltage to an amplifier that translated the signal into a Spike waveform at 5000 Hz. Before parameters were calculated, data was preprocessed using custom-built scripts in MATLAB version 8.2 (see also Kaminski et al., 2016). Data preprocessing included low-pass-filtering at 5 Hz using a 2nd order low-pass Butterworth filter to remove hardware derived artifacts and data resampling to 500 Hz. TiB was then calculated by calculating the total time per trial, subjects spent within a range of ±3° to each side. Additionally, we aimed to decode the kinematic profile of DBT performance using additional variables. Therefore, we calculated the first, second and third derivatives of position representing velocity, acceleration, jerk/smoothness. In addition, the number of zero crossings (ZC) was calculated as the total number of times that signal passed from one side of the horizontal position (0°) to the other. Statistical analyses were performed using IBM SPSS version 22.

Demographics

An independent-samples *t*-test was performed on each demographic variable (age, MMSE-score, total score of physical activity in IPAQ, total score in FAB-scale) to exclude that potential group differences in demographic variables might have influenced task performance. Repeated-measures analysis of variance (RM-ANOVA) with factor GROUP (a-tDCS, s-tDCS) and TIME (pre-post training) were used to assess changes in VAS scores.

Performance Measure Time in Balance (TiB)

Performance data was tested for normality using the Shapiro-Wilk test. As the test showed that the data was not normally distributed, non-parametric tests were used to examine learning improvement.

Training day 1

The Mann-Whitney U Test (MWU) was performed to assess baseline (trial 1) differences between groups. Overall learning was evaluated by performing a Friedman Test on factor TRIAL. First training session improvements were divided in online (trial 1–10) and offline (trial 11–15) learning improvements to disentangle acute tDCS effects and immediate tDCS after effects. Absolute improvement was calculated by subtracting last trial performance from first trial performance (online: t10–t1, offline: t15–t11) and compared between groups using the MWU. Additionally, percentage performance improvement was calculated by subtracting participants first trial performance (t1) from performance of training trial 15 and normalizing the difference to t1 performance and multiplying the term by 100 to create percentage values (online: (t10−t1)/t1*100, offline: (t15−t11)/t11*100). Percentage improvements were compared between groups using the MWU.

Consolidation and training day 2

To investigate skill consolidation from TD1 to TD2, the retention score, calculated as the difference between t15 TD1 performance and t1 TD2 performance, was compared between the two groups using MWU. Overall learning was evaluated by performing a Friedman Test on factor TRIAL. Absolute and percentage performance improvement on TD2 was calculated analogous to TD1 and compared between groups using the MWU.

Predicting DBT Performance by Kinematic Variables

Multiple regression

A partial correlation was performed between each kinematic variable and performance variable TiB. Subsequently, all variables having significant relations with TiB were entered in a regression model. The regression analysis was performed to decode the contribution of specific kinematic variables on overall DBT performance and thereby unravel the predictive power of the kinematic profile for balance performance measures. All variables were log-transformed before entering them into the model, thereby we created residuals with a normal distribution. In the regression model, TiB was defined as the dependent variable and the kinematic variables velocity, acceleration, ZC and trial were predefined as predictor variables. All main variables were entered at the same time and a full-model fit was examined.

tDCS effects on kinematic variables

To evaluate the effect of tDCS on our kinematic data, we calculated the absolute and percentage change of each variable analogous to our absolute and percentage improvement calculation (absolute: t15–t1, percentage: (t15–t1)/t1*100) and compared these values between groups using MWU.

For all analyses, a p-value of < 0.05 was considered to be significant.

RESULTS

Demographics

There were no significant between-group differences in age (independent-samples t-test, $t_{(28)} = -0.82$, $p = 0.42$), MMSE-score (independent-samples t-test, $t_{(28)} = 0.63$, $p = 0.53$), total amount of physical activity (independent-samples t-test, $t_{(28)} = 0.85$, $p = 0.4$) or balance ability on the FAB-scale (independent-samples t-test, $t_{(28)} = 0.13$, $p = 0.9$); see also **Table 1** for mean values of all variables). All participants tolerated the stimulation well. None of the participants reported any side effects from tDCS stimulation but most experienced the tingling sensation on the skin during the ramp-up phase of tDCS. Groups did not differ in their level of attention (RM-ANOVA Time × Group interaction, TD1: $F_{(1,28)} = 2.87$, $p = 0.1$, TD2: $F_{(1,28)} = 1.26$, $p = 0.27$), fatigue (RM-ANOVA Time × Group interaction, TD1: $F_{(1,28)} = 0.19$, $p = 0.67$ TD2: $F_{(1,28)} = 0.05$, $p = 0.98$) or discomfort (RM-ANOVA Time × Group interaction, TD1: $F_{(1,28)} = 0$, $p = 1$, TD2: $F_{(1,28)} = 0.2$, $p = 0.89$) before and after each of the DBT training days (see also **Table 2** for mean values).

TABLE 1 | Group demographics.

Group	Age (years)	MMSE	IPAQ	FAB
a-tDCS, $n = 15$	66.8 ± 5.63	29.33 ± 0.72	6855.6 ± 5682	36.67 ± 2.72
s-tDCS, $n = 15$	68.6 ± 6.00	29.13 ± 0.99	5383.8 ± 3590	36.53 ± 3.02

MMSE: Mini Mental State Examination, total score range of 1–30; cut-off score for exclusion: ≤26. IPAQ: International Physical Activity Questionnaire, total score of physical activity in metabolic equivalent of task minutes per week (MET-minutes), cut-off for high level of physical activity per week: ≥3000. FAB: Fullerton Advanced Balance Scale, total score range of 1–40, cut-off score for higher risk of falls: ≤25. All values are depicted as mean ± standard deviation of the mean.

Performance Measure Time in Balance (TiB)

Training Day 1 (TD1)

There was no baseline difference in TiB between the two groups (MWU: $U = 101.5$, $p = 0.65$), indicating that all participants started at the same performance level. Both groups significantly improved their DBT performance over time (Friedman: $\chi^2_{(14)} = 51.81$, $p < 0.001$, **Figure 1A**). TiB under a-tDCS increased from 2.87 ± 1.09 s at baseline to 3.9 ± 1.74 s, while TiB under s-tDCS increased from 3.13 ± 1.22 s to 5.22 ± 2.77 s. We did not find significant differences between groups regarding their absolute performance improvement neither during tDCS stimulation (online effect, MWU: $U = 106$, $p = 0.78$) nor immediately after tDCS stimulation (offline effect, MWU: $U = 85$, $p = 0.25$). We also did not find significant group differences regarding percentage improvement gain neither during tDCS (MWU: $U = 105$, $p = 0.76$) nor after tDCS (MWU: $U = 103$, $p = 0.69$; see also **Figure 1B**).

TABLE 2 | Visual analog scale (VAS).

	TD1		TD2	
	Before	After	Before	After
a-tDCS				
Attention	9.47 ± 0.74	9.60 ± 0.74	9.27 ± 1.16	9.40 ± 1.18
Fatigue	9.40 ± 1.12	9.47 ± 0.92	9.60 ± 0.74	9.67 ± 0.72
Discomfort	1.20 ± 0.56	1.20 ± 0.56	1.13 ± 0.35	1.20 ± 0.50
s-tDCS				
Attention	9.53 ± 0.74	9.33 ± 1.18	9.47 ± 0.92	9.40 ± 1.12
Fatigue	9.27 ± 1.03	9.28 ± 0.98	9.27 ± 1.44	9.33 ± 1.40
Discomfort	1.13 ± 0.52	1.20 ± 0.53	1.27 ± 1.04	1.21 ± 0.99

Attention, fatigue and discomfort were assessed on a VAS before and after the dynamic balance task (DBT) was performed on TD1 and TD2. Attention scale, ranging from 1 (no attention) to 10 (highest attention level). Fatigue scale, from 1 (high fatigue level) to 10 (no fatigue). Discomfort scale, ranging from 1 (no discomfort) to 10 (highest level of discomfort). All values are expressed as mean ± standard deviation. Please note that there were no changes in attention, fatigue or discomfort within groups (Before vs. After) or between groups (a-tDCS, s-tDCS) on TD1 or TD2.

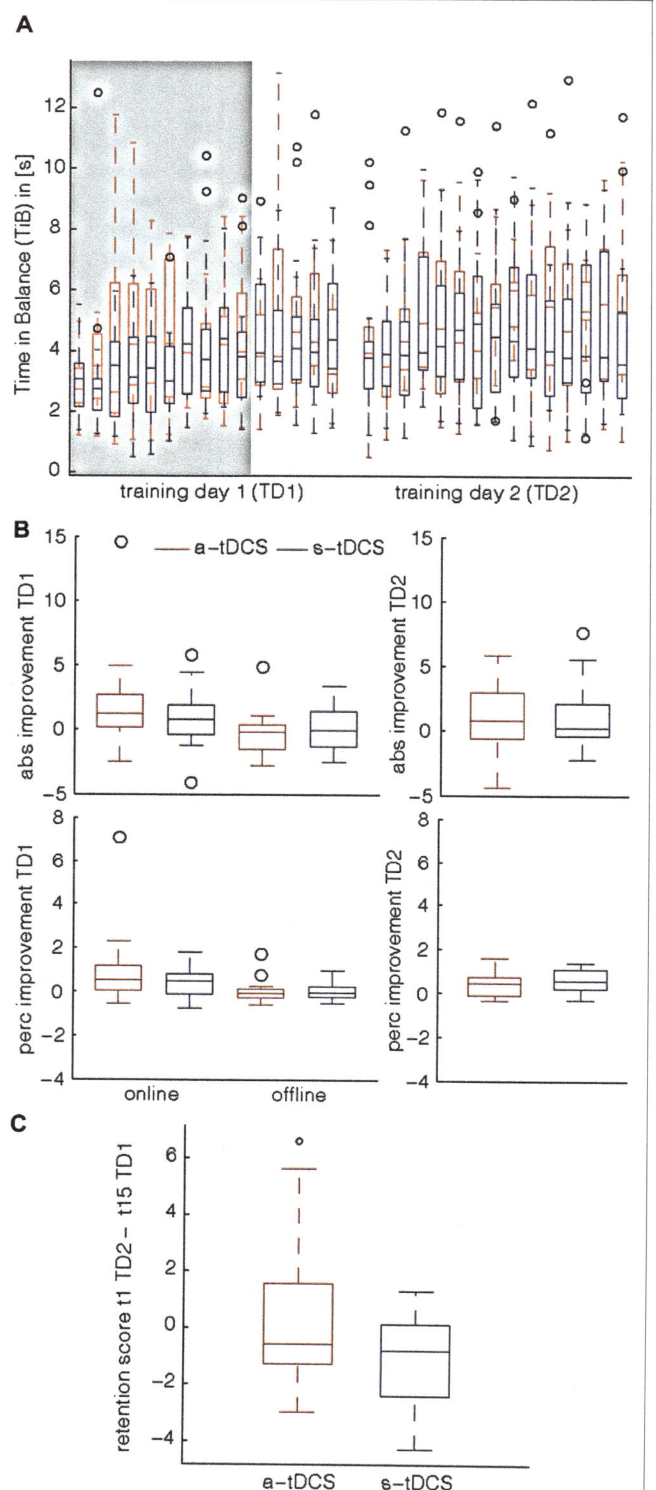

FIGURE 1 | Dynamic balance task (DBT) performance. Results are shown for Training Day 1 (TD1) and Training Day 2 (TD2), which were separated by 24 h. a-tDCS: anodal tDCS, s-tDCS: sham tDCS, abs improvement: absolute improvement, abs improvement TD1: online improvement: trial10–trial1, offline improvement: trial15–trial11, TD2: *(Continued)*

FIGURE 1 | Continued
trial15–trial1, perc improvement: percentage improvement, weighted difference of first and last trial performance multiplied by 100, perc improvement TD1: online improvement: ((t10–t1)/t1*100), offline improvement: ((t15–t11)/t11*100), TD2: ((t15–t1)/t1*100), retention score: difference between trial 15 TD1 and trial 1 TD2 performance (t15TD1–t1TD2). **(A)** Behavioral results for Time in Balance (TiB) performance on both training sessions. There was no baseline difference in TiB between the two groups (trial1, TD1) which indicates that all participants started at the same performance level. Both study groups significantly improved their level of performance over time on TD1 as well as on TD2. Gray shaded box indicates the time of a-tDCS/ s-tDCS stimulation. **(B)** Absolute/Percentage Improvement for TD1. No significant differences between a-tDCS and s-tDCS group were observed when comparing their absolute or percentage improvement gain. On TD1, neither online (t1–10) nor offline effects (t11–15) of tDCS showed a significant group difference. Therefore, one can conclude that the concurrent application of tDCS over M1 leg area did not elicit DBT performance enhancement in our study cohort **(C)** Retention score. There was no significant difference regarding the retention scores of the two groups, which indicates that tDCS did not affect skill retention from TD1 to TD2.

Consolidation and Training Day 2 (TD2)

When comparing the retention scores of the two groups, we found no significant difference (MWU: $U = 76$, $p = 0.13$), which indicates that a-tDCS did not affect skill retention from TD1 to TD2 (**Figure 1C**). Similar to TD1, DBT-learning in both groups improved over time (Friedman: $\chi^2_{(14)} = 34.68$, $p = 0.002$, **Figure 1A**). However, no significant difference regarding the absolute (MWU: $U = 110$, $p = 0.94$) or the percentage improvement gain (MWU: $U = 109$, $p = 0.9$) of the two groups was detected (**Figure 1B**). TiB increased from 4.24 ± 2.87 s to 5.33 ± 2.82 s under a-tDCS, while performance under s-tDCS increased from 3.5 ± 1.03 s to 5.05 ± 3.35 s.

Relationship between Kinematics and Performance

Multiple Regression

Figure 2A depicts the significant partial correlations between our dependent variable TiB and the kinematic variables velocity, acceleration and the number of ZC. As there was no significant correlation between TiB and jerk (see **Figure 2A**), we did not include jerk as a factor in the model. All other kinematic variables and variable trial were included as predictors in the model. The regression model revealed that each independent variable was significantly related to the dependent variable TiB (adjusted $R^2 = 0.72$, $F_{(4,443)} = 285.71$, $p < 0.001$). Larger ZC- and larger acceleration values were associated with greater TiB values (positive correlation), while lower velocity values were associated with higher TiB values (negative correlation). Additionally, TiB and trial showed the expected positive association, indicating that TiB increased with ascending trial numbers (see also **Figure 2B** for regression weights).

tDCS Effects on Kinematic Variables

We did not detect any group difference regarding absolute or percentage change from t1 to t15 in our kinematic variables velocity (abs: $U = 93$, $p = 0.42$, perc.: $U = 103$, $p = 0.69$), acceleration (abs: $U = 78$, $p = 0.15$, perc.: $U = 80$, $p = 0.18$) or the number of ZC (abs: $U = 100$, $p = 0.6$, perc.: $U = 105$,

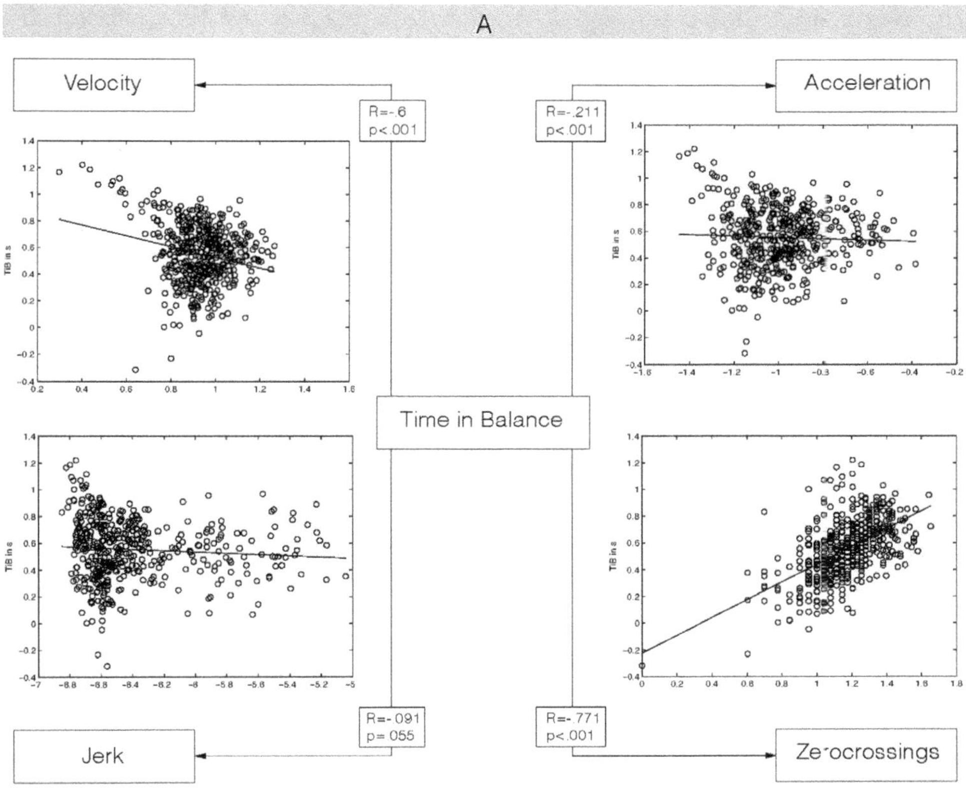

B

Predictor	B	β	t	p
velocity	-1.582	-.918	-15.75	<.001
acceleration	.306	.247	4.02	<.001
ZC	1.08	.891	28.08	<.001
trial	.007	.13	5.09	<.001

FIGURE 2 | Relationship between kinematic variables and balance performance. **(A)** Results of partial correlation analysis, controlling for the other three kinematic variables, respectively. This analysis revealed a specific relationship between time in balance performance and kinematic variables velocity, acceleration and the number of zero crossings (ZC), but not for jerk. Additionally, scatterplots of the relationships between kinematics and performance are added. **(B)** Results from multiple regression analysis, Time in Balance (TiB) as dependent variable, velocity, acceleration, number of ZC and trial as independent predictors. ZC: number of zero crossings, B: unstandardized regression coefficient, β: standardized regression coefficient, t = t test value (t-statistic), p = p-value of t-statistic. Our multiple regression analysis revealed a significant relationship between each of the included variables and our dependent variable TiB. The kinematic variable velocity was negatively correlated with performance, while acceleration and ZC showed a positive relation with TiB. Trial was also positively correlated with TiB.

$p = 0.76$). Interestingly, we found a significant group difference in jerk for absolute ($U = 46$, $p = 0.006$) as well as percentage change ($U = 52$, $p = 0.012$) from t1 to t15, even though the change in jerk was relatively small. While the a-tDCS group showed a small increase in jerk values from t1 to t15 (absolute change: 0.0002 m/s^3, percentage change: 18%), jerk in the s-tDCS group rather decreased from t1 to t15 (absolute change: −0.0035 m/s^3, percentage change: −28%). However, our partial correlation analysis did not reveal a significant association between jerk and TiB; therefore we assume that the group difference in jerk change did not affect our global learning measure TiB.

DISCUSSION

In the present study, our main objective was to examine whether a-tDCS over M1 leg area is capable of enhancing DBT learning in healthy elderly. We expected that, analogous to a younger cohort (Kaminski et al., 2016), targeting the M1 leg area region by means of tDCS would support DBT learning in the elderly and translate into superior learning performance compared to sham stimulation. However, even though both groups successfully increased their level of DBT performance over time, in the present study we found no difference between the a-tDCS and s-tDCS groups' amount of learning. Thus, our results indicate that the application of tDCS over M1 leg area during DBT performance did not elicit performance enhancement in our aged study cohort. But the results also indicate that older adults are able to perform the DBT (Sehm et al., 2014) and significantly improve their performance even within a single training session. Future studies can use this knowledge to directly compare DBT performance between different age cohorts to further investigate age-related deficits in balance learning ability and identify related neural correlates using combined neurophysiological assessments of brain activation with behavioral outcome measures. Furthermore, our results show that a large amount of variance in DBT learning performance can be predicted by kinematic variables, a result that can particularly be important when diagnosing and treating balance and gait disorders.

No Effects of tDCS on Complex Balance Learning in Elderly

Several studies have shown beneficial effects of tDCS over M1 leg area on postural control and locomotion. While Kaski et al. (2012) showed enhanced motor adaptation aftereffects in healthy young adults after using tDCS over M1 leg area, Sohn et al. (2013) were able to demonstrate that tDCS enhanced the overall stability index of hemiplegic stroke patients after only a single session (Sohn et al., 2013). In a previous study, we found that tDCS over M1 leg area does elicit performance improvements in DBT learning in a younger study cohort (Kaminski et al., 2016). However, using the same parameters of tDCS stimulation in our older study sample, we did not see behavioral improvements in DBT learning, a finding that might indicate age-related differences in the capacity for tDCS-induced behavioral changes. One potential explanation for this discrepancy is that the brain regions that are involved in initial DBT learning differ between younger and older adults. In a recent study, it was demonstrated that a single DBT training session results in cortical thickening of M1 leg area in healthy young adults (Taubert et al., 2016). This finding suggests a specific involvement of the leg area sub-region of M1 during initial DBT learning in a younger cohort. However, nothing is known so far about brain activation changes after a single DBT session in older adults. It might be that brain regions other than M1 leg area are more important during initial DBT learning in older age. Another issue that needs to be considered is the timing of the stimulation. It is known that neurophysiological effects of tDCS differ between older and younger adults with older adults showing delayed plasticity of M1 (Fujiyama et al., 2014). Therefore, future studies should consider applying tDCS in older adults before a motor task is performed. What is also known is that older adults exhibit more elaborate brain activation than younger controls when performing a motor task, potentially to compensate for an age-related decline of neuronal efficacy (Heuninckx et al., 2008). Therefore, one could argue that stimulating a single brain region by means of tDCS may not have been sufficient to activate the whole large-scale network responsible for successful performance of this complex task in older adults. This would also be in line with previous studies demonstrating that older individuals show different responses to non-invasive brain stimulation protocols as compared with younger adults (Müller-Dahlhaus et al., 2008; Ridding and Ziemann, 2010). It is also known, that the effects of tDCS on motor outcomes are highly variable (Horvath et al., 2016) and tDCS effects also vary across sessions and individuals (Chew et al., 2015). Additionally, large differences in brain structure as well as in brain function exist in older adults (Stewart et al., 2014), which may also affect task performance and responsiveness to tDCS protocols. Therefore, it may be that the inter-individual variability in older adults is greater than that of younger adults, and may impair our ability to detect differences between groups.

Taken together, we are not able to determine which factor or combination of factors, if any, may have contributed to a facilitatory effect of tDCS on DBT performance in older adults. As argued above, the outcome of tDCS is affected by multiple factors involving task characteristics and individual determinants (Ridding and Ziemann, 2010) and little is known about neuronal correlates of DBT performance in older adults. Therefore, more research is needed to draw a comprehensive picture on dynamic balance ability in the elderly and how non-invasive brain stimulation techniques may interact with such complex coordinative behavior.

Relationship between Kinematic Variables and Balance Control

Previous studies suggest an association between changes in postural control and changes in parameters of movement kinematics. Our regression results are in line with previous findings, showing that the kinematic parameters velocity (Jeka et al., 2004), acceleration (Jeka et al., 2004; Yu et al., 2008) and information on postural sway (Manor et al., 2010) provide important information for maintaining postural control. While velocity showed a strong negative relationship with performance, acceleration and performance were weakly positively correlated. Both velocity and acceleration seem to be sensitive markers of postural stability (Yu et al., 2008), however, we also found that the number of ZC, reflecting postural sway speed, were strongly positively correlated with performance. It has already been shown that greater velocity is associated with higher center of pressure deviation and, thereby, lower postural control (Paillard, 2012). Postural sway velocity, especially in the medial–lateral direction, has high predictive value for individual fall risk (Bigelow and Berme, 2011). As slowing down walking speed can also be an effective strategy to reduce the risk of falls (Roos and Dingwell, 2013), our finding that lower velocity values are associated with higher DBT performance is in good agreement with the literature. Given that DBT learning is associated with higher-frequency movement adjustments, the positive relationship between the postural sway speed and performance is an indicator of greater movement automaticity

(Wulf and Lewthwaite, 2009) and therefore also a marker for learning. Taken together, our data suggest that DBT learning performance can be predicted by the kinematic profile of the movement. This result could be of functional relevance for diagnostics of balance related disorders or individualizing gait retraining or fall prevention treatments.

In a second analysis, we aimed to evaluate the effect of tDCS on our kinematic data. Interestingly, we found a significant effect of tDCS on absolute and percentage change in jerk on training day 1, suggesting that a-tDCS resulted in a small increase of jerk values, while during s-tDCS, jerk was decreased. Higher jerk values reflect "jerkier" movements with more deviation in motion, while lower jerk values represent movements with higher smoothness. However, as we found no correlation between jerk and TiB, we assumed that the effect on jerk did not affect our global learning parameter TiB. While some studies suggested that a decrease in jerk is associated with better performance (e.g., James, 2014), another study rather stated a positive relation of higher jerk values and performance increase (Slaboda, unpublished data). As there are not many studies investigating jerk effects during highly complex, multi-joint movements, the effects of different jerk patterns remain ambiguous and have to be further explored.

Balance and Aging

Older adults show reduced postural stability as declines in muscular strength most severely affect the lower extremities (Frontera et al., 1991; McNeil et al., 2007). However, postural instability also represents an insufficiency of attentional resources since maintaining posture requires the integration of many different modalities of information including vision, proprioception and vestibular feedback (Granacher et al., 2008). In daily life, posture is held during changing environmental conditions, thus making it necessary for the balance system to interact with an external dynamical system (Chagdes et al., 2013). It has been shown that interventions that focus on improving balance in the elderly are most effective when they incorporate more complex exercises (Halvarsson et al., 2015) and also involve cognitive components. The DBT provides a nice setting to evaluate balance ability in older adults as it forces the user to dynamically adjust posture to continuous changes in the environment, thus demanding high attentional resources as well as flexible adaptations. The unstable platform of the balance board nicely mimics continuous changes in the environment and thereby creates an ideal setting for evaluating and training complex postural behavior (Chagdes et al., 2013). Our results show that older adults are able to improve their balance ability during a single session of DBT training and maintain this motor skill at least until a second day of training. Therefore, using the DBT in a longer-term setting may support and improve classical fall prevention trainings and provide an interesting setup for training on instable platforms. However, even though we observed significant learning improvements, DBT learning curves of both groups were characterized by irregular increases and decreases of performance. The underlying mechanism remains unclear, however, one potential explanation might be the difficulty of the motor task. Since we wanted to maintain conditions from our younger study sample (Kaminski et al., 2016), older adults were tested with a TiB range of only 3° while in our previous study, 5° of TiB range were tested (Sehm et al., 2014), thus making it easier for older adults to meet the criterion for successful performance. Therefore, the task may have been more difficult and irregularities in performance may represent difficulties in maintaining better performance over the time course of the training session. On the other hand, decreases in TiB performance may be the result of muscle or cognitive fatigue since the DBT is both physically and attentionally demanding. This, however, seems rather unlikely, since changes in levels of attention but also both muscle and cognitive fatigue were assessed using a VAS and no significant changes were detected.

Study Limitations

In the present study, we used behavioral measurements to assess motor learning in an aging population. However, since no neuroimaging measurements were included, it was not possible to investigate whether specific brain structures or specific brain states may have predicted DBT performance. Additionally, we cannot relate the variance in response to tDCS to a specific brain network. To get a better understanding of the neuronal correlates of DBT learning in older adults and potential tDCS effects on neuronal networks, further studies that combine neurophysiological assessments of brain activation with behavioral outcome measures are needed. Furthermore, our aged study cohort was selected according to relatively strict inclusion criteria and can therefore be considered healthy and active. In the long term, one goal would be to incorporate tDCS-usage as an add-on interventional strategy to treat balance and gait disorders; therefore older adults facing an increased risk of falls should be in the center of interest. Even though we did not detect any tDCS-induced effect on DBT performance in healthy older adults, it is possible that tDCS affects dynamic balance in patients. Additionally, we did not investigate the role of multiple tDCS-sessions on balance performance and did not test for any long-term effects. It is worth considering that multiple tDCS application sessions may have induced stronger behavioral effects that could be more persistent, as suggested by previous studies (Reis et al., 2009; Dell'Osso et al., 2011; Galletly et al., 2012). However, this study was the first step in understanding the role of single-session tDCS during the initial learning phase of a dynamic balancing task in older adults. While we provide initial evidence that tDCS over M1 leg area does not facilitate initial DBT learning in healthy older adults, future studies should be conducted investigating different time scales of DBT learning including also patient populations to draw a comprehensive picture of the effects of tDCS on dynamic balance performance.

CONCLUSION

Combining measures of balance evaluation with methods of non-invasive brain stimulation in older adults is important to advance the knowledge on how to enhance treatment success in terms of fall prevention and gait training. Our results indicate that even though older adults are able to learn a dynamic balancing task over the time course of a single training session, concurrent application of tDCS over M1 leg area did not elicit DBT performance enhancement in our study cohort. More knowledge on neuronal processing of DBT learning in older adults, the influence of tDCS parameters, and the effect of inter-individual differences is required in order to draw a comprehensive picture of whether tDCS can help to enhance older adults dynamic balance learning. However, we also found that balance performance can be predicted by the kinematic movement profile, a result that could be of functional relevance to individualize gait retraining or fall prevention treatments for patients suffering from balance impairments.

AUTHOR CONTRIBUTIONS

EK: study design, study planning, execution, analysis, manuscript writing. MH: study execution, ideas for analysis, suggestions for manuscript writing. VR: study execution, suggestions for manuscript writing. CJS: data analysis, help with figure creation, suggestions for manuscript writing. CG: data analysis. BS: data analysis, suggestions for manuscript writing. AV: suggestions for manuscript writing, study design, interpretation of results. PR: corresponding author, study idea, hypotheses, study design, data analysis, manuscript writing.

ACKNOWLEDGMENTS

We thank the Fazit-Stiftung for funding research conducted by EK.

REFERENCES

Baloh, R. W., Fife, T. D., Zwerling, L., Socotch, T., Jacobson, K., Bell, T., et al. (1994). Comparison of static and dynamic posturography in young and older normal people. *J. Am. Geriatr. Soc.* 42, 405–412. doi: 10.1111/j.1532-5415.1994.tb07489.x

Bigelow, K. E., and Berme, N. (2011). Development of a protocol for improving the clinical utility of posturography as a fall-risk screening tool. *J. Gerontol. A Biol. Sci. Med. Sci.* 66, 228–233. doi: 10.1093/gerona/glq202

Bisson, E. J., Lajoie, Y., and Bilodeau, M. (2014). The influence of age and surface compliance on changes in postural control and attention due to ankle neuromuscular fatigue. *Exp. Brain Res.* 232, 837–845. doi: 10.1007/s00221-013-3795-7

Burke, S. N., and Barnes, C. A. (2006). Neural plasticity in the ageing brain. *Nat. Rev. Neurosci.* 7, 30–40. doi: 10.1038/nrn1809

Chagdes, J. R., Rietdyk, S., Jeffrey, M. H., Howard, N. Z., and Raman, A. (2013). Dynamic stability of a human standing on a balance board. *J. Biomech.* 46, 2593–2602. doi: 10.1016/j.jbiomech.2013.08.012

Chew, T., Ho, K. A., and Loo, C. K. (2015). Inter- and intra-individual variability in response to transcranial direct current stimulation (tDCS) at varying current intensities. *Brain Stimul.* 8, 1130–1137. doi: 10.1016/j.brs.2015.07.031

Craig, C. L., Marshall, A. L., Sjöström, M., Bauman, A. E., Booth, M. L., Ainsworth, B. E., et al. (2003). International physical activity questionnaire: 12-country reliability and validity. *Med. Sci. Sports Exerc.* 35, 1381–1395. doi: 10.1249/01.MSS.0000078924.61453.FB

Dell'Osso, B., Camuri, G., Castellano, F., Vecchi, V., Benedetti, M., Bortolussi, S., et al. (2011). Meta-review of metanalytic studies with repetitive transcranial magnetic stimulation (rTMS) for the treatment of major depression. *Clin. Pract. Epidemiol. Ment. Health* 7, 167–177. doi: 10.2174/17450179011070 10167

Dutta, A., Chugh, S., Banerjee, A., and Dutta, A. (2014). Point-of-care-testing of standing posture with Wii balance board and Microsoft Kinect during transcranial direct current stimulation: a feasibility study. *NeuroRehabilitation* 34, 789–798. doi: 10.3233/NRE-141077

Folstein, M. F., Folstein, S. E., and McHugh, P. R. (1975). "Mini-mental state". A practical method for grading the cognitive state of patients for the clinician. *J. Psychiatr. Res.* 12, 189–198. doi: 10.1016/0022-3956(75) 90026-6

Frontera, W. R., Hughes, V. A., Lutz, K. J., and Evans, W. J. (1991). A cross-sectional study of muscle strength and mass in 45- to 78-yr-old men and women. *J. Appl. Physiol. (1985)* 71, 644–650.

Fujiyama, H., Hyde, J., Hinder, M. R., Kim, S. J., McCormack, G. H., Vickers, J. C., et al. (2014). Delayed plastic responses to anodal tDCS in older adults. *Front. Aging Neurosci.* 6:115. doi: 10.3389/fnagi.2014.00115

Galletly, C., Gill, S., Clarke, P., Burton, C., and Fitzgerald, P. B. (2012). A randomized trial comparing repetitive transcranial magnetic stimulation given 3 days/week and 5 days/week for the treatment of major depression: Is efficacy related to the duration of treatment or the number of treatments? *Psychol. Med.* 42, 981–988. doi: 10.1017/S0033291711001760

Gandiga, P. C., Hummel, F. C., and Cohen, L. G. (2006). Transcranial DC stimulation (tDCS): a tool for double-blind sham-controlled clinical studies in brain stimulation. *Clin. Neurophysiol.* 117, 845–850. doi: 10.1016/j.clinph.2005.12.003

Gardner, M. M., Robertson, M. C., and Campbell, A. J. (2000). Exercise in preventing falls and fall related injuries in older people: a review of randomised controlled trials. *Br. J. Sports Med.* 34, 7–17. doi: 10.1136/bjsm.34.1.7

Granacher, U., Zahner, L., and Gollhofer, A. (2008). Strength, power and postural control in seniors: considerations for functional adaptations and for fall prevention. *Eur. J. Sport Sci.* 8, 325–340. doi: 10.1080/17461390802478066

Halvarsson, A., Oddsson, L., Franzén, E., and Ståhle, A. (2015). Long-term effects of a progressive and specific balance-training programme with multi-task exercises for older adults with osteoporosis: a randomized controlled study. *Clin. Rehabil.* doi: 10.1177/0269215515605553 [Epub ahead of print].

Heuninckx, S., Wenderoth, N., and Swinnen, S. P. (2008). Systems neuroplasticity in the aging brain: recruiting additional neural resources for successful motor performance in elderly persons. *J. Neurosci.* 28, 91–99. doi: 10.1523/JNEUROSCI.3300-07.2008

Horvath, J. C., Vogrin, S. J., Carter, O., Cook, M. J., and Forte, J. D. (2016). Effects of a common transcranial direct current stimulation (tDCS) protocol on motor evoked potentials found to be highly variable within individuals over 9 testing sessions. *Exp. Brain Res.* 234, 2629–2642. doi: 10.1007/s00221-016-4667-8

James, E. G. (2014). Short-term differential training decreases postural sway. *Gait Posture* 39, 172–176. doi: 10.1016/j.gaitpost.2013.06.020

Jeka, J., Kiemel, T., Creath, R., Horak, F., and Peterka, R. (2004). Controlling human upright posture: velocity information is more accurate than position or acceleration. *J. Neurophysiol.* 92, 2368–2379. doi: 10.1152/jn.00983.2003

Kaminski, E., Hoff, M., Sehm, B., Taubert, M., Conde, V., Steele, C. J., et al. (2013). Effect of transcranial direct current stimulation (tDCS) during complex whole body motor skill learning. *Neurosci. Lett.* 552, 76–80. doi: 10.1016/j.neulet.2013.07.034

Kaminski, E., Steele, C. J., Hoff, M., Gundlach, C., Rjosk, V., Sehm, B., et al. (2016). Transcranial direct current stimulation (tDCS) over primary motor cortex leg area promotes dynamic balance task performance. *Clin. Neurophysiol.* 127, 2455–2462. doi: 10.1016/j.clinph.2016.03.018

Kaski, D., Quadir, S., Patel, M., Yousif, N., and Bronstein, A. M. (2012). Enhanced locomotor adaptation aftereffect in the "broken escalator" phenomenon using anodal tDCS. *J. Neurophysiol.* 107, 2493–2505. doi: 10.1152/jn.00223.2011

Krampe, R. T. (2002). Aging, expertise and fine motor movement. *Neurosci. Biobehav. Rev.* 26, 769–776. doi: 10.1016/s0149-7634(02)00064-7

Laczó, B., Antal, A., Rothkegel, H., and Paulus, W. (2014). Increasing human leg motor cortex excitability by transcranial high frequency random noise stimulation. *Restor. Neurol. Neurosci.* 32, 403–410. doi: 10.3233/RNN-130367

Liaw, M. Y., Chen, C. L., Pei, Y. C., Leong, C. P., and Lau, Y. C. (2009). Comparison of the static and dynamic balance performance in young, middle-aged and elderly healthy people. *Chang Gung Med. J.* 32, 297–304.

Liu-Ambrose, T., Khan, K. M., Eng, J. J., Lord, S. R., and McKay, H. A. (2004). Balance confidence improves with resistance or agility training. Increase is not correlated with objective changes in fall risk and physical abilities. *Gerontology* 50, 373–382. doi: 10.1159/000080175

Madhavan, S., and Shah, B. (2012). Enhancing motor skill learning with transcranial direct current stimulation–a concise review with applications to stroke. *Front. Psychiatry* 3:66. doi: 10.3389/fpsyt.2012.00066

Madhavan, S., and Stinear, J. W. (2010). Focal and bi-directional modulation of lower limb motor cortex using anodal transcranial direct current stimulation. *Brain Stimul.* 3, 42–50. doi: 10.1016/j.brs.2009.06.005

Manor, B., Costa, M. D., Hu, K., Newton, E., Starobinets, O., Kang, H. G., et al. (2010). Physiological complexity and system adaptability: evidence from postural control dynamics of older adults. *J. Appl. Physiol. (1985)* 109, 1786–1791. doi: 10.1152/japplphysiol.00390.2010

McNeil, C. J., Vandervoort, A. A., and Rice, C. L. (2007). Peripheral impairments cause a progressive age-related loss of strength and velocity-dependent power in the dorsiflexors. *J. Appl. Physiol. (1985)* 102, 1962–1968. doi: 10.1152/japplphysiol.01166.2006

Müller-Dahlhaus, J. F., Orekhov, Y., Liu, Y., and Ziemann, U. (2008). Interindividual variability and age-dependency of motor cortical plasticity induced by paired associative stimulation. *Exp. Brain Res.* 187, 467–475. doi: 10.1007/s00221-008-1319-7

Nitsche, M. A., Liebetanz, D., Lang, N., Antal, A., Tergau, F., and Paulus, W. (2003). Safety criteria for transcranial direct current stimulation (tDCS) in humans. *Clin. Neurophysiol.* 114, 2220–2222; author reply 2222–2223. doi: 10.1016/s1388-2457(03)00235-9

Nitsche, M. A., and Paulus, W. (2000). Excitability changes induced in the human motor cortex by weak transcranial direct current stimulation. *J. Physiol.* 527, 633–639. doi: 10.1111/j.1469-7793.2000.t01-1-00633.x

Oldfield, R. C. (1971). The assessment and analysis of handedness: the Edinburgh inventory. *Neuropsychologia* 9, 97–113. doi: 10.1016/0028-3932(71)90067-4

Orrell, A. J., Eves, F. F., and Masters, R. S. (2006). Implicit motor learning of a balancing task. *Gait Posture* 23, 9–16. doi: 10.1016/j.gaitpost.2004.11.010

Paillard, T. (2012). Effects of general and local fatigue on postural control: a review. *Neurosci. Biobehav. Rev.* 36, 162–176. doi: 10.1016/j.neubiorev.2011.05.009

Panel on Prevention of Falls in Older Persons, American Geriatrics Society and British Geriatrics Society. (2011). Summary of the updated American Geriatrics Society/British Geriatrics Society clinical practice guideline for prevention of falls in older persons. *J. Am. Geriatr. Soc.* 59, 148–157. doi: 10.1111/j.1532-5415.2010.03234.x

Reis, J., Schambra, H. M., Cohen, L. G., Buch, E. R., Fritsch, B., Zarahn, E., et al. (2009). Noninvasive cortical stimulation enhances motor skill acquisition over multiple days through an effect on consolidation. *Proc. Natl. Acad. Sci. U S A* 106, 1590–1595. doi: 10.1073/pnas.0805413106

Ridding, M. C., and Ziemann, U. (2010). Determinants of the induction of cortical plasticity by non-invasive brain stimulation in healthy subjects. *J. Physiol.* 588, 2291–2304. doi: 10.1113/jphysiol.2010.190314

Roos, P. E., and Dingwell, J. B. (2013). Influence of neuromuscular noise and walking speed on fall risk and dynamic stability in a 3D dynamic walking model. *J. Biomech.* 46, 1722–1728. doi: 10.1016/j.jbiomech.2013.03.032

Rose, D. J., Lucchese, N., and Wiersma, L. D. (2006). Development of a multidimensional balance scale for use with functionally independent older adults. *Arch. Phys. Med. Rehabil.* 87, 1478–1485. doi: 10.1016/j.apmr.2006.07.263

Sawaki, L., Yaseen, Z., Kopylev, L., and Cohen, L. G. (2003). Age-dependent changes in the ability to encode a novel elementary motor memory. *Ann. Neurol.* 53, 521–524. doi: 10.1002/ana.10529

Sehm, B., Taubert, M., Conde, V., Weise, D., Classen, J., Dukart, J., et al. (2014). Structural brain plasticity in Parkinson's disease induced by balance training. *Neurobiol. Aging* 35, 232–239. doi: 10.1016/j.neurobiolaging.2013.06.021

Smith, C. D., Umberger, G. H., Manning, E. L., Slevin, J. T., Wekstein, D. R., Schmitt, F. A., et al. (1999). Critical decline in fine motor hand movements in human aging. *Neurology* 53, 1458–1461. doi: 10.1212/wnl.53.7.1458

Sohn, M. K., Jee, S. J., and Kim, Y. W. (2013). Effect of transcranial direct current stimulation on postural stability and lower extremity strength in hemiplegic stroke patients. *Ann. Rehabil. Med.* 37, 759–765. doi: 10.5535/arm.2013.37.6.759

Stewart, J. C., Tran, X., and Cramer, S. C. (2014). Age-related variability in performance of a motor action selection task is related to differences in brain function and structure among older adults. *Neuroimage* 86, 326–334. doi: 10.1016/j.neuroimage.2013.10.016

Taubert, M., Draganski, B., Anwander, A., Müller, K., Horstmann, A., Villringer, A., et al. (2010). Dynamic properties of human brain structure: learning-related changes in cortical areas and associated fiber connections. *J. Neurosci.* 30, 11670–11677. doi: 10.1523/JNEUROSCI.2567-10.2010

Taubert, M., Mehnert, J., Pleger, B., and Villringer, A. (2016). Rapid and specific gray matter changes in M1 induced by balance training. *Neuroimage* 133, 399–407. doi: 10.1016/j.neuroimage.2016.03.017

Wolf, S. L., Barnhart, H. X., Kutner, N. G., McNeely, E., Coogler, C., and Xu, T. (1996). Reducing frailty and falls in older persons: an investigation of Tai Chi and computerized balance training. Atlanta FICSIT group. Frailty and injuries: cooperative studies of intervention techniques. *J. Am. Geriatr. Soc.* 44, 489–497. doi: 10.1111/j.1532-5415.1996.tb01432.x

Wulf, G., and Lewthwaite, R. (2009). Conceptions of ability affect motor learning. *J. Mot. Behav.* 41, 461–467. doi: 10.3200/35-08-083

Wulf, G., Weigelt, M., Poulter, D., and McNevin, N. (2003). Attentional focus on suprapostural tasks affects balance learning. *Q. J. Exp. Psychol. A* 56, 1191–1211. doi: 10.1080/02724980343000062

Yu, E., Abe, M., Masani, K., Kawashima, N., Eto, F., Haga, N., et al. (2008). Evaluation of postural control in quiet standing using center of mass acceleration: comparison among the young, the elderly and people with stroke. *Arch. Phys. Med. Rehabil.* 89, 1133–1139. doi: 10.1016/j.apmr.2007.10.047

14

Influence of Cervical Spine Mobility on the Focal and Postural Components of the Sit-to-Stand Task

Alain Hamaoui[1,2] and Caroline Alamini-Rodrigues[1]*

[1] Laboratoire de Physiologie de la Posture et du Mouvement, Institut National Universitaire Champollion, Albi, France,
[2] Laboratoire Mouvement, Equilibre, Performance, Santé (EA 4445), Université de Pau et des Pays de l'Adour, Tarbes, France

***Correspondence:**
Alain Hamaoui
alain.hamaoui@univ-jfc.fr

The aim of this study was to determine the influence of cervical spine mobility on the focal and postural components of the sit-to-stand transition, which represent the preparatory and execution phases of the task, respectively. Sixteen asymptomatic female participants (22 ± 3 years, 163 ± 0,06 cm, 57,5 ± 5 kg), free of any neurological or musculoskeletal disorders, performed six trials of the sit-to-stand task at maximum speed, in four experimental conditions varying the mobility of the cervical spine by means of three different splints. A six-channel force plate, which collected the reaction forces and moments applied at its top surface, was used to calculate the center of pressure displacements along the anterior-posterior and medial-lateral axes. The local accelerations of the head, spine, and pelvis, were assessed by three pairs of accelerometers, oriented along the vertical and anterior-posterior axes. Restriction of cervical spine mobility resulted in an increased duration of the focal movement, associated with longer and larger postural adjustments. These results suggest that restricted cervical spine mobility impairs the posturo-kinetic capacity during the sit-to-stand task, leading to a lower motor performance and a reorganization of the anticipatory postural adjustments. In a clinical context, it might be assumed that preserving the articular free play of the cervical spine might be useful to favor STS performance and autonomy.

Keywords: sit-to-stand, postural adjustments, focal movement, posturo-kinetic capacity, cervical spine, mobility

INTRODUCTION

The transition from sitting to standing, commonly named "sit-to-stand (STS)" is a very common daily task. In a study performed on eight wives of physicians and one man, McLeod et al. (1975) found that the STS task is performed four times an hour from 7 am to 10 pm. These results were refined by Dall and Kerr (2010) with an extended study on 140 participants, reporting an average of 60 STS movements per day and 3 per hour.

The STS task implies a rapid transition from a stable seated posture that offers a large contact area between the body and the supporting surfaces, to a less stable standing posture associated with a shorter base of sustentation, a higher location center of gravity and an extended articulated chain to stabilize. The standing posture is frequently a starting point for gait initiation, which involves a complex biomechanical process (Brenière and Do, 1991) preceding the rhythmic pattern of gait. Therefore, the ability to perform the STS movement is instrumental to autonomy, and many studies have been designed to unveil the kinematics and kinetics underlying this self-perturbing task (Burdett et al., 1985; Nuzik et al., 1986; Kralj et al., 1990; Schenkman et al., 1990; Riley et al., 1991; Coghlin and McFadyen, 1994; Roebroeck et al., 1994).

Most authors have divided the STS into two (Nuzik et al., 1986; Rodrigues-de-Paula Goulart and Valls-Solé, 1999), three (Schenkman et al., 1990; Coghlin and McFadyen, 1994; Roebroeck et al., 1994), or four (Kralj et al., 1990) different phases based on kinematics and kinetics data.

When considering the STS within the frame of the posturo-kinetic capacity concept (Bouisset and Zattara, 1983), a distinction should be made between a preparation phase, which corresponds to the anticipatory postural adjustments (APAs), and an execution phase during which the focal movement (FM) is performed. APAs allow for a better performance through a compensation of the disturbing forces associated with the FM (Bouisset and Zattara, 1981) or the generation of propulsive forces (Brenière and Do, 1991), and require postural chain mobility (Bouisset and Le Bozec, 1999). Lower articular free play of the lumbar pelvic area was associated with a reduction of the motor performance in several paradigms such as the pointing task (Lino and Bouisset, 1994), the pushing ramp effort (Le Bozec and Bouisset, 2004) or the STS task (Diakhaté et al., 2013).

However, there is a paucity of information regarding the role of the cervical spine, especially regarding the STS movement. In many kinematic studies of STS, total body movement is represented by a three-segment linkage (trunk-thigh-shank) pivoting about the foot (Shepherd and Gentile, 1994), and the influence of cervical spine mobility is taken into account only in a few experiments. In an earlier study, Jones and Hanson (1970) presented the trajectories of the head during the STS movement, traced from successive frames of motion picture. They constructed triangles from markers placed over the sternum, the seventh cervical vertebra and the head, exhibiting a cervical flexion during the first half of the trajectory. In a video-based kinematic analysis of the STS task, Nuzik et al. (1986) reported an average neck flexion of 8° during the first 35% of the movement cycle, followed by an extension phase. In an electromyographic study of the STS task, Rodrigues-de-Paula Goulart and Valls-Solé (1999) reported an activity of neck motor muscles (trapezius, sternocleidomastoideus) before and after the seat-off instant. Taken all together, these findings lead us to hypothesize that cervical mobility is involved in the preparatory

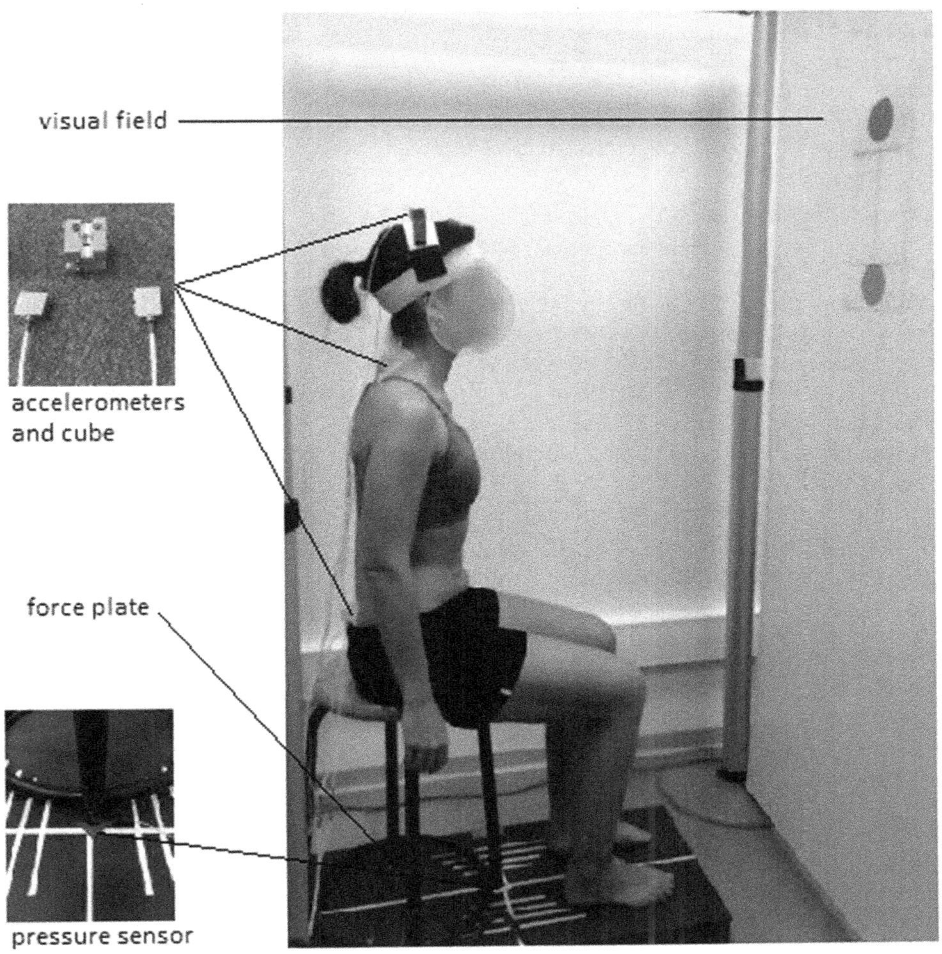

FIGURE 1 | Experimental set-up with force plate, accelerometers, pressure sensor, and visual field.

and in the execution phases of the STS movement, and that a loss of cervical mobility is likely to impair both of them. In a neurophysiological point of view, it must also be noted that the cervical spine controls the orientation of the head, which is a frame of reference for action since it contains the visual and the vestibular systems (Pozzo et al., 1990). The main goal of this study was to assess the effect of cervical mobility restriction on the APAs and on the FM for the STS task. To this aim, biomechanical parameters were analyzed in different conditions varying cervical spine range of motion by means of three different collars.

MATERIALS AND METHODS

Participants

Thirteen asymptomatic female participants (age: 23 ± 3 years; weight: 56 ± 9 kg; height: 163 ± 0,05 cm, BMI: 21 ± 3 kg/m^2), free of any neurological or musculoskeletal disease participated in this study. Only female participants were included in this study to avoid any variation of cervical spine mobility that might be related to gender differences

This study was carried out in accordance with the recommendations of the local "Ethics Committee for Movement Analysis." All subjects gave written informed consent in accordance with the Declaration of Helsinki.

Experimental Set-Up

Force Plate and Stool

A six-channel force plate (Bertec Corp., ref. 6012-15, Columbus, OH, USA), which collected the ground-reaction forces and moments applied at its top surface was used to calculate the coordinates of the center of pressure (CP) along the anterior-posterior axis (Xp), with the following formula: Xp = My/Rz (My is the moment around the medial-lateral axis and Rz is the vertical ground-reaction force).

A stool (height = 48 cm; depth = 39 cm) with four legs and a round wooden top (diameter = 30 cm) was screwed on to the force plate and used for the experiments (**Figure 1**).

To keep constant the friction forces between the stool top and the surface contact of the body, all participants wore the same kind of shorts.

Accelerometers

Three pairs of mono-axial accelerometers (FGP sensors, ref XA1010-B, ± 10g, Les Clayes Sous Bois, France), were used to assess the local accelerations of the pelvis, trunk, and head. Each pair was screwed on to a customized cube (length = 2 cm) with the two active axes located along the anterior-posterior and the vertical axes. The two first cubes were adhered to the skin with double-sided tape, at the level of the first sacral vertebra and first thoracic vertebra. The third cube was placed on top of the head using a system of Velcro bands (**Figure 1**).

Visual Field

The subject's visual field consisted of a frontal white board (72 cm apart from the stool), on which two black disks (diameter = 10 cm) joined by a vertical line were placed at the subject's eye level in the seated (lower disk) and standing (upper disk) postures (**Figure 1**). The participants were requested to focus their gaze on the lower disk at the beginning of the trial, and to follow the vertical line during the ascending phase of the STS, until they reach the upper disk. This visual field was designed to avoid unwanted cervical mobility due to a fixed visual target while the body was ascending. The experimentation room was lit with artificial lighting to obtain constant brightness.

Pressure Sensor

A pressure sensor was placed under the left front leg of the stool (**Figure 1**) to determine the "seat-off" instant.

Data Acquisition System

Data for all the recording devices were collected at 200 Hz with a 16-bit A/D converter board (model CompactDAQ with 9215

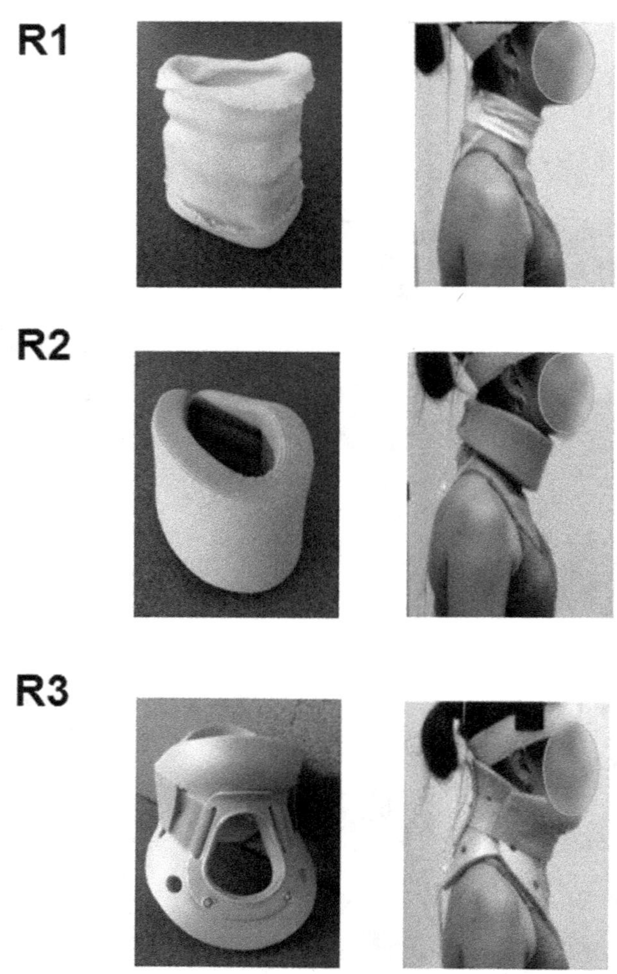

FIGURE 2 | Collars used to gradually restrict the mobility of the cervical spine: jersey tubular bandage (R1), foam cervical collar (R2), Philadelphia collar (R3).

modules, National Instruments, Austin, TX, USA), controlled by a custom code written with Labview software (National Instruments).

Cervical Collar

Three different cervical collars (**Figure 2**) were used to vary the mobility of the cervical spine passively, in accordance with the study of Hartman et al. (1975), who measured cervical spine range of motion in flexion-extension, side bending, and rotation while wearing five commonly used cervical orthoses:

- Jersey tubular bandage (Neuss, Germany): minor restriction of cervical mobility.
- Foam cervical collar (Cooper, Melun, France): medium restriction of cervical mobility.
- Philadelphia collar (Variteks, Istanbul, Turkey): major restriction of cervical mobility.

Procedure

The participants sat on the stool fixed on the platform with their upper limbs relaxed along their trunk, hips, and knees flexed to approximately 90°, barefoot and feet apart. Adhesive tape was put around the feet outline in order to keep the same positioning for every trial.

The subjects had to perform the "STS" task, which consisted in rising from the stool to reach the standing position as fast as possible, in response to a "Go" signal.

The STS was performed in four experimental conditions varying the mobility of the cervical area using the three above-mentioned collars: R0, no collar; R1, jersey tubular bandage; R2, foam cervical collar; R3, Philadelphia collar.

A training period was used to familiarize the subjects with the paradigm before recording.

Ten 3-s runs were performed in every condition, with a rest period of 30 s between runs and of 1 min between series.

The order of the experimental conditions was randomly assigned to avoid any order effect.

Data Analysis

Three parameters were calculated to characterize the APAs and the FM of the STS task along the anterior-posterior axis. These two distinct phases of the task were considered to be separated by the seat-off instant, for which the curve of the pressure sensor begins its fall toward zero (**Figure 3**).

- Duration of anticipatory postural adjustments (*dAPAs*): delay between the instant of seat-off and the first inflection of the CP curve.
- Amplitude of APAs (ΔXp): difference between the maximum and the minimum CP values during the APAs phase.

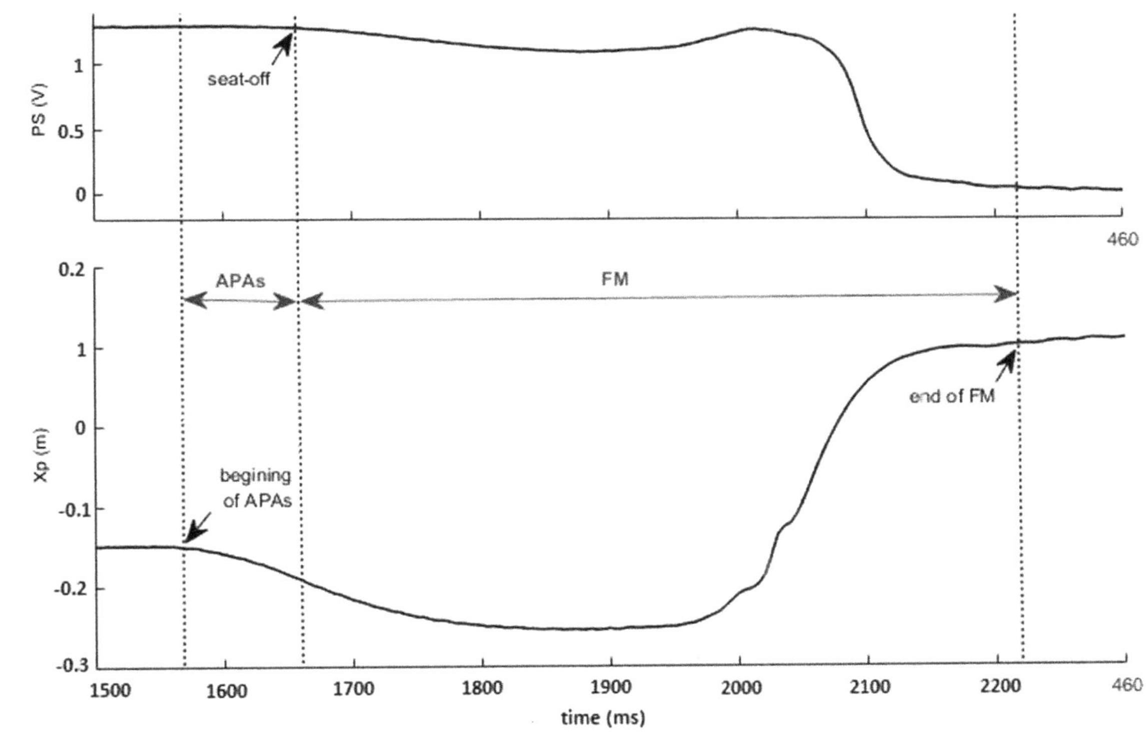

FIGURE 3 | Identification of the anticipatory postural adjustments (APAs) and of the focal movement (FM) phases, using pressure sensor (PS, in V) and anterior-posterior center of pressure (CP) (Xp, in m) traces: the beginning of the APAs and the end of the FM are identified in CP trace, whereas the seat-off is indicated in PS trace. The recording was taken in a representative subject wearing a Philadelphia collar.

- Duration of the focal movement (*dFM*): delay between the seat-off instant and the stabilization of the CP curve (beginning of the plateau region).

The different events (beginning of the APAs, seat-off, end of the FM) were based on the visual inspection of the curves, performed by a fully trained experimenter.

Data from the accelerometers were used to ensure that the head and trunk were kept still before the "Go" signal, and to discard trials in which the participants anticipated the instructions of the experimenter. The accelerometric signals were not used to separate the focal and the postural components of the task, because in complex movements such as the STS, some parts of the bony chain might be involved in both phases, with no clear distinction between the focal and the postural chains.

All parameters were calculated using a customized program written in MatLab software (The MathWorks, Inc., Natick, MA, USA).

A one-way repeated measures analysis of variance (ANOVA) was conducted for each dependent variable, with cervical mobility as a within-subjects factor. When statistical significance was reached, the ANOVA was followed by a within-subjects

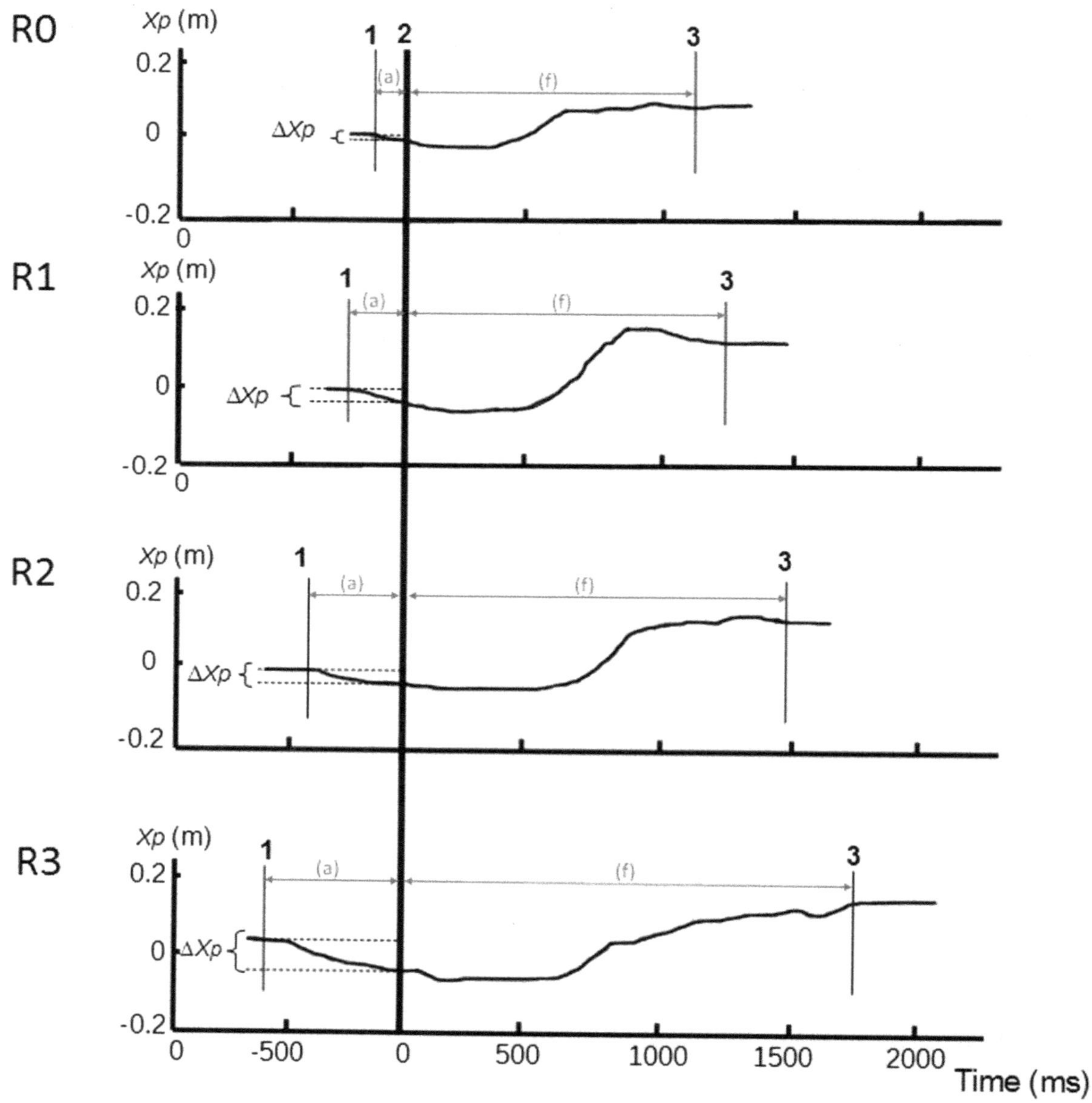

FIGURE 4 | Center of pressure traces along the anterior-posterior axis (Xp, in m) in different conditions of cervical spine mobility: no restriction (R0), jersey tubular bandage (R1), foam cervical collar (R2), Philadelphia collar (R3). Recordings were taken in a representative subject. Line 1: CP onset; line 2: instant of "seat-off"; line 3: CP stabilization. APAs (a) phase is between lines 1 and 2, and focal phase (f) between lines 2 and 3. ΔXp represents the amplitude of the APAs.

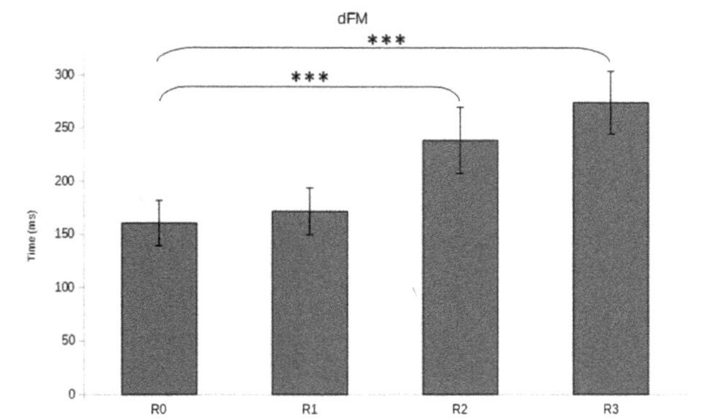

FIGURE 5 | Duration of focal movement (dFM, in ms) as a function of cervical spine mobility. Means and standard deviations are presented in four different conditions varying cervical spine mobility using cervical orthoses: no restriction (R0), jersey tubular bandage (R1, minor restriction), foam cervical collar (R2, medium restriction), Philadelphia collar (R3, major restriction). ***$p < 0.001$.

TABLE 1 | Anticipatory postural adjustments (APAs) and focal mouvement (FM) parameters as a function of cervical spine mobility.

	dAPA (ms)	*Δ Xp (m)*	*dFM (ms)*
RO	14.41 ± 8.04	0.029 ± 0.012	195.3 ± 35.06
R1	15.76 ± 4.16	0.037 ± 0.019	191.42 ± 31.92
R2	22.38 ± 4.51	0.051 ± 0.023	241.66 ± 42.97
R3	27.77 ± 6.83	0.059 ± 0.022	268.29 ± 40.63
Overall effect	$p < 0.01$	$p < 0.001$	$p < 0.001$
p(RO/R1)	*NS*	*NS*	*NS*
p(RO/R2)	$p < 0.05$	$p < 0.01$	$p < 0.001$
p(RO/R3)	$p < 0.001$	$p < 0.001$	$p < 0.001$

Mean ± SD of APAs duration (dAPAs), APAs amplitude (ΔXp), and focal movement duration (dMF) are presented in the different conditions varying cervical spine mobility: jersey tubular bandage (R1), foam cervical collar (R2), Philadelphia collar (R3).

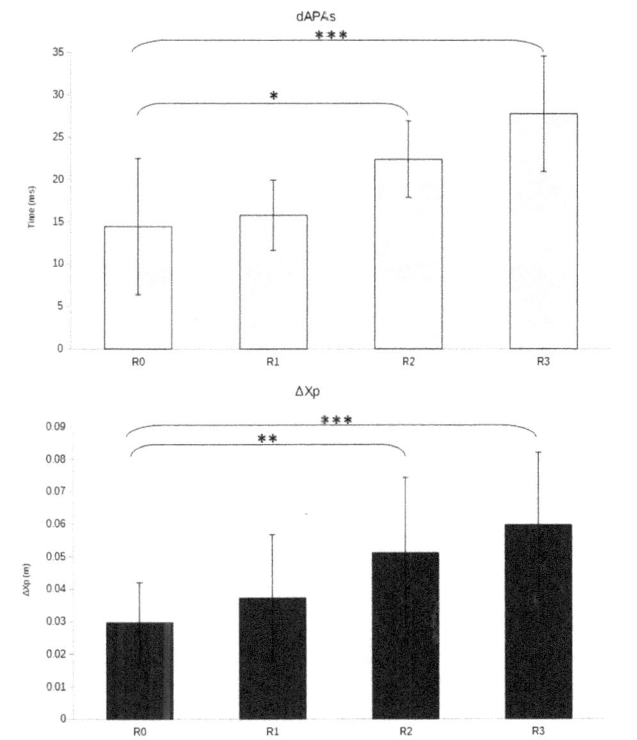

FIGURE 6 | Duration (dAPAs, in ms) and amplitude (ΔXp, in m) of anticipatory adjustments as a function of cervical spine mobility. Means and standard deviations are presented in four different conditions varying cervical spine mobility using cervical orthoses: no restriction (R0), jersey tubular bandage (R1, minor restriction), foam cervical collar (R2, medium restriction), Philadelphia collar (R3, major restriction). *$p < 0.05$; **$p < 0.01$; ***$p < 0.001$.

analysis of contrasts to compare the levels of the independent variable. As we presumed a significant difference between a reference condition (R0, no collar) and the three others ones (R1, R2, and R3), we used a simple contrast which compared R0 to each category (R1, R2, and R3). All statistical analysis were performed using the Statistical Package for Social Sciences (SPSS) software V22 (Chicago, IL, USA).

RESULTS

The visual inspection of CP traces along the anterior-posterior axis showed a gradual increase of APAs duration, APAs amplitude, and FM from R0 to R3 (**Figure 4**), which was confirmed by the statistical analysis. Indeed, the ANOVA revealed that the duration of the FM increased with the restriction of cervical spine mobility induced by the three collars ($p < 0.001$ for the overall effect) with significant variations in R2 and R3 relative to R0 (**Figure 5** and **Table 1**).

Similar variations were observed for the APAs, which presented higher duration ($p < 0.01$ for the overall effect) and magnitude ($p < 0.001$ for the overall effect) when cervical spine mobility was restricted (**Figure 5** and **Table 1**). The within-subjects contrast analysis showed significant differences between the R0 and R2 conditions ($p < 0.05$ for APAs duration and $p < 0.01$ for APAs amplitude) and between the R0 and R3 conditions ($p < 0.001$ for APAs duration and APAs amplitude) (**Figure 6**).

It must be noted that no significant variation was observed between R0 (no collar) and R1 (jersey tubular bandage) for any of the three analyzed parameters.

DISCUSSION

Cervical Spine Mobility Is a Significant Parameter in the STS Task

The statistical analysis of the biomechanical parameters revealed that the FM duration of the STS task increased stepwise with the restriction of cervical spine mobility. As the subjects were requested to perform the task as fast as possible, it can be assumed that lower cervical spine mobility results in poorer performance for the STS task. This phenomenon could firstly be related to a lower ability to perform the FM when the articular free play of the cervical spine is restricted, in accordance with literature depicting the mobilization of this area during the focal phase of the STS. Indeed, Nuzik et al. (1986) reported a neck extension after the first 35% of the movement cycle, and Rodrigues-de-Paula Goulart and Valls-Solé (1999) showed that two motor muscles of the neck, namely trapezius and sternocleidomastoideus, present a noticeable EMG activity during the focal phase of the movement.

Secondly, the loss of cervical mobility may also impair the ability to perform efficient APAs, which represent a part of the central motor program that tends to reduce the early perturbations induced by the FM. In the paradigm of STS (Diakhaté et al., 2013) as in gait initiation (Brenière and Do, 1991), which include a shift of the center of mass (CM), APAs also contribute to the generation of the propulsive forces. It is assumed that APAs must be developed for the movement to be performed efficiently (Bouisset and Zattara, 1981). APAs involve postural chain mobility, and restricted articular free play has been shown to induce poorer performance in various paradigms, such as manual pointing or pushing (Bouisset and Le Bozec, 1999). The implication of cervical spine mobility during the anticipatory phase of the STS task is supported by existing literature, with Jones and Hanson (1970) representing a cervical flexion at the beginning of the STS trajectory in accordance with Nuzik et al. (1986). In the study by Rodrigues-de-Paula Goulart and Valls-Solé (1999), early EMG activity of the sternocleidomastoideus prior to the seat-off instant, very close to the onset of tibialis anterior that is the first muscle to be activated, has been reported. As the motor pattern of the APAs, including the motor muscles and the mobilized joints, is task specific (Bouisset and Zattara, 1981), the restriction of cervical spine mobility might not be easily compensated for. Consequently, APAs will become less efficient and require a significant increase of their amplitude and duration to counterbalance the disturbances associated with the FM, or to generate the propulsive forces. This adaptation of APAs programming is in line with a previous study exploring the effect of support base surface on the paradigm of shoulder flexion at maximum velocity while standing (Zattara and Bouisset, 1992). In this study, the authors showed that restricted support surface was associated with longer APAs and a lower performance of the FM (represented by the angular velocity peak).

Cervical Spine as a Possible Guide for STS Kinematics

Beyond its key role as a part of the postural chain whose mobility reduces the disturbance associated with the FM in the STS, the cervical spine may also have other functions due to its upper location along the bony chain and articulation with the head. The early head flexion followed by an extension (Jones and Hanson, 1970), with a similar pattern for the trunk and pelvis (Nuzik et al., 1986), might provide the head and cervical spine with a guide function for STS kinematics. This function was suggested in a series of pictures taken in the burst mode in a few trials, with head mobility apparently starting and guiding the whole body trajectory. These hypotheses require an extended EMG and kinematic study to be assessed.

This specific role of the cervical spine could also be considered from a neurophysiological point of a view, as these vertebrae determines head orientation in space, and may vary visual field, vestibular activity, and cervical proprioception, which all provide substantial input for motor control (Paulus et al., 1984; Roll et al., 1989; Cullen, 2012). In the performance of complex tasks such as jumping, it has been shown that the head is sequentially stabilized in different positions, during several successive time periods (Pozzo et al., 1990). Hence, restricted articular free play in the cervical area might also impair the sensitive and sensory flow used by the CNS to control the STS task.

APAs Are Adaptable

The analysis of CP displacements according to the seat-off instant showed that APAs duration and magnitude increased stepwise with the restriction of cervical spine mobility, suggesting that the local variations of the articular free play were integrated in the central programming of the task. This fine tuning of APAs is in line with literature demonstrating their adaptability to different biomechanical parameters, such as the size of the base of support (Yiou et al., 2007), or additional loads (Bouisset and Zattara, 1981). It may now be assumed that APAs are also adaptable to spine mobility variations.

Clinical Implications

To date, little attention has been paid to cervical spine mobility in the STS task, either in a physiological perspective or in treatment and prevention strategies. It is well know that restriction of cervical spine mobility is frequent in the elderly (Lansade et al., 2009) or in neck pain syndroms (Cagnie et al., 2007), and results from this study suggest that it may impair the ability to perform the STS task. As a consequence, preserving or extending the cervical articular free play in these cases, using rehabilitation techniques or adapted physical programs, may be useful to preserve functional autonomy. Indeed, it must be recalled that the STS, which is considered a fundamental prerequisite for daily activities (Boukadida et al., 2015), is performed in mean 60 times per day (Dall and Kerr, 2010).

Elsewhere, the prescription of cervical collars, although they may represent an efficient tool to relieve pain or to favor cervical spine recovery (Muzin et al., 2007), should take into account their negative effect on the STS task, especially for patients presenting a loss of functional autonomy.

CONCLUSION

This study has shown that passive restriction of cervical mobility results in a lower motor performance in the STS task, with an adaptation of the APAs, which become longer and larger. It is assumed that cervical spine mobility is an integral part of both the postural and the focal components of the STS task, with potential implications in rehabilitation strategies and adapted physical activity programs.

AUTHOR CONTRIBUTIONS

AH contributed with project creation, data analysis, and drafted the manuscript. CA-R contributed with project creation, data collection, and data analysis. AH and CA-R discussed the results and revised the manuscript.

FUNDING

This work was funded by University JF Champollion and Conseil Régional Occitanie, France.

ACKNOWLEDGMENT

The authors thank Vérane Faure for her valuable help in the analysis of the results.

REFERENCES

Bouisset, S., and Le Bozec, S. (1999). "Body balance stability and postural adjustments associated with voluntary movement," in *Motor Control: Today and Tomorrow*, eds G. N. Gantchev, S. Mori, and J. Massion (Sofia: Academic Publishing House "Prof. M. Drinov").

Bouisset, S., and Zattara, M. (1981). A sequence of postural movements precedes voluntary movement. *Neurosci. Lett.* 22, 263–270. doi: 10.1016/0304-3940(81)90117-8

Bouisset, S., and Zattara, M. (1983). "Anticipatory postural movements related to a voluntary movement," in *Space Physiology* (Toulouse: Cepadues Publisher), 137–141.

Boukadida, A., Piotte, F., Dehail, P., and Nadeau, S. (2015). Determinants of sit-to-stand tasks in individuals with hemiparesis post stroke: a review. *Ann. Phys. Rehabil. Med.* 58, 167–172. doi: 10.1016/j.rehab.2015.04.007

Brenière, Y., and Do, M. C. (1991). Control of gait initiation. *J. Mot. Behav.* 23, 235–240. doi: 10.1080/00222895.1991.9942034

Burdett, R. G., Habasevich, R., Pisciotta, J., and Simon, S. R. (1985). Biomechanical comparison of rising from two types of chairs. *Phys. Ther.* 65, 1177–1183. doi: 10.1093/ptj/65.8.1177

Cagnie, B., Cools, A., De Loose, V., Cambier, D., and Danneels, L. (2007). Reliability and normative database of the Zebris cervical range-of-motion system in healthy controls with preliminary validation in a group of patients with neck pain. *J. Manipulative Physiol. Ther.* 30, 450–455. doi: 10.1016/j.jmpt.2007.05.003

Coghlin, S. S., and McFadyen, B. J. (1994). Transfer strategies used to rise from a chair in normal and low back pain subjects. *Clin. Biomech.* 9, 85–92. doi: 10.1016/0268-0033(94)90029-9

Cullen, K. E. (2012). The vestibular system: multimodal integration and encoding of self-motion for motor control. *Trends Neurosci.* 35, 185–196. doi: 10.1016/j.tins.2011.12.001

Dall, P. M., and Kerr, A. (2010). Frequency of the sit to stand task: an observational study of free-living adults. *Appl. Ergon.* 41, 58–61. doi: 10.1016/j.apergo.2009.04.005

Diakhaté, D. G., Do, M. C., and Le Bozec, S. (2013). Effects of seat–thigh contact on kinematics performance in sit-to-stand and trunk flexion tasks. *J. Biomech.* 46, 879–882. doi: 10.1016/j.jbiomech.2012.12.022

Hartman, J. T., Palumbo, F., and Hill, B. J. (1975). Cineradiography of the braced normal cervical spine. A comparative study of five commonly used cervical orthoses. *Clin. Orthop. Relat. Res.* 97–102. doi: 10.1097/00003086-197506000-00012

Jones, F. P., and Hanson, J. A. (1970). Postural set and overt movement: a force-platform analysis. *Percept. Mot. Skills* 30, 699–702. doi: 10.2466/pms.1970.30.3.699

Kralj, A., Jaeger, R. J., and Munih, M. (1990). Analysis of standing up and sitting down in humans: definitions and normative data presentation. *J. Biomech.* 23, 1123–1138. doi: 10.1016/0021-9290(90)90005-N

Lansade, C., Laporte, S., Thoreux, P., Rousseau, M.-A., Skalli, W., and Lavaste, F. (2009). Three-dimensional analysis of the cervical spine kinematics: effect of age and gender in healthy subjects. *Spine* 34, 2900–2906. doi: 10.1097/BRS.0b013e3181b4f667

Le Bozec, S., and Bouisset, S. (2004). Does postural chain mobility influence muscular control in sitting ramp pushes? *Exp. Brain Res.* 158, 427–437. doi: 10.1007/s00221-004-1918-x

Lino, F., and Bouisset, S. (1994). Effect of seat contact area on the velocity of a pointing task. *J. Biomech.* 27, 733. doi: 10.1016/0021-9290(94)91153-3

McLeod, P. C., Kettelkamp, D. B., Srinivasan, V., and Henderson, O. L. (1975). Measurements of repetitive activities of the knee. *J. Biomech.* 8, 369–373. doi: 10.1016/0021-9290(75)90072-X

Muzin, S., Isaac, Z., Walker, J., Abd, O. E., and Baima, J. (2007). When should a cervical collar be used to treat neck pain? *Curr. Rev. Musculoskelet. Med.* 1, 114–119. doi: 10.1007/s12178-007-9017-9

Nuzik, S., Lamb, R., VanSant, A., and Hirt, S. (1986). Sit-to-Stand Movement Pattern. *Phys. Ther.* 66, 1708–1713. doi: 10.1093/ptj/66.11.1708

Paulus, W. M., Straube, A., and Brandt, T. (1984). Visual stabilization of posture. Physiological stimulus characteristics and clinical aspects. *Brain* 107(Pt 4), 1143–1163. doi: 10.1093/brain/107.4.1143

Pozzo, T., Berthoz, A., and Lefort, L. (1990). Head stabilization during various locomotor tasks in humans. I. Normal subjects. *Exp. Brain Res.* 82, 97–106. doi: 10.1007/bf00230842

Riley, P. O., Schenkman, M. L., Mann, R. W., and Hodge, W. A. (1991). Mechanics of a constrained chair-rise. *J. Biomech.* 24, 77–85. doi: 10.1016/0021-9290(91)90328-K

Rodrigues-de-Paula Goulart, F., and Valls-Solé, J. (1999). Patterned electromyographic activity in the sit-to-stand movement. *Clin. Neurophysiol.* 110, 1634–1640. doi: 10.1016/S1388-2457(99)00109-1

Roebroeck, M. E., Doorenbosch, C. A. M., Harlaar, J., Jacobs, R., and Lankhorst, G. J. (1994). Biomechanics and muscular activity during sit-to-stand transfer. *Clin. Biomech.* 9, 235–244. doi: 10.1016/0268-0033(94)90004-3

Roll, J. P., Vedel, J. P., and Roll, R. (1989). Eye, head and skeletal muscle spindle feedback in the elaboration of body references. *Prog. Brain Res.* 80, 113–123; discussion57–60. doi: 10.1016/s0079-6123(08)62204-9

Schenkman, M., Berger, R. A., Riley, P. O., Mann, R. W., and Hodge, W. A. (1990). Whole-body movements during rising to standing from sitting. *Phys. Ther.* 70, 638–648. doi: 10.1093/ptj/70.10.638

Shepherd, R. B., and Gentile, A. M. (1994). Sit-to-stand: functional relationship between upper body and lower limb segments. *Hum. Mov. Sci.* 13, 817–840. doi: 10.1016/0167-9457(94)90020-5

Yiou, E., Hamaoui, A., and Le Bozec, S. (2007). Influence of base of support size on arm pointing performance and associated anticipatory postural adjustments. *Neurosci. Lett.* 423, 29–34. doi: 10.1016/j.neulet.2007.06.034

Zattara, M., and Bouisset, S. (1992). "Influence of a reduction of postural base configuration on the velocity of unilateral and bilateral upper limbs movements," in *Proceedings of the VIIIth Meeting of the European Society of Biomechanics*, (Rome: Bellotti P and Cappozzo A), 226.

15

Sensory Integration during Vibration of Postural Muscle Tendons When Pointing to a Memorized Target

Normand Teasdale [1,2], Mariusz P. Furmanek [3], Mathieu Germain Robitaille [1], Fabio Carlos Lucas de Oliveira [1] and Martin Simoneau [1]*

[1]Département de Kinésiologie, Faculté de Médecine, Université Laval, Quebec City, QC, Canada, [2]Centre de Recherche sur les Soins et les Services de Première Ligne de l'Université Laval (CERSSPL-UL), Quebec City, QC, Canada, [3]Human Motor Behavior Laboratory, Department of Human Motor Behavior, The J. Kukuczka Academy of Physical Education, Katowice, Poland

***Correspondence:**
Normand Teasdale
normand.teasdale@kin.ulaval.ca*

Vibrating ankle muscles in freely standing persons elicits a spatially oriented postural response. For instance, vibrating the Achilles tendons induces a backward displacement of the body while vibrating the tibialis anterior muscle tendons induces a forward displacement. These displacements have been called vibration induced falling (VIF) responses and they presumably are automatic. Because of the long delay between the onset of the vibration and the onset of the VIF (about 700 ms), and the widespread cortical activation following vibration, there is a possibility that the sensory signals available before the VIF can be used by the central nervous system to plan a hand pointing action. This study examined this suggestion. Ten healthy young participants stood on a force platform and initially were trained to point with and without vision to a target located in front of them. Then, they were exposed to conditions with vibration of the Achilles tendons or tibialis anterior muscle tendons and pointed at the target without vision. The vibration stopped between each trial. Trials with vision (without vibration) were given every five trials to maintain an accurate perception of the target's spatial location. Ankle vibrations did not have an effect on the position of the center of foot pressure (COP) before the onset of the pointing actions. Furthermore, reaction and movement times of the pointing actions were unaffected by the vibration. The hypotheses were that if proprioceptive information evoked by ankle vibrations alters the planning of a pointing action, the amplitude of the movement should scale according to the muscle tendons that are vibrated. For Achilles tendon vibration, participants undershot the target indicating the planning of the pointing action was influenced by the vibration-evoked proprioceptive information (forward displacement of the body). When the tibialis anterior were vibrated (backward displacement of the body), however, shorter movements were also observed. Longer movements would have increased the backward response of the sensed body movement. Thus, it is possible that pointing actions were adjusted on the basis of the expected consequences of the planned pointing action to avoid a response that could have compromised postural stability.

Keywords: sensory integration, posture, vibration, vibration induced falling response, hand pointing

INTRODUCTION

Since the pioneering work of Goodwin et al. (1972), we know that vibrations to the tendon of a muscle produce sensations of limb movements. The vibration activates mainly the muscle spindle primary endings and gives rise to an instantaneous afferent pattern (Goodwin et al., 1972; Burke et al., 1976; Roll and Vedel, 1982). The primary endings respond to low amplitude vibrations in a one-to-one manner for vibration frequencies as low as 3 Hz up to 80 Hz. Cutaneous receptors also can contribute to the sensation (Collins and Prochazka, 1996; Aimonetti et al., 2007, 2012).

When a person stands freely with the eyes closed, vibrating the Achilles tendons generate sensory signals similar to those that would be observed if the body would be moving forward (Eklund, 1972; Gurfinkel et al., 1988; Roll et al., 1989a,b). The postural response following the onset of the vibration is in the opposite direction, towards the back as if it was generated to compensate the stretching signals of the calf muscles generated by the vibration of the Achilles tendons. A similar, but reversed response occurs when vibrating the tibialis anterior muscle tendons; the sensory signal indicates the body is moving backward and a forward postural response is observed. These postural responses have been described as "vibration induced falling" responses (VIF; Eklund, 1972, 1973). It is believed that VIF responses are involuntary and represent an automatic reaction originating from supraspinal centers (e.g., Eklund, 1972; Gurfinkel et al., 1988; Roll et al., 1989b). Several recent cerebral imaging studies have shown that a widespread cortical activity is observed when a muscle tendon is vibrated (for a review, Naito et al., 2016). The areas activated include the primary motor cortex, dorsal premotor cortex, supplementary motor area. Activation also occurs in somatosensory areas. The time course of VIF responses is quite slow. For instance, Quoniam et al. (1995) reported that the VIF response starts about 700 ms after the onset of the vibration on the tendon of the tibialis anterior. There are also reports of an initial faster (within 200 ms after vibration onset) but small center of foot pressure (COP) response in the direction opposite to that of the following (and related) main evoked postural displacement (Caudron et al., 2008). It has been suggested this initial response is automatic because it was observed when subjects self-triggered the vibration stimuli or when they could expect the onset of the stimuli through specific timing cues.

Because of the observed delay and the widespread cortical activation, there is a possibility that before the VIF response (which presumably is also automatic), an internal representation of the body (body scheme) is updated to indicate a change in the postural orientation. To examine this possibility, we asked subjects to point at a memorized target (hence without vision) from a standing posture. Specifically, if signals arising from vibrating the tendons reach higher level structures during the planning phase of the pointing movement, the motor commands for the upper arm should scale according to the muscles being vibrated when the movement is produced before the onset of the VIF. Hence, vibrating the Achilles tendons, because it gives rise to afferent signals indicating a forward displacement of the body, should lead to shorter movements than those without vibration. Alternately, vibrating the tibialis anterior tendons, because it gives rise to afferent signals indicating a backward displacement of the body, should lead to longer movements than those without vibration. Such results would provide strong support to the hypothesis that the sensory signals arising from the vibration induce an update of the internal representation of the body. This representation of the spatial position of the body could be available for the planning of motor commands of upper arm goal-directed movements.

MATERIALS AND METHODS

Participants

Prior to commencing, participants were briefed about the experiment and provided a written informed consent. All forms and procedures were approved by the Human Research Ethics Committee of Université Laval. A total of 10 right-handed volunteers (6 males, 4 females; mean age: 24.3 ± 4.1 years old; mean body mass: 70.3 ± 11.9 kg; mean height 1.70 ± 0.10 m) with no known history of neurological or motor disorders participated in this investigation. After an initial analysis, data for one male participant were discarded because of systematic large overshooting of the target, even with vision of the target location.

Task and Procedures

Participants stood barefoot on a force platform with their feet externally rotated by 10° and their heels 10 cm apart. Landmarks on the platform allowed maintaining a relatively constant position for all trials. In the start position, the participant's right index finger touched the xiphoid process of the sternum with the elbow flexed and the arm at, approximately, 60° abduction. The contralateral arm was along the body. A target was located in front of the participant at about 80% of each participant's arm length just below the height of the xiphoid process. For all trials, the task was to move rapidly the arm across the transverse plane and to stop with the right index finger just over the target with as much accuracy as possible. Participants were told to hold their index over the target for approximately 1 s before returning to the start position.

For each trial, a ready signal indicated the subjects to adopt the starting posture. The approximate initial anterior-posterior position and stability of the COP was verified visually on an oscilloscope (Hewlett-Packard 54601A) through monitoring the platform force moment around the mediolateral axis. For trials with vibration of the ankle muscle tendons, vibrators on both gastrocnemii or tibialis anterior muscles tendons were activated once the participant adopted a stable starting posture and the vibration lasted until the end of the trial. An auditory stimulus (4 kHz, 250 ms) presented 400 ms after the onset of the vibration was the imperative signal to point at the target. Assuming a mean reaction time of 300 ms, we postulated that most pointing actions would be planned before or around the onset of the VIF response. This is so because Quoniam et al. (1995) reported that the VIF response starts approximately 700 ms after the onset of vibration.

Each participant performed a total of 45 pointing movements with an interval of approximately 30 s between trials. All participants first pointed to the target without any vibration with full vision (Vision, five trials), and without vision (No Vision, five trials). Then, before each subsequent block of five trials, two trials with vision and without vibration were given to recalibrate the participants (i.e., to maintain an accurate perception of the target location). After another block without vision and without vibration, two blocks of five trials with vibration of the Achilles tendons and two blocks of five trials with vibration of the tibialis anterior muscle tendons followed. Trials with ankle vibration were performed without vision. Hereafter, the four experimental conditions are named Vision, No-vision, Vibration Achilles and Vibration TA.

Instrumentation

Two custom-made vibrators served to stimulate the muscle proprioceptors. Each vibrator is made of a small DC motor inserted into a plastic cylinder (10 cm long, 3 cm in diameter). They generate a mechanical oscillation of 1-mm amplitude at a frequency of 80 Hz. The vibrators were securely fixed with rubber bands over the Achilles or tibialis anterior tendon.

A force platform (AMTI, OR-6 with MSA-6 MiniAmp, Watertown, MA, USA) fixed on the floor allowed recording the ground reaction force (Fz) and the moments around the sagittal (Mx) and frontal (My) axis. The platform was surrounded by a large wooden base (1.5 m wide × 2 m long) leveled with the platform. All signals were filtered (fourth-order zero-lag Butterworth filter, 7 Hz cut-off frequency) prior to calculating the COP.

An 8-camera video system (MaxPRO ver. 1.4.2.2, Innovision Systems Inc., Columbiaville, MI, USA) allowed recording the three-dimensional position of reflective markers placed bilaterally on the acromion, greater trochanter, lateral epicondyle of femur, lateral malleolus, and unilaterally (right side) on the lateral epicondyle of the elbow, styloid process of ulna and tip of the index finger. A target also was placed on a tripod in front of each participant just below the height of the xiphoid process at about 80% of each participant's arm length. For the first two subjects, the markers were sampled at 100 Hz. Because the data processing increased the delay between trials, we then collected all subsequent data at 30 Hz.

Disposable self-adhesive surface electromyography (EMG) electrodes (Thought Technology Ltd., Uni-Gel™ Single electrodes T3425, Montreal West, QC, Canada) were placed on the right side of the body on the anterior portion of the deltoid (AD), biceps brachi (BB), triceps brachii (TB), gluteus maximus (GM), semitendinosus (SEM) and on the left side for the tensor fasciae latae (TFL), biceps femoris (BF) and rectus femoris (RF). The ground electrode was placed at the olecranon process. The placements were defined in accordance the Surface EMG for Noninvasive Assessment of Muscles (SENIAM) guidelines (Hermens et al., 2000). All EMG signals were amplified at subject dependent gains (Octopus Bortec Biomedical Ltd., Calgary, AB, Canada) and analog band-pass filtered from 10 Hz to 1000 Hz.

A microcontroller (Basic Stamp® BS2sx, Parallax Inc., Rocklin, CA, USA) served to control the timeline of each trial, the activation of the vibrators and the piezoelectric buzzer, and to synchronize recording of all data. All signals, but the kinematics, were recorded at 1 kHz with a 16-bit A/D converter (PCI-DAS6031, Measurement Computing, Norton, MA, USA).

Data Analysis

Data were analyzed using custom Matlab software (Matlab, the Mathworks Inc., Natick, MA, USA). **Figure 1** presents the timeline for a trial with vibration. Reaction time was defined as the delay between the onset of the auditory stimulus and that of the index finger. The onset of the index was defined using a custom made algorithm detecting the first change in the signal above a baseline level (Teasdale et al., 1993). For each trial, the COP position of the participants along the antero-posterior axis was rebased using the mean position of the COP for a 500 ms period at the onset of a trial. To document the occurrence of the VIF response, the mean COP position then was computed for three different periods of 500 ms (a, b, c on **Figure 1**): (a) before the onset of the vibration (about 1.5 s before the onset of the movement for conditions without vibration); (b) just before the onset of the movement; and (c) when the participant's index finger was stabilized at the endpoint. We hypothesized that the VIF response would be observed only during the third period (a backward position of the COP when the Achilles tendons were vibrated and a forward position when the tibialis tendons were vibrated).

The 3D positions of all markers were obtained using MaxPro (Innovision Systems Inc. Columbiaville, MI, USA). All kinematic signals were then imported in Matlab and synchronized with all other signals prior to further processing (fourth order low-pass zero-phase lag Butterworth filter with a cutoff frequency of 7 Hz). Constant error (CE) and absolute error (AE) were computed by comparing the end position of the index finger with that of the target. All statistical tests were performed with Statistica (version 12.0, StatSoft, Tulsa, OK, USA). Mean and standard error of the mean (SE) are presented throughout the manuscript.

RESULTS

Reaction Time and Movement Time for the Pointing Movements

As stated above, for trials with vibration of the ankle tendons, an auditory stimulus to indicate participants to point at the target was given 400 ms after the onset of the vibration. With this procedure, we wanted participants to plan and initiate their pointing action before the VIF response. On average, reaction time was 419 ± 30 ms and it was unaffected by any of the vision or vibration conditions ($F_{(3,24)} = 1.84$, $p = 0.165$, $\eta^2 = 0.19$). This indicates that on average, the delay between the onset of the vibration and that of the pointing action was 819 ms. Movement time for the pointing action also was not different across all conditions (on average, 353 ± 30 ms, $F_{(3,24)} = 7.73$, $p = 0.067$, $\eta^2 = 0.25$).

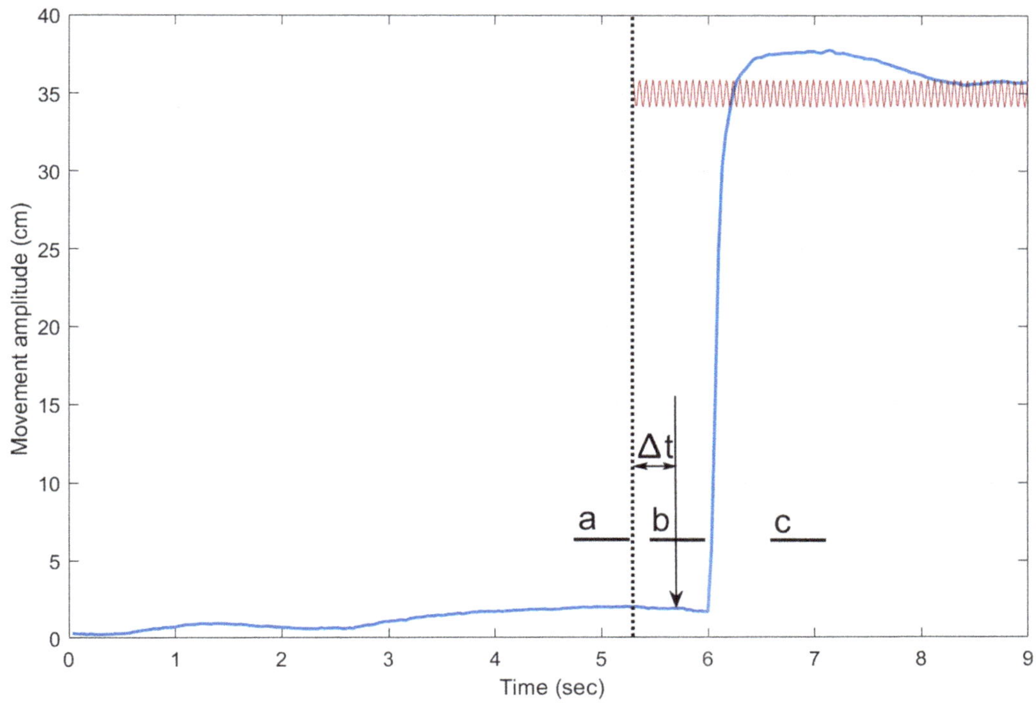

FIGURE 1 | Timeline of a trial with vibration. The thick blue line illustrates the index finger displacement. The dotted vertical line shows the onset of the vibration. The sound (vertical arrow pointing down) arrived 400 ms after the onset of the vibration. The small thick horizontal lines indicate the three 500-ms periods where the mean center of foot pressure (COP) position along the antero-posterior axis was computed (a: before the onset of the vibration, b: before the onset of the pointing movement and c: at the end of the pointing). For trials without vibration, a similar timeline was adopted.

COP Along the Antero-Posterior Axis

Figure 2 presents the mean COP position along the antero-posterior axis for the No-vibration (Vision and No-vision) and Vibration (Vibration Achilles, Vibration TA) conditions for the three periods analyzed (i.e., a, b and c on **Figure 1**). The ANOVA revealed a significant interaction of Condition × Period ($F_{(6,42)} = 6.61$, $p = 0.000$, $\eta^2 = 0.48$). A difference between the conditions was observed for the last period only, that is, once the subjects had reached the target (i.e., after the end of the pointing action). As expected, the COP moved forward when the tibialis anterior tendons were vibrated while it moved backward when the Achilles tendons were vibrated (see **Figure 2**). It is important to note that, as expected, no difference in the COP position was observed before the onset of the pointing action. This suggests participants planned their movement before the VIF response had occurred.

Amplitude and Accuracy of the Pointing Movements

To test our main hypothesis, for the pointing actions, we calculated both the CE and the AE. The ANOVA for CE (**Figures 3**—upper panel) showed a significant effect of Condition ($F_{(3,27)} = 3.79$, $p = 0.023$, $\eta^2 = 0.32$). As hypothesized, when the Achilles tendons were vibrated, the CE was negative (undershoot of the target). On the other hand, we did not observe a positive CE when the tibialis anterior tendons were vibrated as the CE was negative as well. For the AE (**Figure 3**—lower panel), the error was smaller with vision than for all other conditions but this difference was not significant ($F_{(3,27)} = 2.27$, $p = 0.10$, $\eta^2 = 0.22$).

It could be argued that the negative CE observed when the Achilles tendons were vibrated resulted from a backward displacement of the body arising from the VIF response and not from a planned shorter hand movement. To verify this possibility, we computed the distance between the right acromion and the index finger. A shorter amplitude when the Achilles tendons were vibrated would indicate that the pointing response was shorter since the amplitude is now referenced to the body and not to an external referential. On average, the amplitude for the Vision, No-vision and re-calibration trials were 56.4, 55.6 and 55.8 cm, respectively. Mean values for these control conditions were compared using T-tests and all differences were non-significant ($t_{(8)} = 1.03$, $p = 0.33$ for the comparison between the Vision and No-vision conditions; $t_{(8)} = -0.99$, $p = 0.35$ for the comparison between the Vision and the re-calibration trials). The mean amplitude when the Achilles tendons were vibrated was significantly shorter than the mean amplitude of the preceding trials (on average, 53.97 cm when the Achilles were vibrated; $t_{(8)} = 4.60$, $p = 0.001$). This suggests that the negative CE (shorter amplitude) did not result from a backward movement of the

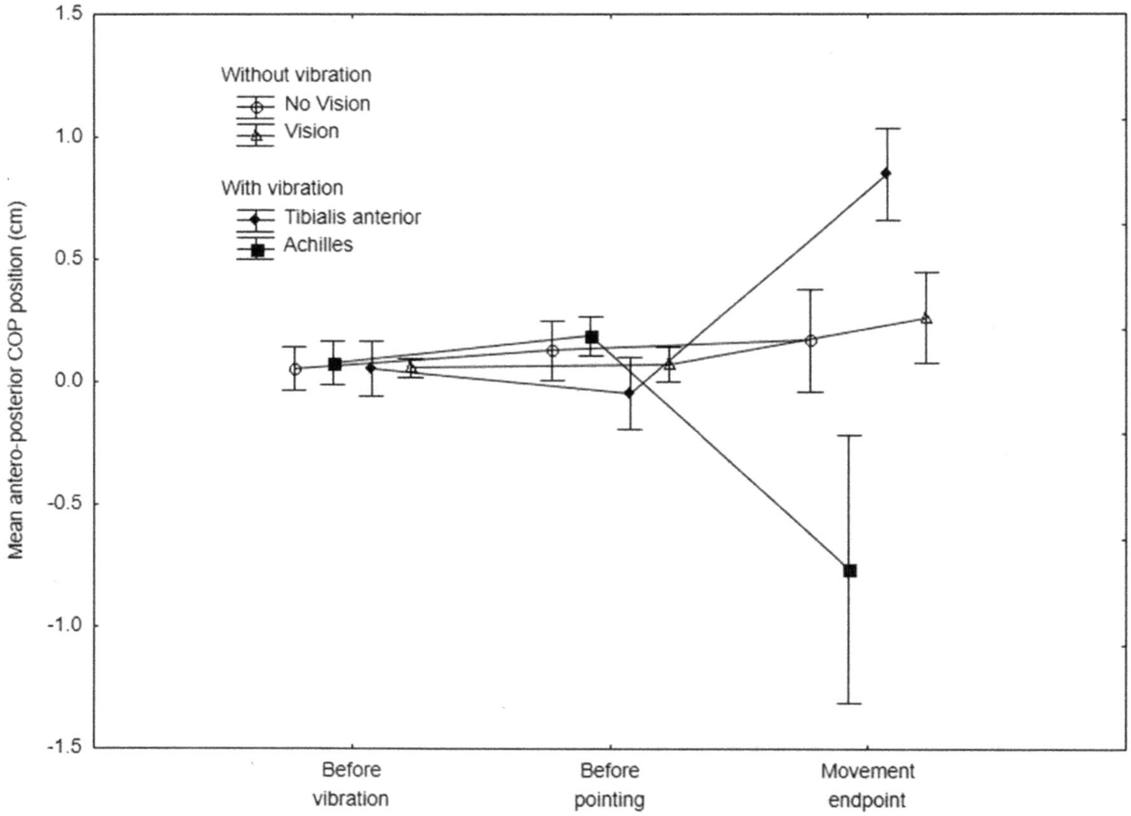

FIGURE 2 | Mean COP position along the antero-posterior axis at three different periods for the no-vibration (vision and no-vision) and vibration (Achilles and tibialis anterior) conditions. The mean COP was calculated for the three 500-ms periods (i.e., before the vibration, before the onset of the pointing movement and at the end of the movement). Positive values indicate a forward COP position with reference to baseline values (that is, once a participant adopted the initial posture and showed a stable COP position within the first 4 s). Negative values indicate a backward COP position with reference to baseline values.

body associated with the VIF but from a shorter pointing action with respect to the shoulder joint. The analyses for trials when the tibialis tendons were vibrated also showed a shorter pointing amplitude with respect to the shoulder joint (on average, 53.8 cm when the tibialis tendons were vibrated; $t_{(8)} = 4.25$, $p = 0.002$).

We also compared CE for the first pointing movement with vibration to subsequent trials. None of the participants had experimented the vibration before the first trial and a shorter amplitude for this trial could not be associated with a feedforward motor plan to avoid a potential destabilization. Specifically, we compared CE for the first trial with a vibration of the Achilles tendons (-3.4 ± 0.9 cm) to the mean of trials with (-0.4 ± 0.4 cm) and without vision (-0.6 ± 1.0 cm) preceding the first trial with vibration. Compared to trials with vision, the CE was negative (i.e., systematic undershoot of the target) and significantly smaller for the first trial with vibration of the Achilles tendons ($F_{(1,8)} = 11.896$, $p = 0.008$, $\eta^2 = 0.85$). A similar result was observed when comparing the CE for the first trial with vibration of the Achilles tendons to those without vision ($F_{(1,8)} = 7.29$, $p = 0.027$, $\eta^2 = 0.65$). These results suggest the vibration-evoked sensory information was integrated into the motor plan for the pointing action of the very first trial with vibration.

We conducted similar analyses for trials with vibration of the TA tendons, although participants had already experienced 10 trials with vibration of the Achilles tendons when they first were submitted to the first trial with the vibration of the TA tendons. The first trial with vibration of the TA tendons also showed a negative CE (-3.1 ± 1.1 cm), but the comparisons with trials without vision and with vision showed that these differences were not significant ($F_{(1,8)} = 4.69$, $p = 0.064$, $\eta^2 = 0.37$, and $F_{(1,8)} = 1.8$, $p = 0.216$, $\eta^2 = 0.18$, respectively for the comparisons with the Vision and No Vision conditions).

EMG Activity

Finally, we examined the EMG activity for three muscles involved in the pointing action, the anterior deltoid, the biceps and TB. We specifically wanted to determine if the activity of the main agonist (TB) and antagonist (BB) muscles would show any modulation associated with the vibration of ankle tendons (for instance, smaller activity for the triceps and greater activity for the biceps when the Achilles tendons were vibrated). After

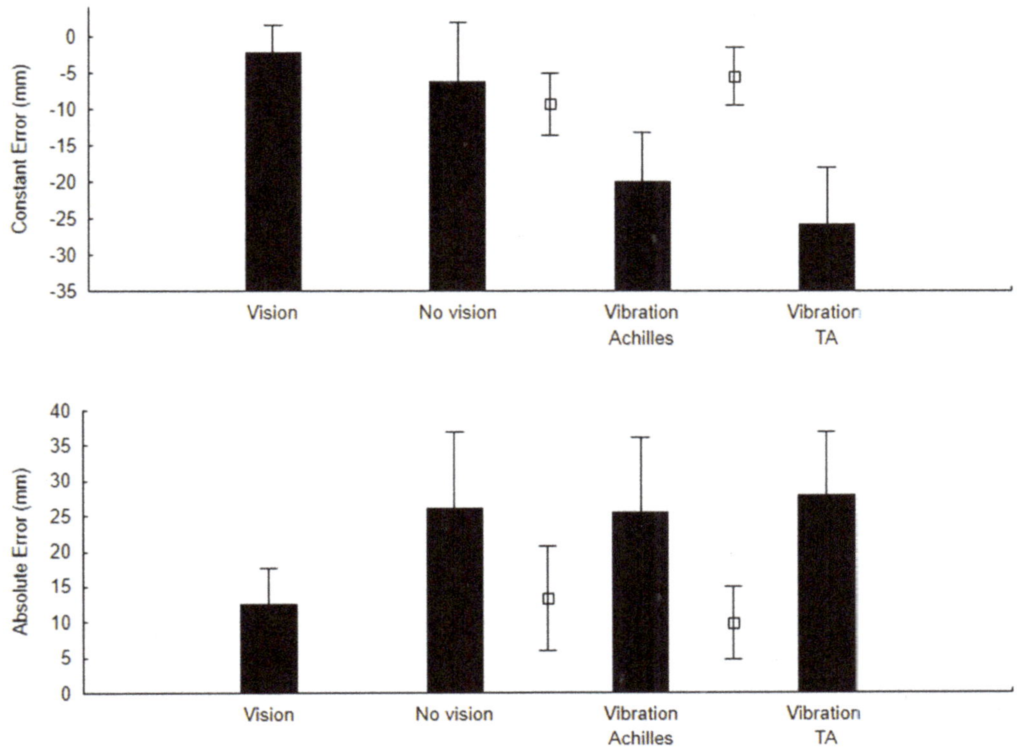

FIGURE 3 | Constant error (CE) and variable error (VE) for the no-vibration (vision and no-vision) and vibration (Achilles and tibialis anterior) conditions. For comparison purposes, open square symbols depict mean values for the re-calibration trials (i.e., trials when pointing was performed with vision before each block of trials with vibration and without vision).

a visual inspection of all data to insure EMG signals were normal within this period, data for one participant were removed because of irregular triceps signals. For the remaining eight participants, we calculated the $\int_{-50}^{100} EMG$ from 50 ms before the onset of the hand movement to 100 ms after the onset for each conditions. To allow between-subjects comparisons, the $\int_{-50}^{100} EMG$ obtained for the conditions No Vision, Vibration Achilles and Vibration TA were normalized using the same period from the condition Vision. Then, for each muscle, data for these three conditions were submitted to a one-way ANOVA. All ANOVAs were non-significant ($F_{(2,14)} = 0.29$, $p = 0.75$, $\eta^2 = 0.04$, $F_{(2,14)} = 2.46$, $p = 0.12$, $\eta^2 = 0.26$ and $F_{(2,14)} = 1.75$, $p = 0.21$, $\eta^2 = 0.20$ for the anterior deltoid, BB and TB, respectively).

DISCUSSION

Vibration applied to ankle tendons is known to induce a body displacement in freely standing subjects and an illusory body tilt in restrained subjects. For instance, vibrating the Achilles tendon induces a backward body displacement in freely standing subjects and an illusory forward tilt when the body is restrained (Eklund, 1972; Kavounoudias et al., 2001; Adamcova and Hlavacka, 2007; Ceyte et al., 2007). The body displacement observed in freely standing subjects is presumed to represent an automatic reaction (e.g., Eklund, 1972; Gurfinkel et al., 1988; Roll et al., 1989b). In the present study, and as observed previously in freely standing subjects, vibrating the Achilles tendons led to a backward body displacement and conversely vibrating the TA tendons led to a forward body displacement. Importantly, in our study, whole body large displacements were observed after the pointing action and not before. No large VIF response was noted between the onset of the vibration and the onset of the pointing action. On average, the delay between these two events was 819 ms which is slightly longer than the latency of the body displacement after a tendon vibration (VIF response) reported by Quoniam et al. (1995). This first observation is important as it clearly suggests that the planning of the pointing action was made while vibration-evoked proprioceptive information could be interpreted by the central nervous system as a change in the postural orientation while this was not the case yet. The key question of this study was whether this information was included in the motor plan of the pointing action. Our hypothesis was that if this sensory information reaches higher level structures and is interpreted as a change in postural orientation during the planning phase of the pointing action, the amplitude of the movement should scale according to the muscles being vibrated. As expected, the amplitude of the pointing actions was shorter when Achilles tendons were vibrated. Vibrating the TA tendons, however, also yielded shorter movements while we expected longer movements.

There is a possibility that the shorter movements were not the result of integrating the postural orientation *per se* but rather a general response to conditions of postural instability. This has been proposed by Slijper and Latash (2004). In their study, they observed an increased co-contraction of distal muscles and reciprocal adjustments in trunk muscles when subjects were submitted to vibration of the Achilles tendons. They suggested these adjustments served to ensure equilibrium when subjects were submitted to conditions of postural instability (vibrating Achilles tendons being one of their conditions). In our study, movements of shorter amplitude and lower speed could have served to limit the instability induced by the pointing action. There are some arguments against this possibility, however. First, if the shorter amplitudes were a strategic response to control postural instability, slower movements could have been observed for the vibration conditions. This was not the case as movement times were similar for all conditions. Another argument is based on the lack of difference between the amplitude of the first trial with vibration of the Achilles tendons and the amplitude of pointing actions with and without vision. None of the participants had experimented the vibration before this first trial and a shorter amplitude for this first trial could not be associated with a feedforward motor plan to avoid potential destabilization.

The suggestion that sensory information from ankle proprioception and plantar sole mechanoreceptors serve to estimate body orientation when planning a motor response is in agreement with recent observations by Mouchnino et al. (2015). In this study, the authors measured the cortical response to somatosensory stimulation of cutaneous inputs during the planning phase of a step initiation and during its execution. They observed a facilitation of the P50-N80 SEP component in the early planning phase of the step initiation. The authors suggested that this mechanism could enhance the perception of cutaneous input leading to a more accurate planning and execution of the forces needed to unload the moving limb. In their study, the cutaneous inputs were directly involved in the motor action. Here, our results suggest that similar mechanisms may exist to update the motor plan of an upper-limb goal directed movement. For instance, the control of posture does not only serve the motor planning of an upper limb action by receiving feedforward commands and contributing through feedback processes once the movement is initiated. Rather, sensory information about body orientation during the actual planning of the upper arm movement can be integrated rapidly to modify and update the motor plan of the upper limb movement.

There is also a possibility that foot pressure distributions affected this result as it has been shown that vibration induced postural responses are dependent on the pressure distributions (Kavounoudias et al., 2001; Thompson et al., 2011). These authors proposed that ankle proprioception and plantar sole mechanoreceptors might be processed simultaneously following a vector addition mode to determine body orientation. For example, in Thompson et al. (2011) study, participants were submitted to a support platform perturbation (toes up or toes down) and the concurrent application of a vibration to the Achilles tendon and to the rear foot had differential effect on posture. Vibration of the Achilles tendon increased the influence of the rear foot vibration for toes up perturbations. On the other hand, it decreased the influence of the rear foot vibration when toes down perturbations were given. The authors suggested that this indicates the central nervous system uses both sources of sensory information to build a reference of verticality influencing the control of equilibrium during quiet and perturbed stance. A similar mechanism may have occurred in the present study and this could explain why we did not observe any overshoot when the TA muscle tendons were vibrated. In this particular case, the sensory signals from the TA (before the onset of the pointing action) suggested a backward movement of the body. A rapid pointing response of a greater amplitude would have produced a greater backward body movement that could have compromised postural stability. This was not the case when the Achilles tendons were vibrated as the sensory signals (before the onset of the movement) indicated a forward movement of the body allowing to produce a pointing movement of a shorter amplitude that did not compromise postural stability. Additional studies will be needed to examine if this could explain the shorter amplitudes observed when the TA tendons were vibrated (for example, by using movements of shorter amplitudes that would be less likely to destabilize subjects).

As for all studies, there are some limitations to this study. Presentation of the vibration conditions was not randomized. The main dependent variable in this study was the amplitude of the pointing action. The pointing action was made to a memorized target and included the usual motor variability associated with producing fast goal-directed motor actions (Schmidt et al., 1979; Harris and Wolpert, 1998; Scott, 2004). We felt that randomizing conditions could add some additional undesirable variability. This has been observed in several postural studies. For instance, Horak et al. (1989) showed that the scaling of a postural response (muscle and torque responses) to postural perturbation amplitudes disappeared when perturbation amplitudes were randomized. Martin et al. (2000) also reported that the uncertainty about a visual perturbation (double-step paradigm) modified the planning of pointing actions to a target.

In conclusion, our results suggest that the sensory signals evoked by vibrating Achilles tendons prior to the VIF responses are integrated into the motor plan of a pointing action. We did not observe longer movements when the tibialis anterior tendons were vibrated. This indicates subjects integrated both the sensory signals evoked by vibrating muscle tendons and the expected consequences of the planned pointing action.

AUTHOR CONTRIBUTIONS

NT and MS contributed to conception, design, preparation, analysis and interpretation of the data and writing. MPF contributed to conception, data collection and analysis and writing. FCLO contributed to data collection and analysis. MGR contributed to preparation and data analysis. All authors approved the final version.

FUNDING

This research was supported by funding from the Natural Sciences and Engineering Research Council of Canada to MS and NT.

ACKNOWLEDGMENTS

Special thanks to Laurence Mouchnino for several discussions on the effect of vibrating muscle tendons on balance control.

REFERENCES

Adamcova, N., and Hlavacka, F. (2007). Modification of human postural responses to soleus muscle vibration by rotation of visual scene. *Gait Posture* 25, 99–105. doi: 10.1016/j.gaitpost.2006.01.008

Aimonetti, J. M., Hospod, V., Roll, J.-P., and Ribot-Ciscar, E. (2007). Cutaneous afferents provide a neuronal population vector that encodes the orientation of human ankle movements. *J. Physiol.* 580, 649–658. doi: 10.1113/jphysiol.2006.123075

Aimonetti, J. M., Roll, J. P., Hospod, V., and Ribot-Ciscar, E. (2012). Ankle joint movements are encoded by both cutaneous and muscle afferents in humans. *Exp. Brain Res.* 221, 167–176. doi: 10.1007/s00221-012-3160-2

Burke, D., Hagbarth, K. E., Löfstedt, L., and Wallin, B. G. (1976). The responses of human muscle spindle endings to vibration of non-contracting muscles. *J. Physiol.* 261, 673–693. doi: 10.1113/jphysiol.1976.sp011580

Caudron, S., Boy, F., Forestier, N., and Guerraz, M. (2008). Influence of expectation on postural disturbance evoked by proprioceptive stimulation. *Exp. Brain Res.* 184, 53–59. doi: 10.1007/s00221-007-1079-9

Ceyte, H., Cian, C., Zory, R., Barraud, P. A., Roux, A., and Guerraz, M. (2007). Effect of Achilles tendon vibration on postural orientation. *Neurosci. Lett.* 416, 71–75. doi: 10.1016/j.neulet.2007.01.044

Collins, D. F., and Prochazka, A. (1996). Movement illusions evoked by ensemble cutaneous input from the dorsum of the human hand. *J. Physiol.* 496, 857–871. doi: 10.1113/jphysiol.1996.sp021733

Eklund, G. (1972). General features of vibration-induced effects on balance. *Ups. J. Med. Sci.* 77, 112–124. doi: 10.1517/03009734000000016

Eklund, G. (1973). Further studies of vibration-induced effects on balance. *Ups. J. Med. Sci.* 78, 65–72.

Goodwin, G. M., McCloskey, D. I., and Matthews, P. B. (1972). Proprioceptive illusions induced by muscle vibration: contribution by muscle spindles to perception? *Science* 175, 1382–1384. doi: 10.1126/science.175.4028.1382

Gurfinkel, V. S., Levik, Y. S., Popov, K. E., Smetanin, B. N., and Shlikov, V. Y. (1988). "Body scheme in the control of postural activity," in *Stance and Motion*, eds V. S. Gurfinkel, M. E. Ioffe, J. Massion and J. P. Roll (Boston, MA: Springer US), 185–193.

Harris, C. M., and Wolpert, D. M. (1998). Signal-dependent noise determines motor planning. *Nature* 394, 780–784. doi: 10.1038/29528

Hermens, H. J., Freriks, B., Disselhorst-Klug, C., and Rau, G. (2000). Development of recommendations for SEMG sensors and sensor placement procedures. *J. Electromyogr. Kinesiol.* 10, 361–374. doi: 10.1016/s1050-6411(00)00027-4

Horak, F. B., Diener, H. C., and Nashner, L. M. (1989). Influence of central set on human postural responses. *J. Neurophysiol.* 62, 841–853.

Kavounoudias, A., Roll, R., and Roll, J. P. (2001). Foot sole and ankle muscle inputs contribute jointly to human erect posture regulation. *J. Physiol.* 532, 869–878. doi: 10.1111/j.1469-7793.2001.0869e.x

Martin, O., Teasdale, N., Simoneau, M., Corbeil, P., and Bourdin, C. (2000). Pointing to a target from an upright position in human: tuning of postural responses when there is target uncertainty. *Neurosci. Lett.* 281, 53–56. doi: 10.1016/s0304-3940(00)00801-6

Mouchnino, L., Fontan, A., Tandonnet, C., Perrier, J., Saradjian, A. H., Blouin, J., et al. (2015). Facilitation of cutaneous inputs during the planning phase of gait initiation. *J. Neurophysiol.* 114, 301–308. doi: 10.1152/jn.00668.2014

Naito, E., Morita, T., and Amemiya, K. (2016). Body representations in the human brain revealed by kinesthetic illusions and their essential contributions to motor control and corporeal awareness. *Neurosci. Res.* 104, 16–30. doi: 10.1016/j.neures.2015.10.013

Quoniam, C., Hay, L., Roll, J. P., and Harlay, F. (1995). Age effects on reflex and postural responses to propriomuscular inputs generated by tendon vibration. *J. Gerontol. A Biol. Sci. Med. Sci.* 50, B155–B165. doi: 10.1093/gerona/50a.3.b155

Roll, J. P., and Vedel, J. P. (1982). Kinaesthetic role of muscle afferents in man, studied by tendon vibration and microneurography. *Exp. Brain Res.* 47, 177–190. doi: 10.1007/bf00239377

Roll, J. P., Vedel, J. P., and Ribot, E. (1989a). Alteration of proprioceptive messages induced by tendon vibration in man: a microneurographic study. *Exp. Brain Res.* 76, 213–222. doi: 10.1007/bf00253639

Roll, J.-P., Vedel, J.-P., and Roll, R. (1989b). Eye, head and skeletal muscle spindle feedback in the elaboration of body references. *Prog. Brain Res.* 80, 113–123; Discussion 57–60. doi: 10.1016/s0079-6123(08)62204-9

Schmidt, R. A., Zelaznik, H., Hawkins, B., Frank, J. S., and Quinn, J. T. (1979). Motor-output variability: a theory for the accuracy of rapid motor acts. *Psychol. Rev.* 47, 415–451. doi: 10.1037/0033-295x.86.5.415

Scott, S. H. (2004). Optimal feedback control and the neural basis of volitional motor control. *Nat. Rev. Neurosci.* 5, 532–546. doi: 10.1038/nrn1427

Slijper, H., and Latash, M. L. (2004). The effects of muscle vibration on anticipatory postural adjustments. *Brain Res.* 1015, 57–72. doi: 10.1016/j.brainres.2004.04.054

Teasdale, N., Bard, C., Fleury, M., Young, D. E., and Proteau, L. (1993). Determining movement onsets from temporal series. *J. Mot. Behav.* 25, 97–106. doi: 10.1080/00222895.1993.9941644

Thompson, C., Bélanger, M., and Fung, J. (2011). Effects of plantar cutaneo-muscular and tendon vibration on posture and balance during quiet and perturbed stance. *Hum. Mov. Sci.* 30, 153–171. doi: 10.1016/j.humov.2010.04.002

16

Physical and Psychological Factors Associated with Walking Capacity in Patients with Lumbar Spinal Stenosis with Neurogenic Claudication

Mariève Houle [1], Jean-Daniel Bonneau [2], Andrée-Anne Marchand [2] and Martin Descarreaux [3]*

[1] Department of Anatomy, Université du Québec à Trois-Rivières, Trois-Rivières, QC, Canada, [2] Department of Chiropractic, Université du Québec à Trois-Rivières, Trois-Rivières, QC, Canada, [3] Department of Human Kinetics, Université du Québec à Trois-Rivières, Trois-Rivières, QC, Canada

***Correspondence:**
Mariève Houle
marieve.houle@uqtr.ca

Objective: The purpose of this study was to evaluate the current state of scientific knowledge regarding physical and psychological factors associated with walking capacity in patients with lumbar spinal stenosis (LSS) with neurogenic claudication.

Design: Systematic scoping review.

Literature Search: We searched CINAHL (Cumulative Index to Nursing and Allied Health Literature), MEDLINE, Cochrane, PsycINFO, and SPORTDiscus databases.

Study Selection Criteria: Cohorts and cross-sectional studies reporting on associations between physical or psychological factors and impaired walking capacity in patients with symptomatic LSS were included.

Data Synthesis: Data were synthetized to identify associations between physical or psychological factors and either walking capacity, gait pattern characteristics, or functional tasks.

Results: Twenty-four studies were included. Walking capacity was significantly correlated with several pain outcomes, disability, estimated walking distance, and cross-sectional area of the lumbar spine. Gait pattern characteristics such as speed and stride were strongly and positively correlated with disability outcomes. Functional tasks were significantly correlated with lower back and upper limb disability, lower limb endurance strength, ranges of motion, and speed. Associations with psychological factors were mostly conflicting except for the Rasch-based Depression Screener and the Pain Anxiety Symptom Scale (PASS-20) questionnaire that were associated with a decreased performance in functional tasks.

Conclusion: Physical and psychological factors that are associated with walking capacity in patients with symptomatic LSS were identified. However, many associations reported between physical or psychological factors and walking capacity were conflicting, even more so when correlated with walking capacity specifically.

Keywords: lumbar spinal stenosis, neurogenic claudication, walking capacity, gait pattern characteristics, functional task

INTRODUCTION

Symptomatic lumbar spinal stenosis (LSS), characterized by a limited walking capacity due to leg pain, is a leading cause of disability in the elderly (1, 2). Narrowing of the lumbar spinal canal or lateral foramina, as well as compression or decreased blood flow to the nerve roots (3, 4) are considered the main causes of pain in this musculoskeletal condition. Lumbar spinal stenosis is affecting between 11 and 39% (5, 6) of the global population, especially people over the age of 65 (6, 7). The acquired form of LSS arises from degenerative changes, including disc degeneration (herniation or bulging), hypertrophy of the ligamentum flavum, and spondylolisthesis and/or facet osteoarthritis (3, 4, 8) and can involve the central canal, lateral recess, foramina, or any combination of these anatomical sites (8). Congenital LSS is due to abnormalities during development, leading up to smaller pedicles length, which directly affects the antero-posterior diameter of the spinal canal (9).

In patients with LSS, self-reported symptoms combined with a physical examination represent the main assessment components of the clinical portrait severity, considering that symptoms and associated disability do not always correlate with results from magnetic resonance imaging (MRI). Advanced imaging provides information on the presence and extent of lumbar spine degenerative changes and on the lumbar spinal canal size, but does not translate information on functional capacity (6). Indeed, a number of patients will show clear and severe signs of stenosis on imaging but will experience few or no symptoms. Commonly reported symptoms of LSS include leg pain, numbness, cramps, fatigue, and weakness (8, 10). These symptoms can be grouped under one appellation: neurogenic claudication (NC). The presence of NC is modulated by the patient's posture, as it is brought on by lumbar extension when standing or walking and relieved by lumbar flexion (i.e., sitting or bending forward) (8).

Neurogenic claudication is triggered by performing daily activities that require prolonged standing postures such as walking, and patients often face a decrease in quality of life (QoL) due to important walking and functional limitations. The assessment of walking limitations plays a central role in LSS management, both in the decision-making process regarding the diagnosis (11) and treatment options (12). Most recent studies evaluating treatment effects in patients with LSS have measured walking abilities using different assessment methods. Some of these studies focused on walking distance (13–15), while others focused on walking time (16, 17), or both (18, 19) to report on walking capacity. Indeed, severe symptoms combined with a decrease in walking capacity, and subsequently in QoL, prompt neurosurgeons to opt for surgery in patients with LSS (20, 21).

Walking impairment is a major issue in LSS, and many physical and psychological factors are related to this decrease in functional capacity. Several gait measures such as step length, cadence, step width, and gait cycle have been assessed in LSS patients, but it is not clear if and how they relate to the decline in walking capacity. It is also known that walking limitations can negatively influence or be influenced by psychological factors such as a perceived low QoL and self-efficacy, and increased anxiety and kinesiophobia (22, 23). Assessing physical and psychological factors may provide relevant information that would improve our understanding of how LSS affects daily activities.

The purpose of this study was to evaluate the current state of scientific knowledge regarding physical and psychological factors associated with walking capacity in patients with LSS and associated NC.

METHODS

As systematic scoping reviews are used to inform future research directions, this study design was deemed the most appropriate to capture information from heterogeneous studies, map existing literature and identify knowledge gaps (24). This scoping review was based on the framework of Levac et al. using a 5-step review method (25) and on the framework of Peters et al. for the systematic aspect of the study conduct (24). This study was registered on Open Science Framework (https://osf.io/6az7c/?view_only=15ad45d1f1f14517b3706b154af12bb6).

Step 1: Identifying the Research Question

This scoping review was conducted to answer the following question: What are the physical and psychological factors associated with walking capacity in patients with LSS and associated NC?

The main focus of this systematic scoping review was walking capacity in patients with LSS and associated NC. Exploring associations between physical or psychological factors and walking capacity or performance in functional tasks should provide critical information regarding the impact of LSS on daily functioning. Interventions targeting physical and psychological factors associated with the decline in walking capacity could improve patients' walking capacity and QoL and support surgical decision-making.

Step 2: Identifying Relevant Studies

The search strategy was elaborated in collaboration with a university librarian and was conducted using CINAHL (Cumulative Index to Nursing and Allied Health Literature), MEDLINE, Cochrane, PsycINFO, and SPORTDiscus databases from inception to October 4, 2019. Then, an update of the literature was completed on June 18, 2020. A combination of keywords and MeSH terms was used to identify relevant studies. The lead investigator (MH) conducted the literature search. The search strategy was first developed for MEDLINE and adapted to other databases when needed (see **Supplement Material 1**). Other sources such as Google Scholar and reference lists of relevant studies were hand-searched to ensure a comprehensive overview of the subject. An EndNote library (version X9, Clarivate Analytics, Boston, MA, USA) was created to import all citations from the search strategy. Then, all duplicates were identified and removed.

Step 3: Study Selection

Definitions of Key Concepts

Symptomatic LSS was defined as back and/or leg pain causing NC in patients diagnosed with degenerative LSS. The targeted outcome was walking capacity which was considered from two different perspectives: walking capacity defined as a distance or time spent walking, and walking capacity defined as performance during a functional task that repetitively involve lower limbs and/or trunk movement (e.g., the Timed Up and Go test or stairs climbing). Associated factors of walking capacity were regarded as either physical or psychological. Physical factors were divided into patient-reported outcome measures (PROMs) [e.g., pain, disability and QoL] and objectives measures [e.g., gait pattern characteristics (e.g., speed, cadence, and step width), lower limb strength and range or motion (ROM)] while psychological factors of interest included anxiety, depression, kinesiophobia, frailty, and self-efficacy.

Inclusion and Exclusion Criteria

To be included in this scoping review, studies had to be limited to human participants and be published in peer-reviewed scientific journals in either French, English, or Spanish language. Study designs were limited to cohort, and cross-sectional studies. Randomized controlled trials were also considered provided that they present baseline data of participants with LSS and associated NC and reported on correlation or regression prior to the beginning of the intervention. In addition, assessments had to include at least one physical and/or psychological outcome measures. To be include, studies needed to fulfill inclusion criteria regarding the specific populations (P), intervention (I), and outcomes measures (O) that are presented in **Table 1**. In addition, studies that included participants with congenital LSS, scoliosis, or vascular claudication were excluded. The following types of publication were also excluded: validation study, case study, cases series, systematic review and meta-analysis, gray literature, and governmental documents.

Screening

All potentially eligible articles were independently screened by a pair of reviewers (MH, MERP) in two phases, using a standardized Excel spreadsheet. In phase one screening, titles and abstracts were classified as relevant, possibly relevant, or irrelevant according to the eligibility criteria. Then during phase two screening, the full text of possibly relevant articles was reviewed by the same pair of reviewers for final determination of eligibility. Reviewers discussed disagreement to reach consensus for both phases of screening and a third independent reviewer (AAM) was consulted to achieve consensus if needed.

Step 4: Charting the Data

The following descriptive variables were extracted from all relevant studies using a standardized extraction form: authors, year of publication, title, country, study design, sample size, definitions of both LSS and NC, description of the study population (number of participants with LSS, LSS type, age, and gender ratio), independent variables, dependent variables, and key findings from study results. A pair of researchers independently extracted data (MH, JDB) and if necessary, a third person (AAM) was involved to resolve disagreements.

Step 5: Collating, Summarizing, and Reporting Results

Study Designs and Participants

Data regarding study designs, sample sizes, and patients' characteristics were summarized to provide an overall picture of the populations studied.

Quality Assessment

Quality assessment of all eligible studies was independently completed by two reviewers (MH, JDB) using the Appraisal tool for Cross-sectional Studies (AXIS) (26). When a disagreement between the two reviewers occurred, a third person (AAM) was involved to reach consensus. The AXIS tool contains 20 questions that address three different domains: study design (7 questions), study quality (7 questions) and risk of bias (6 questions). Each question is answered by either "yes" (1 point), "no" (0 point), or "do not know" (0 point). A sum of all "yeses" is calculated to provide an overall score with higher scores indicating higher quality. As none of the studies reported a description of the non-responders (question 7), question 14 ("If appropriate, was information about non-responders described?") became non-applicable and therefore was removed from the quality assessment checklist, bringing the maximum possible score to 19. Furthermore, question 19 ("Were there any funding sources or conflicts of interest that may affect the authors' interpretation of the result?") was given one point when it was specified that there were no conflicts of interest.

TABLE 1 | Inclusion criteria regarding population, intervention, and outcomes measures.

Inclusion criteria	P	I	C	O
	• Patients with LSS: Localization: - Central - Foraminal - Lateral • With or without spondylolisthesis • Coexisting LSS types (e.g., central + foraminal) • Presenting with NC • Having at least 18 years old	• Associations provided before any medical intervention is initiated • Data collected during one of these situations: - Walking - Climbing stairs - Running - Functional tasks	• Non-applicable	• Physical and psychological factors related to: - Walking capacity - Functional tasks - Gait pattern characteristics

If there was a mixed sample (e.g., LSS and healthy participants), the study was kept only if data from patients with LSS could be extracted separately.
P, Population; I, Intervention; C, Comparison; O, Outcome measures; LSS, lumbar spinal stenosis; NC, neurogenic claudication.

Results Organization

Results were first organized into two broad categories based on the nature of the reported associations. The categories were defined as follow: associations in relation to [1] walking capacity, and [2] functional tasks. Then, within each category, results were organized based on outcome measure types (i.e., PROMs, objective outcome measures, and any other relevant outcome whenever applicable).

RESULTS

The initial literature search identified 6,034 possible studies for inclusion in the scoping review. Following the removal of duplicates ($n = 1{,}665$), 4,369 studies remained. Initial screening of titles and abstracts resulted in the exclusion of 4315 articles that did not meet inclusion criteria. Out of the remaining 54 full-text articles, 21 fulfilled the inclusion criteria. Frequent updates of the search strategy were conducted during the review process. In light of the last update conducted on July 15, 2021, three additional articles fulfilling inclusion criteria were found bringing the final number of included studies to 24. All studies were published between 2007 and 2020 from 11 different countries over 3 continents (see **Supplement Material 2** *for more details*). **Figure 1** presents the study selection flowchart.

Participants

Out of the 24 studies, seventeen were cross-sectional studies, five were prospective observational studies, one was a secondary analysis of a RCT, and one was a retrospective observational study. Sample sizes ranged from 12 to 1009 participants. In

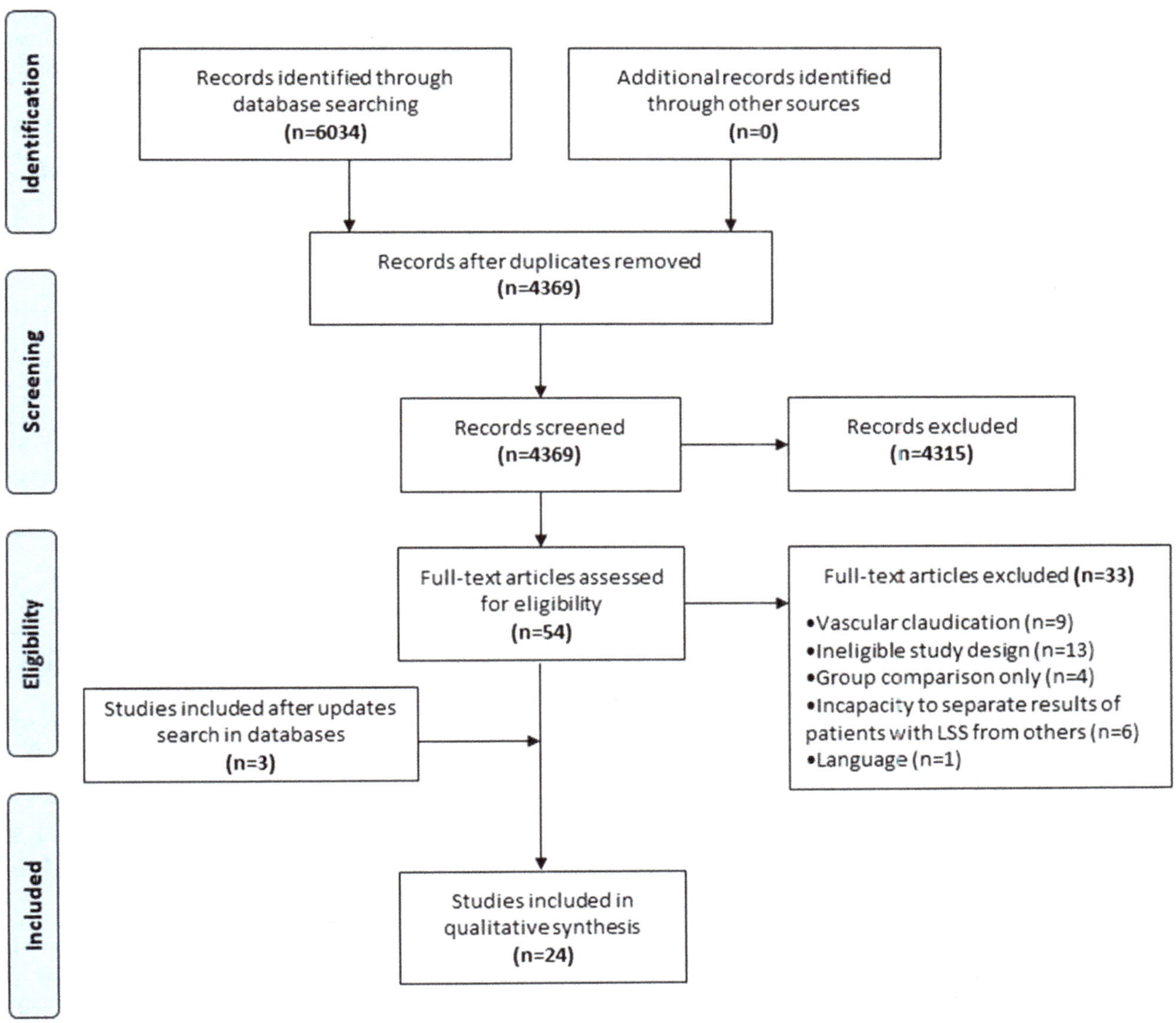

FIGURE 1 | PRISMA flowchart.

addition, out of the 2,973 participants included in the 24 studies, 1,694 had symptomatic LSS with NC. In most studies ($n = 17$), LSS was diagnosed using a combination of clinical assessment such as patient's history and/or physical examination, and findings of MRI. Regarding NC, only seven studies described NC as pain, numbness, weakness, or tingling in the lower extremity brought on by lumbar extension, standing, or walking. Based on criteria provided for inclusion of participants (or introduction section when inclusion criteria prevented the definitive identification of LSS subtypes), 974 presented with central LSS, 246 presented with combined central LSS and spondylolisthesis, 66 presented with either central or foraminal stenosis, 54 with either central or lateral stenosis, 49 with either central LSS or a combination of central and foraminal stenosis or lateral stenosis and 14 presented with lateral LSS. Finally, there were 291 patients for which the exact LSS type (e.g., central) was not explicitly described. Mean age of participants ranged from 58 to 76.9 years old across studies. Extracted data regarding population are presented in **Supplement Material 2**.

Quality Assessment

The 24 studies were assessed for quality using the AXIS tool. Two studies (27, 28) scored between 6 and 10, 14 studies (15, 19, 21, 29–39) scored between 11 and 15, and 8 studies (40–47) scored between 16 and 19. The items from the AXIS tool are reported in **Supplement Material 3**.

Associations

Surprisingly, no study investigated associations between gait pattern characteristics and walking capacity or functional tasks. However, a few studies reported associations between either physical or psychological factors and gait pattern characteristics. Considering that gait pattern characteristics do have a direct impact on walking capacity, these unplanned associations have been extracted and are now presented as a third category of associations along with walking capacity and functional tasks. All reported associations (significant or not) between either physical or psychological factors, and measures of walking capacity, functional tasks, or gait pattern characteristics are presented in **Supplementary Table 1**.

There was significant heterogeneity within both PROMs and objective measures used to assess physical and psychological factors for each category of outcome measures among the studies. **Figure 2** illustrates the range of outcome measures reported.

As a large range of associated factors were retrieved from the 24 studies, only significant associations with walking capacity, functional tasks, and gait pattern characteristics are reported herein. Additional details regarding non-significant associations are reported in **Supplement Material 4**. All associations are illustrated in **Figure 3**.

Physical and Psychological Factors Associated With Walking Capacity

PROMs

Pain. Overall, conflicting results were found based on the four studies reporting on the association between leg and/or back pain and walking capacity (distance or time). More specifically, Ishimoto et al. reported a weak positive association between symptomatic LSS (lower limb and/or buttock pain) and the 6-m walking time at maximal pace (vs. usual pace) (31). Tomkins-Lane and Battie (15) reported moderate positive correlations between walking distance and number of years with back pain and number of years with leg pain. They also reported moderate negative associations between walking capacity and intensity of leg pain before walking, and the items 8 (pain and discomfort over the past week affecting activities) and 15 (pain and discomfort over the past week requiring medication) of the Health Utilities Index Mark 3 (HUI) questionnaire (15). The other two studies did not report significant associations between pain and walking capacity (28, 40).

Disability. Overall, conflicting results were found based on the six studies reporting on the association between disability and walking capacity (distance or time).

Three studies (28, 40, 44) measured disability using the Quebec Back Pain Disability Scale (QBPDS), of which only one showed a strong negative correlation between the total QBPDS score and walking distance (40). When looking at the questionnaire individual subscales, four (walk, reach, run, and groceries) were strongly and negatively correlated with total walking distance and one (stand) was strongly and negatively correlated with walking time to first symptoms.

All four studies using the Swiss Spinal Stenosis Questionnaire found moderate to strong negative correlations with walking capacity (15, 40, 41, 46). Specifically, Drury et al. reported a moderate association between walking distance and the SSSQ total score. Regarding the SSSQ individual subscales, results among the four studies were conflicting. Drury et al. reported moderate to strong negative correlations between walking capacity and the physical function and each component of the symptom subscale (pain, sensory and neuroischemic) (41). Thornes et al. reported a moderate negative correlation between walking capacity and the physical function subscale and Tomkins and Battie reported a moderate negative correlation between walking capacity and the symptom subscale. However, two studies also reported no correlation between walking capacity and some SSSQ subscales (40, 46).

All three studies using the Oswestry Disability Index (ODI) found weak to strong correlations with total walking distance (15, 40, 44). However, Conway et al. reported a non-significant correlation between the ODI and walking capacity regarding time to first symptoms (40).

Quality of Life. Overall, conflicting results were found based on the five studies reporting on the association between quality of life and walking capacity (distance or time) (15, 37, 40, 41, 44).

All three studies reporting on QoL using the 36-item Short Form Health Survey (SF-36) reported at least one significant associations of varying strength with walking distance (37, 40, 41). Of these, one reported a strong positive correlation between SF-36 and walking distance (41). When looking at the questionnaire individual subscales, three studies reported moderate to strong positive correlations between the physical functioning (PF) subscale and walking distance (37, 40, 41). Moreover, Drury et al. (41) reported moderate positive correlations between four of the subscales (role physical, bodily

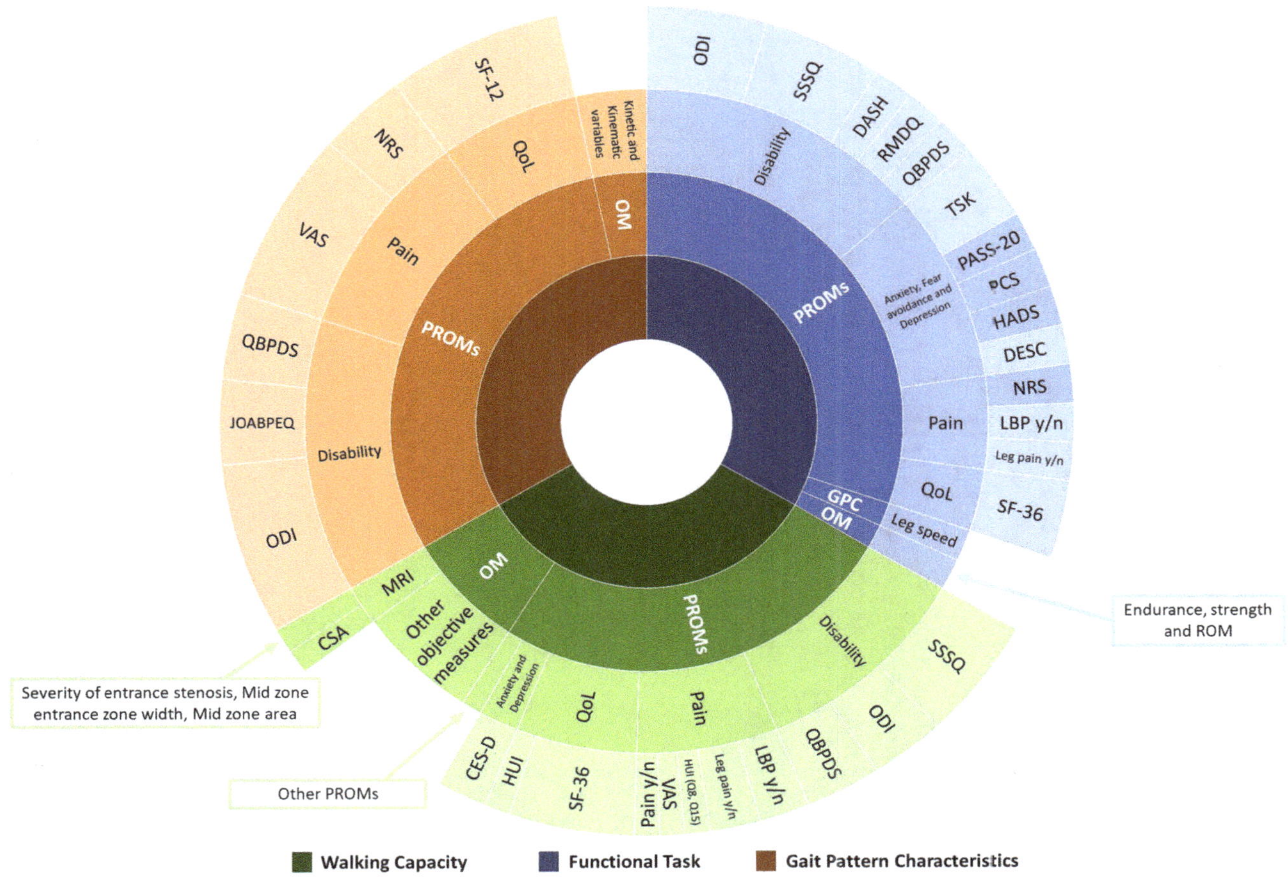

FIGURE 2 | Range and proportion of tools used to assess physical and psychological factors associated with walking capacity, functional task, and gait pattern characteristics. PROMs, Patient-Reported Outcome Measures; OM, Objective Measures; GPC, Gait Pattern Characteristics; QoL, Quality of Life; MRI, Magnetic Resonance Imaging; ODI, Oswestry Disability Index; SSSQ, Swiss Spinal Stenosis Questionnaire; DASH, Disability of the Arm, Shoulder and Hand questionnaire; RMDQ, Roland-Morris Disability Questionnaire; QBPDS, Quebec Back Pain Disability Scale; TSK, Tampa Scale of Kinesiophobia; PASS-20, Pain Anxiety Symptoms Scale; PCS, Pain Catastrophizing Scale; HADS, Hospital Anxiety and Depression Scale; DESC, Rasch-based Depression Screener; NRS, Numeric Rating Scale; LBP, Low Back Pain; SF-36, 36-item Short Form Health Survey; SF-12, Medical Outcomes Short-Form 12; HUI, Health Utilities Index Mark 3; VAS, Visual Analog Scale; CES-D, Center of Epidemiological Studies Depression Scale; CSA, Cross-sectional area; JOABPEQ, Japanese Orthopedic Association Back Pain Evaluation Questionnaire.

pain, general health index and social functioning) and walking distance whereas they reported a weak positive correlation between the vitality subscale and walking distance. Out of the two studies reporting on the association between the mental health subscale and walking distance (37, 41), only one reported a moderate positive correlation (37). One study used a shorter version of the SF-36 (SF-12) and reported no significant association (44). Finally, one study reported a moderate positive correlation between health-related QoL using the HUI questionnaire and walking capacity (15).

Anxiety and Depression. One study assessed depression using the CES-D and reported no significant correlation between depression status and walking distance (19).

Estimated Walking Distance. One study assessed estimated walking distance and showed a strong significant correlation between this estimated and measured walking distances (40).

Objective Outcome Measures

MRI Findings. Overall, conflicting results were found based on the three studies reporting on the association between MRI characteristics and walking capacity (distance or time) (19, 27, 33). One study reported a negative association between the cross-sectional area of the dural tube measured at L1/L2 and walking distance (19). Two studies reported no significant correlation between MRI findings and walking distance (27, 33).

Other Objective Outcome Measures. Overall, conflicting results were found based on the six studies reporting on the association between other objective measures and walking capacity (15, 19, 30, 36, 40). Specifically, one study reported a strong positive correlation between maximum time of continuous activity per day over a 7-day period (at a minimum of low intensity) and walking distance (40), and another study reported a moderate positive correlation between daily step count and walking

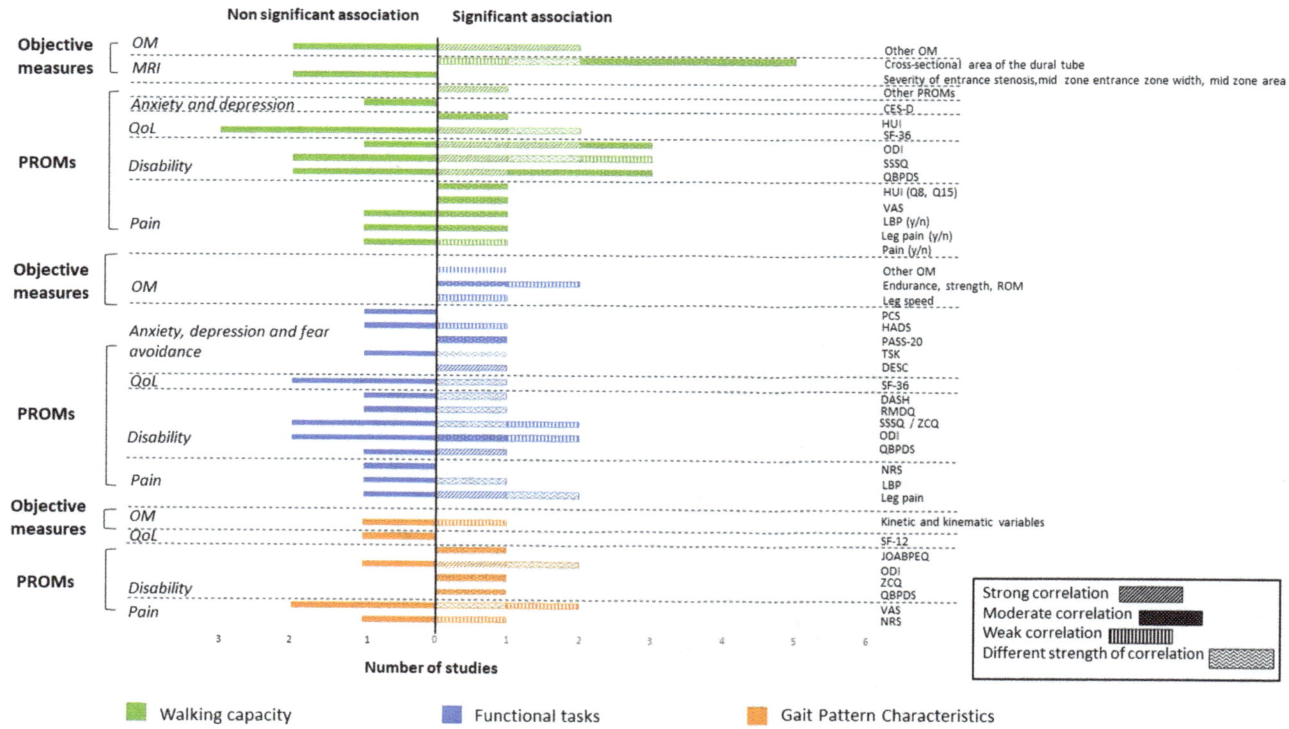

FIGURE 3 | Associations between walking capacity, gait pattern characteristics, functional tasks, and PROMs and objective measures expressed in number of studies. PROMs, Patient-Reported Outcome Measures; OM, Objective Measures; QoL, Quality of Life; MRI, Magnetic Resonance Imaging; CES-D, Center of Epidemiological Studies Depression Scale; HUI, Health Utilities Index Mark 3; SF-36, 36-item Short Form Health Survey; SF-12, Medical Outcomes Short-Form 12; ODI, Oswestry Disability Index; SSSQ, Swiss Spinal Stenosis Questionnaire; ZCQ, Zurich Claudication Questionnaire; QBPDS, Quebec Back Pain Disability Scale; LBP, Low Back Pain; VAS, Visual Analog Scale; ROM, Range of Motion; PASS-20, Pain Anxiety Symptoms Scale; PCS, Pain Catastrophizing Scale; HADS, Hospital Anxiety and Depression Scale; TSK, Tampa Scale of Kinesiophobia; DESC, Rasch-based Depression Screener; DASH, Disability of the Arm, Shoulder and Hand questionnaire; RMDQ, Roland-Morris Disability Questionnaire; NRS, Numeric Rating Scale; JOABPEQ, Japanese Orthopedic Association Back Pain Evaluation Questionnaire.

distance (35). One study showed a moderate negative correlation between balance problems and walking capacity (15). One study reported a negative association between BMI and walking distance, and a positive association between functional status (combination of tests) and walking distance (19). One study reported a strong negative correlation between trunk postural sway and maximum walking distance (36). Two of these studies also showed no significant association between other objectives measures and walking capacity (36, 40). Finally, one study reported a moderate negative correlation between handgrip strength and walking time and a weak positive correlation between handgrip strength and walking distance (30).

Physical and Psychological Factors Associated With Functional Tasks

PROMs

Pain. Overall, conflicting results were found based on the four studies reporting on the association between pain outcomes and functional tasks (31, 35, 38, 40). More specifically, strong positive correlations were found between leg pain severity and overall activity per day measured with an activity monitor, as well as maximum time of continuous activity per day (40).

Pryce et al. reported moderate to strong correlations between back pain (intensity and related function), leg pain (related function), and physical activity (volume and duration). Physical activity intensity was not associated with either back or leg pain intensity and function. They also reported moderate to strong negative correlations between back or leg pain intensity and bout length or maximum bout length of meaningful activity. However, back pain intensity was negatively correlated with bout length and maximum bout length only at meaningful physical activity intensity, while leg pain intensity was only correlated at moderate intensity (between 1.5 and 2.99 METs) (38). All other associations between pain and functional tasks were non-significant (31, 35).

Disability. Overall, conflicting results were found based on the five studies reporting on the association between disability and functional tasks (32, 35, 38, 40, 46, 47).

Conway et al. reported strong negative correlations between disability, measured using the run subscale of the QBPDS questionnaire, and overall activity per day, as well as between disability and time of continuous activity. All other correlations between the QBPDS and functional tasks were not significant (40).

Four studies conducted correlation analyses between the ODI and functional tasks (32, 38, 40, 47). Results from Pryce et al. (38) showed moderate to strong negative correlations between disability and physical activity volume, intensity, and duration. They also showed moderate to strong negative correlations between disability and maximum bout length at meaningful intensity and at moderate intensity during ambulatory behavior. The ODI was only correlated with bout length during ambulatory behavior at moderate intensity. Thornes et al. reported an association between stability in gait and the total ODI score. All other associations between ODI and functional tasks were not significant (32, 40).

The Roland-Morris Disability Questionnaire (RMDQ) was used in the study by Pryce et al. (38) to assess disability. In this study, authors reported moderate to strong negative correlations between disability and physical activity volume, intensity, and duration. They also reported moderate to strong negative correlations between disability and bout length and maximum bout length during ambulatory behavior (38).

Three studies reported on the correlation between the SSSQ [also known as the Zurich Claudication Questionnaire (ZCQ)] total score or subscales and functional tasks (35, 46, 47). The results of Thornes et al. (46) showed negative moderate correlations between the symptoms subscale and the 30-second Sit-to-Stand test, and the One Leg Stance test while they showed a positive moderate correlation between the symptoms subscale and the stair climbing test. The authors also reported a moderate correlation between the physical function subscale and stair climbing (46) and a weak association between the physical function subscale and the score of the Mini-BESTest (47). However, Minetama et al. (35) reported non-significant correlations between daily step count and the symptom subscale or the physical function subscale of the SSSQ.

Finally, Price et al. reported moderate to strong negative correlations between disability measured using the DASH questionnaire and physical activity volume, intensity, and duration, as well as bout length and maximum bout length during ambulatory behavior (38).

Quality of Life. Overall, conflicting results were found based on the two studies reporting on the association between QoL and functional tasks (38).

Pryce et al. reported moderate to strong positive correlations between the SF-36 total score and physical activity (volume, duration, intensity), and ambulatory behavior (bout length and maximum bout length) at both meaningful and moderate intensity (38). Further details about correlations between functional task and all SF-36 subscales are presented in **Supplementary Table 1**.

Depression, Anxiety, and Fear Avoidance. Two studies reported on the association between either depression or fear avoidance and functional tasks (21, 35). Depression was strongly and negatively correlated with the patient's participation in social, daily and work-related activities using the Aachen Activity and Participation Index (AAPI). Depression was also moderately and positively correlated with lower extremity function using the RehaCAT lower extremity subscale and with activities of daily living when using the RehaCAT lower extremity subscale. Minetama et al. (35) reported moderate negative correlations between daily step count and the total score, the cognitive anxiety subscale, the escape/avoidance subscale, and the fear subscale of the Pain Anxiety Symptom Scale (PASS-20). The authors also reported a weak negative correlation between daily step count and depression as measured by the Hospital Anxiety and Depression Scale (HADS) but no correlation with anxiety also measured by the HADS (35).

Furthermore, two studies reported on the association between kinesiophobia and functional tasks (21, 35). The somatic focus subscale of the Tampa Scale of Kinesiophobia (TSK) was strongly and positively correlated with the RehaCAT lower extremity subscale while the activity avoidance subscale was moderately and positively correlated with the RehaCAT lower extremity subscale. The score of the RehaCAT activities of daily living subscale was moderately and positively correlated with the somatic focus and the activity avoidance subscales of the TSK (21). The correlation between daily step count and kinesiophobia was not significant (35).

Finally, one study reported a correlation between daily step count and pain catastrophizing as measured with the Pain Catastrophizing Scale (PCS) (35). However, the correlations between each subscale of the PCS were not significantly correlated with daily step count

Objective Outcome Measures

Other Objective Outcome Measures. Two studies reported on the associations between other objective measures and functional tasks performance. Schmidt et al. (39) reported weak associations between either trunk extensor muscle endurance, leg strength asymmetry, or leg speed during a leg press and the Short Physical Performance Battery score. They also reported weak associations between either trunk extensor muscle endurance, knee flexion ROM, or knee extension strength asymmetry and the Habitual Gait Speed test, and a weak association between leg strength and the Chair Stand test (39). Finally, one study reported a moderate negative correlation between handgrip strength and walking steps (30).

Physical and Psychological Factors Associated With Gait Pattern Characteristics

PROMs

Pain Severity. Overall, conflicting results were found based on the three studies reporting on the association between pain severity and gait pattern characteristics (29, 34, 43). To assess pain severity, one study used the 11-point Numeric Rating Scale (NRS) and two studies used a Visual Analog Scale (VAS) (29, 34, 43). Only back pain, measured using the NRS, was weakly and positively correlated to walking velocity (29). Regarding leg pain, Kuwahara et al. (34) reported a moderate negative correlation between leg pain and peak trunk tilt during walking (34). Other significant correlations were reported between pain severity (location unspecified) and width of base of support, the Gait Disability Index (GDI), peak lumbar tilt pre- and post-walking, and changes in pelvis tilt variation during stance (43). All other gait pattern characteristics measured in these studies were non-significant.

Disability. Overall, conflicting results were found based on the three studies reporting on the association between disability and gait pattern characteristics (29, 42, 44).

Out of two studies using the ODI to assess disability (29, 44), one study reported strong positive correlations between disability and gait velocity and step length, as well as a weak positive correlation between disability and base of support (29). The same authors also reported that other gait pattern characteristics such as cadence, lumbar proprioception (except for left lateral bending) and ROM were not correlated with the ODI score. The second study reported a strong correlation between disability and free walking speed (44).

One study reported a moderate correlation between disability, measured using the QBPDS, and free walking speed (44).

Finally, one study reported weak positive associations between disability, measured using the JOABPED total score or its individual subscales, and short stride when walking (42).

Quality of Life. One study reported non-significant correlations between QoL using the SF-12 and gait pattern characteristics (29).

Objective Outcome Measures

Other Objective Outcome Measures. One study reported weak positive correlations between anterior trunk flexion angle during walking and step length as well as maximum ankle plantar flexion moment (45).

DISCUSSION

This systematic scoping review explored the current state of scientific knowledge regarding the associations between physical or psychological factors and walking capacity in patients with LSS. Results show that physical factors are more commonly studied than psychological factors with 22 studies reporting on physical factors and 3 reporting on psychological factors. The systematic scoping review highlighted the use of a wide range of PROMs and objective measures, with disability being the most frequently reported outcome measure followed by pain. Among objective measures, reported tools were heterogenous with most used in no more than one study. A third outcome category (gait pattern characteristics) was added following data extraction given that no study directly assessed gait pattern characteristics in relation to walking capacity. Considering the impact of gait pattern characteristics on decreased walking capacity, associations between physical or psychological factors and gait pattern characteristics were reported. Results among studies were conflicting regarding associations between PROMs and either walking capacity, functional tasks, or gait pattern characteristics. Results were also conflicting for associations between objective measures and either walking capacity, functional tasks, or gait pattern characteristics. Some outcome measures, however, were clearly associated with several measures related to walking capacity. For instance, walking capacity was significantly associated with pain outcomes, disability, estimated walking distance, and cross-sectional area of the dural tube in the lumbar spine L1/L2. Among the included studies, functional tasks were associated with physical factors such as lower back and upper limb disability, and lower limb endurance, strength, ROM, and speed. Strong significant correlations were also found between gait pattern characteristics (speed and stride) and disability outcomes. These results clearly highlight the intricate and heterogeneous presentation of symptomatic LSS.

Conflicting results can possibly be explained by the heterogeneity of walking capacity tests used across studies. Most tests were not validated in people with symptomatic LSS (28, 31–33, 36, 41, 44, 46), although a few were validated in elderly individuals (31, 32, 44). Out of nine walking tests, only four (Self-Pace walking tests, Shuttle walking test, Treadmill walking test and 6-meter walking test) were validated and/or reliable specifically for patients with LSS (see **Supplement Material 5** for further details). Further studies are needed to assess the validity of commonly used walking tests in patients with symptomatic LSS. Validated walking test for patient with LSS should be used to better understand walking limitations caused by LSS.

The most commonly reported psychological factor was depression and results were conflicting. The Rasch-based Depression Screener (DESC) and PASS-20 questionnaire were associated with decreased performance in functional tasks. Other psychological factors including anxiety, depression and kinesiophobia were either not associated or showed conflicting evidence of association with walking capacity, functional tasks, or gait pattern characteristics. A comprehensive assessment of walking capacity combined with a better knowledge of the physical and psychological factors associated with walking capacity will help health care professionals identified targeted rehabilitation strategies.

The present systematic scoping review highlighted conflicting results among studies reporting on the association between PROMs or objectives measures and measures related to walking capacity (i.e., walking capacity, functional tasks, and gait pattern characteristics). The wide range of questionnaires used to assess the same outcome could also explain some of these conflicting results. For instance, disability was reported using 6 different questionnaires, with only one being specifically validated for LSS (the SSSQ). Low back pain and/or leg pain were also reported among studies using different tools (presence or absence thereof, VAS, NRS, or HUI). The most commonly reported QoL questionnaire used was the SF-36. However, its association with walking capacity and functional tasks was unclear. On the other hand, the HUI, also used to assess QoL, was associated with greater walking capacity. Objective measures were all different across studies and such heterogeneity impeded our ability to determine whether specific outcome measures are related to walking capacity in patients with LSS. In addition, no study specifically assessed gait pattern characteristics such as stride, walking phases, or walking velocity in relation to walking distance or walking time. It seems important to evaluate these characteristics in order to establish if deviations from normal gait pattern are present in patients with symptomatic LSS. Knowing that risk of fall is increased in populations with mobility impairment (32), a better understanding of walking gait characteristics that can modify walking capacity is needed to know if these walking parameters can also contribute to an increased risk of fall. As such, slower walking speed seems to be related to increased fear of falling (48). Given that some changes in gait pattern normally occur with aging, it is important to know if additional changes are brought on by symptomatic LSS.

Another possible explanation for the conflicting results is the lack of a clear definition for LSS in the studies. Diagnostic ascertainment for inclusion of participants was not clearly mentioned in some studies. Furthermore, many studies reported only the range of included LSS subtypes among participant instead of providing the exact number of individuals per subtype. They also did not clearly describe affected levels.

Clinical Implications

For clinicians, understanding which walking parameters are modified in patients with LSS would provide new insights on the consequences brought on by LSS on gait. If any of these parameters are identified as associated factors, clinicians will be able to establish a treatment plan and monitor clinical evolution more closely over time. Clinicians are also aware that the patient's psychological state can have an impact on the prognosis of musculoskeletal disorders. For instance, patients with LSS reporting depression or at high risk of developing depression show poorer outcomes over time (49). However, more studies are needed to inform the possible implications of psychological status on walking-related functions in patients with LSS.

The Self-Paced Walking Test (SPWT) was the most used test to assessed walking capacity in patients with LSS and was the only reliable and validated one for this specific population. Results from the present systematic scoping review suggest that subjective evaluation tools such as the SSSQ and ODI were the disability-related questionnaires the most used and for which there were many significant associations with the three domains (walking capacity, functional tasks, and gait pattern characteristics). Regarding QoL, the most used questionnaire was the SF-36 but results were conflicting across studies. MRI findings (cross-sectional area) were associated with walking capacity. Regarding objective measures and psychological factors, current evidence suggests that further studies are needed to be able to better formulate recommendations for clinicians. Exploring other biomechanical walking parameters such as minimal toe clearance, speed, simple and double stance and step width can be interesting indicators to consider when assessing walking capacity in future studies.

Strengths and Limitations

To our knowledge, this is the first systematic scoping review to assess physical and psychological factors associated with walking capacity in patients with LSS. One strength of this review is that every step was consistent with the current standards for conducting a systematic scoping review (24, 25). It is not, however, without limitation. The first limitation of our study was the low number of studies that provided a direct evaluation of walking capacity. Only studies published in English, French or Spanish were considered for this scoping review. We cannot rule-out that additional relevant evidence may have been published in other languages. Moreover, most of the studies did not specify the level and location of the LSS limiting the clinical interpretation of the results with regards to distinction of LSS subtypes.

CONCLUSION

The present systematic scoping review allowed to identify physical and psychological factors that are associated with walking capacity in patients with symptomatic LSS. However, a large number of associations reported between walking capacity and physical or psychological factors were conflicting especially when correlated directly with the assessment of walking capacity.

AUTHOR CONTRIBUTIONS

MH was the principal investigator of this scoping review, participated in the study design, literature search, data extraction, results formatting, and as well as the manuscript writing. JBD participated in the data extraction and results formatting. AAM and MD participated in the study design, overall supervision of the project, and manuscript writing and revision. AAM was also involved in the screening process as the third person to obtain consensus (sorting and quality rating). All authors read and approved the final manuscript.

FUNDING

The study was funded by the Chaire de recherche internationale en santé neuromusculosquelettique and its partner the Centre intégré universitaire de santé et de services sociaux de la Mauricie-et-du-Centre-du-Québec.

ACKNOWLEDGMENTS

Thanks to the laboratory assistant Marie-Élisabeth Roy-Poulin for her help at different stages of the screening process.

REFERENCES

1. Ammendolia C, Côté P, Southerst D, Schneider M, Budgell B, Bombardier C, et al. Comprehensive nonsurgical treatment versus self-directed care to improve walking ability in lumbar spinal stenosis: a randomized trial. *Arch Phys Med Rehabil.* (2018) 99:2408–19 e2. doi: 10.1016/j.apmr.2018.05.014
2. Budithi S, Dhawan R, Cattell A, Balain B, Jaffray D. Only walking matters-assessment following lumbar stenosis decompression. *Eur Spine J.* (2017) 26:481–7. doi: 10.1007/s00586-016-4881-x
3. Kobayashi S. Pathophysiology, diagnosis and treatment of intermittent claudication in patients with lumbar canal stenosis. *World J Orthop.* (2014) 5:134–45. doi: 10.5312/wjo.v5.i2.134
4. Hartvigsen J, Hancock MJ, Kongsted A, Louw Q, Ferreira ML, Genevay S, et al. What low back pain is and why we need to pay attention. *Lancet.* (2018) 391:2356–67. doi: 10.1016/S0140-6736(18)30480-X
5. Kalichman L, Cole R, Kim DH, Li L, Suri P, Guermazi A, et al. Spinal stenosis prevalence and association with symptoms: the Framingham Study. *Spine J.* (2009) 9:545–50. doi: 10.1016/j.spinee.2009.03.005
6. Jensen RK, Jensen TS, Koes B, Hartvigsen J. Prevalence of lumbar spinal stenosis in general and clinical populations: a systematic review and meta-analysis. *Eur Spine J.* (2020) 29:2143–63. doi: 10.1007/s00586-020-06339-1
7. Comer CM, Redmond AC, Bird HA, Conaghan PG. Assessment and management of neurogenic claudication associated with lumbar spinal stenosis in a UK primary care musculoskeletal service: a survey of current practice among physiotherapists. *BMC Musculoskelet Disord.* (2009) 10:121. doi: 10.1186/1471-2474-10-121
8. Genevay S, Atlas SJ. Lumbar spinal stenosis. *Best Pract Res Clin Rheumatol.* (2010) 24:253–65. doi: 10.1016/j.berh.2009.11.001
9. Singh K, Samartzis D, Vaccaro AR, Nassr A, Andersson GB, Yoon ST, et al. Congenital lumbar spinal stenosis: a prospective, control-matched, cohort radiographic analysis. *Spine J.* (2005) 5:615–22. doi: 10.1016/j.spinee.2005.05.385
10. Lurie J, Tomkins-Lane C. Management of lumbar spinal stenosis. *BMJ.* (2016) 352:h6234. doi: 10.1136/bmj.h6234
11. Tomkins-Lane C, Melloh M, Wong A. Diagnostic tests in the clinical diagnosis of lumbar spinal stenosis: consensus and results of an International Delphi Study. *Europ Spine J.* (2020) 29:2188–97. doi: 10.1007/s00586-020-06481-w
12. Tomkins-Lane CC, Holz SC, Yamakawa KS, Phalke VV, Quint DJ, Miner J, et al. Predictors of walking performance and walking capacity in people with lumbar spinal stenosis, low back pain, and asymptomatic controls. *Arch Phys Med Rehabil.* (2012) 93:647–53. doi: 10.1016/j.apmr.2011.09.023
13. Williamson E, Ward L, Vadher K, Dutton SJ, Parker B, Petrou S, et al. Better Outcomes for Older people with Spinal Trouble (BOOST) trial: a randomised controlled trial of a combined physical and psychological intervention for older adults with neurogenic claudication, a protocol. *BMJ Open.* (2018) 8:e022205. doi: 10.1136/bmjopen-2018-022205
14. Barz T, Melloh M, Staub L, Roeder C, Lange J, Smiszek F-G, et al. The diagnostic value of a treadmill test in predicting lumbar spinal stenosis. *Europ Spine J.* (2008) 17:686–90. doi: 10.1007/s00586-008-0593-1
15. Tomkins-Lane CC, Battie MC. Predictors of objectively measured walking capacity in people with degenerative lumbar spinal stenosis. *J Back Musculoskelet Rehabil.* (2013) 26:345–52. doi: 10.3233/BMR-130390
16. Ammendolia C, Côté P, Rampersaud YR, Southerst D, Budgell B, Bombardier C, et al. The boot camp program for lumbar spinal stenosis: a protocol for a randomized controlled trial. *Chiropr Man Therap.* (2016) 24:25. doi: 10.1186/s12998-016-0106-y
17. Marchand AA, Suitner M, O'Shaughnessy J, Chatillon CE, Cantin V, Descarreaux M. Feasibility of conducting an active exercise prehabilitation program in patients awaiting spinal stenosis surgery: a randomized pilot study. *Sci Rep.* (2019) 9:12257. doi: 10.1038/s41598-019-48736-7
18. Rainville J, Childs LA, Peña EB, Suri P, Limke JC, Jouve C, et al. Quantification of walking ability in subjects with neurogenic claudication from lumbar spinal stenosis–a comparative study. *Spine J.* (2012) 12:101–9. doi: 10.1016/j.spinee.2011.12.006
19. Zeifang F, Schiltenwolf M, Abel R, Moradi B. Gait analysis does not correlate with clinical and MR imaging parameters in patients with symptomatic lumbar spinal stenosis. *BMC Musculoskelet Disord.* (2008) 9:89. doi: 10.1186/1471-2474-9-89
20. Takenaka H, Sugiura H, Kamiya M, Nishihama K, Ito A, Suzuki J, et al. Predictors of walking ability after surgery for lumbar spinal canal stenosis: a prospective study. *Spine J.* (2019) 19:1824–31. doi: 10.1016/j.spinee.2019.07.002
21. Quack V, Boecker M, Mueller C, Mainz V, Geiger M, Heinemann A, et al. Psychological factors outmatched morphological markers in predicting limitations in activities of daily living and participation in patients with lumbar stenosis. *BMC Musculoskelet Disord.* (2019) 20:1–9. doi: 10.1186/s12891-019-2918-0
22. Mullen SP, McAuley E, Satariano WA, Kealey M, Prohaska TR. Physical activity and functional limitations in older adults: the influence of self-efficacy and functional performance. *J Gerontol B Psychol Sci Soc Sci.* (2012) 67:354–61. doi: 10.1093/geronb/gbs036
23. Ammendolia C, Schneider M, Williams K, Zickmund S, Hamm M, Stuber K, et al. The physical and psychological impact of neurogenic claudication: the patients' perspectives. *J Can Chiropr Assoc.* (2017) 61:18–31.
24. Peters MD, Godfrey CM, Khalil H, McInerney P, Parker D, Soares CB. Guidance for conducting systematic scoping reviews. *Int J Evidence-Based Healthcare.* (2015) 13:141–6. doi: 10.1097/XEB.0000000000000050
25. Levac D, Colquhoun H, O'Brien KK. Scoping studies: advancing the methodology. *Implement Sci.* (2010) 5:69. doi: 10.1186/1748-5908-5-69
26. Downes MJ, Brennan ML, Williams HC, Dean RS. Development of a critical appraisal tool to assess the quality of cross-sectional studies (AXIS). *BMJ Open.* (2016) 6:e011458. doi: 10.1136/bmjopen-2016-011458
27. Sigmundsson FG, Kang XP, Jönsson B, Strömqvist B. Correlation between disability and MRI findings in lumbar spinal stenosis: a prospective study of 109 patients operated on by decompression. *Acta Orthopaed.* (2011) 82:204–10. doi: 10.3109/17453674.2011.566150
28. Tong HC, Haig AJ, Geisser ME, Yamakawa KS, Miner JA. Comparing pain severity and functional status of older adults without spinal symptoms, with lumbar spinal stenosis, and with axial low back pain. *Gerontology.* (2007) 53:111–5. doi: 10.1159/000096861
29. Conrad BP, Shokat MS, Abbasi AZ, Vincent HK, Seay A, Kennedy DJ. Associations of self-report measures with gait, range of motion and proprioception in patients with lumbar spinal stenosis. *Gait Posture.* (2013) 38:987–92. doi: 10.1016/j.gaitpost.2013.05.010
30. Inoue H, Watanabe H, Okami H, Shiraishi Y, Kimura A, Takeshita K. Handgrip strength correlates with walking in lumbar spinal stenosis. *Eur Spine J.* (2020) 29:2198–204. doi: 10.1007/s00586-020-06525-1
31. Ishimoto Y, Yoshimura N, Muraki S, Yamada H, Nagata K, Hashizume H, et al. Prevalence of symptomatic lumbar spinal stenosis and its association with physical performance in a population-based cohort in Japan: the Wakayama Spine Study. *Osteoarthritis Cartilage.* (2012) 20:1103–8. doi: 10.1016/j.joca.2012.06.018
32. Kim H-J, Chun H-J, Han C-D, Moon S-H, Kang K-T, Kim H-S, et al. The risk assessment of a fall in patients with lumbar spinal stenosis. *Spine.* (2011) 36:E588–E92. doi: 10.1097/BRS.0b013e3181f92d8e
33. Kuittinen P, Sipola P, Aalto TJ, Määttä S, Parviainen A, Saari T, et al. Correlation of lateral stenosis in MRI with symptoms, walking capacity and EMG findings in patients with surgically confirmed lateral lumbar spinal canal stenosis. *BMC Musculoskelet Disord.* (2014) 15:247. doi: 10.1186/1471-2474-15-247
34. Kuwahara W, Kurumadani H, Tanaka N, Nakanishi K, Nakamura H, Ishii Y, et al. Correlation between spinal and pelvic movements during gait and aggravation of low back pain by gait loading in lumbar spinal stenosis patients. *J Orthopaed Sci.* (2019) 24:207–13. doi: 10.1016/j.jos.2018.09.002
35. Minetama M, Kawakami M, Teraguchi M, Kagotani R, Mera Y, Sumiya T, et al. Associations between psychological factors and daily step count in patients with lumbar spinal stenosis. *Physiother Theory Pract.* (2020). doi: 10.1080/09593985.2020.1855685. [Epub ahead of print].
36. Nagai K, Aoyama T, Yamada M, Izeki M, Fujibayashi S, Takemoto M, et al. Quantification of changes in gait characteristics associated with intermittent claudication in patients with lumbar spinal stenosis. *J Spinal Disord Tech.* (2014) 27:E136–42. doi: 10.1097/BSD.0b013e3182a2656b
37. Özdemir E, Paker N, Bugdayci D, Tekdos DD. Quality of life and related factors in degenerative lumbar spinal stenosis: a controlled study. *J Back Musculoskelet Rehabil.* (2015) 28:749–53. doi: 10.3233/BMR-140578

38. Pryce R, Johnson M, Goytan M, Passmore S, Berrington N, Kriellaars D. Relationship between ambulatory performance and self-rated disability in patients with lumbar spinal stenosis. *Spine.* (2012) 37:1316–23. doi: 10.1097/BRS.0b013e31824a8314
39. Schmidt CT, Ward RE, Suri P, Kiely DK, Ni P, Anderson DE, et al. Association of neuromuscular attributes with performance-based mobility among community-dwelling older adults with symptomatic lumbar spinal stenosis. *Arch Phys Med Rehabil.* (2017) 98:1400–6. doi: 10.1016/j.apmr.2017.02.028
40. Conway J, Tomkins CC, Haig AJ. Walking assessment in people with lumbar spinal stenosis: capacity, performance, and self-report measures. *Spine J.* (2011) 11:816–23. doi: 10.1016/j.spinee.2010.10.019
41. Drury T, Ames SE, Costi K, Beynnon B, Hall J. Degenerative spondylolisthesis in patients with neurogenic claudication effects functional performance and self-reported quality of life. *Spine.* (2009) 34:2812–7. doi: 10.1097/BRS.0b013e3181b4836e
42. Fujita N, Sakurai A, Miyamoto A, Michikawa T, Otaka Y, Suzuki S, et al. Stride length of elderly patients with lumbar spinal stenosis: multi-center study using the Two-Step test. *J Orthopaed Sci.* (2019) 24:787–92. doi: 10.1016/j.jos.2019.01.006
43. Garbelotti SA Jr, Lucareli PRG, Ramalho A Jr, de Godoy W, Bernal M, Greve JMDA. An investigation of the value of tridimensional kinematic analysis in functional diagnosis of lumbar spinal stenosis. *Gait Posture.* (2014) 40:150–3. doi: 10.1016/j.gaitpost.2014.03.013
44. Grelat M, Gouteron A, Casillas J-M, Orliac B, Beaurain J, Fournel I, et al. Walking speed as an alternative measure of functional status in patients with lumbar spinal stenosis. *World Neurosurg.* (2019) 122:e591–e7. doi: 10.1016/j.wneu.2018.10.109
45. Igawa T, Katsuhira J, Hosaka A, Uchikoshi K, Ishihara S, Matsudaira K. Kinetic and kinematic variables affecting trunk flexion during level walking in patients with lumbar spinal stenosis. *PLoS ONE.* (2018) 13:e0197228. doi: 10.1371/journal.pone.0197228
46. Thornes E, Robinson HS, Vøllestad NK. Degenerative lumbar spinal stenosis and physical functioning: an exploration of associations between self-reported measures and physical performance tests. *Disabil Rehabil.* (2018) 40:232–7. doi: 10.1080/09638288.2016.1250123
47. Thornes E, Robinson HS, Vøllestad NK. Dynamic balance in patients with degenerative lumbar spinal stenosis; a cross-sectional study. *BMC Musculoskelet Disord.* (2018) 19:192. doi: 10.1186/s12891-018-2111-x
48. Chamberlin ME, Fulwider BD, Sanders SL, Medeiros JM. Does fear of falling influence spatial and temporal gait parameters in elderly persons beyond changes associated with normal aging? *J Gerontol A Biol Sci Med Sci.* (2005) 60:1163–7. doi: 10.1093/gerona/60.9.1163
49. Hébert JJ, Abraham E, Wedderkopp N, Bigney E, Richardson E, Darling M, et al. Preoperative factors predict postoperative trajectories of pain and disability following surgery for degenerative lumbar spinal stenosis. *Spine.* (2020) 45:E1421–30. doi: 10.1097/BRS.0000000000003587

17

APAs Constraints to Voluntary Movements: The Case for Limb Movements Coupling

Fausto G. Baldissera[1]* *and Luigi Tesio*[2, 3]*

[1] Retired, Milan, Italy, [2] Department of Biomedical Sciences for Health, Università degli Studi di Milano, Milan, Italy,
[3] Department of Neuro-Rehabilitation Sciences, Istituto Auxologico Italiano-IRCCS, Milan, Italy

Correspondence:
Fausto G. Baldissera
fausto.baldissera@unimi.it
Luigi Tesio
luigi.tesio@unimi.it

When rhythmically moving two limbs in either the same or in opposite directions, one coupling mode meets constraints that are absent in the other mode. Isodirectional (ISO) flexion-extensions of the ipsilateral hand and foot can be easily performed with either the hand prone or supine. Instead, antidirectional (ANTI) movements require attentive effort and irresistibly tend to reverse into ISO when frequency increases. Experimental evidence indicates that the direction dependent easy-difficult dichotomy is caused by interference of the anticipatory postural commands associated to movements of one limb with voluntary commands to the other limb. Excitability of the resting wrist muscles is subliminally modulated at the period of ipsilateral foot oscillations, being phase-opposite in the antagonists and distributed so as to facilitate ISO and obstacle ANTI coupling of the hand (either prone or supine) with the foot. Modulation is driven by cortical signals dispatched to the forearm simultaneously with the voluntary commands moving the foot. If right foot oscillations are performed when standing on the left foot with the right hand touching a fixed support, the subliminal excitability modulation is replaced by overt contractions of forearm muscles conforming the APAs features. This suggests that during hand-foot ANTI coupling the voluntary commands to forearm muscles are contrasted by APAs commands of opposite sign linked to foot oscillations. Correlation between the easy-difficult dichotomy and the APAs distribution is also found in coupled adduction-abduction of the arms or hands in the transverse plane and in coupled flexion-extension of the arms in the parasagittal plane. In all these movements, APAs commands linked to the movement of each limb reach the motor pathways to the contralateral muscles homologous to the prime movers and can interfere during coupling with their voluntary activation. APAs are also generated in postural muscles of trunk and lower limbs and size-increase when the movement frequency is incremented. The related increase in postural effort apparently contributes in destabilizing the difficult coupling mode. Motor learning may rely upon more effective APAs. APAs and focal contraction are entangled within the same voluntary action. Yet, neural diseases may selectively impair APAs, which represent a potential target for rehabilitation.

Keywords: APAs, limb movements coupling, in phase and antiphase coupling, direction principle, APAs destabilizing effects on coupling, coupled movements synchronization, motor learning/training

INTRODUCTION

This review is concerned with a so far neglected aspect of the interaction between Anticipatory Postural Adjustments, APAs, and voluntary movements. Beside the APAs main function of assisting the execution of voluntary movements of any particular body segment, under defined circumstances APAs may result in the impairment of body movements. In particular, this occurs during coupled movements of the limbs and is especially apparent in rhythmic cyclic movements.

In many gestures of everyday life, e.g., handiworks, sport activities or music playing, the voluntary movements of different limb segments may be coupled into a variety of combinations. It is common experience that when oscillating a given couple of limbs in either the same or in opposite directions (in external coordinates), movements are easily performed in one coupling mode whereas coupling in the other mode is hampered. The evidence summarized here strongly suggests that the constraints selectively hindering one specific coupling mode, either the iso- or the antidirectional one, are generated by the APAs associated with the same voluntary limb movements.

The review is structured as follows. Sections *The "Direction Principle" in Coupling Flexion-Extension of the Ipsilateral Hand and Foot. Easy vs. Difficult Coupling Modes* and *Role of Kinesthetic Afferents from the Moving Segments in Controlling the Hand-Foot Synchronism during Coupled Movements: An Interlimb or Intralimb Feedback?* will describe the features of the hand-foot coupled movements and the mechanisms providing the control of movements synchronization. In turn, Sections *Neural Mechanisms Underlying the "Direction Principle" in Hand-Foot Coupling* and *Role of APAs in Differentiating ISO vs. ANTI Coupling Modes in Other Types of Limb Movements* will discuss experimental evidence of the selective APAs effects on coupling coordination in the above as well as in other couples of limbs. Section *Postural Constraints from Neuroscience to Sports and Rehabilitation Medicine* will discuss some potential implications of this knowledge in motor learning, force training, and rehabilitation.

Direction-Dependent Differential Coordination of Coupled Movements of the Limbs

The early observations on limb movements coupling [Müller, 1840; Meige, 1901; Noica (Bucarest), 1912] report that, when performing mirror movements like drawing circles in the air with the two hands in the parasagittal plane, it is quite easy to rotate the hands in the same direction, whereas circling the hands in opposite directions is difficult or even impossible.

For several decades this phenomenon did not attract further interest. On occasion of a seminar held by the first author over 30 years ago, Pietro Civaschi, a physiatrist at the Neurological Institute Carlo Besta in Milan, asked for some explanation about the striking preference of normal individuals to move two ipsilateral body segments together (for instance, the ipsilateral hand and foot in the parasagittal plane) in the same rather than in opposite directions. Having no explanation at that moment, the answer was to analyze the matter together, in the hope of gaining a deeper insight.

This review will summarize the results of the experimental series stemmed from that proposal. The successive steps of this research entered different fields of motor neurosciences and were reported in an irregular series of separate papers. Because of the time dispersion of the reports and the variety of methodological and conceptual approaches utilized, it seemed convenient to facilitate the interested reader by tracing in one review the logic route connecting the successive experiments, interpretations and hypotheses.

Three different combinations of coupled limb movements were studied (**Figure 1**): (1) coupled flexion-extension of ipsilateral hand and foot in the parasagittal plane; (2) coupled

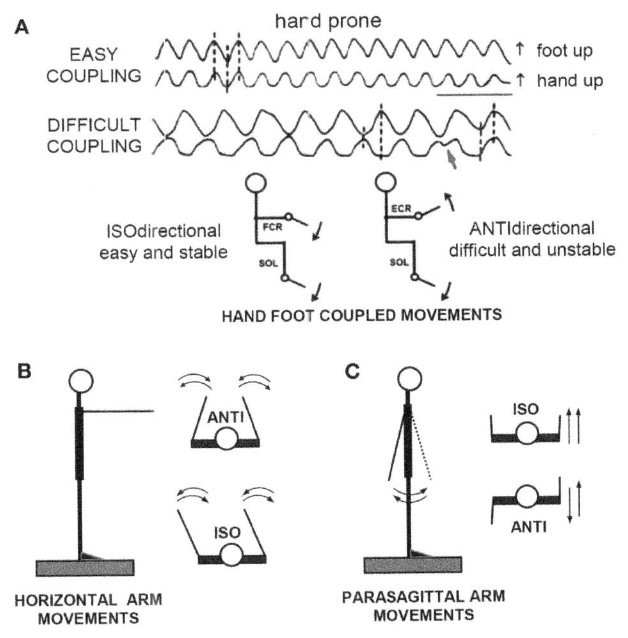

FIGURE 1 | The "direction principle" in hand-foot coupling. (A) Subjects seated on an armchair, with the forearms supported in horizontal position, either prone, or supine. The right hand and foot were fixed to basculating supports, free to cover full-range flexion-extensions of the wrist and ankle. Despite their lower frequency, the ANTIdirectional (difficult) oscillations spontaneously reverse (blue arrow) to the easier ISOdirectional coupling. Time calibration, 1 s. **(B,C)** Schematic illustration of ISO and ANTI coupling of the arm cyclic movements in the horizontal and parasagittal plane, respectively. Reproduced from Baldissera et al. (1982) © Elsevier 1982, with permission of Elsevier.

Abbreviations: Muscles: ECR, Extensor Carpi Radialis; FCR, Flexor Carpi Radialis; RPM, right Pectoralis Major; LPM, left Pectoralis Major; LFCR, right Infraspinatus; LIS, left Infraspinatus; RAD, right Anterior Deltoid; LAD, left Anterior Deltoid; RPD, right Posterior Deltoid; RLD, right Latissimus Dorsi; LPD, left Latissimus Dorsi; RES, right Erector Spinae; LES, left Erector Spinae; RIC, right Ischiocruralis; LIC, left Ischiocruralis; SOL, Soleus; TA, Tibialis Anterior. Neurophysiologic and mechanical variables: CMAPs, Compound Muscle Action Potentials; TMS, Transcranial Magnetic Stimulation; CoP, Center of Pressure; $\Delta\dot{V}O_2$, oxygen uptake; $\Delta\Phi$, interlimb relative phase; SD$\Delta\Phi$, Standard Deviation of the $\Delta\Phi$ variability.

adduction-abduction movements of the arms in the horizontal (transverse) plane and (3) coupled flexion-extension movements of the arms in the parasagittal plane.

The preferred coupling mode is isodirectional in movement types 1 and 3, and antidirectional in type 2. Substantial evidence was found that in all three movement types the direction-dependent dichotomy between preferred and non-preferred modes correlates with the distribution of the Anticipatory Postural Adjustments associated with the same movements.

For methodological, technical, and statistical details the original papers should be consulted.

THE "DIRECTION PRINCIPLE" IN COUPLING FLEXION-EXTENSION OF THE IPSILATERAL HAND AND FOOT. EASY vs. DIFFICULT COUPLING MODES

When asked to perform simultaneous rhythmic flexions-extension movements of the extremities in the parasagittal plane, in the way they feel the most easy and spontaneous, all subjects normally choose to keep the forearm prone and to rotate the extremities in the same angular direction[1] (isodirectional coupling, ISO), by synchronizing hand extension with foot dorsal flexion and hand flexion with foot plantar flexion (**Figure 1A**, uppermost traces).

If asked to increase the oscillations rate, all subjects are able to maintain the ISO coupling for more than 1 min even at the maximal possible rate (3–4 Hz). When requested to reverse the phase between the limbs (antidirectional coupling, ANTI, lower traces), the subjects generally stop briefly, restore the movements with some initial hesitation and/or errors, and are afterwards compelled to pay continuous attention to maintain the phase opposition. Any attention release, as well as any attempt to increase the movement frequency, eventually leads to a breaking point, beyond which the association reverses to the isodirectional pattern (blue arrow). Transitions is abrupt or preceded by a progressive shift of the interlimb phase difference, and occurs after a time that progressively shortens as the movement frequency increases: continuing for more than 10 s is impossible beyond a critical frequency that ranges between 1.2 and 2.5 Hz in different individuals.

Finally, when invited to repeat the task with the hand supine, all subjects confirm their preference for ISO coupling, now associating hand flexion to foot dorsal flexion and hand extension to foot plantar flexion. The determinant factor of coupling preference seems therefore to be the movements reciprocal direction (*direction principle*, Baldissera et al., 1982) and not a stable pattern of parallel innervation of specific muscles in the forearm and the leg.

Coupling Coordination: Accuracy and Stability of the Interlimb Relative Phase

In the following years studies on limb coupled movements increased in number and the "direction principle" was found to hold in many other types of coupled movements of ipsilateral limbs (cfr Baldissera et al., 1982, 1991, 1994, 2000; Baldissera and Cavallari, 2001; Kelso and Jeka, 1992; Carson et al., 1995; Jeka and Kelso, 1995; Swinnen et al., 1995; Serrien and Swinnen, 1998), bilateral limbs (cfr. Kelso, 1984; Carson, 1993; Swinnen et al., 1995; Serrien and Swinnen, 1998; Swinnen, 2002) and also different segments within one limb (for instance flexion-extension of the wrist with flexion-extension of the elbow, as earlier recognized by Kots et al., 1971). As a general rule, one given coupling mode, in some occasions ISO and in others ANTI, is easily performed, subjectively preferred and better co-ordinated; whereas the opposite mode is difficult to perform (thus, non-preferred) and less coordinated. *Easy* and *preferred*, as well as *difficult* and *non-preferred* will be used hereafter as synonyms.

Kelso's theoretical elaboration (Haken et al., 1985, see Presentation 1 in the Supplementary Material) assimilates the coupled oscillations of two limbs to those of a system of non-linear oscillators moving in one of two stable states (in phase or in phase opposition) with different levels of stability. This model stresses the centrality of the *interlimb relative phase*, $\Delta\Phi$, as being the collective variable that describes the qualitative changes in pattern coordination. In real movements the $\Delta\Phi$ variability, i.e., the coupling instability, is expressed by its standard deviation, SD$\Delta\Phi$. The latter is positively related to the oscillation frequency and it is higher in the difficult (non-preferred) compared to the easy (preferred) coupling mode. Based on this observation, when the movement frequency, and thus SD$\Delta\Phi$, reaches to a critical level, the model shifts by 180° from the unstable to the stable state. Accordingly, the values of SD$\Delta\Phi$ indicate for each value of the movement frequency the degree of coupling instability, and thus the difficulty in contrasting the phase reversal.

Mechanical Differences between the Limbs and Neural Compensation for Their Desynchronizing Effect on Coupled Movements

In order to understand the mechanistic origin of the differences in coordination stability between the two coupling modes, two interlaced aspects needed to be analyzed. First, how synchronization between the limbs is achieved and how this is influenced by the limb mechanical properties; second, why the interlimb coordination varies when the coupling mode is reversed. A response to the first question is proposed in Section *Role of Kinesthetic Afferents from the Moving Segments in Controlling the Hand-Foot Synchronism during Coupled Movements: An Interlimb or Intralimb Feedback?*. In Sections *Neural Mechanisms Underlying the "Direction Principle" in Hand-Foot Coupling and Role of APAs in Differentiating ISO vs. ANTI Coupling Modes in Other Types of Limb Movements* evidence will be presented suggesting that the constraints to the "difficult" mode depend on the directional distribution of the anticipatory postural adjustments associated with the primary movements.

Mechanical Characteristics of the Hand and Foot Oscillations

The oscillations of the hand (Stark, 1968; Stiles et al., 1983; Lakie et al., 1984; Lehman and Calhoun, 1990) and foot

[1]Throughout this review the movement direction will always be referred to external coordinates.

(Hunter and Kearney, 1982) can be satisfactorily modeled by a 2nd-order system (a pendulum) with lumped parameters (mass, stiffness, and viscosity). During passive oscillations, the unloaded hand behaves like a simple mass (negligible elastic and viscous momenta) but when the wrist is pre-loaded it behaves like a mass-spring system (Lehman and Calhoun, 1990). Also during voluntary cyclic flexion-extension of the wrist (Bobet and Norman, 1990) and elbow (Viviani et al., 1976), the phase relationships between the movers EMGs and the joint position approximate those of an ideal pendulum.

Accordingly, should two limbs share identical mechanical properties and be moved by homologous muscles (e.g., flexion-extension of the two hands), a common rhythm generator sending one and the same motor command in parallel to both segments (Schmidt et al., 1979; Turvey et al., 1989) would obtain a correct coupling at all frequencies. If instead the two limbs have different mechanical features, as it is the case for the hand and foot, the oscillations of the two limbs induced by a parallel synchronous command will have different phase delays with respect to the command itself. Moreover, the interlimb phase difference would increase as the movement frequency is raised.

Based on the greater mass of the foot compared to the hand, one would predict that, when driven by a common command, the foot oscillations are phase-delayed with respect to the hand by an extent proportionate to the movement frequency. In fact (Baldissera et al., 2000), the hand movements cycle slightly lags the required synchronism with the foot cycle (namely 0° in ISO and 180° in ANTI) by an almost constant value over the entire frequency range (**Figure 2A**). Correspondingly (compare **Figure 2B** and **Figure 2C**), as the frequency is raised the onset of the EMG activity in forearm muscles (*Extensor Carpi Radialis,* ECR) progressively phase-advances the EMG onset in leg muscles (*Tibialis Anterior*, TA). This occurs in both coupling modes.

These findings would indicate that: (1) the mechanical impedance is greater for the hand than for the foot, despite the smaller mass of the hand; and (2) when the movement frequency is raised, the increase of the hand-foot delay is avoided by a progressive phase advance of the EMG burst in ECR with respect to TA, demonstrating that a neural mechanisms has intervened to counteract the desynchronizing effects of the mechanical disparities.

In conformity with the afore mentioned pendulum model (see features and details in Presentation 2 in Supplementary Material), the input-output phase relations of each limb were derived (Baldissera et al., 2000, 2004; Esposti et al., 2005) from the frequency-dependent changes of the phase delay between the onset of the EMG activity in the movement prime movers (input) and the homologous instant of the related movements (output).

The frequency responses of both the hand and the foot fit the pendulum equation. The foot response, however, shows a slower decay and a higher value of the ratio $\sqrt{K/I}$ (the resonant frequency) compared to the corresponding response of the hand, indicating that the larger mass of the foot is naturally associated with an even larger active stiffness. This difference will justify the smaller EMG-movement lag in the foot than the in hand illustrated in **Figure 2C**.

ROLE OF KINESTHETIC AFFERENTS FROM THE MOVING SEGMENTS IN CONTROLLING THE HAND-FOOT SYNCHRONISM DURING COUPLED MOVEMENTS: AN INTERLIMB OR INTRALIMB FEEDBACK?

The neural control mechanisms that compensates for the desynchronizing effects of the mechanical disparities between

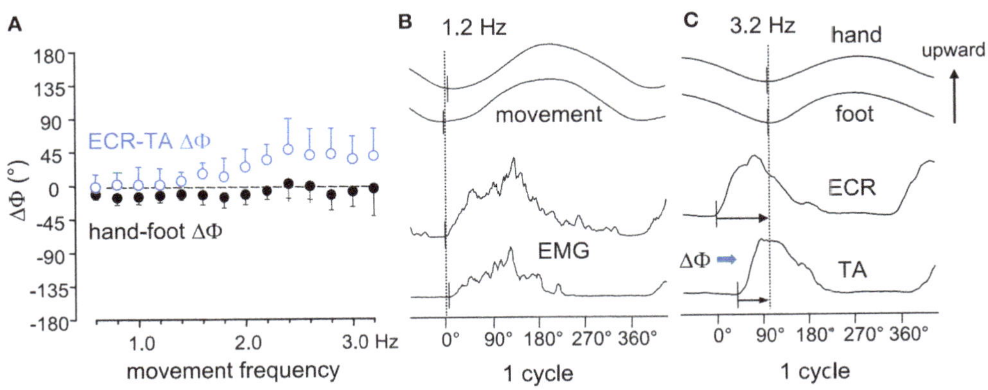

FIGURE 2 | (A) the phase difference between the two movements (*hand-foot ΔΦ*, filled black circles) remains mostly unmodified over the entire frequency range. **(B)** at 1.2 Hz the upward rotation of the two limbs and the onset of the integrated EMGs in the respective movers *ECR, Extensor Carpi Radialis*; *TA, Tibialis Anterior*, all start synchronously. **(C)** at 3.2 Hz, both movements lag the EMG burst onsets, the hand to a larger extent than the foot (black arrows), revealing that the two limbs have different mechanical features. This difference, however, is compensated for by a calibrated advance of the ECR on the TA burst (*ECR-TA ΔΦ*, blue arrow) which increases with frequency (open circles in A) and maintains the movements synchronism.

the limbs might theoretically monitor the deviations of the instantaneous hand-foot relative phase, $\Delta\Phi$, from the programmed value (0° or 180°) and use these error signal for recovering the intended synchronism. Alternatively, each oscillating limb might be provided with an independent neural control which monitors the position of that limb and reacts so as to eliminate any phase mismatch between the rhythmic central command and the actual movement. The functional difference between these two mechanisms lies in the fact that the first one would tend to keep the interlimb relative phase constant whilst being unable to control the synchronization of the limbs oscillations with the central rhythm generator; while the second mechanism would simultaneously achieve both results. Distinguishing between these two mechanisms was attempted by two complementary approaches.

First, the existence of a crossed kinesthetic feedback between the limbs was explored by testing whether the afferent signals generated during voluntary oscillations of one limb may induce excitability changes in the motor structures innervating the second, resting limb. Second, the phase synchronization of the hand and foot oscillations with an external clock signal was measured both when the two segments were moved in isolation and when they were coupled, either iso- or antidirectionally. This allowed to test whether the clock-movement phase-delay, measured when one limb is moved alone, changed as the two limbs were coupled, thus proving that one limb can influence the other in controlling the interlimb synchronization.

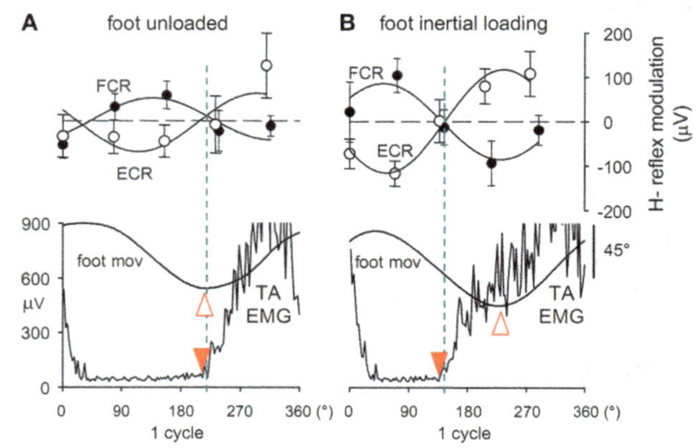

FIGURE 3 | (A) Cyclic modulation the H-reflex size, phase-opposite in the two forearm antagonists *ECR* (open circles) and *FCR* (filled circles), at 5 delays during ipsilateral foot oscillations.Modulation is expressed as the absolute deviation of the reflex size from the cycle mean value and is plotted together with the angular position of the ipsilateral foot (*foot mov*, dorsal flexion up) and the EMG activity in TA muscle (*TA EMG*). Best-fit sinusoidal functions (solid lines) with the same period as movement are superimposed to the H-reflex plots. Crossing between the two H modulation sine waves (dashed blue line) occurs almost synchronously with both the foot flexion peak (open arrowhead) and the onset of TA activation (filled arrowhead). After foot inertial loading **(B)** the foot flexion peak lags the onset of the TA burst by about 90°, while the H-reflex modulation remains phase-linked to the TA activation, showing to be insensitive to the afferent signals monitoring the phase shift of the foot position. Figure assembled with data from Cerri et al. (2003) and Borroni et al. (2004).

Modulation of Motoneuronal Excitability in the Resting Forearm Muscles during Voluntary Oscillations of the Ipsilateral Foot

The excitability of wrist flexor and extensor muscles in the resting forearm was tested during voluntary oscillations of the ipsilateral foot, so as to ascertain whether it was modified by the foot movements (Baldissera et al., 2002).

Indeed, during foot oscillations the size of the H-reflex evoked in the resting *Flexor Carpi Radialis* (FCR) undergoes a sine-wave modulation with the same period as the foot movements (**Figure 3A**). With the forearm in prone position, the FCR H-reflex (filled circles) is facilitated during foot plantar flexion and dis-facilitated during dorsiflexion, while a phase-opposite H-modulation is seen in the antagonist *Extensor Carpi Radialis*, ECR (open circles). Moreover, when the forearm position is changed from prone to supine, the modulation in both ECR and FCR shifts by 180° with respect to the foot movement, thus maintaining the phase opposition in the two antagonists (Borroni et al., 2004; Byblow et al., 2007).

Should these subliminal excitability changes in forearm flexor and extensor motoneurons occur when the hand is moved together with the foot, they would have the same sign (excitatory or inhibitory) as the simultaneous voluntary commands to forearm muscles during ISO coupling; and an opposite sign in ANTI coupling, thus favoring the former and contrasting the latter coupling mode. Moreover, this pattern would hold both when the hand is prone and when it is supine, in agreement with the "direction principle" of hand-foot coupling.

The compound muscle action potentials (CMAPs) evoked in FCR and ECR muscles by transcranial magnetic stimulation (TMS) of the primary motor cortex are also modulated in size during foot oscillations, with the same time course of, but more strongly than, the H-reflex. Finally, interactions between the corticospinal and the Ia afferent effects (Baldissera et al., 2002) convincingly prove that the changes in motoneurons excitability associated with foot oscillations have a cortical origin.

Similar results were also obtained by other investigators in the context of bimanual coupling. In sitting subjects with the hands in semiprone position, Carson et al. (2004) found that the amplitude of the H-reflex and CMAPs in the resting FCR muscle is cyclically modulated during rhythmic oscillations of the contralateral wrist in the horizontal plane. Further, by analysing the EMG spectrogram, Ridderikhoff et al. (2005) found evidence for bursting activity in the resting ECR that occurs in phase with the extension of the contralateral wrist. Also in these cases the excitability modulation would favor the preferred coupling mode, which is mirror symmetrical (ANTI in external coordinates) in these hand movements.

Altogether, these results seemingly supported the working hypothesis that the kinesthetic signals for position (and/or velocity) from one limb cyclically activate the corticospinal projections to the other limb, thereby modulating the motoneuron excitability. Through this mechanism, the afferent signals from the foot might in fact interfere—either positively or negatively according to the coupling mode—with the generation of the voluntary cortical commands to the hand.

This conclusion was soon falsified, however. Since application of an inertial load to the foot, as well as raising the frequency of foot movements, both increase the phase-delay of the foot oscillations with respect to the motor commands (Section *The "Direction Principle" in Coupling Flexion-Extension of the Ipsilateral Hand and Foot. Easy vs. Difficult Coupling Modes* and Presentation 2 in Supplementary Material), it was argued that if the H-reflex modulation at the forearm was driven by the kinesthetic information from the moving foot, if would remain phase linked to the foot rotation. Instead (Cerri et al., 2003), after both loading (**Figure 3B**) and/or increasing the oscillation frequency, the H-modulation in the forearm muscles remains tightly linked to the voluntary motor command, thus anticipating the foot movement. This finding disproves that the cyclic excitability modulation in forearm motoneurons is elicited by the afferent signals that transduce the foot rotation and suggests that it is instead generated in the forearm area of the primary motor cortex simultaneously with the voluntary commands dispatched to the foot. The view that the interlimb relative phase is controlled through an interlimb afferent feedback is then seriously challenged. The possibility remains, however, that the hypothesized crossed feedback was hidden in this experiment because it is only activated when both limbs are oscillated together.

If this were to be the case, however, the different mechanical properties of the two segments would imply that, when each segment is moved alone, the movement phase delay with respect to an external clock (*clock-mov delay)* is different in each limb, and that such difference increases as the oscillation frequency is raised. Consequently, achieving the movements synchronization during coupling through a crossed kinesthetic feedback would necessarily modify the "intrinsic" *clock mov-delay* of either one of the two limbs or both.

Independent Position Control of Each Limb by a "Private" Kinesthetic Feedback

As depicted in **Figure 4A** (Baldissera et al., 2006), the *clock-mov delay* of both the hand and the foot remains almost constant when the frequency is increased (negative values = movement delay) and is not significantly different when the limbs are moved in isolation (green solid and dashed lines) or when they are isodirectionally coupled (hand: blue circles, foot: red triangles). Enhancing the mechanical difference between the limbs, e.g., by connecting the hand to an inertial load (**Figure 4B**), does increase the hand phase delay with respect to the foot but is ineffective in dividing the phase curves obtained when the hand is moved alone and when it is coupled. All this holds true for antidirectional coupling too. Further details on these measurements are given in Presentation 3 in Supplementary Material.

In conclusion, the phase delay with respect to a common time-giver is apparently controlled in each limb independently from what simultaneously occurs in the other limb, even after artificially enhancing the mechanical disparity between the limbs.

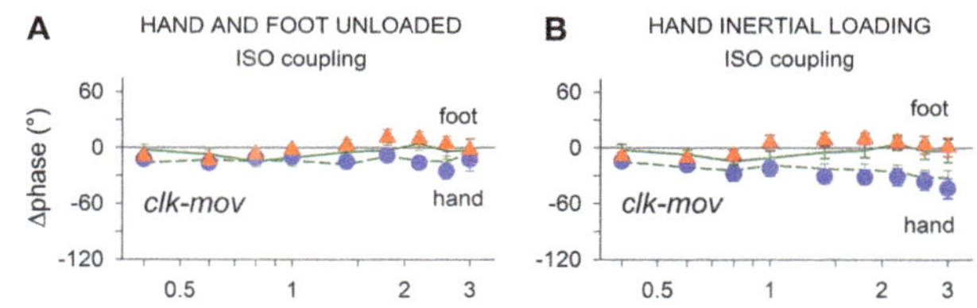

FIGURE 4 | Frequency dependent changes of the *clock-mov* phase-delay during separate oscillations of the hand and foot (green dashed and continuous lines, respectively) and during hand-foot ISO coupling (hand, blue circles; foot, red triangles). (A) When both limbs are unloaded the *clk-mov* delay of each limb, no matter whether isolated or coupled, remains nearly constant over the whole frequency range. **(B)** same relations as in **(A)** but obtained after applying an inertial load to the hand. Loading induced the expected increase of the hand *clk-mov* delay as the frequency is raised but in either limb the frequency relations obtained during separate and coupled movements still superimpose.

The control of the interlimb relative phase will thus directly result from the efficacy of the separate phase controllers of each limb.

The synchronism control of each individual limb may possibly be operated through a "private" kinesthetic feedback which provides matching of the limb movements with the motor commands linked to the central time giver. A neuro-mechanical model that faithfully simulates the operations of such a feedback (Esposti et al., 2007) is illustrated in Presentation 4 in Supplementary Material.

Added to the previously discussed evidence that the excitability changes in forearm motoneurons during foot movements are not generated by afferent signals, these last results should definitely rule out the hypothesis that the coupling coordination is achieved by a crossed kinesthetic feedback between the limbs.

NEURAL MECHANISMS UNDERLYING THE "DIRECTION PRINCIPLE" IN HAND-FOOT COUPLING

Altogether, the results reported in Section *Role of Kinesthetic Afferents from the Moving Segments in Controlling the Hand-Foot Synchronism during Coupled Movements: An Interlimb or Intralimb Feedback?* enlighten both issues presented in Section *Mechanical Differences between the Limbs and Neural Compensation for their Desynchronizing Effect on Coupled Movements.* On one side, they indicate, in a way consistent with basic physical and neurophysiological concepts, that the limbs relative phase results from an independent synchronization of each limb movement with the common clock signal. On the other side, these results also show that during foot voluntary oscillations the commands that move the foot are associated with descending subliminal commands to the "isodirectional" muscles in the resting forearm, distributed so as to facilitate ISO and contrast ANTI coupling both in the prone and supine forearm position.

Once excluded that the effects onto the resting forearm are generated by the kinesthetic afferents that monitor the foot movements, it remained to understand which physiological role these effects may have within the frame of motor control. A survey of the known motor mechanisms led to the idea that they may carry Anticipatory Postural Adjustments, APAs.

Anticipatory Postural Adjustments (APAs) as Possible Candidates for Generating the Subliminal Excitability Modulation in Forearm Muscles during Foot Oscillations

Albeit in different conceptual and experimental contexts, the modulation of motoneuron excitability in one limb during voluntary movements of another limb had been described since several years, and explicitly discussed in many instances as due to APAs (Kasai and Komiyama, 1996; Kawanishi et al., 1999; Hiraoka, 2001).

APAs (Marsden et al., 1978, 1981; Cordo and Nashner, 1982; Bouisset and Zattara, 1987; Zattara and Bouisset, 1988; Bouisset and Do, 2008), are unconscious muscle contractions aimed at preparing fixation chains linking the segment(s) to be consciously moved to one or more firm supports, where the reaction forces to the prime movers contraction can develop (third Newton's principle) without producing any displacement. In this way it is determined which of the body segments connected by the prime movers will actually move. In the absence of a firm support, APAs will produce counter-movements that contrast the postural unbalance produced by the consciously intended movement (also said the "focal" movement). However counterintuitive it may appear, the unconscious APAs are yet a necessary and fundamental component in the generation and control of the "willed" movements.

In EMG recordings, APAs are characterized by the combined activation of muscles in one or more fixation chains, simultaneously with, or in slight advance to, the prime movers contraction. APAs scale in size with the magnitude of the primary movement (Aruin and Latash, 1996), they are influenced by the position and number of the fixation points (Slijper and Latash, 2000) and by tactile and proprioceptive information (Slijper and Latash, 2004). Also, their timing and spatial distribution may vary when the surround conditions or some feature of the movement (e.g., the direction) are changed (Cordo and Nashner, 1982; Nashner and Forssberg, 1986; Aruin and Latash, 1995). Of direct relevance in the present context are the facts that during flexion/extension of the wrist the APAs in proximal arm muscles are directionally organized (Chabran et al., 1999, 2001) and, even more interesting, that they are generated in elbow flexors when the forearm is supine but in elbow extensors when it is prone (Aoki, 1991), showing that APAs action is "isodirectional" with the primary "focal" movement whatever the forearm position.

In the past years, interest for APAs has been mainly focused on their role in stabilizing the body equilibrium, while a minor attention was devoted to their general function of providing firm support to any moving segment. For instance, the interactions between coupled limb movements and the overall body posture have been examined looking at the effects exerted by the coordinated movements on the stability of body balance (Ferry et al., 2004; Ustinova et al., 2004; Forner-Cordero et al., 2007). Here, instead, we will focus on the less investigated effects of postural anticipatory adjustments on coordination of voluntary movements (cfr. Yiou, 2005; Yiou and Schneider, 2007; Yiou et al., 2007, for the interactions between the postural dynamics elicited by arm pointing and the step initiation).

APAs Generated in Forearm Muscles during Movements of the Ipsilateral Foot Reproduce the Same Distribution Pattern as the Subliminal Modulation

Convincing experimental evidence supports the hypothesis that the subliminal excitability changes in forearm muscles linked to the ipsilateral foot oscillation should be recognized as APAs.

When sitting on an armchair, as in the standard experiments on hand-foot coupling, body fixation is mainly obtained through the large contact surface of the posterior aspect of trunk and thighs with the seat. This would strongly attenuate the postural role of the forearm contact with its support, so that only small or subliminal APAs should develop in forearm muscles, perhaps corresponding to the excitability changes described in Section *Neural Mechanisms Underlying the "Direction Principle" in Hand-Foot Coupling.* Enhancing the forearm postural role might then transform those subliminal changes into manifest contractions.

Consider the following experiment. The subject stands upright, with the left foot on a stable surface, the right foot on a pivoting platform and the right arm protracted with the hand contacting a rigid support (inset of **Figure 5**) so as to increase the postural role of the right arm. In this asset, the cyclic flexion-extension of the right foot, which entails the risk of a forward/backward fall, is indeed counteracted by a cyclic activation of the forearm flexor and extensor motoneurons which has the same period as the foot movement (Baldissera and Esposti, 2005). If the hand is prone and in palmar contact with the support (**Figure 5A**), the positive phase of the modulation in FCR is coincident with the contraction of the plantar flexor SOL. Conversely, if the hand contact is dorsal (**Figure 5B**), activity is modulated in ECR and its positive phase coincides with the activation of TA. With the hand supine the above pattern reverses (**Figures 5C,D**).

If cyclic foot oscillations are replaced by fast flexion or extension movements, single EMG bursts fulfilling the APAs requisites develop in the "isodirectional" forearm muscles, together with a simultaneous depression of the background activity (when present) in the antagonists (**Figure 6**).

The strict topographical superimposition of these canonically identified APAs with the cyclic EMG activities and the subliminal excitability modulation observed when sitting would indicate that they share the same nature, even if one cannot exclude that the cyclic effects include reflex components too (see also later).

In summary, during single and cyclic foot movements and irrespective of the movement direction (plantar or dorsal flexion) and forearm position (prone or supine), excitatory burst or cyclic contractions, respectively, arise in those forearm muscles that rotate the hand isodirectionally with the foot, providing a subsidiary postural support at the hand contact. Matching these overt activities with the subliminal excitability modulation observed in the sitting position suggests that they represent two grades of one and the same event, i.e., the preparation of a fixation chain connecting the moving foot to the firm hand support. It seems therefore apparent that even when a manifest intervention of anticipatory postural adjustments is not required, subthreshold APAs may nevertheless develop, which can only be disclosed by instrumental excitability testing; and that, depending on the body postural needs, the subliminal changes can be transformed into overt APAs and viceversa.

To mechanistically explain this APAs flexibility it was imagined (Baldissera and Esposti, 2005) that any given voluntary movement is associated with the co-activation of an arborized pattern of postural commands directed toward a number of possible fixation points; and that activation of the arborization branches is supraliminal in those directed to the segments providing actual support and subliminal in those not involved at the moment in that function. Within this organization, the control of APAs might consist, from time to time, in amplifying transmission to certain targets and attenuate transmission to others, a task that could be automatically accomplished by low-level mechanisms based on afferent information.

Indeed two experimental observations support this view. On one side, studies on the feline reticulospinal neurons candidate for APA transmission (Schepens and Drew, 2004, 2006; Schepens et al., 2008) disclosed that on occasion of single forelimb movements a widespread postural activity is induced from the motor cortex in reticulospinal neurons. Such activity is then restricted to the motoneurons actually involved in postural support by selectively gating (inhibiting) at the spinal level the transmission of the APA commands to the other motoneurons, so that they remain available for voluntary activation. On the other side, in man, when two supports are available and one of the two fixation chains is voluntarily privileged, activation of the second chain is proportionally attenuated (Esposti and Baldissera, 2011) This shows that gating of the APAs commands does not take place in all-or-none fashion but is modulated in a coordinated way in the different chains.

This organization would create a pattern of subliminal activation of the motor pathways to those body segments that are not (but may potentially be) used for postural support. Even when they are subliminal, the forearm APAs described

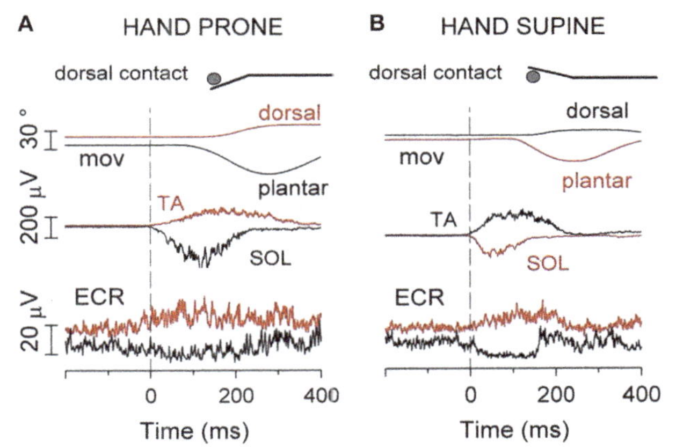

FIGURE 6 | (A) Hand prone, dorsal contact. Red traces: TA contraction and the ensuing foot dorsal flexion are preceded by an excitatory APA in ECR, the "isodirectional" mover of the hand. Black traces: contraction of SOL and foot plantar flexion are preceded by an inhibitory APA in ECR. **(B)** Hand supine, dorsal contact. Red traces: an excitatory APA in ECR precedes contraction of the "isodirectional" SOL and foot plantar flexion. Black traces: when the movement direction is inverted to dorsal, ECR becomes "antidirectional" to SOL and the APA changes to inhibitory. Reproduced from Baldissera and Esposti (2005) © Wolters Kluwer Health, Inc. 2005, with permission of Wolters Kluwer Health, Inc..

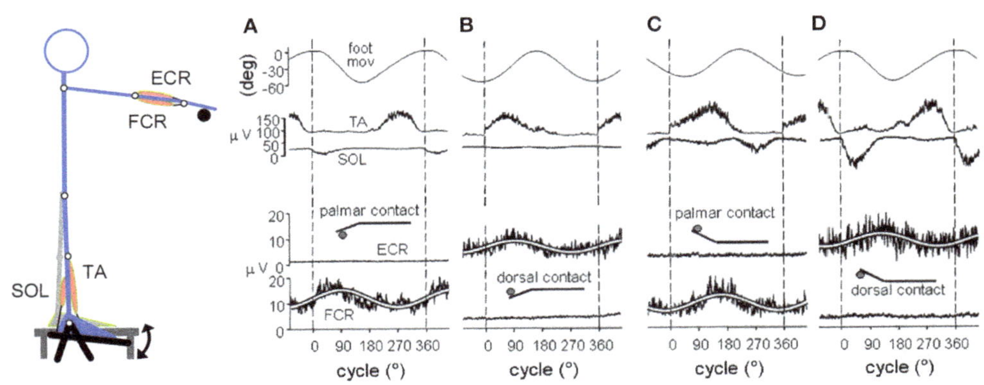

FIGURE 5 | When standing on the left foot, with the right hand touching a fixed support (inset), cyclic oscillations of right foot modulate sinusoidally the EMG activity of ipsilateral wrist muscles at the frequency of the foot movement (1.5 Hz). Soleus (SOL) EMG reversed. **(A)** hand prone, palmar contact; FCR EMG is cyclically modulated, the positive phase coincides with SOL activation. **(B)** dorsal contact; the positive phase of the ECR EMG modulation coincides with TA activation. **(C,D)** hand supination reverses the above pattern. In this and the following figures the white lines superimposed to the EMG recordings are the best fit sine-waves with the same period as the movements. Reproduced from Baldissera and Esposti (2005) © Wolters Kluwer Health, Inc. 2005, with permission of Wolters Kluwer Health, Inc.

above might selectively contrast the voluntary co-activation of "antidirectional" foot and hand movers: hence the necessity of suppressing APAs by gating. In this perspective, the gating mechanism would be central in determining the hand-foot coupling preference since its attenuation or default would selectively hamper the ANTI movements.

Imagine that during flexion-extension of the right foot one needs, or wants, to simultaneously move a body segment—for instance the right hand—that belongs to one of the fixation chains that actually assist the foot movement. Following this decision, the forearm muscles would be simultaneously targeted by both the voluntary command moving the hand and the APAs command linked to the foot movement, thus being called to function as prime movers and as postural muscles at the same time.

Being dispatched to the same target, the voluntary and the APAs commands will converge at some, yet unknown, level of the motor pathways to forearm muscles. When voluntary and APA actions are isodirectional, i.e., when the postural and the voluntary commands have the same sign (either excitatory or inhibitory) this convergence will favor both actions and the previously described double goal will be met. Conversely, when the voluntary and the postural actions have opposite directions, a conflict will be generated, which may be avoided only if either the voluntary command or the APA command is suppressed. An example of voluntary movement suppression is the irresistible transition from the difficult to the easy coupling mode (Section *The "Direction Principle" in Coupling Flexion-Extension of the Ipsilateral Hand and Foot. Easy vs. Difficult Coupling Modes*). The alternative intervention, i.e., the APAs suppression aimed to free the voluntary mobilization, cannot regard a main fixation chain without challenging the steady equilibrium but it might allow voluntary activation of those muscles that actually have a minor postural function (like forearm muscles when sitting on a chair).

In conclusion, in hand-foot coupling a neural conflict between APAs and voluntary commands may occur in the motor pathways to the prime movers when the two segment are moved in opposite angular directions. The entity of the conflict should in turn depend on the APAs size, i.e, on the functional relevance of the fixation chain in which the prime movers are actually included.

ROLE OF APAS IN DIFFERENTIATING ISO vs. ANTI COUPLING MODES IN OTHER TYPES OF LIMB MOVEMENTS

In the practical impossibility of collecting from human experiments more detailed and direct evidence concerning the intimate neuronal mechanisms of the interaction between postural and voluntary actions, it seemed reasonable to search for further indirect evidence supporting the interpretation proposed for hand-foot coupling. Considering that APAs generation is intrinsic to every voluntary movement, it was decided to test whether the correlation between APAs distribution and coupling preference is also observed in other types of coupled limb movements, so as to represent a general rule of motor control.

A suitable experimental model to start exploring the reliability of this idea are the coupled movements of the arms, performed in either the horizontal (transverse) or the vertical (parasagittal) plane. Indeed, in both types of movements the moving masses and the available fixation chains remain the same, but changing the plane of arms motion would produce a topographical re-distribution of the reaction forces and moments and, consequently, of the APAs. Assuming the coupling stability to be correlated with the APAs distribution and size, it would be expected to observe stability to vary in agreement with the intervening changes in the APAs pattern.

Verifying the above idea implied measuring in the four coupling combinations, i.e., horizontal ISO (*hISO*) and ANTI (*hANTI*) and parasagittal ISO (*pISO*) and ANTI (*pANTI*), (1) the variability of the movements relative phase, $SD\Delta\Phi$ (i.e., the reciprocal of coupling stability, see Section *The "Direction Principle" in Coupling Flexion-Extension of the Ipsilateral Hand and Foot. Easy vs. Difficult Coupling Modes*), to be matched, in each coupling combination, with (2) the distribution of the postural adjustments associated with unidirectional and cyclic arm movements.

Coupling Coordination of ISO vs. ANTI Cyclic Movements of the Arms in the Horizontal and Parasagittal Planes

A directional easy-vs.-difficult polarization is found in arm coupled movements performed in either plane of motion, being however opposite in horizontal movements (ANTI vs. ISO) with respect to parasagittal movements (ISO vs. ANTI) (Baldissera et al., 2008b; Baldissera and Esposti, 2013). Indeed $SD\Delta\Phi$ is lower (i.e., coupling stability is higher) in *hANTI* and *pISO* than in both *hISO* and *pANTI*. No significant $SD\Delta\Phi$ difference is found between the two easy modes while $SD\Delta\Phi$ is higher in *hISO* than in *pANTI*. Consequently, the stability loss between easy and difficult coupling is larger in horizontal than in parasagittal movements. Summing up, the instability (difficulty) of the four movement combinations, as evaluated by $SD\Delta\Phi$, increases along the scale $hANTI \neq pISO < pANTI < hISO$.

APAs Associated with Arm Movements in the Horizontal and Parasagittal Plane

The reaction forces to movements of one arm in either the horizontal or parasagittal planes, are discharged by two main fixation chains, to the contralateral arm and to the ground, respectively (cfr. **Figure 7** for horizontal movements).

The relative engagement of each chain varies according to the body asset. In the standing position, the major anticipatory postural activation usually develops in muscles of the chain to the ground, but when the ground surface is slippery (e.g., iced), or when sitting on a turnable chair, the role of APAs in muscles of the contralateral arm becomes relevant.

Distribution of the muscular and mechanical APAs linked to unidirectional movements of one and, more rarely, both arms was already reported by several authors (e.g., Belen'kii et al., 1967; Friedli et al., 1984; Bouisset and Zattara, 1987; Zattara and Bouisset, 1988; Aruin and Latash, 1995; Hodges

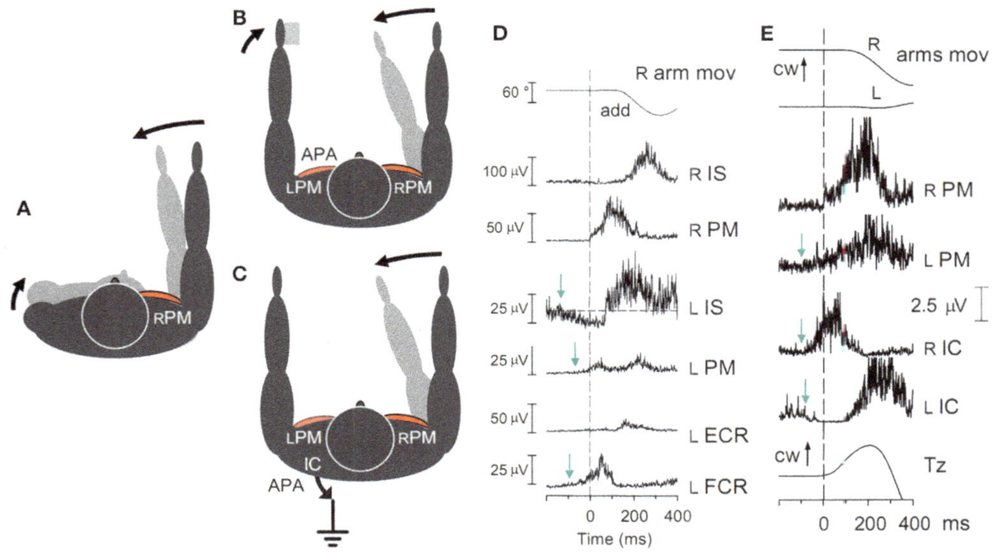

FIGURE 7 | (A) Contraction of the right RPM in the absence of any fixation chain would counter-rotate the right arm and the trunk. A pure arm movement is obtained if the trunk rotation is opposed by APAs in the fixation chain between the arms **(B)** and/or to the ground **(C)**. **(D)** Fast adduction of the right arm in the horizontal plane, prime mover right RPM. Subject sitting on a turnable chair, palmar surface of the left hand touching a fixed support. Excitatory APAs develop in left arm muscles LPM and LFCR, inhibitory APAs in LIS. All APAs precede the prime mover contraction (dashed line). No inhibition is seen in LECR, due to the absence of any background activity. **(E)** Activation of the RPM is preceded by excitatory APAs in both the LPM and the RIC, while LIC is simultaneously inhibited. The related change of Tz starts simultaneously with the RPM activation. cw, clock-wise.

et al., 1999, 2000; Shiratori and Aruin, 2004; Bouisset and Do, 2008; Tomita et al., 2010). In the perspective discussed here, however, these data had to be supplemented with some further observation.

APAs in Arm Adduction-Abduction in the Horizontal Plane

Fast unidirectional movements of the right arm

When standing upright, the voluntary adduction of the right arm in the horizontal plane (prime mover right *Pectoralis Major*, RPM) exerts at the shoulder a torque that tends to rotate the trunk clockwise (**Figure 7A**). This torque is contrasted by the body inertia and actively counteracted by a counterclockwise torque simultaneously generated by the two fixation chains mentioned above (**Figures 7B,C**), in different proportions in the various contexts (Baldissera et al., 2008a,b).

Fixation chain between the arms. During a fast adduction of the right arm, if a rigid support is available to the left hand (**Figure 7B**) APAs develop in the homologous left-side adductor, LPM, and in the wrist flexor LFCR (**Figure 7D**); meanwhile in the left *Infraspinatus*, LIS, the background EMG activity (if present) is reciprocally depressed. These APAs discharge the primary rotational perturbation onto the support and arrest the clockwise rotation of the trunk. When no support is available, APAs in LPM fixate the left arm to the trunk, thus increasing the overall inertia, or even produce an adduction of the left arm and a mirror reaction torque, in either case attenuating the trunk rotation.

Fixation chain to the ground. A counterclockwise torque is also exerted on the thorax by APAs in the trunk and lower limb muscles (**Figure 7C**), an example of which are the prominent burst in the right *Ischiocruralis* muscle, RIC, and the simultaneous anticipatory depression of LIC (**Figure 7E**). These asymmetric APAs generate at the ground a clockwise reaction torque about the vertical axis, *Tz*, in the direction opposite to the arm acceleration.

When the right arm is cyclically oscillated, in both fixation chains the above APAs are replaced (**Figure 8A**) by a sinusoidal EMG modulation with the same period as the right arm oscillations (Baldissera et al., 2008b). In both arm (LPM) and leg (RIC) muscles, the modulation phase-advances the RPM cyclic activity, its absolute timing being quantitatively congruent with the time-anticipation of the APAs linked to unidirectional movements.

Cyclic coupled adduction-abduction of both arms

During coupled arm movements, APAs in arms muscles cannot be distinguished from the voluntary activation, and only APAs in the fixation chain to the ground can be analyzed.

When cyclic movements are mirror symmetrical (ANTI), EMG modulation in LIC and RIC is absent or marginal over the whole frequency range (1.0–3.0 Hz), justifying the virtual annihilation of *Tz* (**Figure 8B**). Conversely, during arms ISO movements (**Figure 8C**), the amplitude of the phase-opposite modulation of RIC and LIC EMG and the size of *Tz* are much larger than in one-arm movements and this difference steeply increases when the frequency is raised (see also Section *Effects of APAs in the Fixation Chain to the Ground on Coupling Coordination of Horizontal and Parasagittal Arm Movements*).

The view that the APAs and the sinusoidal EMG modulation share the same nature is not only suggested by the identical distribution and the temporal compatibility of the two events, but it is also supported by the observation (Leonard et al., 2011) that when the target of a pointing task is unexpectedly shifted after the movement had started, the correction movement is preceded by legs postural adjustments in the same way as at the movement initiation, showing that the online correction of voluntary finalized movements includes both the conscious and the associated APA commands. If one considers that cyclic movements are continuously changing in velocity and direction so as to require uninterrupted control of trajectory and timing, it is reasonable that the related APA commands are continuously updated over the entire sinusoidal course of movements. Thus, although the possibility exists that these cyclic postural activities may include reflex components too, we will continue hereafter to name the cyclic postural activities as APAs.

APAs in Arm Flexion-Extension in the Parasagittal Plane

Fast unidirectional flexion or extension

The reaction forces to arm movements in the parasagittal plane are discharged by APAs in the same two fixation chains as horizontal movements, but with a different topographical distribution. For a mechanical analysis of these effects, see Esposti and Baldissera (2013).

APAs in the fixation chain between the arms

Supplementing the scanty data available in the literature (Zattara and Bouisset, 1988) it was disclosed (Esposti and Baldissera, 2013) that a fast flexion (**Figures 9A,B**) or extension of the right arm (prime movers right *Anterior Deltoid*, RAD, and *Posterior Deltoid* RPD, respectively) elicits APAs in the left side homologous LAD and LPD so as to replicate the excitation and inhibition pattern of RAD and RPD. In the left extensor

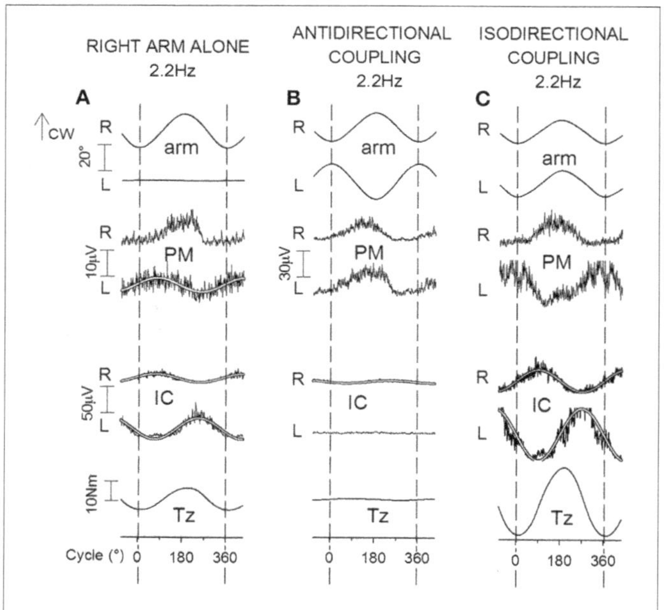

FIGURE 8 | Cyclic postural adjustments during rhythmic oscillations in the horizontal plane of the right arm alone (A) and of both arms in ANTI and ISO coupling **(B,C)**. Prime movers, RPM in **(A)**, RPM and LPM in **(B,C)**. During one arm movements, cyclic APAs develop both in LPM and, phase-opposite, in RIC andLIC. This same pattern of EMG modulation, but doubled in size, is present in IC muscles during ISO (difficult) coupling **(C)**. During ANTI coupling, instead, activity is absent in LIC and minimal in RIC **(B)**. In all coupling modes, *Tz* undergoes changes parallel to the IC activities; cw, clock-wise.

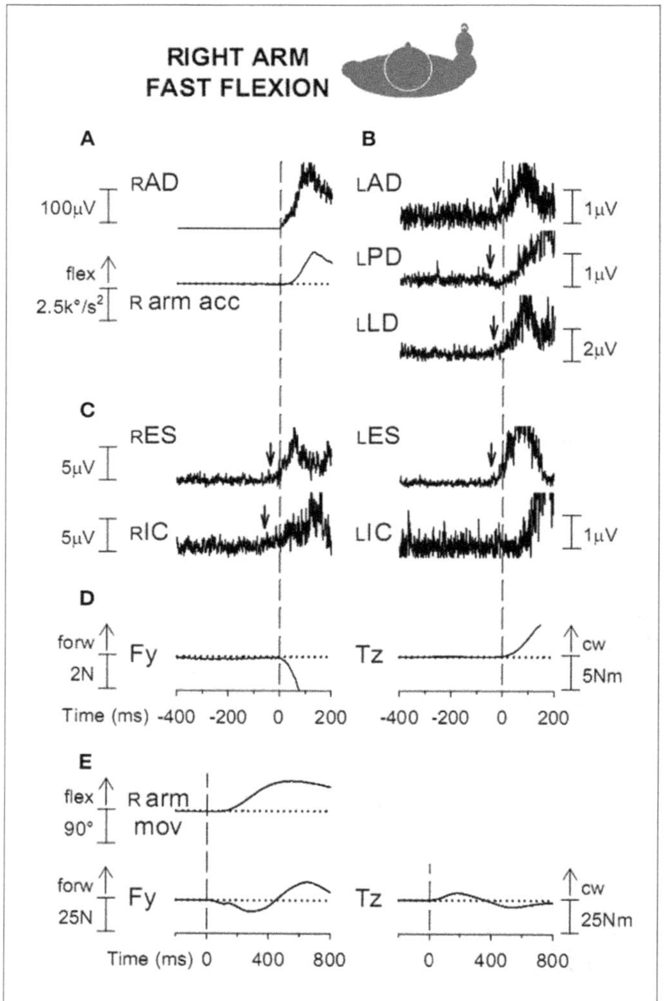

FIGURE 9 | (A) Voluntary activation of RAD and acceleration (R arm acc) of the ensuing arm flexion. Vertical dashed line: onset of the RAD EMG burst. **(B)** APAs in the left arm muscles, excitatory in LAD and LLD and inhibitory in LPD. **(C)** excitatory APAs in trunk muscles RES and LES and in the right leg muscle RIC. **(D)** anterior-posterior force *Fy* and clockwise moment about the body vertical axis *Tz*, discharged to the ground. **(E)**. *Fy* and *Tz* changes are displayed on a longer time base. Dashed line: onset of prime mover burst; cw, clock-wise.

Latissimus Dorsi, LLD, APAs are instead opposite to the voluntary actions in RLD.

APAs in the fixation chain to the ground

Many details of the APAs in trunk and legs associated with flexion-extension of one or both arms had been previously reported (see above for references, cfr. also Zattara and Bouisset, 1988; Shiratori and Aruin, 2004; Bleuse et al., 2005; Bouisset and Do, 2008; Morris et al., 2013) and some were confirmed. Fast flexion of the right arm (**Figure 9C**) is associated with symmetric APAs in the right and left *Erector Spinae* (RES and LES) and asymmetric APAs in RIC and LIC, excitatory on the right side during arm flexion (cfr. Zattara and Bouisset, 1988; Bleuse et al., 2005) and on the left side during extension. An anticipatory change of the anterior-posterior force *Fy* and of the torque *Tz* are meanwhile discharged to the ground (**Figures 9D,E**). During single arm oscillations all the above APAs are replaced by EMG modulation cycles with the same period as the arm movement and increasing in size when the movement frequency is raised (Baldissera and Esposti, 2013).

Cyclic coupled flexion-extension of both arms

During ISO arms oscillations (**Figure 10A**) cyclic APAs develop symmetrically both in RES and LES and in RIC and LIC (**Figure 10B**), as requested to cope with the anterior-posterior perturbation. When frequency is raised, APAs in both muscles pairs increase in size remaining synchronous on the two sides. The anterior-posterior reaction force *Fy* undergoes a sinusoidal modulation with the same period as the arm movements (**Figure 10C**) and significantly increases in size when the frequency increases. Conversely, the size of *Tz* remains negligible throughout the whole frequency range.

During ANTI coupling (**Figures 10D–F**) the APAs modulation in RES and LES is significantly smaller than in ISO, but it increases in either mode as the frequency is raised. The phase difference between the two sides is highly variable among subjects and, on the average, half-way between 0° and −180°. Cyclic APAs activation is phase-opposite in RIC and LIC and, when the frequency is raised, it increases in size to a greater extent than in ISO. Concerning the ground reactions, the sinusoidal modulation of *Fy* remains very low over all the frequency range, while the torque *Tz* significantly increases between 1.0 and 2.2 Hz but progressively decreases by about the same amount between 2.2 and 3.4 Hz (see later). The phase of *Tz* oscillations during ANTI is opposite to that of the right arm movements and is not significantly affected by frequency.

In summary, the coupled arm oscillations in the horizontal and parasagittal plane are distinguished because the preferred (more stable) coupling mode is ANTI in horizontal and ISO in parasagittal movements. Both movement types, however, share the common feature that the unstable coupling mode is the one in which: (1) in the motor pathways to the prime movers of each arm the voluntary commands have opposite sign with respect of the APAs commands linked to the voluntary activation of the contralateral arm (cfr. Section *APAs Associated with Arm Movements in the Horizontal and Parasagittal Plane*); and, (2)

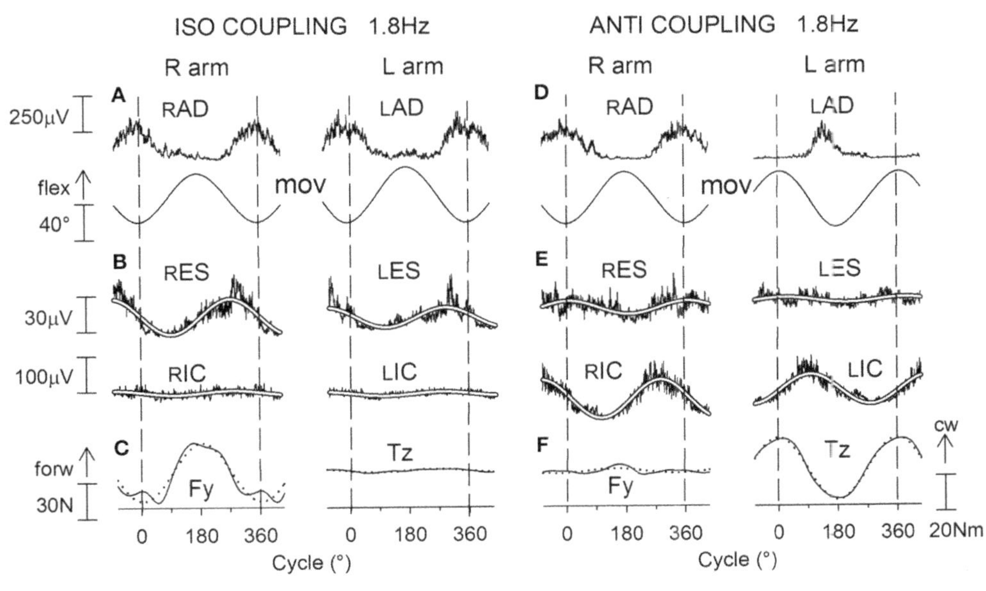

FIGURE 10 | Voluntary oscillations of both arms in the parasagittal plane. ISO and ANTI coupling. Same labels as in **Figure 9**. **(A,D)**: cyclic voluntary EMG activity in RAD and LAD muscles and ensuing oscillations of the right and left arms. In ISO coupling the activation of both trunk (ES) and thigh (IC) postural muscles is synchronous on the two sides **(B)** and corresponds **(C)** to a clear-cut anterior-posterior ground reaction *Fy* while the torque *Tz* is marginal. **(E)** in ANTI coupling, the EMG modulation in RES and LES remains synchronous but consistently lower with respect to ISO, whereas the IC activation s increased in size and is phase-opposite in RIC and LIC. Correspondingly **(F)**, a large reaction torque *Tz* is generated while *Fy* is strongly reduced.

the prime movers generate torsional perturbations, which are discharged by APAs to the ground by producing a reactive torque *Tz.*

Interactions betweeen APAs and Voluntary Commands during Coupled Arm Movements

Combining the results presented in Sections *Coupling Coordination of ISO vs. ANTI Cyclic Movements of the Arms in the Horizontal and Parasagittal Planes and APAs Associated with Arm Movements in the Horizontal and Parasagittal Plane* suggests that the selective constraints affecting the two difficult modes, *hISO* and *pANTI*, may be related to the APAs that occur in both the fixation chains, between the arms and to the ground.

In the following, the two mechanisms will be discussed separately.

Neural Interference between APAs and Voluntary Commands in the Motor Pathways to the Prime Movers in Horizontal and Parasagittal Arm Movements

Horizontal movements

During ANTI (mirror symmetrical) coupling, voluntary, and postural commands to the prime movers have the same sign (i.e., both excitatory or inhibitory). Accordingly, they should potentiate each other. However, it should be noted that in ANTI coupling the two arms exert on the trunk opposite torques that physically cancel each other, so that no postural adjustment is needed. Indeed, no APAs are generated during ANTI in the fixation chain to the ground (**Figure 8B**) and, reasonably, APAs should be absent in the contralateral arm too, thus leaving movement coupling unaffected.

During ISO coupling the APAs elicited in the prime movers of either arm are opposite in sign with respect to the voluntary commands. Hence, maintaining the movement amplitude, as done in the experiments described here, would require that either the voluntary commands are increased or APAs are actively suppressed (gated). The former intervention, however, would be doomed to fail since when the frequency (velocity) of the arm movements increases, the size of APAs also increases (Baldissera et al., 2008b, see also Shiratori and Aruin, 2007).

Parasagittal arm movements

The interaction between voluntary and APAs commands is somewhat more complex in parasagittal than in horizontal oscillations (cfr. discussion in Baldissera and Esposti, 2013).

In the motor pathways to *Anterior* and *Posterior Deltoid*, the voluntary commands and the APAs linked to the movement of the contralateral arm have the same sign during ISO, thus facilitating or leaving unaffected (see above) the coupled movements. Conversely, during ANTI coupling, voluntary commands and APAs have opposite sign and maintaining the movement amplitude requires APAs to be actively suppressed (gated).

In the motor pathways to *Latissimus Dorsi*, instead, APAs and voluntary commands have opposite sign during ISO (see Section *APAs in Arm Flexion-Extension in the Parasagittal Plane*), thus creating a local neural conflict during the preferred mode.

Escape from APAs suppression

As discussed in Section *Anticipatory Postural Adjustments (APAs) as Possible Candidates for Generating the Subliminal Excitability Modulation in Forearm Muscles during Foot Oscillations for hand-foot coupling,* the conflict arising in both horizontal and parasagittal movements when APAs and voluntary commands have opposite signs can be solved with the intervention of the control mechanism that provides gating of transmission of the APAs commands (Schepens and Drew, 2004, 2006; Schepens et al., 2008). One sign of such intervention may be the higher increase of cerebral activation during non-preferential coupling compared to preferential coupling (Sadato et al., 1997; Debaere et al., 2001, 2004; Immisch et al., 2001; Ullen et al., 2003).

However, as the oscillation frequency increases, the size of APAs also increases, implying that the gating mechanism for APAs suppression must be intensified in parallel. Descriptively, the decay in coupling stability observed when either the movement frequency is raised or the exercise duration is prolonged, fits the general description of fatiguing systems. It may therefore be supposed that during "difficult" coupling the gating system undergoes neural "fatigue" (linked to the turnover of synaptic transmitters, adaptation, or potentiation phenomena, etc.) proportionate to the frequency and duration of the exercise, so as to progressively attenuate the suppression of APAs transmission. This, in turn, would increase the coupling instability and favor the transition to the opposite coupling mode.

Effects of APAs in the Fixation Chain to the Ground on Coupling Coordination of Horizontal and Parasagittal Arm Movements

The major clue suggesting that in both movement types APAs in the chain to the ground may exert an indirect influence on coupling coordination is the increase of the chained postural actions observed when passing from the more stable to the less stable coupling mode (Sections *APAs in Arm Adduction-Abduction in the Horizontal Plane and APAs in Arm Flexion-Extension in the Parasagittal Plane*). Evidence for such an effect has also been reported by Van der Woude et al. (2008) for synchronous and alternate hand cycling. Aimed to better elucidate this correlation, the effort sustained by the postural chain to the ground was tentatively quantified (1) by the forces discharged to the ground and (2) by the energy cost of the chain actions.

Ground reactions Fy and Tz

Each of the EMG and mechanical variables pertaining to the fixation chain to the ground is exclusively related to either *Fy* or *Tz* (Esposti et al., 2013). The latter can then be taken as indicators of the overall entity of postural actions occurring in the chain.

In a group of subjects performing both horizontal and parasagittal movements in the same experimental session, no significant *Tz* changes are observed (**Figure 11B**) at any frequency in the two more stable "easy" modes (*pISO* and *hANTI*). Conversely, *Tz* is large and increases with frequency in

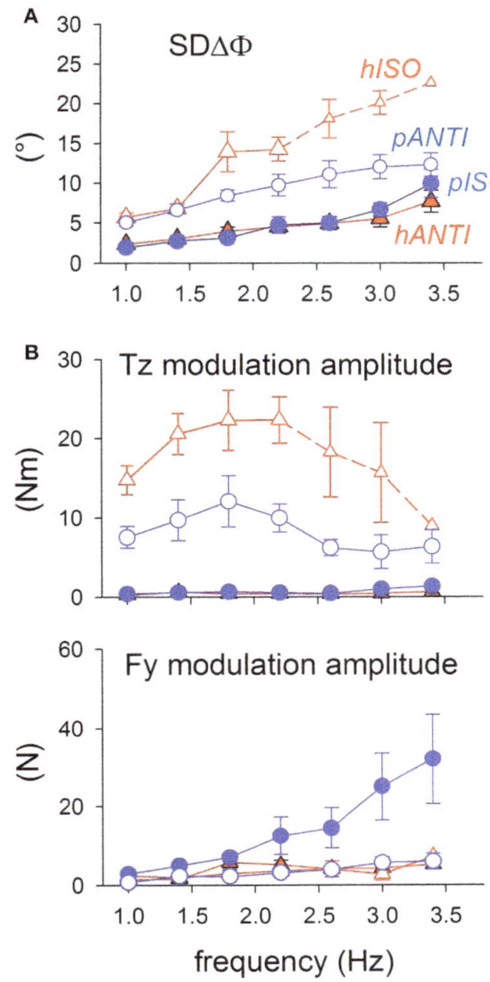

FIGURE 11 | Coordination marker SDΔΦ and postural markers *Fy* and *Tz* recorded during coupled arm movements performed by the same subjects in both the horizontal and parasagittal planes (red triangles and blue circles, respectively). Filled symbols, stable (easy) modes; open symbols, unstable (difficult) modes. **(A)** SDΔφ is identical in the easy modes *pISO* and *hANTI*, larger in *pANTI* and even more so in *hISO*. Small symbols and dashed lines: values obtained in only part of the subjects. **(B)** *Tz* is virtually null in the two easy modes (filled symbols) and not significantly different between the two movement types. Instead, it increases with frequency in the two difficult modes (open symbols), more in *hISO* than in *pANTI*. Above 2.0–2.4 Hz, *Tz* starts however to decrease progressively. Size of *Fy* increases monotonically with frequency up to 3.4 Hz in *pISO* while it remains negligible in the other three movement combination.

both the "difficult" modes, significantly more in *hISO* than in *pANTI*. Thus, the distribution gradient for *Tz* among the four movements combinations is: *hANTI* ≠ *pISO* < *pANTI* < *hISO*, i.e., just the same as for SDΔΦ.

The anterior-posterior force *Fy* is appreciable and increases significantly with frequency only during ISO parasagittal movements (**Figure 11B**) thus appearing as unsuitable for discriminating among the four movement conditions.

Note, however, that in both movement types *Tz* decreases above 2.0–2.5 Hz while SDΔΦ continues to grow (compare **Figure 11A** and **Figure 11B**). This discrepancy might disprove the existence of a causal link between postural effort and coupling stability but it may also indicate that in the high frequency range *Tz* does not express all the forces generated for postural aims because part of them are "absorbed" within the different chained segments of the trunk by opposite muscular actions.

Oxygen uptake during coupling of horizontal and parasagittal movements

Theoretically, in both horizontal or parasagittal movements the mechanical work for voluntarily oscillating the two arms together should be equal in ISO and in ANTI, insofar as the movements amplitude and frequency are identical in the two modes. Since these two last conditions were respected in the present experiments, the muscle force and the metabolic consumption for moving the arms should be the same in ISO and ANTI modes. If so, for each movement type, the difference in energy consumption between the stable and unstable coupling modes should represent the cost of the global postural effort in the fixation chain to the ground.

The energy cost of each exercise, $\Delta\dot{V}O_2$ (i.e., the difference between the steady-state oxygen uptake at rest and during the exercise) was evaluated in two groups of subjects during arm oscillations in the horizontal and parasagittal plane, respectively, and normalized for both the body mass and movements amplitude (Esposti et al., 2010, 2013).

In *horizontal movements* (**Figure 12A**, blue triangles) $\Delta\dot{V}O_2$ is quite larger in *hISO* (difficult) than *hANTI* (easy) and increases in both modes when the frequency is raised from 1.4 to 2.0 Hz, to a larger extent in ISO than in ANTI. The related values of SDΔΦ are distributed following the same pattern (**Figure 12B**).

In *parasagittal movements* (**Figure 12A**, black circles), $\Delta\dot{V}O_2$ is higher in *pANTI* (difficult) than in *pISO* (easy) and shows a highly significant linear correlation with frequency in both coupling modes, with a higher slope in ANTI than in ISO. The corresponding changes of SDΔΦ also show a highly significant linear correlation with frequency (**Figure 12B**).

In conclusion, the normalized $\Delta\dot{V}O_2$ varies across the four movement combinations along the gradient: *hANTI* ≠ *pISO* > *pANTI* > *hISO*, analogously to the gradient for SDΔΦ measured in these and previous experiments.

Figure 12C relates SDΔΦ with $\Delta\dot{V}O_2$ and shows that in *parasagittal movements* at any given level of $\Delta\dot{V}O_2$, SDΔΦ is definitively higher (i.e., coordination is worse) in *pANTI* than in *pISO*, signaling that a quote of the ISO vs. ANTI stability loss is not related to a change in oxygen uptake, (i.e., to the postural effort), but to some non-metabolic factor(s), presumably to the neural conflict between APAs and voluntary commands.

The metabolic and non-metabolic quotes can be separated from each other. On one side, the quote of the stability loss independent from the oxygen uptake is calculated by subtracting from each other the ISO and ANTI linear relations in plot **Figure 12C**. On the other side, subtraction of the ISO and ANTI linear relations in plot **Figure 12B** measures the total stability loss, due to both the metabolic and the non-metabolic

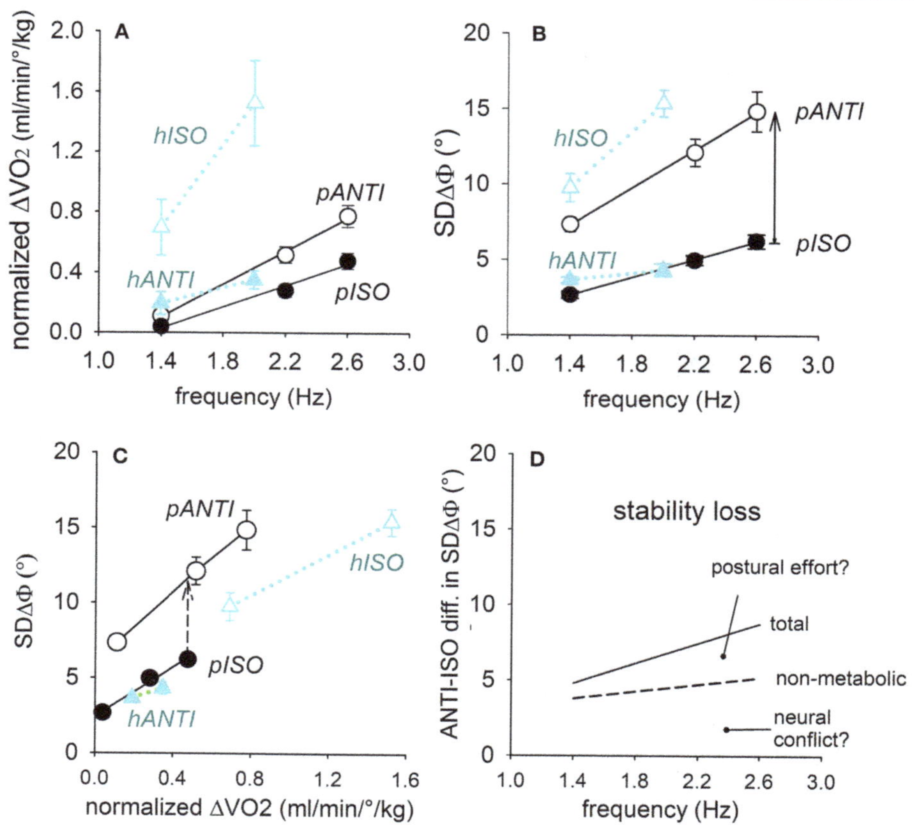

FIGURE 12 | Relations of the oscillation frequency with the normalized oxygen uptake $\Delta\dot{V}O_2$ (A) as well as with the coupling variability SDΔΦ **(B)**, in either coupling mode of the horizontal and parasagittal movements (black and blue symbols, respectively). In **(C)**, direct correlation between SDΔΦ and $\Delta\dot{V}O_2$. The SDΔΦ-$\Delta\dot{V}O_2$ relation in the two difficult modes (*pANTI* and *hISO*) runs higher and has a higher slope than in the respective easy modes (*pISO* and *hANTI*). Continuous arrow in **(B)**: total ISO-vs.-ANTI stability loss; dashed arrow in **(C)**: stability loss independent from $\Delta\dot{V}O_2$. Both are marked at 2.6 Hz. In **(D)** the total and the non-metabolic stability losses in parasagittal movements are plotted by a continuous and dashed lines, respectively, so as to separate the two components of the stability loss, namely the *neural conflict* and the *postural effort*.

components. The total and the non-metabolic losses are shown in plot **Figure 12D** (continuous and dashed lines, respectively) over the range of the frequencies tested, allowing to identify the quote of the stability loss linked to the increase of $\Delta\dot{V}O_2$, i.e., to the postural effort of the fixation chain to the ground.

Mechanism for the coupling destabilizing effect of the postural effort

Hypothesizing a causal relationships between SDΔΦ and the oxygen uptake is possibly supported by the repeated observation that fatigue of either postural or focal muscles modifies APAs timing and size (Morris and Allison, 2006; Strang and Berg, 2007; Kanekar et al., 2008; Strang et al., 2008, 2009). Even if the fatigue levels attained in the cited experiments were not reached in the present exercises, one might argue that the intensified recruitment of both the prime and the postural muscles of trunk and legs during the non-preferred coupling may tend to alter the phase relationships of APAs with respect to the prime movers activity. A control mechanism for maintaining the synchronization between the voluntary and postural components of the movements should then be required, which would progressively become more expensive as the movement frequency increases, giving rise to fatigue phenomena similar to those proposed for the decay of APAs gating in the motor pathways to arm muscles (Baldissera et al., 2008b; Baldissera and Esposti, 2013). If this were to be the case, the stability loss in the less-coordinated coupling mode may result from a unique phenomenon, i.e., the exhaustion of the control mechanisms that govern the interferences arising at different neuronal levels between postural and conscious voluntary commands.

Flexion-Extension Movements of the Hand in the Horizontal Plane

In a group of subjects whose horizontal movements of the arms had been previously analyzed, the same experimental scheme was followed to investigate coupled flexion-extension movements of the hands in the horizontal plane (Baldissera et al., 2008b). As for arm horizontal movements, SDΔΦ of the hand oscillations is significantly higher (i.e., coupling stability is lower) in ISO than in ANTI coupling, in conformity with the APAs distribution in the two modes.

Rules of Interlimb Coupling: A Special Case of APAs Physiology

The ensemble of the above results demonstrates that the easiness/difficulty of coupled limb movements does not depend on the associated muscles, neither on the ISO or ANTI modality *per se,* nor on the limbs being ipsilateral or symmetric. It strongly suggests, instead, that the coupling preference depends, for each type of coupled movements, on the distribution and size of the anticipatory postural adjustments that assist those movements. While performing their fundamental function of body fixation and stabilization during voluntary movements, APAs fatally generate some undesired "side effect" too. This happens when, during a certain focal movement, one simultaneously wants to move another body segment, belonging to a fixation chain, in the direction opposite to the APAs actions on that same segment. If a main chain reaching the ground is involved, where APAs are strong, performing the voluntary movement would require the APAs to be suppressed (gated) but, in this way, the static equilibrium would be lost. If instead the chain is a secondary one, APAs can be reduced via gating to a weak or subliminal level so that coupling of the two movements becomes possible while the movements are slow. Increasing the movement frequency, then coupling becomes unstable, difficult or even impossible, supposedly due to the exhaustion of the gating mechanism (Section *Neural Interference between APAs and Voluntary Commands in the Motor Pathways to the Prime Movers in Horizontal and Parasagittal Arm Movements*) and to the increased postural effort (Section *Effects of APAs in the Fixation Chain to the Ground on Coupling Coordination of Horizontal and Parasagittal Arm Movements*).

Since APAs are excitatory or inhibitory depending on the direction (in extrinsic coordinates) of the focal movement, this would explain why a "direction principle" rules the dichotomy of easy vs. difficult coupling.

Finally, it has to be expected that any factor that modifies the generation, execution, and organization of the APAs (for instance factors depending on the individual variability, on changes in the sensory context or in the body attitude, on training or on pathological events, see Section *Postural Constraints from Neuroscience to Sports and Rehabilitation Medicine*), will affect the coordination of limb coupled movements too. It cannot of course be excluded that other yet unknown factors may add to the APAs in destabilizing limbs coupling.

POSTURAL CONSTRAINTS FROM NEUROSCIENCE TO SPORTS AND REHABILITATION MEDICINE

In the above Chapters some of the rules of the anticipatory postural control were elucidated, with special reference to the APAs interference with interlimb coordination. Which is the potential translation of this knowledge beyond theoretical neuroscience?

"Will" Develops by Entangling Focal and Postural Movements

APA control is an intrinsic component of voluntary movement, not an "external" phenomenon: by definition, APAs exist as far as a movement is voluntary. Yet, APA develop quite independently and much later with respect to the capacity to imagine a voluntary movement. APA control is only primitively organized in the newborn (see Girolami et al., 2010 for references), consistently with the immature myelination of the central nervous system at birth. Once their neurobiological substrate is mature, focal, and postural movements remain entangled during further motor learning.

The APA component of learning is more relevant the more the movement involves long chains of muscles for within-body and body-ground stabilization.

APA as a Candidate "Neural Factor" in Force Development and Loss

The APA physiology provides a promising model for the explanation of the well-known, yet not entirely understood, "neural" mechanisms underlying the effect of resistance/power training. "Resistance" training, aimed at improving force and power in voluntary movements through muscle hypertrophy, is most commonly based on exercises of heavy lifting efforts which, despite high risk to destabilize the body system, are usually perceived as rather simple to learn and perform. Yet, unspecified "neural" factors (Sale, 1988) have long been postulated to explain (a) why force gains anticipate (even by many weeks) muscle hypertrophy (Clark et al., 2008) and (b) why, although the focal main muscles may stay the same in different exercises, the force gain is higher for the trained and very similar movements (Wirth et al., 2016). Consistently enough, force training with fast movements entails the highest force gain in movements performed at the trained speed; unilateral training allows higher unilateral force gains, compared to bilateral training, etc. (Jones and Rutherford, 1987). Unspecified "neural" factors, supported by TMS (Pearce et al., 2013) and fMRI (Farthing et al., 2011) findings, have also been claimed to subtend cross-education, i.e., force gains on the same movement of the untrained side, or force maintenance after immobilization, thanks to force training of the opposite side, as well as force gains achievable after pure mental practice (Yue and Cole, 1992; Reiser et al., 2011). In all cases, results may depend on the specific postural chains engaged, and thus unconsciously trained or not, in different exercises. De-training leads to force loss higher than the loss in muscle mass (Narici et al., 1989).

APA as a Candidate Ingredient of Skill Acquisition and Loss and Motor Learning

Recent studies evidenced that APA efficiency actually subtends also skill, and not only force, of voluntary movements. For instance, earlier APAs in shoulder muscles have been shown to be associated with higher accuracy in pointing tasks (Caronni et al.,

2013), and in the greater accuracy of pointing with the dominant, compared to the non-dominant upper limb (Bruttini et al., 2016).

De-training also conceals a loss of APAs efficiency. After only a 12 h wrist and fingers immobilization a simple finger tapping task is altered, due to insufficient stabilization of the elbow, reflecting delayed activation or inhibition of proximal muscles (Bolzoni et al., 2012). In general, an improvement of APAs has long been suspected as a potential component of learning of voluntary movements (Rutherford and Jones, 1986).

Yet the relationships between APAs and learning were not extensively investigated in the subsequent literature. It was shown, however, that exercises requiring high motor skills rapidly lead to improvements in balance (Aruin et al., 2015; Kanekar and Aruin, 2015) and in a reaching task while standing (Saito et al., 2014). Improvements were invariably associated with an earlier recruitment of the APAs in lower limb muscles.

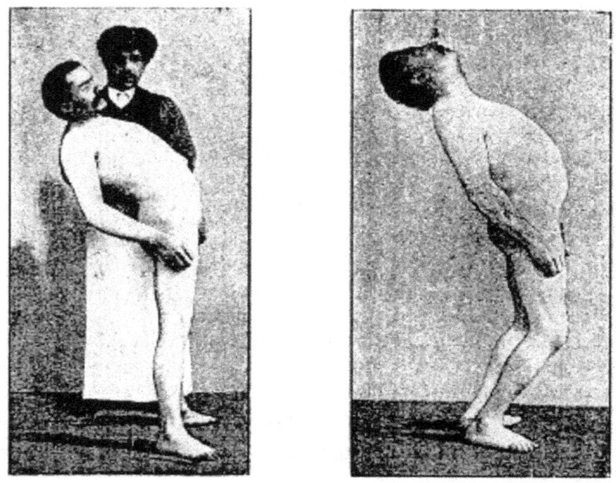

FIGURE 13 | A cerebellar patient (left panel) is requested to lean backward (focal movement) while standing. If not supported by the assistant, he will fall. The right panel shows the correct movement, in which knee flexion (APA) precedes the trunk extension, so that the body center of mass will be projected within the base of support ("cerebellar asynergy," after Babinski, 1899). This established clinical finding was confirmed by later, refined neurophysiologic research. Yet, after nearly 120 years this still remains one of the brightest demonstrations that the postural component of a voluntary moment can be impaired independently from its focal component.

APA Can be Specifically Affected in Neural Diseases: Hints to Clinical Diagnostics

Postural and focal movements can be de-coupled in case of nervous diseases. There seems to be no single "APA organ" within the central nervous system: rather, many CNS structures are involved. These include hemispheric cortex, cerebellum, basal ganglia, brain stem, and spinal cord (for a quick overview, see Discussion in Ioffe et al., 2007).

The cerebellum is certainly a key node of the network of postural control (Ioffe et al., 2007). The fact that cerebellar damage entails "postural" consequences was already acknowledged, as shown in **Figure 13** by a famous Babinski's example of a "postural" alteration after cerebellar lesion leaving the "focal" movement unaffected (Babinski, 1899). Cerebellar lesions may selectively impair also the APAs subtending within-limb movements. For instance, in patients with cerebellar ataxia, simple brisk movements of the finger are associated with alterations of the APAs engaging proximal arm muscles (Bruttini et al., 2015; Cavallari et al., 2016).

Recent research also showed that the lesion of many other cerebral structures (e.g., of the supplementary motor area (Viallet et al., 1992) or of the basal ganglia (Viallet et al., 1987) can lead to selective alterations of APAs, thus affecting within-limb and/or body-ground chaining. With respect to the "easy" and "difficult" hand-foot coupling described above, it has been shown that after hemispheric stroke, the "difficult" coupling is selectively impaired (or even impossible) on the unaffected side, which retains an otherwise skilled motricity (Baldissera et al., 1994). The frame of APAs physiology offers an explanation.

As illustrated in Section Role of APAs in Differentiating ISO vs. ANTI Coupling Modes in Other Types of Limb Movements, APAs may well-spread contralaterally to a focal movement; further, the successful completion of the APA "arborization" is a pre-requisite for the subsequent contraction of focal muscles (Cordo and Nashner, 1982; Brown and Frank, 1987). Hence, any impairment of APA commands on the paretic side may impair or even prevent a focal movement on the unaffected side. Not surprisingly, in hemiparetic patients, strength and coordination are affected on the "healthy" side, too (Santos et al., 2016). While overt postural disturbances may not appear, yet the hand-foot coupling test may reveal that they stand subliminal in the background. Therefore, asking for anti-phase coupling of the unimpaired hand and foot can be proposed as a simple, yet highly sensitive bedside test of hemispheric damage. The test is not specific to hemispheric lesions, however. All of the above considerations stimulate clinical reasoning. The studies on APAs in cerebellar patients suggest that ataxia can be seen as a typical consequence of APAs disorders, not less than of the programming of focal movements. Limb ataxia (commonly evidenced by dismetry in the classic index-to-nose or heel-to-knee tests), the incapacity to maintain a stable level of isometric force ("dys-stenia," Tesio, 2010), as well as trunk ataxia with balance deficits can all be interpreted as primarily caused by APAs disturbances. The subject knows what the focal movement should be but is unable to avoid position and/or force errors due to altered APAs.

The capacity of disease to affect selectively focal rather than postural movements is demonstrated by the case of survival of APAs after loss of its related focal movement. This observation is common in clinical practice but only exceptionally reported in the literature. For instance, ischemic or anesthetic block of the hand does not abolish APAs in proximal muscles (Bruttini et al., 2014). Brachial plexus lesions may entail the complete loss of shoulder abduction, yet the "luxury" of a fixation chain crossing the midline during a voluntary effort is preserved. Thus, the very existence of APA warrants the presence of genuine "will," thus providing a useful clinical sign. Fixation chains can only be rarely lost: they may disappear in case of cognitive deficits (e.g., hemineglect or apraxia), chronic "learned non-use" in deep-seated palsies (Taub et al., 2014) or conditions such as simulation and conversion disorders (Tesio and Colombo, 1992).

APA Can be Selectively Trained in Sports and Rehabilitation Medicine

Motor training science (Magill and Anderson, 2014) has long acknowledged that "coupling" some movements is much more difficult to be trained and learned, compared to other. For instance, teaching how to de-couple the upper limbs in bimanual activities, usually a difficult challenge, is made more effective by dedicated training techniques (Walter and Swinnen, 1994).

Although training a "voluntary" movement is usually explicitly addressed to its focal component, yet it entails an unconscious and indirect training of its postural component (Mouchnino et al., 1992; Ioffe et al., 2007). As a rule, training can be addressed to the desired focal movement (explicit training) or another actual or imagined movement to which the desired one is unconsciously associated (implicit training). This holds also for skilled exercises improperly claimed to directly train the APAs (Aruin et al., 2015; Kanekar and Aruin, 2015). Actually, neither approach targets explicitly the APAs. Specific APA training paradigms are still missing. First, the APA chains subtending the normal voluntary movements must be predicted: although they mostly spread along the plane of the focal movement (Gabbett and Masters, 2011; Bruttini et al., 2014) a detailed "atlas" of expected APAs in various motor tasks is far from being developed. Second, APAs disorders usually consist in incomplete chaining and/or delayed timing/phasing between focal and various postural muscles. The between-muscle delays are in the order of tenths of milliseconds, depending on the muscles involved. In a clinical environment, a very skilled palpation of tendon tension can often succeed in capturing such between-muscle delays. A much easier and sharper temporal discrimination, in the order of few milliseconds, can be reached, both by patient and therapist, by binaural listening of sharp tones generated by transduction of the surface EMG from a focal and a postural muscle, and separately sent to the right and left ears (Tesio et al., 1996). This form of augmented feedback can be said to explicitly target the APAs and to provide a "knowledge of result" fostering the learning of the correct APA (Schmidt and Lee, 2005).

Despite the examples given above, the diagnosis and the treatment of APAs' deficits, both in sports and rehabilitation sciences, is still at the frontiers of physiology and represent a promising field of research.

AUTHOR CONTRIBUTIONS

All authors contributed in collecting the literature, critically analyzing it, and writing the manuscript. All authors approved the final version and agree to be accountable for all aspects of this work.

REFERENCES

Aoki, F. (1991). Activity patterns of upper arm muscles in relation to direction of rapid wrist movement in man. *Exp. Brain Res.* 83, 679–682. doi: 10.1007/BF00229847

Aruin, A. S., and Latash, M. L. (1995). Directional specificity of postural muscles in feed-forward postural reactions during fast voluntary arm movements. *Exp. Brain Res.* 103, 323–332. doi: 10.1007/BF00231718

Aruin, A. S., and Latash, M. L. (1996). Anticipatory postural adjustments during self-initiated perturbations of different magnitude triggered by a standard motor action. *Electroencephalogr. Clin. Neurophysiol.* 101, 497–503. doi: 10.1016/S0013-4694(96)95219-4

Aruin, A. S., Kanekar, N., Lee, Y. J., and Ganesan, M., (2015). Enhancement of anticipatory postural adjustments in older adults as a result of a single session of ball throwing exercise. *Exp. Brain Res.* 233, 649–655. doi: 10.1007/s00221-014-4144-1

Babinski, J. (1899). De l' asynergie cérébelleuse. *Rev. Neurol.* 7, 806–816.

Baldissera, F. G., and Esposti, R. (2013). The role of anticipatory postural adjustments in interlimb coordination of coupled arm movements in the parasagittal plane: II. Postural activities and coupling coordination during cyclic flexion-extension arm movements, ISO- and ANTI-directionally coupled. *Exp. Brain. Res.* 229, 203–219. doi: 10.1007/s00221-013-3605-2

Baldissera, F. G., Cavallari, P., and Esposti, R. (2006). Synchrony of hand-foot coupled movements: is it attained by mutual feedback entrainment or by independent linkage of each limb to a common rhythm generator *BMC Neurosci.* 7:70. doi: 10.1186/1471-2202-7-70

Baldissera, F., and Cavallari, P. (2001). Neural compensation for mechanical loading of the hand during coupled oscillations of the hand and foot. *Exp. Brain Res.* 139, 18–29. doi: 10.1007/s002210100762

Baldissera, F., and Esposti, R. (2005). Postural constraints to coupling of ipsilateral hand-foot movements. *Neuroreport* 16, 1615–1619. doi: 10.1097/01.wnr.0000181586.49130.48

Baldissera, F., Borroni, P., and Cavallari, P. (2000). Neural compensation for mechanical differences between hand and foot during coupled oscillations of the two segments. *Exp. Brain Res.* 133, 165–177. doi: 10.1007/s002210000368

Baldissera, F., Cavallari, P., and Civaschi, P. (1982). Preferential coupling between voluntary movements of ipsilateral limbs. *Neurosci. Lett.* 34, 95–100. doi: 10.1016/0304-3940(82)90098-2

Baldissera, F., Cavallari, P., and Esposti, R. (2004). Foot equilibrium position controls partition of voluntary command to antagonists during foot oscillations. *Exp. Brain Res.* 155, 274–282. doi: 10.1007/s00221-003-1723-y

Baldissera, F., Rota, V., and Esposti, R. (2008a). Anticipatory postural adjustments in arm muscles associated with movements of the contralateral limb and their possible role in interlimb coordination. *Exp. Brain Res.* 185, 63–74. doi: 10.1007/s00221-007-1131-9

Baldissera, F., Rota, V., and Esposti, R. (2008b). Postural adjustments in arm and leg muscles associated with isodirectional and antidirectional coupling of upper limb movements in the horizontal plane. *Exp. Brain Res.* 190, 289–305. doi: 10.1007/s00221-008-1470-1

Baldissera, F., Borroni, P., Cavallari, P., and Cerri, G. (2002). Excitability changes in human corticospinal projections to forearm muscles during voluntary movement of ipsilateral foot. *J. Physiol.* 539, 903–911. doi: 10.1113/jphysiol.2001.013282

Baldissera, F., Cavallari, P., Marini, G., and Tassone, G. (1991). Differential control of in-phase and anti-phase coupling of rhythmic movements of ipsilateral hand and foot. *Exp. Brain Res.* 83, 375–380.

Baldissera, F., Cavallari, P., and Tesio, L. (1994). "Coordination of cyclic coupled movements of hand and foot in normal subjects and on the healthy side of hemiplegic patients," in *Interlimb Coordination: Neural, Dynamical and*

Cognitive Constraints, eds S. P. Swinnen, H. Heuer, J. Massion, and P. Casaer (San Diego, CA: Academic Press), 229–242.

Belen'kii, V. E., Gurfinkel', V. S., and Pal'tsev, E. I. (1967). [Control elements of voluntary movements]. *Biofizika* 12, 135–141.

Bleuse, S., Cassim, F., Blatt, J. L., Defebvre, L., Derambure, P., and Guieu, J. D. (2005). Vertical torque allows recording of anticipatory postural adjustments associated with slow, arm-raising movements. *Clin. Biomech.* 20, 693–699. doi: 10.1016/j.clinbiomech.2005.03.005

Bobet, J., and Norman, R. W. (1990). Least-squares identification of the dynamic relation between the electromyogram and joint moment. *J. Biomech.* 23, 1275–1276. doi: 10.1016/0021-9290(90)90386-H

Bolzoni, F., Bruttini, C., Esposti, R., and Cavallari, P. (2012). Hand immobilization affects arm and shoulder postural control. *Exp. Brain Res.* 220, 63–70. doi: 10.1007/s00221-012-3115-7

Borroni, P., Cerri, G., and Baldissera, F. (2004). Excitability changes in resting forearm muscles during voluntary foot movements depend on hand position: a neural substrate for hand-foot isodirectional coupling. *Brain Res.* 1022, 117–125. doi: 10.1016/j.brainres.2004.07.003

Bouisset, S., and Do, M. C. (2008). Posture, dynamic stability, and voluntary movement. *Neurophysiol. Clin.* 38, 345–362. doi: 10.1016/j.neucli.2008.10.001

Bouisset, S., and Zattara, M. (1987). Biomechanical study of the programming of anticipatory postural adjustments associated with voluntary movement. *J. Biomech.* 20, 735–742. doi: 10.1016/0021-9290(87)90052-2

Brown, J. E., and Frank, J. S. (1987). Influence of event anticipation on postural actions accompanying voluntary movement. *Exp. Brain Res.* 67, 645–650.

Bruttini, C., Esposti, R., Bolzoni, F., and Cavallari, P. (2016). Higher Precision in pointing movements of the preferred vs. non-preferred hand is associated with an earlier occurrence of anticipatory postural adjustments. *Front. Hum. Neurosci.* 10:365. doi: 10.3389/fnhum.2016.00365

Bruttini, C., Esposti, R., Bolzoni, F., and Cavallari, P. (2014). Ischemic block of the forearm abolishes finger movements but not their associated anticipatory postural adjustments. *Exp. Brain Res.* 232, 1739–1750. doi: 10.1007/s00221-014-3866-4

Bruttini, C., Esposti, R., Bolzoni, F., Vanotti, A., Mariotti, C., and Cavallari, P. (2015). Temporal disruption of upper-limb anticipatory postural adjustments in cerebellar ataxic patients. *Exp. Brain Res.* 233, 197–203. doi: 10.1007/s00221-014-4103-x

Byblow, W. D., Coxon, J. P., Stinear, C. M., Fleming, M. K., Williams, G., Müller, J. F., et al. (2007). Functional connectivity between secondary and primary motor areas underlying hand-foot coordination. *J. Neurophysiol.* 98, 414–422. doi: 10.1152/jn.00325.2007

Caronni, A., Bolzoni, F., Esposti, R., Bruttini, C., and Cavallari, P. (2013). Accuracy of pointing movements relies upon a specific tuning between anticipatory postural adjustments and prime mover activation. *Acta Physiol.* 208, 111–124. doi: 10.1111/apha.12081

Carson, R. G. (1993). Manual asymmetries: old problems and new directions. *Hum. Mov. Sci.* 12, 479–506. doi: 10.1016/0167-9457(93)90001-6

Carson, R. G., Goodman, D., Kelso, J. A., and Elliott, D. (1995). Phase transitions and critical fluctuations in rhythmic coordination of ipsilateral hand and foot. *J. Mot. Behav.* 27, 211–224. doi: 10.1080/00222895.1995.9941711

Carson, R. G., Riek, S., Mackey, D. C., Meichenbaum, D. P., Willms, K., Forner, M., et al. (2004). Excitability changes in human forearm corticospinal projections and spinal reflex pathways during rhythmic voluntary movement of the opposite limb. *J. Physiol.* 560, 929–940. doi: 10.1113/jphysiol.2004.069088

Cavallari, P., Bolzoni, F., Bruttini, C., and Esposti, R. (2016). The organization and control of intra-limb anticipatory postural adjustments and their role in movement performance. *Front. Hum. Neurosci.* 10:525. doi: 10.3389/fnhum.2016.00525

Cerri, G., Borroni, P., and Baldissera, F. (2003). Cyclic H-reflex modulation in resting forearm related to contractions of foot movers, not to foot movement. *J. Neurophysiol.* 90, 81–88. doi: 10.1152/jn.00030.2003

Chabran, E., Fourment, A., Maton, B., and Ribreau, C. (1999). Chronology of upper limb anticipatory postural adjustments associated with voluntary wrist flexions and extensions in humans. *Neurosci. Lett.* 268, 13–16. doi: 10.1016/S0304-3940(99)00354-7

Chabran, E., Maton, B., Ribreau, C., and Fourment, A. (2001). Electromyographic and biomechanical characteristics of segmental postural adjustments associated with voluntary wrist movements. Influence of an elbow support. *Exp. Brain Res.* 141, 133–145. doi: 10.1007/s002210100823

Clark, B. C., Issac, L. C., Lane, J. L., Damron, L. A., and Hoffman, R. L. (2008). Neuromuscular plasticity during and following 3 wk of human forearm cast immobilization. *J. Appl.Physiol.* 105, 868–878. doi: 10.1152/japplphysiol.90530.2008

Cordo, P. J., and Nashner, L. M. (1982). Properties of postural adjustments associated with rapid arm movements. *J. Neurophysiol.* 47, 287–302.

Debaere, F., Swinnen, S. P., Beatse, E., Sunaert, S., van Hecke, P., and Duysens, J. (2001). Brain areas involved in interlimb coordination: a distributed network. *Neuroimage* 14, 947–958. doi: 10.1006/nimg.2001.0892

Debaere, F., Wenderoth, N., Sunaert, S., van Hecke, P., and Swinnen, S. P. (2004). Cerebellar and premotor function in bimanual coordination parametric neural responses to spatiotemporal complexity and cycling frequency. *Neuroimage* 21, 1416–1427. doi: 10.1016/j.neuroimage.2003.12.011

Esposti, R., and Baldissera, F. (2011). Combined recruitment of two fixation chains during cyclic movements of one arm. *Hum. Mov. Sci.* 30, 213–226. doi: 10.1016/j.humov.2010.02.005

Esposti, R., and Baldissera, F. G. (2013). The role of anticipatory postural adjustments (APAs) in interlimb coordination of coupled arm movements in the parasagittal plane: I. Apas associated with fast discrete flexion and extension movements of one arm or of both arms ISO- and ANTI-directionally coupled. *Exp. Brain. Res.* 228, 527–539. doi: 10.1007/s00221-013-3584-3

Esposti, R., Cavallari, P., and Baldissera, F. (2005). Partition of voluntary command to antagonist muscles during cyclic flexion–extension of the hand. *Exp. Brain Res.* 162, 436–448. doi: 10.1007/s00221-004-2120-x

Esposti, R., Cavallari, P., and Baldissera, F. (2007). Feedback control of the limbs position during voluntary rhythmic oscillation *Biol. Cybern.* 97, 123–136. doi: 10.1007/s00422-007-0159-z

Esposti, R., Esposito, F., Ce, E., and Baldissera, F. (2010). Difference in the metabolic cost of postural actions during iso- and antidirectional coupled oscillations of the upper limbs in the horizontal plane. *Eur. J. Appl. Physiol.* 108, 93–104. doi: 10.1007/s00421-009-1193-4

Esposti, R., Limonta, E., Esposito, F., and Baldissera, F. G. (2013). The role of anticipatory postural adjustments in interlimb coordination of coupled arm movements in the parasagittal plane: III. Difference in the energy cost of postural actions during cyclic flexion–extension arm movements, ISO- and ANTI-directionally coupled. *Exp. Brain. Res.* 231, 293–303. doi: 10.1007/s00221-013-3691-1

Farthing, J. P., Krentz, J. R., Magnus, C. R. A., Barss, T. S., Lanovaz, J. L., Cummine, J., et al. (2011). Changes in fMRI cortical activation with cross-education to an immobilized limb. *Med. Sci. Sports Exerc.* 43, 1394–1405. doi: 10.1249/MSS.0b013e318210783c

Ferry, M., Martin, L., Termoz, N., Côté, J., and Prince, F. (2004). Balance control during an arm rising movement in bipedal stance: which biomechanical factor is controlled? *Biol. Cybern.* 91, 104–114. doi: 10.1007/s00422-004-0501-7

Forner-Cordero, A., Levin, O., Li, Y., and Swinnen, S. P. (2007). Posture control and complex arm co-ordination: analysis of multijoint coordinative movements and stability of stance. *J. Mot.Behav.* 39, 215–226. doi: 10.3200/JMBR.39.3.215-226

Friedli, W. G., Hallett, M., and Simon, S. R. (1984). Postural adjustments associated with rapid voluntary arm movements 1. Electromyographic data. *J. Neurol. Neurosurg. Psychiatry* 47, 611–622.

Gabbett, T., and Masters, R. (2011). Challenges and solutions when applying implicit motor learning theory in a high performance sport environment: examples from rugby league. *Int. J. Sports Sci. Coach.* 6, 567–575. doi: 10.1260/1747-9541.6.4.567

Girolami, G. L., Stiratori, T., and Aruin, A. S. (2010). Anticipatory postural adjustments in children with typical motor development. *Exp. Brain Res.* 205, 153–165. doi: 10.1007/s00221-010-2347-7

Haken, H., Kelso, J. A., and Bunz, H. (1985). A theoretical model of phase transitions in human hand movements. *Biol. Cybern.* 51, 347–356. doi: 10.1007/BF00336922

Hiraoka, K. (2001). Phase-dependent modulation of the soleus H-reflex during rhythmical arm swing in humans. *Electroen. Clin. Neuro.* 41, 43–47.

Hodges, P. W., Cresswell, A. G., Daggfeldt, K., and Thorstensson, A. (2000). Three dimensional preparatory trunk motion precedes asymmetrical upper limb movement. *Gait Posture* 11, 92–101. doi: 10.1016/S0966-6362(99)00055-7

Hodges, P., Cresswell, A., and Thorstensson, A. (1999). Preparatory trunk motion accompanies rapid upper limb movement. *Exp. Brain Res.* 124, 69–79. doi: 10.1007/s002210050601

Hunter, I. W., and Kearney, R. E. (1982). Dynamics of human ankle stiffness: variation with men ankle torque. *J. Biomech.* 15, 747–752. doi: 10.1016/0021-9290(82)90089-6

Immisch, I., Waldvogel, D., van Gelderen, P., and Hallett, M. (2001). The role of the medial wall and its anatomical variations for bimanual antiphase and in-phase movements. *Neuroimage* 14, 674–684. doi: 10.1006/nimg.2001.0856

Ioffe, M. E., Chernikova, L. A., and Ustinova, K. I. (2007). Role of cerebellum in learning postural tasks. *Cerebellum* 6, 87–94. doi: 10.1080/14734220701216440

Jeka, J. J., and Kelso, J. A. (1995). Manipulating symmetry in the coordination dynamics of human movement. *J. Exp. Psychol. Hum. Percept. Perform.* 21, 360–374. doi: 10.1037/0096-1523.21.2.360

Jones, D. A., and Rutherford, O. M. (1987). Human muscle strength training: the effects of three different regimens and the nature of the resultant changes. *J. Physiol. (Lond).* 391, 1–11. doi: 10.1113/jphysiol.1987.sp016721

Kanekar, N., and Aruin, A. S. (2015). Improvement of anticipatory postural adjustments for balance control: effect of a single training session. *J. Electromyogr. Kinesiol.* 25, 400–4005. doi: 10.1016/j.jelekin.2014.11.002

Kanekar, N., Santos, M. J., and Aruin, A. S. (2008). Anticipatory postural control following fatigue of postural and focal muscles. *Clin. Neurophysiol.* 119, 2304–2313. doi: 10.1016/j.clinph.2008.06.015

Kasai, T., and Komiyama, T. (1996). Soleus H-reflex depression induced by ballistic voluntary arm movement in human. *Brain Res.* 714, 125–134. doi: 10.1016/0006-8993(95)01508-6

Kawanishi, M., Yahagi, S., and Kasai, T. (1999). Neural mechanisms of soleus H-reflex depression accompanying voluntary arm movement in standing humans. *Brain Res.* 832, 13–22. doi: 10.1016/S0006-8993(99)01454-7

Kelso, J. A. (1984). Phase transitions and critical behavior in human bimanual coordination. *Am. J. Physiol.* 246, R1000–R1004.

Kelso, J. A., and Jeka, J. J. (1992). Symmetry breaking dynamics of human multilimb coordination. *J. Exp. Psychol. Hum. Percept. Perform.* 18, 645–668. doi: 10.1037/0096-1523.18.3.645

Kots, Y. M., Krinskiy, V. I., Naydin, V. L., and Shik, M. L. (1971). "The control of movements of the joints and kinesthetic afferentation," in *Models of Structural Functional Organization of Certain Biological Systems*, eds I. M. Gel'fand, V. S. Gurfinkei, S. V. Fomin, and M. L. Tsetlin (Cambridge: MIT Press), 37–52.

Lakie, M., Walsh, E. G., and Wright, G. W. (1984). Resonance at the wrist demonstrated by the use of a torque motor: an instrumental analysis of muscle tone in man. *J. Physiol. (Lond).* 353, 265–285, doi: 10.1113/jphysiol.1984.sp015335

Lehman, S. L., and Calhoun, B. M. (1990). An identified model for human wrist movements. *Exp. Brain Res.* 81, 199–208. doi: 10.1007/BF00230116

Leonard, J. A., Gritsenko, V., Ouckama, R., and Stapley, P. J. (2011). Postural adjustments for online corrections of arm movements in standing humans. *J. Neurophysiol.* 105, 2375–2388. doi: 10.1152/jn.00944.2010

Magill, R. A., and Anderson, D. I. (2014). *Motor Learning and Control: Concepts and Applications.* New York, NY: McGraw-Hill.

Marsden, C. D., Merton, P. A., and Morton, H. B. (1978). Anticipatory postural responses in the human subject [proceedings]. *J. Physiol.* 275, 47P–48P.

Marsden, C. D., Merton, P. A., and Morton, H. B. (1981). Human postural responses. *Brain* 104, 513–534. doi: 10.1093/brain/104.3.513

Meige, H. (1901). Les mouvements en miroir: leurs applications pratiques et thérapeutiques. *Rev. Neurol.* 19, 780.

Morris, S. L., and Allison, G. T. (2006). Effects of abdominal muscle fatigue on anticipatory postural adjustments associated with arm raising. *Gait Posture* 24, 342–348. doi: 10.1016/j.gaitpost.2005.10.011

Morris, S. L., Lay, B., and Allison, G. T. (2013). Transversus abdominis is part of a global not local muscle synergy during arm movement. *Hum. Mov. Sci.* 32, 1176–1185. doi: 10.1016/j.humov.2012.12.011

Mouchnino, L., Aurenty, R., Massion, J., and Pedotti, A. (1992). Coordination between equilibrium and head-trunk orientation during leg movement: a new strategy build up by training. *J. Neurophysiol.* 67, 1587–1598.

Müller, J. (1840). *Handbuch der Physiologie des Menschen.* Koblenz: Hòlscher.

Narici, M. V., Roi, G. S., Landoni, L., Minetti, A. E., and Cerretelli, P. (1989). Changes in force, cross-sectional area and neural activation during strength training and detraining of the human quadriceps. *Eur. J. Appl. Physiol. Occup. Physiol.* 59, 310–319. doi: 10.1007/BF02388334

Nashner, L. M., and Forssberg, H. (1986). Phase-dependent organization of postural adjustments associated with arm movements while walking. *J. Neurophysiol.* 55, 1382–1394.

Noica (Bucarest) (1912). Étude sur les mouvements associé de l'homme normal et des malades. *L'Encéphale* 3, 201–221.

Pearce, A. J., Hendy, A., Bowen, W. A., and Kidgell, D. J. (2013), Corticospinal adaptations and strength maintenance in the immobilized arm following 3 weeks unilateral strength training. *Scand. J. Med. Sci. Sports* 23, 740–748. doi: 10.1111/j.1600-0838.2012.01453.x

Reiser, M., Büsch, D., and Munzert, J. (2011). Strength gains by motor imagery with different ratios of physical to mental practice. *Front. Psychol.* 2:194. doi: 10.3389/fpsyg.2011.00194

Ridderikhoff, A., Daffertshofer, A., Peper, C. L., and Beek, P. J. (2005). Mirrored EMG activity during unimanual rhythmic movements. *Neurosci. Lett.* 381, 228–233. doi: 10.1016/j.neulet.2005.02.041

Rutherford, O. M., and Jones, D. A. (1986). The role of learning and coordination in strength training. *Eur. J. Appl. Physiol. Occup. Physiol.* 55, 100–105. doi: 10.1007/BF00422902

Sadato, N., Yonekura, Y., Waki, A., Yamada, H., and Ishii, Y. (1997). Role of the supplementary motor area and the right premotor cortex in the coordination of bimanual finger movements. *J. Neurosci.* 17, 9667–9674.

Saito, H., Yamanaka, M., Kasahara, S., and Fukushima, J. (2014). Relationship between improvements in motor performance and changes in anticipatory postural adjustments during whole-body reaching training. *Hum. Mov. Sci.* 37, 69–86. doi: 10.1016/j.humov.2014.07.001

Sale, D. G. (1988). Neural adaptation to resistance training. *Med. Sci. Sports Exerc.* 20, S135–S145. doi: 10.1249/00005768-198810001-00009

Santos, G. L., García-Salazar, L. F., Souza, M. B., Oliveira, A. B., Camargo, P. R., and Russo, T. (2016). Torque steadiness and muscle activation are bilaterally impaired during shoulder abduction and flexion in chronic post-stroke subjects.*J. Electromyogr. Kinesiol.* 30, 151–160. doi: 10.1016/j.jelekin.2016.07.003

Schepens, B., and Drew, T. (2004). Independent and convergent signals from the pontomedullary reticular formation contribute to the control of posture and movement during reaching in the cat. *J. Neurophysiol.* 92, 2217–2238. doi: 10.1152/jn.01189.2003

Schepens, B., and Drew, T. (2006). Descending signals from the pontomedullary reticular formation are bilateral, asymmetric, and gated during reaching movements in the cat. *J. Neurophysiol.* 96, 2229–2252. doi: 10.1152/jn.00342.2006

Schepens, B., Stapley, P., and Drew, T. (2008). Neurons in the pontomedullary reticular formation signal posture and movement both as an integrated behavior and independently. *J. Neurophysiol.* 100, 2235–2253. doi: 10.1152/jn.01381.2007

Schmidt, A. S., and Lee, T. D. (2005). "Augmented feedback," in *Motor Control and Learning*, eds A. S. Schmidt and T. D.Lee (Champaigne, IL: Human Kinetics), 364–400.

Schmidt, R. A., Zelaznik, H., Hawkins, B., Frank, J. S., and Quinn, J. T. J. (1979). Motor-output variability: a theory for the accuracy of rapid motor acts. *Psychol. Rev.* 86, 415–451. doi: 10.1037/0033-295x.86.5.415

Serrien, D. J., and Swinnen, S. P. (1998). Load compensation during homologous and non-homologous coordination. *Exp. Brain Res.* 121, 223–229. doi: 10.1007/s002210050455

Shiratori, T., and Aruin, A. (2007). Modulation of anticipatory postural adjustments associated with unloading perturbation: effect of characteristics of a motor action. *Exp. Brain Res.* 178, 206–215. doi: 10.1007/s00221-006-0725-y

Shiratori, T., and Aruin, A. S. (2004). Anticipatory postural adjustments associated with rotational perturbations while standing on fixed and free-rotating supports. *Clin. Neurophysiol.* 115, 797–806. doi: 10.1016/j.clinph.2003.11.015

Slijper, H., and Latash, M. (2000). The effects of instability and additional hand support on anticipatory postural adjustments in leg, trunk, and arm muscles during standing. *Exp. Brain Res.* 135, 81–93. doi: 10.1007/s002210000492

Slijper, H., and Latash, M. L. (2004). The effects of muscle vibration on anticipatory postural adjustments. *Brain Res.* 1015, 57–72. doi: 10.1016/j.brainres.2004.04.054
Stark, L. S. (1968). *Neurological Control Systems. Studies in Bioengineering.* New York, NY: Plenum Press.
Stiles, R. N. (1983). Lightly damped hand oscillations: acceleration-related feedback and system damping. *J. Neurophysiol.* 50, 327–343.
Strang, A. J., and Berg, W. P. (2007). Fatigue-induced adaptive changes of anticipatory postural adjustments. *Exp. Brain Res.* 178, 49–61. doi: 10.1007/s00221-006-0710-5
Strang, A. J., Berg, W. P., and Hieronymus, M. (2009). Fatigue-induced early onset of anticipatory postural adjustments in non-fatigued muscles: support for a centrally mediated adaptation. *Exp. Brain Res.* 197, 245–254. doi: 10.1007/s00221-009-1908-0
Strang, A. J., Choi, H. J., and Berg, W. P. (2008). The effect of exhausting aerobic exercise on the timing of anticipatory postural adjustments. *J. Sports Med. Phys. Fitness* 48, 9–16.
Swinnen, S. P. (2002). Intermanual coordination: from behavioural principles to neural-network interactions. *Nat. Rev. Neurosci.* 3, 348–359. doi: 10.1038/nrn807
Swinnen, S. P., Dounskaia, N., Verschueren, S., Serrien, D. J., and Daelman, A. (1995). Relative phase destabilization during interlimb coordination: the disruptive role of kinesthetic afferences induced by passive movement. *Exp. Brain Res.* 105, 439–454.
Taub, E., Uswatte, G., and Mark, V. W. (2014). The functional significance of cortical reorganization and the parallel development of CI therapy. *Front. Hum. Neurosci.* 8:396. doi: 10.3389/fnhum.2014.00396
Tesio, L. (2010). "Ataxia," in *Multiple Sclerosis. Recovery of Function and Neurorehabilitation*, eds J. Kesselring, G. Comi, and A. Thompson (Cambridge, UK: Cambridge University Press), 201–213.
Tesio, L., and Colombo, B. (1992). "Luxury" recruitment of remote fixator muscle: a sign of organic weakness. *Mov. Disord.* 7, 156
Tesio, L., Gatti, R., Monzani, M., and Franchignoni, F. P. (1996). EMG-Feedback from two muscles in postural reactions: a new pocket device for the patient-therapist pair. *J. Electromyogr. Kinesiol.* 6, 277–279. doi: 10.1016/S1050-6411(96)00013-2
Tomita, H., Fukaya, Y., Homma, S., Ueda, T., Yamamoto, Y., and Shionoya, K. (2010). Anticipatory postural muscle activity associated with bilateral arm flexion while standing in individuals with spastic diplegic cerebral palsy: a pilot study. *Neurosci. Lett.* 479, 166–170. doi: 10.1016/j.neulet.2010.05.059
Turvey, M. T., Schmidt, R. C., and Rosenblum, L. D. (1989). 'Clock' and 'motor' components in absolute coordination of rhythmic movements. *Neuroscience* 33, 1–10. doi: 10.1016/0306-4522(89)90305-9
Ullen, F., Forssberg, H., and Ehrsson, H. H. (2003). Neural networks for the coordination of the hands in time. *J. Neurophysiol.* 89, 1126–1135. doi: 10.1152/jn.00775.2002
Ustinova, K. I., Goussev, V. M., Balasubramaniam, R., and Levin, M. F. (2004). Disruption of coordination between arm, trunk and center of pressure displacement in patients with hemiparesis. *Motor Control* 8, 139–159. doi: 10.1123/mcj.8.2.139
Van der Woude, L. H., Horstman, A., Faas, P., Mechielsen, S., Bafghi, H. A., and de Koning, J. J. (2008). Power output and metabolic cost of synchronous and asynchronous submaximal and peak level hand cycling on a motor driven treadmill in able-bodied male subjects. *Med. Eng. Phys.* 30, 574–580. doi: 10.1016/j.medengphy.2007.06.006
Viallet, F., Massion, J., Massarino, R., and Khalil, R. (1987). Performance of a bimanual load-lifting task by parkinsonian patients. *J. Neurol. Neurosurg. Psychiatry* 50, 1274–1283. doi: 10.1136/jnnp.50.10.1274
Viallet, F., Massion, J., Massarino, R., and Khalil, R. (1992). Coordination between posture and movement in a bimanual load lifting task: putative role of a medial frontal region including the supplementary motor area. *Exp. Brain Res.* 88, 674–684. doi: 10.1007/BF00228197
Viviani, P., Soechting, J. F., and Terzuolo, C. A. (1976). Influence of mechanical properties on the relation between EMG activity and torque. *J. Physiol.* 72, 45–58.
Walter, C. B., and Swinnen, S. P. (1994). "The formulation ad dissolution of "bad habits" during the acquistion of coordinations kills," in *Interlimb Coordination: Neural, Dynamical and Cognitive Constraints*, eds S. P. Swinnen, H. Heuer, J. Massion, and P. Casaer (San Diego, CA: Academic Press), 491–513.
Wirth, K., Hartmann, H., Sander, A., Mickel, C., Szilvas, E., and Keiner, M. (2016). The impact of back squat and leg-press exercises on maximal strength and speed-strength parameters. *J. Strength Cond. Res.* 30, 1205–1212. doi: 10.1519/JSC.0000000000001228
Yiou, E. (2005). Performance and postural interactions during synchronous pointing and leg flexion. *Med. Sci. Sports Exerc.* 37, 91–99. doi: 10.1249/01.MSS.0000150019.39648.01
Yiou, E., and Schneider, C. (2007). Coordination of pointing and stepping: do postural phenomena result from the juxtaposition of the dynamics of each task? *Neurosi. Lett.* 425, 63–68. doi: 10.1016/j.neulet.2007.08.012
Yiou, E., Schneider, C., and Roussel, D. (2007). Coordination of rapid stepping with arm pointing: anticipatory changes and step adaptation. *Hum. Mov. Sci.* 26, 357–375. doi: 10.1016/j.humov.2007.03.003
Yue, G., and Cole, K. J. (1992). Strength increases from the motor program: comparison of training with maximal voluntary and imagined muscle contractions. *J. Neurophysiol.* 67, 1114–1123.
Zattara, M., and Bouisset, S. (1988). Posturo-kinetic organisation during the early phase of voluntary upper limb movement. 1. Normal subjects. *J. Neurol. Neurosurg. Psychiatry* 51, 956–965. doi: 10.1136/jnnp.51.7.956

18

Proof-of-Concept of the Virtual Reality Comprehensive Balance Assessment and Training for Sensory Organization of Dynamic Postural Control

Sanghee Moon[1,2], Chun-Kai Huang[2], Maryam Sadeghi[2], Abiodun E. Akinwuntan[2,3] and Hannes Devos[2]**

[1] Department of Physical Therapy, Ithaca College, Ithaca, NY, United States, [2] Laboratory for Advanced Rehabilitation Research in Simulation, Department of Physical Therapy, Rehabilitation Science, and Athletic Training, University of Kansas Medical Center, Kansas City, KS, United States, [3] Office of the Dean, School of Health Professions, University of Kansas Medical Center, Kansas City, KS, United States

***Correspondence:**
Sanghee Moon
smoon2@ithaca.edu
Hannes Devos
hdevos@kumc.edu

Accurate quantification of the impact of visual, somatosensory, and vestibular systems on postural control may inform tailor-made balance intervention strategies. The aim of this proof-of-concept study was to determine the safety, sense of presence, system usability, and face validity of a newly developed Virtual Reality Comprehensive Balance Assessment and Training (VR-ComBAT) in healthy young individuals. The VR-ComBAT included six balance condition: (1) stable surface with fixed virtual reality (VR) surroundings; (2) stable surface with blacked out VR surroundings; (3) stable surface with VR visual conflict; (4) unstable surface with fixed VR surroundings; (5) unstable surface with blacked out VR surroundings; and (6) unstable surface with VR visual conflict. Safety was evaluated using the number of adverse events, including scores on the Simulator Sickness Questionnaire. Sense of presence was evaluated using the igroup Presence Questionnaire (iPQ). System usability was assessed using the Systems Usability Scale (SUS). Friedman analyses with *post hoc* Wilcoxon Signed Rank tests were employed to demonstrate face validity by quantifying center of pressure (COP) changes in mean distance, mean velocity, and mean frequency in the anteroposterior (AP) and mediolateral (ML) direction across the six conditions. Twenty-three participants (27.4 $\pm$ 8.0 years old; 13 women) reported no adverse events. Participants scores on average 44.9 $\pm$ 9.6 on the iPQ and 79.7 $\pm$ 9.9 on the SUS. *Post hoc* analyses showed significant changes in COP-based measures when compared to baseline. The mean frequency change of COP showed direction-dependence in which increased frequency change in AP was observed while decreased change in ML was noted. The VR-ComBAT provides a safe, feasible, and cost-effective VR environment that demonstrates consistent sensory re-weighting between visual, somatosensory, and vestibular systems. Future studies should investigate whether VR-ComBAT can be used to inform precision rehabilitation of balance and fall prevention in older adults without and with neurological conditions.

Keywords: virtual reality, balance, sensory organization test, postural control, center of pressure

INTRODUCTION

Postural control requires the brain to integrate information from vision, somatosensory, and vestibular cues in order to respond timely and accurately to changes in the body's alignment and tone with respect to visual surroundings, support surface, internal references, and gravity (Alcock et al., 2018; Ivanenko and Gurfinkel, 2018). These sensory systems sometimes provide conflicting information (Nashner and Peters, 1990). To illustrate, while sitting on a moving bus, the eyes inform the brain that the surroundings appear to be moving whereas the somatosensory system provides information that the body is stationary. In such cases, the brain needs to ignore or prioritize conflicting information to accomplish postural control (Gaerlan, 2010). Discrepancies in these systems become even more apparent in individuals with neurological conditions, resulting in increased postural imbalance, a higher risk of falls, and, in many cases, a higher fear of falling (Horak, 2006; Cronin et al., 2017). Accurate detection of the system that affects postural control in neurological conditions is key to tailor balance intervention and fall prevention programs to the needs of individuals at risk of falls.

Several computerized balance assessment tools have been developed, including dynamic posturography [e.g., Neurocom® SMART EquiTest®, Bertec® computerized dynamic posturography (CDP/IVR), Biodex® Balance] or wearable motion sensors (e.g., APDM Opal). These computerized balance assessment tools enable quantitative assessment of postural control (Mancini and Horak, 2010), reduce test performance variability, increase sensitivity to subtle changes (Visser et al., 2008), and determine the systems that may underly impaired postural control (Mancini and Horak, 2010). Of those, the Neurocom® SMART EquiTest® system (Natus, San Carlos, CA, United States) and Bertec computerized dynamic posturography (Bertec®, Columbus, OH, United States) are considered the gold standard of dynamic posturography assessment. These computerized sensory organization tests (SOT) challenge the visual, somatosensory, and vestibular systems to provide a detailed assessment of the underlying sensory deficits affecting balance. Although effective in evaluating and treating balance disorders (Alahmari et al., 2014), the high cost ($80,000–$180,000), space needs for the equipment, lack of portability, and time needed for training, have limited the use of the computerized SOT in clinical practice (Visser et al., 2008). The Clinical Test of Sensory Interaction on Balance (CTSIB) was developed to discern the relative contributions of the visual, somatosensory, and vestibular systems to postural control (Shumway-Cook and Horak, 1986). This test includes six static balance conditions with eyes open, eyes closed, and the use of a dome to create visual conflict combining with feet on firm or foam surface. This test was later modified to only four conditions, excluding the visual dome from the test procedures as the balance tasks with the visual dome did not differ from those in the eyes closed conditions (Cohen et al., 1993). Although clinically useful, the scoring system is crude, semi-objective, and may not be sensitive enough to detect subtle changes in postural control in neurodegenerative conditions (Suttanon et al., 2011).

The advent of portable force platforms with head-mounted virtual reality (VR) technology may provide a clinical, cost-effective, and user-friendly dynamic posturography assessment without compromising the evaluative and rehabilitative effectiveness of current computerized SOT. Although VR technology has emerged in the rehabilitation realm as a promising intervention tool to improve balance and gait (de Rooij et al., 2016; Cano Porras et al., 2018, 2019; Massetti et al., 2018; Chen et al., 2020), only few studies utilized VR to assess the sensory organization of postural balance (Lubetzky et al., 2018, 2019; Trueblood et al., 2018; Wittstein et al., 2020). However, it is not clear whether the SOT administered using a head-mounted VR set is safe and easy to use, provides a realistic experience to the user, and discriminates between postural control conditions that test different balance systems.

Unlike the Equilibrium Score calculated from the force platform of the Equitest® that evaluates postural balance through center of pressure (COP) displacement only in the anteroposterior (AP) direction, portable force platforms provide a multidimensional assessment of postural control. Quiet standing on a foam increased COP displacement in the AP direction by 8%, and in the mediolateral (ML) direction by 21% (Reynard et al., 2019). Adding assessment of ML sway and sway area has shown to quantify fall risk in neurological conditions, such as changes in postural sway characteristics while standing with eyes closed in Parkinson's disease (Błaszczyk et al., 2007). Additionally, measuring COP frequency in AP and ML directions brings perspective of adopting different strategies to maintain balance. For example, evidence suggests that changes in perturbation conditions alter COP AP or ML frequency characteristics (Creath et al., 2005). Previous study also noted that postural sway in AP and ML directions can be attributed to ankle and hip control, respectively (Saffer et al., 2008).

The aim of this proof-of-concept study was to demonstrate the safety, sense of presence, system usability, and face validity of the Virtual Reality Comprehensive Balance Assessment and Training (VR-ComBAT) in healthy individuals. The overall hypothesis was that the VR-ComBAT will provide a safe and standardized VR-based balance testing environment in the healthy population. To test our hypothesis, we gauged sense of presence and system usability in the VR environment and satisfaction with our novel VR-based test. Face validity of the VR-ComBAT was evaluated by comparing multidirectional COP displacement and frequency measures across different postural control conditions.

MATERIALS AND EQUIPMENT

Hardware and Software Specifications

The VR-ComBAT consists of a computer that processes the VR input and output [Alienware (Intel® Core™ i7-7800X CPU @ 3.50GHz; 16.0 GB RAM), Dell USA Corporation, Round Rock, TX, United States], a commercially available, head-mounted device (HMD) with integrated VR (HTC VIVE Pro Eye, HTC, Taoyuan, Taiwan), and two VR tracking sensors (Steam VR Base Stations, HTC, Taoyuan, Taiwan). The HTC VIVE Pro Eye headset includes dual-OLED 3.5-inch displays with a combined resolution of 2,880 × 1,600 pixels. The refresh rate of the screen is 90 Hz. The field of view is 110 degrees. The Steam VR (version 1.13, Valve, Bellevue, WA, United States) was used to simultaneously link the computer and the VR headset.

The VR headset was integrated with a force plate (AMTI Optima, Watertown, MA, United States) to measure the displacement and velocity of COP. The sampling frequency of the force plate was 200 Hz. The force plate was manually synchronized with the VR system by simultaneously starting the VR conditions and force plate measurement at each trial. The experimental setup is shown in **Figure 1**.

Unity 3D (version 2019.3.0; San Francisco, CA, United States) was utilized to create the VR-ComBAT environment. The executable application is available at http://bit.ly/VR-ComBAT (github). The basic setup of the VR environment includes three panels (one front, and two side panels), positioned at 90-degree angle to each, with multi-colored triangular patterns to help participants with visual fixation on the VR environment (**Figure 2**).

Balance Conditions

The VR-ComBAT emulates six different conditions, that, in combination, test visual, somatosensory, and vestibular systems of balance (**Figure 2**). These conditions mimic the six conditions in the SOT of the Equitest®: (1) stable surface with fixed VR surrounding; (2) stable surface with blacked out VR surroundings; (3) stable surface with VR visual conflict; (4) unstable surface with fixed VR surroundings; (5) unstable surface with blacked out VR surroundings; and (6) unstable surface with VR visual conflict.

Condition 1 is a baseline that measures static balance on a fixed surface. The surrounding panels in the VR environment remain stationary. Participants can use input from visual, somatosensory, and vestibular systems to maintain balance. In condition 2, participants cannot rely on vision to remain upright since the VR surroundings are blackened out. Condition 3 creates a conflict between normal input from the somatosensory and vestibular systems and the visual information from the moving VR panels. The surrounding panels are moving in the anteroposterior direction with a maximum of 20 degrees and a maximum velocity of 15 degrees/s. Conditions 4, 5, and 6 are identical to 1, 2, and 3, respectively. However, in conditions 4, 5, and 6, a foam (Amazon Basics Balance Pad for Exercise Training, 35 cm × 5 cm × 40 cm, density = 0.04 g/cm^3) is placed between the feet and the force plate, thus challenging the somatosensory system.

METHODS

Participants

This study was conducted in the Laboratory for Advanced Rehabilitation Research in Simulation, at the University of Kansas Medical Center. This proof-of-concept study recruited 23 healthy participants if they were (1) between 19 and 65 years of age; (2) had no walking or balance impairment [>45 in Berg Balance Scale (BBS; Berg et al., 1992) and >20 in Mini Balance Evaluation Systems Test (Mini-BESTest; Leddy et al., 2011)]; and (3) were able to understand and follow instructions in English. We excluded individuals who (1) had a history of neurological or vestibular conditions and (2) had visual acuity or visual field impairment that could not be resolved by corrective lenses. All participants signed written informed consent. The study ethics was approved by the Institutional Review Board at the University of Kansas Medical Center (#STUDY00145395).

Study Protocol

Following written consent, demographic information (age, sex, and education) was collected. The BBS (total score: 56, lower score indicating higher risk of balance problems) and Mini-BESTest (total score: 28, lower score indicating the higher risk of balance problems) were administered to confirm the absence of any balance impairments. Cognitive impairments were ruled out using the Montreal Cognitive Assessment (MOCA; Nasreddine et al., 2005). Next, participants were fitted with the VR headset and asked to step on the force plate. Then, participants stood on the force plate (conditions 1–3) or on the foam surface (conditions 4–6) with their feet shoulder width apart and hands naturally placed at their sides. Participants were asked to remain in the same position during each VR-ComBAT task (**Figure 3**). All participants were newly recruited and had no previous exposure to the VR-ComBAT system. There was no practice or learning trial before the recording, since all the conditions in VR-ComBAT were thoroughly explained by the lead researcher and were easy to perform for healthy young participants. Participants with glasses wore the VR headset without taking their glasses off, which allowed participants to experience the VR environment with their normal vision or corrected-to-normal vision. Participants were instructed to stand as still as possible. Each condition consisted of three trials that lasted 20 s per trial. Between each trial, a 5-s break was given. For conditions 2 and 4 (blacked out VR surroundings), the light of the testing room was also turned off to create a completely dark VR environment by removing any lights coming from the gaps of the VR headset. During the experiment, safety was assured by a gait belt and a research team member next to a participant in case of a fall or near-fall event. The experimental protocol is shown in **Figure 4**.

Outcome Measures

Safety

The number of adverse events (e.g., falls) was recorded. VR HMD is believed to increase simulator sickness (similar to motion sickness) compared to remote VR displays (Kim et al., 2014; Dennison et al., 2016). This increased proneness to simulator sickness is thought to stem from the high-fidelity, stereoscopic rendering of VR images. The realistic images displayed in VR HMD can create discrepancies between the perceived and expected visual sensory information, leading to increased symptoms of simulator sickness (Chang et al., 2020). We administered the Simulator Sickness Questionnaire (SSQ) after condition 6, which is the condition that was expected to induce

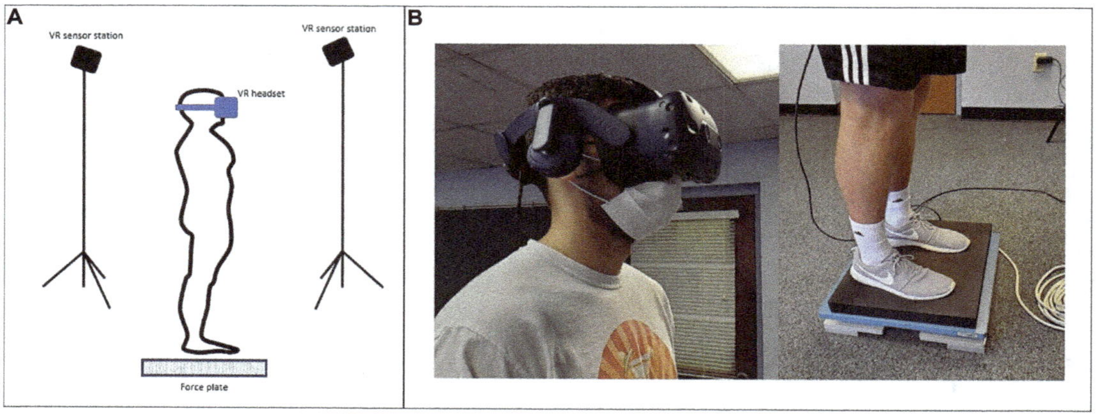

FIGURE 1 | (A) Virtual Reality Comprehensive Balance Assessment and Training (VR-ComBAT) setup; **(B)** A participant wears the VR headset and stands on the foam surface placed over the force plate.

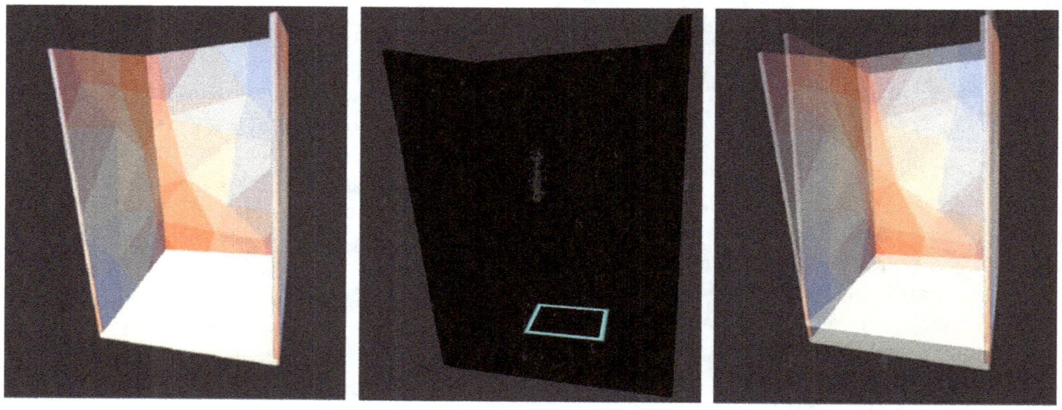

FIGURE 2 | Six VR-ComBAT conditions. (1) stable surface with fixed virtual reality (VR) surroundings; (2) stable surface with blacked out VR surroundings; (3) stable surface with VR visual conflict; (4) unstable surface with fixed VR surroundings; (5) unstable surface with blacked out VR surroundings; and (6) unstable surface with VR visual conflict.

most simulator sickness. The SSQ is regarded as the current gold standard in calculating simulator sickness in research (Kennedy et al., 1993; Jinjakam and Hamamoto, 2012). The SSQ is accurate and reliable to measure simulator sickness in high-fidelity VR environments such as driving simulators, flight simulators, and other VR systems (Kennedy et al., 1993). The score is comprised of three subsections, each with seven symptoms, in which there is some overlap: disorientation, nausea, and oculomotor. The symptoms include general discomfort, fatigue, headache, eyestrain, difficulty focusing, increased salivation, sweating, nausea, difficulty concentrating, the fullness of head, blurred vision, dizziness (eyes open and closed), vertigo, stomach awareness, and burping. The weighted score formula was used to calculate the global index, which reflects the total discomfort level, as well as the scores for the three subsections.

According to previous research (Kennedy et al., 1993), the three subscale scores were calculated by summing scores associated with each subscale and multiplying them by an appropriate weighting factor (9.54 for SSQ-Nausea, 7.58 for SSQ-Oculomotor, and 13.92 for SSQ-Disorientation). To calculate the total score of SSQ, the result was equal to the sum of the three unweighted subscale scores, multiplied by 3.74. A person with a total score of >100 is considered actively ill due to simulator sickness (Kennedy et al., 1993).

Sense of Presence

Sense of presence was evaluated using the iPQ. The iPQ is a multidimensional scale assessing the sense of presence in a VR environment. Sense of presence refers to the subjective feeling of being in a virtual environment. The reliability and validity of the iPQ have been established in previous work (Panahi et al., 2009). The 14 items of the questionnaire are scores on questionnaire contains 14 items, scored on an ordinal scale ranging from 1 to 5. One item reflects general sense of presence. The other items are categorized into sense of spatial presence (5 items), involvement (4 items), and experienced realism (4 items) (Hein et al., 2018).

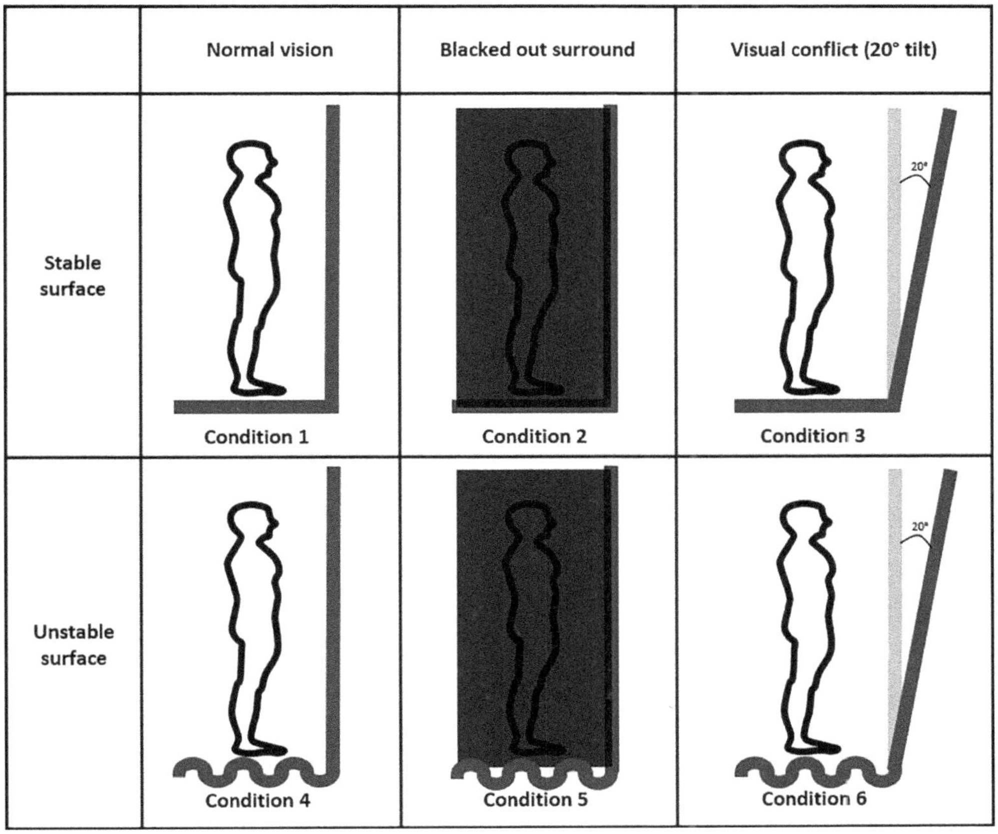

FIGURE 3 | Six VR-ComBAT conditions in the virtual environment. Conditions 1 and 4, conditions 2 and 5, and conditions 3 and 6 share the same VR balance testing environments.

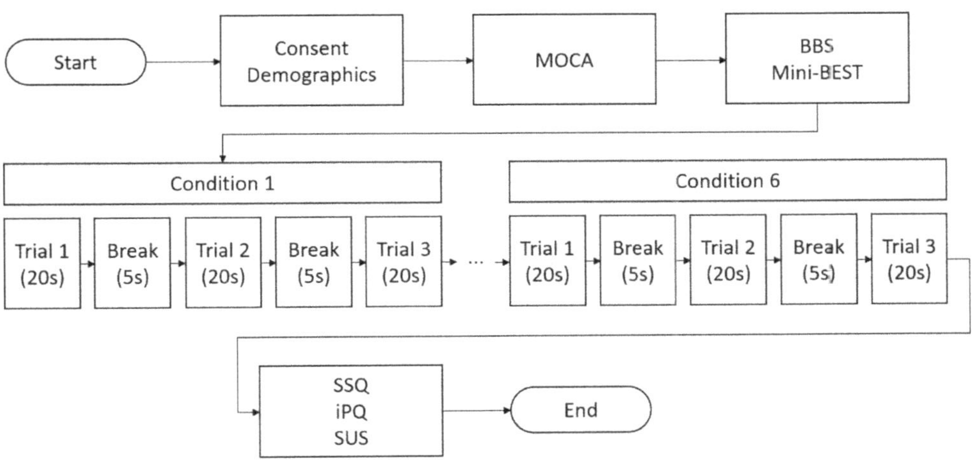

FIGURE 4 | A flow chart of VR-ComBAT experimental procedure (BBS = Berg Balance Scale; iPQ = igroup Presence Questionnaire; Mini-BEST = Mini Balance Evaluation Systems Test; MOCA = Montreal Cognitive Assessment; SSQ = Simulator Sickness Questionnaire; SUS = System Usability Scale).

System Usability

The SUS was administered to capture participants' viewpoints on effectiveness, efficiency, and satisfaction levels of the VR-ComBAT (Brooke, 1996; Bangor et al., 2008). The questionnaire contains 10 items, each scored on a range from ranges from 0 to 100. The SUS total scores representing a composed measure of the system's overall usability on a scale from 0 to 100.

Face Validity

Face validity evaluates the extent to which the measured variable appears to adequately measure the conceptual variable (Thomas et al., 1992). The face validity of VR-ComBAT to discriminate between different postural control conditions was evaluated using quantitative COP measures. These COP data were extracted from the force plate and processed using the MATLAB application (MathWorks, Natick, MA, United States) to calculate the following outcomes (Prieto et al., 1996):

- Mean distance in the AP (MeanAP) or ML (MeanML) direction: The average distance in the AP/ML direction from the mean COP.
- Mean velocity in the AP (VelAP) or ML (VelML) direction: The average velocity of COP in the AP/ML direction.
- 95% confidence ellipse area (95%Area): The area that encloses approximately 95% of the points on the COP path.
- Mean frequency in the AP (MfAP) or ML (MfML) direction: The frequency (Hz) of a sinusoidal oscillation with an average value of total path length of excursions in AP (or ML) over MeanAP (or MeanML).

Statistical Analysis

All statistical analyses were performed using SPSS (version 26, IBM Corporation, Armonk, NY, United States). The distribution of data was examined for normality using the Shapiro–Wilk test. Since the number of participants of this study was small and almost all data were not normally distributed, the Friedman test was conducted to examine the differences between conditions followed by *post hoc* Wilcoxon Signed Rank test. We identified *a priori* four pairwise comparisons to minimize committing type 1 error. We compared (1) condition 2 to condition 1 to tease out somatosensory system contributions; (2) condition 4 to condition 1 to tease out visual system contributions; and (3) condition 5 to condition 1 and (4) condition 6 to condition 5 to tease out vestibular system contributions (Shumway-Cook, 2011; Pletcher et al., 2017). The effect size ($r = \frac{Z}{\sqrt{n}}$) was adopted to indicate the strength of two conditions of VR-ComBAT. Of note, given that Wilcoxon Signed-rank test was conducted in this study, to more accurately reflect this non-parametric approach, we calculated the effect size (r) according to Rosenthal et al. instead of Cohen's d effect size (Rosenthal et al., 1994). The significance levels of all analyses were set $\alpha = 0.05$.

RESULTS

Participants (13 women and 10 men) were on average 27.4 ± 8 years old and reported 19.2 ± 2.5 years of education. None of the participants showed any impairment in static or dynamic balance, as evidenced by maximum scores on the BBS (56 ± 0) and on the Mini-BESTest (28 ± 0). Participants scored on average 28.3 ± 1.4 on the MOCA, indicating no cognitive impairments (**Table 1**).

Safety

No adverse events were reported during or after the study visit. SSQ total scores were on average 33.3 ± 66.1. Average SSQ average subscores were 2.9 ± 6.1 for nausea, 3 ± 5.9 for oculomotor, and 3 ± 7.2 for disorientation. Participants either scored none or slight on each item of the SSQ.

Sense of Presence

The average iPQ score of total iPQ was 44.9 ± 9.6 with average subscores of 18.8 ± 3.7 for spatial presence, 11.3 ± 3.5 for involvement, and 10.7 ± 2.7 for experienced realism.

System Usability

The SUS demonstrated nearly a total score of 80 in system usability (79.7 ± 9.9).

Face Validity

The Friedman test revealed significant differences across the six conditions for all COP-based measures ($p < 0.01$). *Post hoc* analyses (**Table 2**) showed that participants exhibited worse performance on most COP measures in conditions 2, 4, and 5 compared to condition 1.

In the frequency-based analysis, an inverse trend between MfAP and MfML was observed across the conditions. Pairwise comparisons showed that MfAP increased while MfML decreased with respect to increased task difficulty (**Figure 5**).

DISCUSSION

The aim of this proof-of-concept study was to determine the safety, sense of presence, systems usability, and face validity of the newly developed VR-ComBAT in healthy young individuals. We gauged sense of presence in the VR environment and satisfaction with our novel VR-based system as important outcomes of sense of presence. We also included comprehensive quantitative comparisons of multidirectional COP outcomes across the six conditions. The results of this study support our hypotheses that the VR-ComBAT is safe, highly acceptable, and able to detect multidirectional changes of postural control in terms of COP amid different conditions from healthy young participants.

The VR-ComBAT provided a safe and feasible virtual balance testing environment. As Howarth and Costello noted (Howarth and Costello, 1997), VR environments can induce temporary side effects such as general discomfort, fatigue, headache, nausea, and irritating eyes. However, in our study, no adverse events were reported by participants. In addition, the results of SSQ suggested that the VR-ComBAT did not cause any adverse effects of VR throughout the experiment.

Our findings on the sense of presence of the VR-ComBAT measured by iPQ and SUS demonstrated that our novel VR system was well accepted by participants. The total iPQ (44.9) was 9.9-point above neutral presence (35 = 70/2), demonstrating that participants indicated being present in the VR-ComBAT environment. The means of the three subscales of iPQ all contributed to the averaged overall score [spatial

TABLE 1 | Demographic and clinical characteristics.

	Age	Sex	BBS	Mini-BESTest	MOCA
Participants (N = 23)	27.4 ± 8.0	13 female,10 male	56 ± 0	28 ± 0	28.3 ± 1.4

BBS, Berg Balance Scale; Mini-BESTest, Mini Balance Evaluation Systems Test; MOCA, Montreal Cognitive Assessment.

TABLE 2 | COP-based measures across the six VR-ComBAT conditions (N = 23).

	Condition 1	Condition 2	Condition 3	Condition 4*	Condition 5*	Condition 6
MeanAP (mm)	3.71 (1.02)	4.17 (1.90) *0.21 [0.12–0.36]*	3.90 (1.26) *0.18 [0.13–0.22]*	5.50 (1.57) *0.61 [0.49–0.74]*	5.92 (1.83) *0.62 [0.78–0.46]*	5.92 (2.16) *0.62 [0.46–0.78]*
MeanML (mm)	1.33 (0.65)	1.61 (0.82)* *0.34 [0.3–0.38]*	1.73 (1.41) *0.37 [0.32–0.42]*	3.15 (1.08) *0.62 [0.49–0.75]*	3.24 (1.19) *0.62 [0.48–0.75]*	3.12 (1.19) *0.62 [0.49–0.75]*
VelAP (mm/s)	17.31 (3.46)	18.71 (4.03)* *0.4 [0.25–0.56]*	18.89 (3.22) *0.42 [0.25–0.58]*	29.73 (7.56) *0.62 [–0.25 to 1.49]*	32.96 (8.19) *0.62 [–0.49 to 1.72]*	29.59 (7.61)** *0.62 [–0.24 to 1.49]*
VelML (mm/s)	9.22 (1.21)	9.82 (1.65)* *0.38 [0.31–0.45]*	9.56 (1.74) *0.20 [0.12–0.27]*	15.40 (3.93) *0.62 [0.18–1.05]*	15.88 (3.30) *0.62 [0.15–1.09]*	14.39 (3.02) ** *0.62 [0.25–0.98]*
95%Area (mm^2)	148.99 (102.53)	190.46 (152.39)* *0.26 [–10.1 to 10.61]*	209.30 (239.64) *0.21 [–13.14 to 13.56]*	530.12 (314.76) *0.62 [–23.99 to 25.23]*	574.78 (342.18) *0.62 [–29.91 to 31.15]*	569.81 (450.65) *0.62 [–29.24 to 30.48]*
MfAP (Hz)	0.92 (0.29)	0.96 (0.37) *0.05 [0.01–0.09]*	0.96 (0.27) *0.1 [0.09–0.12]*	1.03 (0.32) *0.31 [0.3–0.33]*	1.06 (0.27) *0.41 [0.4–0.43]*	0.98 (0.30) ** *0.23 [0.22–0.24]*
MfML (Hz)	1.49 (0.56)	1.39 (0.64) *0.25 [0.23–0.27]*	1.38 (0.63) *0.34 [0.34–0.35]*	0.96 (0.28) *0.6 [0.56–0.76]*	0.96 (0.29) *0.58 [0.53–0.61]*	0.91 (0.25) ** *0.59 [0.55–0.64]*

Each cell represents the mean (standard deviation) on top and effect size r [95% CI] compared to condition 1 at bottom in italics.
**Significant differences when compared to condition 1 ($p < 0.05$).*
***Significant decrease when compared to condition 5 ($p < 0.05$).*
MeanAP/MeanML, Mean distance of COP in the anteroposterior/mediolateral direction; VelAP/VelML, Mean velocity of COP in the anteroposterior/mediolateral direction; 95%Area, 95% confidence ellipse area of COP; MfAP/MfML, Mean rotational frequency of COP in the anteroposterior/mediolateral direction.

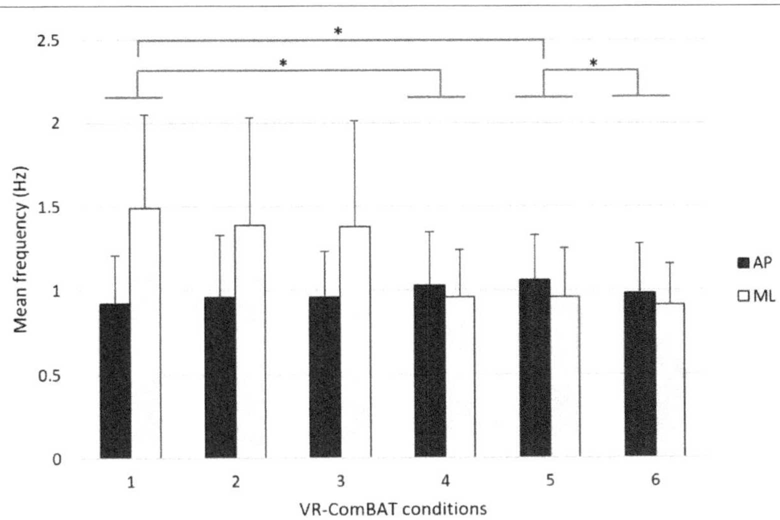

FIGURE 5 | Mean rotational frequency of COP in anteroposterior (black) and mediolateral (gray) directions across the 6 VR-ComBAT conditions. *Significant differences ($p < 0.05$).

presence (18.8 out of 25), involvement (11.3 out of 20), and experience realism (10.7 out of 20)]. The average total score of SUS was approximately 80 out of 100, which demonstrated high effectiveness, efficiency, and satisfaction levels of the VR-ComBAT. The high system usability of VR was also reported in a VR-based rehabilitation study (Meldrum et al., 2012).

The six conditions of the VR-ComBAT emulate an environment equivalent to the SOT. Combined, they are purported to evaluate the sensory systems involved in postural control. Comparing conditions 2, 4, and 5 versus condition 1, our findings are consistent with results from previous SOT studies in healthy younger and older adults (Cohen et al., 1996;

Pletcher et al., 2017). When the somatosensory system is confronted with a challenging environment (e.g., conditions 4 and 5), healthy young participants reweighted appropriately to their vision and vestibular systems to maintain postural control. The large effect sizes observed in condition 4 vs. 1 and condition 5 vs. 1 support postural control reliance on vision and vestibular systems, respectively (Pletcher et al., 2017). When comparing condition 6 (unstable surface with VR visual conflict) to condition 5 (unstable surface with blacked out VR surroundings), the significant decreased mean velocity and mean frequency indicate that blacking out the VR surroundings compromised postural control more so than providing conflicting visual information through a moving VR surround. Our results demonstrate that the perturbed somatosensory system might be compensated for by the visual-guided scene through the VR-ComBAT. Vision contributes to balance during quiet standing, and a previous study showed that individuals with impaired vision failed to maintain their postural stability in challenging conditions (Ray et al., 2008). To this end, future studies identifying the changes of COP-based measures in patients with sensory deficits using VR-ComBAT are warranted.

In addition to the findings in the AP direction, the COP-based measures in the ML direction (e.g., MeanML, VelML, and MfML) demonstrated significant changes in this study (e.g., conditions 2, 4, 5 vs. condition 1). Specifically, the change of mean COP frequency of this study is direction-dependent where the mean frequency increases in the AP direction while it decreases in the ML direction with respect to increased task difficulty (**Figure 5**). While confronted with a challenging environment, healthy young adults seem to restrict ML movement to maintain postural control. This direction-dependent phenomenon was in line with current evidence that additional energy expenditure, such as muscular effort, is required to maintain lateral stability during walking (Kuo and Donelan, 2010). More evidence is required to elucidate whether there is a relationship between COP frequency changes in different directions and energy expenditure. Future studies using the VR-ComBAT will examine whether this direction-dependent phenomenon of COP frequency alters in older adults or patients with deficits in sensory integration.

A previous study that integrated VR HMD with posturography provided similar conditions as the Equitest® SOT (Wittstein et al., 2020) and demonstrated a moderate reliability and a weak correlation between the developed VR SOT and the EquiTest® (Wittstein et al., 2020). The VR-ComBAT of this study emulates conditions that are equivalent to those in the EquiTest® as illustrated in **Figure 2**. In addition, our study provided a quantitative analysis of COP distance, velocity, area, and frequency in the anteroposterior and mediolateral direction. The importance of including multidirectional COP outcomes was illustrated in our direction-dependent phenomenon of frequency changes in the anteroposterior and mediolateral direction.

There are limitations to this proof-of-concept study. The current study included a relatively small number of healthy young adults. Therefore, we did not adjust for multiple comparisons in the *post hoc* analyses. Although we established the safety of the VR-ComBAT in healthy individuals, further studies are warranted to validate the VR-ComBAT in people with balance impairments. In addition, the balance testing conditions in the VR-ComBAT system were based on the testing conditions that originate from the EquiTest®. Although the current study demonstrated the face validity of the novel system, our new test requires validation against the EquiTest®. We list future directions of work to overcome the limitations observed in the current work and optimize the utilization of the VR-ComBAT. First, we plan to integrate the VR-ComBAT with a cognitive assessment to evaluate the effect of dual-tasking on reweighting for postural control. The eye-tracking integrated VR system such as HTC VIVE Pro Eye can be used to extract pupillary response, which is a valid measure of cognitive workload in demanding postural conditions (Orlosky et al., 2017). Second, we will employ the VR-ComBAT in older and/or patient populations to confirm the sensitivity of the VR-ComBAT in evaluating sensory organization of postural control. Third, not all clinical settings can afford a relatively expensive force plate system. One of the overarching goals of the VR-ComBAT development is to provide a cost-effective system. We developed the VR-ComBAT for research purposes. Thus, the cost of the current setup including force platform system ($10,000–$20,000) and VR HMD system ($500–$2,000) may be expensive for most clinics. However, we plan to create a clinically affordable VR-ComBAT by replacing the force plate with cost-effective COP measures such as Nintendo Wii Fit or gyroscope/accelerometers in smartphones. Lastly, our study found meaningful outcomes of COP changes in ML direction. Future VR-ComBAT conditions should include ML tilting in VR to further elucidate the effect of visual conflict on ML postural control.

In conclusion, this current proof-of-concept study demonstrates the safety, sense of presence, and face validity of the VR-ComBAT integrated with a COP measuring system.

ETHICS STATEMENT

The studies involving human participants were reviewed and approved by IRB at University of Kansas Medical Center. The patients/participants provided their written informed consent to participate in this study.

AUTHOR CONTRIBUTIONS

SM and HD designed the study. SM performed the experiments. SM, C-KH, MS, and HD analyzed the collected data. All authors wrote the manuscript, discussed the results, and commented on the manuscript.

REFERENCES

Alahmari, K. A., Marchetti, G. F., Sparto, P. J., Furman, J. M., and Whitney, S. L. (2014). Estimating postural control with the balance rehabilitation unit: measurement consistency, accuracy, validity, and comparison with dynamic posturography. *Arch. Phys. Med. Rehabil.* 95, 65–73. doi: 10.1016/j.apmr.2013.09.011

Alcock, L., O'brien, T. D., and Vanicek, N. (2018). Association between somatosensory, visual and vestibular contributions to postural control, reactive balance capacity and healthy ageing in older women. *Health Care Women Int.* 39, 1366–1380. doi: 10.1080/07399332.2018.1499106

Bangor, A., Kortum, P. T., and Miller, J. T. (2008). An empirical evaluation of the system usability scale. *Int. J. Hum. Comp. Interact.* 24, 574–594. doi: 10.1080/10447310802205776

Berg, K. O., Wood-Dauphinee, S. L., Williams, J. I., and Maki, B. (1992). Measuring balance in the elderly: validation of an instrument. *Can. J. Public Health* 83(Suppl. 2), S7–S11.

Błaszczyk, J. W., Orawiec, R., Duda-Kłodowska, D., and Opala, G. (2007). Assessment of postural instability in patients with Parkinson's disease. *Exp. Brain Res.* 183, 107–114. doi: 10.1007/s00221-007-1024-y

Brooke, J. (1996). "Sus: a "quick and dirty'usability," in *Usability Evaluation in Industry*, eds P. W. Jordan, B. Thomas, I. McLelland, and B. A. Weerdmeester (London: Taylor and Francis), 189.

Cano Porras, D., Sharon, H., Inzelberg, R., Ziv-Ner, Y., Zeilig, G., and Plotnik, M. (2019). Advanced virtual reality-based rehabilitation of balance and gait in clinical practice. *Ther. Adv. Chronic Dis.* 10:2040622319868379.

Cano Porras, D., Siemonsma, P., Inzelberg, R., Zeilig, G., and Plotnik, M. (2018). Advantages of virtual reality in the rehabilitation of balance and gait. *Syst. Rev.* 90, 1017–1025. doi: 10.1212/wnl.0000000000005603

Chang, E., Kim, H. T., and Yoo, B. (2020). Virtual reality sickness: a review of causes and measurements. *Int. J. Hum. Comput. Interact.* 36, 1658–1682. doi: 10.1080/10447318.2020.1778351

Chen, Y., Gao, Q., He, C. Q., and Bian, R. (2020). Effect of virtual reality on balance in individuals with Parkinson disease: a systematic review and meta-analysis of randomized controlled trials. *Phys. Ther.* 100, 933–945. doi: 10.1093/ptj/pzaa042

Cohen, H., Blatchly, C. A., and Gombash, L. L. (1993). A study of the clinical test of sensory interaction and balance. *Phys. Ther.* 73, 346–351; discussion 351–344.

Cohen, H., Heaton, L. G., Congdon, S. L., and Jenkins, H. A. (1996). Changes in sensory organization test scores with age. *Age Ageing* 25, 39–44. doi: 10.1093/ageing/25.1.39

Creath, R., Kiemel, T., Horak, F., Peterka, R., and Jeka, J. (2005). A unified view of quiet and perturbed stance: simultaneous co-existing excitable modes. *Neurosci. Lett.* 377, 75–80. doi: 10.1016/j.neulet.2004.11.071

Cronin, T., Arshad, Q., and Seemungal, B. M. (2017). Vestibular deficits in neurodegenerative disorders: balance, dizziness, and spatial disorientation. *Front. Neurol.* 8:538. doi: 10.3389/fneur.2017.00538

de Rooij, I. J., Van De Port, I. G., and Meijer, J. G. (2016). Effect of virtual reality training on balance and gait ability in patients with stroke: systematic review and meta-analysis. *Phys. Ther.* 96, 1905–1918. doi: 10.2522/ptj.20160054

Dennison, M. S., Wisti, A. Z., and D'zmura, M. (2016). Use of physiological signals to predict cybersickness. *Displays* 44, 42–52. doi: 10.1016/j.displa.2016.07.002

Gaerlan, M. G. (2010). *The Role of Visual, Vestibular, and Somatosensory Systems in Postural Balance.* Ph. D. thesis. Las Vegas, NV: University of Nevada.

Hein, D., Mai, C., and Hußmann, H. (2018). "The usage of presence measurements in research: a review," in *Proceedings of the International Society for Presence Research Annual Conference (Presence)*, (Prague: The International Society for Presence Research), 21–22.

Horak, F. B. (2006). Postural orientation and equilibrium: what do we need to know about neural control of balance to prevent falls? *Age Ageing* 35(Suppl. 2), ii7–ii11.

Howarth, P. A., and Costello, P. J. (1997). The occurrence of virtual simulation sickness symptoms when an HMD was used as a personal viewing system. *Displays* 18, 107–116. doi: 10.1016/s0141-9382(97)00011-5

Ivanenko, Y., and Gurfinkel, V. S. (2018). Human postural control. *Front. Neurosci.* 12:171. doi: 10.3389/fnins.2018.00171

Jinjakam, C., and Hamamoto, K. (2012). "Simulator sickness in immersive virtual environment," in *Proceedings of the 5th 2012 Biomedical Engineering International Conference*, Muang, 1–4.

Kennedy, R. S., Lane, N. E., Berbaum, K. S., and Lilienthal, M. G. (1993). Simulator sickness questionnaire: an enhanced method for quantifying simulator sickness. *Int. J. Aviat. Psychol.* 3, 203–220. doi: 10.1207/s15327108ijap0303_3

Kim, K., Rosenthal, M. Z., Zielinski, D. J., and Brady, R. (2014). Effects of virtual environment platforms on emotional responses. *Comput. Methods Programs Biomed.* 113, 882–893. doi: 10.1016/j.cmpb.2013.12.024

Kuo, A. D., and Donelan, J. M. (2010). Dynamic principles of gait and their clinical implications. *Phys. Ther.* 90, 157–174. doi: 10.2522/ptj.20090125

Leddy, A. L., Crowner, B. E., and Earhart, G. M. (2011). Utility of the Mini-BESTest, BESTest, and BESTest sections for balance assessments in individuals with Parkinson disease. *J. Neurol. Phys. Ther.* 35, 90–97. doi: 10.1097/npt.0b013e31821a620c

Lubetzky, A. V., Harel, D., Kelly, J., Hujsak, B. D., and Perlin, K. (2019). Weighting and reweighting of visual input via head mounted display given unilateral peripheral vestibular dysfunction. *Hum. Mov. Sci.* 68:102526. doi: 10.1016/j.humov.2019.102526

Lubetzky, A. V., Kary, E. E., Harel, D., Hujsak, B., and Perlin, K. (2018). Feasibility and reliability of a virtual reality oculus platform to measure sensory integration for postural control in young adults. *Physiother. Theory Pract.* 34, 935–950. doi: 10.1080/09593985.2018.1431344

Mancini, M., and Horak, F. B. (2010). The relevance of clinical balance assessment tools to differentiate balance deficits. *Eur. J. Phys. Rehabil. Med.* 46, 239–248.

Massetti, T., Da Silva, T. D., Crocetta, T. B., Guarnieri, R., De Freitas, B. L., Bianchi Lopes, P., et al. (2018). The clinical utility of virtual reality in neurorehabilitation: a systematic review. *J. Cent. Nerv. Syst. Dis.* 10:1179573518813541.

Meldrum, D., Glennon, A., Herdman, S., Murray, D., and Mcconn-Walsh, R. (2012). Virtual reality rehabilitation of balance: assessment of the usability of the Nintendo Wii® Fit Plus. *Disabil. Rehabil. Assist. Technol.* 7, 205–210. doi: 10.3109/17483107.2011.616922

Nashner, L. M., and Peters, J. F. (1990). Dynamic posturography in the diagnosis and management of dizziness and balance disorders. *Neurol. Clin.* 8, 331–349. doi: 10.1016/s0733-8619(18)30359-1

Nasreddine, Z. S., Phillips, N. A., Bédirian, V., Charbonneau, S., Whitehead, V., Collin, I., et al. (2005). The montreal cognitive assessment, MoCA: a brief screening tool for mild cognitive impairment. *J. Am. Geriatr. Soc.* 53, 695–699. doi: 10.1111/j.1532-5415.2005.53221.x

Orlosky, J., Itoh, Y., Ranchet, M., Kiyokawa, K., Morgan, J., and Devos, H. (2017). Emulation of physician tasks in eye-tracked virtual reality for remote diagnosis of neurodegenerative disease. *IEEE Trans. Vis. Comput. Graph.* 23, 1302–1311. doi: 10.1109/tvcg.2017.2657018

Panahi, S. M., Fathi, A. A., Azad, F. P., and Montazer, G. A. (2009). Reliability and validity of igroup presence questionnaire (ipq). *J. Behav. Sci.* 3, 27–34.

Pletcher, E. R., Williams, V. J., Abt, J. F., Morgan, P. M., Parr, J. J., Wohleber, M. F., et al. (2017). Normative data for the NeuroCom sensory organization test in US military special operations forces. *J. Athl. Train.* 52, 129–136. doi: 10.4085/1062-6050-52.1.05

Prieto, T. E., Myklebust, J. B., Hoffmann, R. G., Lovett, E. G., and Myklebust, B. M. (1996). Measures of postural steadiness: differences between healthy young and elderly adults. *IEEE Trans. Biomed. Eng.* 43, 956–966. doi: 10.1109/10.532130

Ray, C. T., Horvat, M., Croce, R., Mason, R. C., and Wolf, S. L. (2008). The impact of vision loss on postural stability and balance strategies in individuals with profound vision loss. *Gait Posture* 28 58–61. doi: 10.1016/j.gaitpost.2007.09.010

Reynard, F., Christe, D., and Terrier, P. (2019). Postural control in healthy adults: determinants of trunk sway assessed with a chest-worn accelerometer in 12 quiet standing tasks. *PLoS One* 14:e0211051. doi: 10.1371/journal.pone.0211051

Rosenthal, R., Cooper, H., and Hedges, L. (1994). Parametric measures of effect size. *Handb. Res. Synth.* 621, 231–244.

Saffer, M., Kiemel, T., and Jeka, J. (2008). Coherence analysis of muscle activity during quiet stance. *Exp. Brain Res.* 185, 215–226.

Shumway-Cook, A. (2011). *Motor control.* Alphen aan den Rijn: Wolters Kluwer press.

Shumway-Cook, A., and Horak, F. B. (1986). Assessing the influence of sensory interaction of balance. Suggestion from the field. *Phys. Ther.* 66, 1548–1550. doi: 10.1093/ptj/66.10.1548

Suttanon, P., Hill, K. D., Dodd, K. J., and Said, C. M. (2011). Retest reliability of balance and mobility measurements in people with mild to moderate Alzheimer's disease. *Int. Psychogeriatr.* 23, 1152–1159. doi: 10.1017/s1041610211000639

Thomas, S. D., Hathaway, D. K., and Arheart, K. L. (1992). Face validity. *West. J. Nurs. Res.* 14, 109–112.

Trueblood, P. R., Rivera, M., Lopez, C., Bentley, C., and Wubenhorst, N. (2018). Age-based normative data for a computerized dynamic posturography system that uses a virtual visual surround environment. *Acta Otolaryngol.* 138, 597–602. doi: 10.1080/00016489.2018.1429653

Visser, J. E., Carpenter, M. G., Van Der Kooij, H., and Bloem, B. R. (2008). The clinical utility of posturography. *Clin. Neurophysiol.* 119, 2424–2436.

Wittstein, M. W., Crider, A., Mastrocola, S., and Gonzalez, M. G. (2020). Use of virtual reality to assess dynamic posturography and sensory organization: instrument validation study. *JMIR Serious Games* 8:e19580. doi: 10.2196/19580

19

Normative Data for the NeuroCom® Sensory Organization Test in Subjects Aged 80–89 Years

Laura Perucca[1,2†], Antonio Robecchi Majnardi[1†], Silvia Frau[2] and Stefano Scarano[1,2]*

[1] Department of Neurorehabilitation Sciences, IRCCS Istituto Auxologico Italiano, Milan, Italy, [2] Department of Biomedical Sciences for Health, University of Milan, Milan, Italy

***Correspondence:**
Laura Perucca
l.perucca@auxologico.it*

† These authors have contributed equally to this work and share first authorship

Aging is known to increase the risk of falling. In older people, whose share in the total population is rising sharply, the Sensory Organization Test (SOT, Equitest NeuroCom) is a useful tool during rehabilitation and in clinical research for assessing postural stability, risk of falling, and balance improvement. Normative data for the SOT in the healthy population older than 79 years have not been previously published. We recruited 53 recreationally active healthy subjects aged 80 years and older from the general population in a cross-sectional study. We presented the normative data for SOT for the 80–84 and 85–89 years groups. Our results showed that the "vestibular" balance control tended to be affected by aging more than the vision and proprioception-based systems. A striking reduction in performance after the age of 85 years was observed. These findings will be useful for clinical and research purposes.

Keywords: normative data, balance, posturography, EquiTest®, Sensory Organization Test, aging

INTRODUCTION

Humankind is experiencing constant lengthening in life and healthy years. In recent decades, the percentage of the older population has been rising sharply. According to data from the World Population Prospect (2019 Revision), the number of people aged 80 years or older tripled between 1990 and 2019, growing up to 143 million, and this number will triple by 2050, reaching 426 million (United Nations Department of Economic and Social Affairs [UNDESA], 2020). The World Health Organization defines an older person as one with a chronological age of 65 years or older (World Health Organization [WHO], 2013). Various subgroupings have been proposed by gerontologists to distinguish the diversity of older age (Forman et al., 1992; Zizza et al., 2009). The simplest criteria distinguish young old (60–69 years), middle old (70–79 years), and very old (80+ years) (Forman et al., 1992). This subdivision is further articulated by defining the oldest old (OO) as those aged 85+ years (Garfein and Herzog, 1995), thus implicitly limiting the very old (VO) to a 5-year wide group. However, these definitions are frequently updated as life expectancy continues to rise. The old population is the most susceptible to illness and disability (Christensen et al., 2009): the risk of falling increases with aging and is a major risk after 85 years old (Ferrer et al., 2012), becoming one of the main problems associated with aging (Rogers and Mille, 2003).

In physical and rehabilitation medicine, a large variety of clinical and instrumental tests are used to evaluate postural stability, that is, the ability to control the position of the center of mass in relation to a person's base of support, during either static or dynamic tasks. The computed dynamic posturographic EquiTest® System (NeuroCom® International, Inc., Clackamas, OR,

United States) (NeuroCom® International Inc., 2003) provides qualitative and quantitative analysis of balance control performance through the description of the center of gravity (COG) sway during standing (Nashner and Peters, 1990). Within the EquiTest® System, the Sensory Organization Test (SOT) creates sensory-conflict conditions, making the visual and/or the proprioceptive balance control systems unreliable. Scores are assigned to the oscillation of the subject (the higher, the greater the stability). In essence, the reliable system(s), including the vestibular one, are stressed in order to substitute the unreliable ones. Based on the SOT scores in the various conditions, "sensory analysis" (SA) scores are provided. SOT and SA norms are provided for age groups up to 79 years (20–59, 60–69, 70–79) (NeuroCom® International Inc., 2003). Those for subjects aged 80+ years are lacking.

From a quantitative point of view, normative data are crucial in the understanding of balance performance in healthy subjects (Guskiewicz et al., 1997; Ferber-Viart et al., 2007), in patients affected by vestibular (Pedalini et al., 2009; Alahmari et al., 2014) or other neurological disorders (Voorhees, 1990), and in the aging population as such (Anacker and Di Fabio, 1992; Buatois et al., 2007). Since healthy elderly people are known to show greater body sways during balance tasks with respect to younger individuals (Murray et al., 1975; Forth et al., 2007), a tool to assess whether these augmented oscillations have to be considered physiological or not is necessary, for both clinical and research purposes. The SOT has shown a decline in performance with increasing age in healthy adults (Forth et al., 2007). This study aimed to provide normative data for EquiTest SOT and SA for VO (aged 80–84 years) and OO subjects, with the latter group defined for this study in the 85–89 years range.

MATERIALS AND METHODS

Participants

Subjects aged 80+ years were recruited from a general healthy Italian population. To be included, subjects older than 79 years old and younger than 90 years old had to be able to walk without aid for at least 50 m, provide informed consent, and understand the instructions given during clinical and instrumental evaluations. We excluded individuals with diseases affecting the nervous system, both central and/or peripheral (e.g., Parkinson's disease, previous traumatic brain injury, pallesthesia < 4/8), previous hip or knee joint replacement or other major surgeries or pathologies affecting the lower limbs or the spine, and acute or chronic pain. Mild visual impairment and mild hearing loss that did not affect activities of daily living were not considered as exclusion criteria. We investigated medication intake to rule out interactions with balance. All participants underwent a standardized neurological examination and structured medical interviews.

The study enrolled 53 subjects fitting the inclusion/exclusion criteria for T0 evaluation. We performed the second evaluation (T1) 2 weeks after T0 to assess the stability and reproducibility of the measurements. Of the 53 subjects, 39 carried out both test sessions. 14 participants dropped out after performing T0 evaluation, for the following reasons: $n = 2$ nausea or dizziness occurred after T0, $n = 1$ gym exercises performed between T0 and T1, $n = 4$ onset of acute pathologies after T0, $n = 3$ reported the testing session as too tiring and refused to participate to the follow-up, and $n = 4$ unsuitable climatic conditions at T1 date (hot summer temperatures).

Motor and cognitive status of the sample was assessed using validated instruments for the main functional domains: Mini Mental State Examination adjusted for age and schooling for cognitive status (Folstein et al., 1975; Magni et al., 1996), Functional Independence Measure for the overall degree of motor and cognitive independence (Linacre et al., 1994), 10-m Walking Test for gait (Brandstater et al., 1983), Equiscale (Tesio et al., 1997), and Dizziness Handicap Inventory short form (Tesio et al., 1999) for balance.

All tests were conducted at the Department of Neurorehabilitation of the Istituto Auxologico Italiano Research Hospital (Milan, Italy). All subjects were informed of the testing procedures and signed a written consent form approved by the hospital's ethics committee, which also approved the study. This trial has been registered at ClinicalTrials.gov (Identifier: NCT04773496).

To assess postural stability, we used an EquiTest System equipped with the Data Acquisition Toolkit (software version 8.6.1). Data on patients' age and height (measured on a precision scale) were provided at the beginning of the test as required by the device software. The EquiTest uses a mobile visual surrounding and a support surface containing a dual-force plate, consisting of two 23 × 46 cm footplates connected by a pin joint that can rotate in the sagittal plane following the patient's anteroposterior sway, thus systematically altering the visual and somatosensory environments. We asked the subjects to stand upright on the instrument support without wearing footwear, with foot placement standardized relative to their height and with arms relaxed at their sides. They had to look straight forward and stand as still as possible during the trials. The SOT measures the sway of the COG under six different conditions (**Table 1**). The visual surround and the force plate, separately or together, may move in a sway-referenced manner, following the patient's own anteroposterior sway, thus delivering inaccurate information to the eyes, feet, and joints. Subjects wore a safety jacket hanging from the top of the instrument frame. Data were recorded during three trials for each condition. Each trial lasted 20 s. The sway gain setting was fixed at 1.00, making the support surface and/or visual surround matching the patient's sway exactly.

In the EquiTest System the amount of sway of the COG is expressed in degrees to allow comparison of scores between individuals of different heights. The angular limits of stability are nearly the same for all normal adults, regardless of height (NeuroCom® International Inc., 2003). The equilibrium score compares the patient's anteroposterior (AP) sway during each trial to a theoretical sway stability limit of 12.5 degrees (NeuroCom® International Inc., 2003). SOT Scores for each condition are given in the range of 0–100, with higher scores representing better performance and participants swaying to the limits of stability receiving low scores (NeuroCom® International Inc., 2003). Score 0 is assigned to a trial marked as "fall" (a

TABLE 1 | The six conditions of the Sensory Organization Test [Adapted from Instructions for Use: EQUITEST® SYSTEM OPERATOR'S MANUAL, Clackamas, OR (United States): NeuroCom® International Inc., 2003].

	Condition 1	Condition 2	Condition 3	Condition 4	Condition 5	Condition 6
Eyes	Open	Closed	Open	Open	Closed	Open
Surroundings	Fixed	n.a.	Sway-referenced	Fixed	n.a.	Sway-referenced
Platform	Fixed	Fixed	Fixed	Sway-referenced	Sway-referenced	Sway-referenced
Sensory System used	Somatosensory	Somatosensory	Somatosensory	Vision	Vestibular	Vestibular

n.a., not applicable.

stepping reaction, hands touching the surround or, in extreme cases, subject being supported by the safety jacket). Score 100 is assigned to full stability (never achievable in practice). A cumulative 0–100 SOT score (composite SOT) is also assigned to the overall test. Normative data are given as age-specific 95th percentile limits.

The SA scores (0–100, the higher the better the condition) were computed as ratio between the mean scores of specific conditions: SOM represents the ratio of the second to the first condition (if reduced it suggests a somatosensory impairment is present); VIS is the ratio of the fourth condition to the first (if reduced i.e., inability to use vision for compensatory purposes); VEST is the ratio of the fifth to the first condition (if reduced i.e., a possible vestibular deficit as in condition 5 balance is entrusted exclusively to the vestibular system). PREF highlights the visual preference (ratio of conditions with unreliable vision compared to those where vision is absent—i.e., conditions (3 + 6) to (2 + 5), when reduced it implies the subject relies on visual information even when those are unreliable (NeuroCom® International Inc., 2003).

The first evaluation (T0) (subject's history, functional scales, and instrumental evaluation) took approximately 90 min for each subject. To assess the reliability of the measurement, we repeated all six conditions of the SOT (T1) 2 weeks later (± 2 days). We asked the participants not to train or practice any kind of exercise between T0 and T1. Data collection was carried out by operators with experience in this assessment or trained for this purpose.

Statistical Analysis

We performed data analysis using STATA statistical software, version 11 (Computing Resource Center, Los Angeles, CA, United States, 2011). Descriptive statistics (mean ± SD, median) for each SOT condition and composite scores were generated. The SOT's score distributions for the entire sample and for the two different populations (VO and OO) were tested for normality (skewness and kurtosis test). Data are represented using bar charts and box plots. To allow comparison with the normative data of the previous 10-year age group, we set the level of significance at $p < 0.05$. We calculated the normative data as stated by NeuroCom, setting the limits of normality at the 5th percentile by applying the following equation: *SOT norms = mean - (SD * 1.67)* (NeuroCom® International Inc., 2003).

To assess the test-retest reliability, we used intraclass correlation coefficients (ICC 3.1, two-way random-effect model, absolute agreement) for the composite SOT and for each condition evaluated at T0 and T1. According to the literature (Koo and Li, 2016), reproducibility is labeled as poor when ICC < 0.5, moderate if between 0.5 and 0.75, good if between 0.75 and 0.9, excellent when > 0.90.

RESULTS

53 subjects participated in the study (25 women, 47%). The mean ± SD age of the entire sample was 83.4 ± 3 years (median: 82 years), with a range of 80–89 years. The mean and median ages did not differ substantially between men (83 ± 3.2 years, median: 81.5 years, range: 80–89 years) and women (83.88 ± 6 years, 84 years, 80–89 years). By applying the stated definition of VO (80–84 years) and OO (for this study 85–89 years), we divided the sample into two populations, as follows: VO, $n = 35$ (66%), and OO, $n = 18$ (34%). For both VO and OO, descriptive statistics for demographics and functional tests are provided in **Table 2**. The subjects were cognitively intact and had no balance, walking, or global functional impairments. T1 assessment was performed by 26 VO and 13 OO participants.

The SOT scores for the entire sample and for the two different groups (VO and OO) were not normally distributed, according to the skewness and kurtosis test. The bimodal distribution of the observed scores seemed to fit the study's originally proposed division between two different populations (VO and OO). The non-parametric Mann–Whitney test confirmed that the scores for each condition (except conditions 3 and 6) and composite SOT were statistically different between the two groups.

Descriptive data (median and interquartile range) for the six conditions and the composite SOT for the two groups are shown as box plots in **Figure 1**, while mean scores for each condition and for the composite SOT are presented in **Figure 2**. **Table 3** summarizes the descriptive statistics (mean ± SD and median), normative data, and variance analysis for SOT. Descriptive statistics (mean ± SD and median) and normative data for SA are presented in **Table 4**. Normative data for each condition and composite SOT are reported in **Figure 3**, while normative data for SA are in **Figure 4**. In **Tables 3, 4** and **Figures 2–4** the data on the 70–79 years age group, as provided by NeuroCom in the User's manual, are reported in order to give the reader a quick comparison among the different age groups. The NeuroCom's sample was composed of 29 participants (14 women and 15 men). No further statistical analysis has been performed on the NeuroCom's sample data.

We tested the test-retest reliability of our sample and the ICC values provided good reproducibility of the Composite SOT

TABLE 2 | Descriptive data on very old (VO) and oldest old (OO) groups.

		VO (80–84 years old) (n = 35)	OO (85–89 years old) (n = 18)
	Score range (better score)	**Mean ± SD (Median)**	**Mean ± SD (Median)**
Age	n.a.	81.5 ± 1.4 (81)	87.1 ± 1.7 (87)
Male	n.a.	57.1% (n = 20)	44.4% (n = 8)
Number of medications	n.a.	2.5 ± 2.3 (2)	3.0 ± 2 (3)
MMSE(*)	0–30 (30)	28.6 ± 1.8 (29.1)	29.6 ± 2.4 (30.3)
FIM® – Comprehensive	18–126 (126)	125 ± 1.4 (126)	123.9 ± 2.4 (124)
FIM® – Motor	13–91 (91)	90.1 ± 1.4 (91)	89.6 ± 0.8 (90)
FIM® – Cognitive	5–35 (35)	35 ± 0.16 (35)	34.3 ± 2.4 (35)
Equiscale	0–16 (16)	15.3 ± 1 (16)	14.5 ± 1 (15)
DHI	0–13 (0)	0.6 ± 0.94 (0)	0.8 ± 0.8 (1)
Step length cm	Ability to perform the 10 mWT	64.9 ± 7.6 (65)	57.5 ± 6.9 (58)
Gait speed m/s		1.17 ± 0.2 (1.18)	1.1 ± 0.1 (1.1)

n.a., not applicable; MMSE, Mini Mental State Examination; FIM, Functional Independence Measure; DHI, Dizziness Handicap Inventory short form; 10 mWT, 10-m Walking Test.
(*) MMSE scores have been corrected for age and schooling. The number of medications taken by subjects ranged from 0 to 10 and were mostly in the three main categories of anti-hypertensives, proton-pump inhibitors, and those for benign prostate hypertrophy. Among the subjects, 17% (n = 9) did not take any medication, 17% (n = 9) took only one medication, and 34% (n = 18) took a maximum of two or three drugs per day. Only four subjects used more than six medications per day.

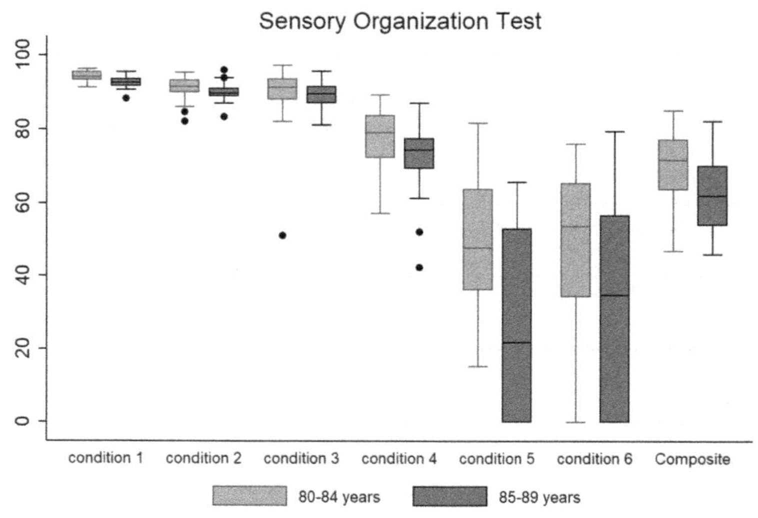

FIGURE 1 | Box plots (median and interquartile range; outliers are represented as dots) for the six testing conditions and for the composite Sensory Organization Test for the very old (80–84 years) and oldest old (85–89 years) groups.

and moderate to good reproducibility for each of the six SOT condition scores. ICC values are reported in **Table 5**.

DISCUSSION

The study of SOT in the healthy population has recently developed (Guskiewicz et al., 1997; Ferber-Viart et al., 2007; Pierchała et al., 2012; Pletcher et al., 2017), but not yet in the population aged 80–89 years. As suggested by the increased incidence of falls in the elderly, one or more of the systems involved in postural control lose efficiency with age (Peterka and Black, 1990). Our results showed that balance control in VO and OO is less effective when vestibular information is the only one available, in particular above 84 years of age. This finding is consistent with previous clinical observations (Ferrer et al., 2012). The older adults of the third millennium are the healthiest, most active, and longest-living in human history and are now a demographic phenomenon in most countries (United Nations Department of Economic and Social Affairs [UNDESA], 2020). The literature deals comprehensively with the concept of healthy aging and the interaction between physiological age-related deficits and actual neurological pathology (Morris and McManus, 1991; Kaye et al., 1994; Nardone et al., 2000; Papegaaij et al., 2014). Aging involves the degeneration of various central nervous system (CNS) and peripheral nervous system (PNS) structures, with a loss in brain volume and weight around 5% per decade after age 40 and possible more above age 70

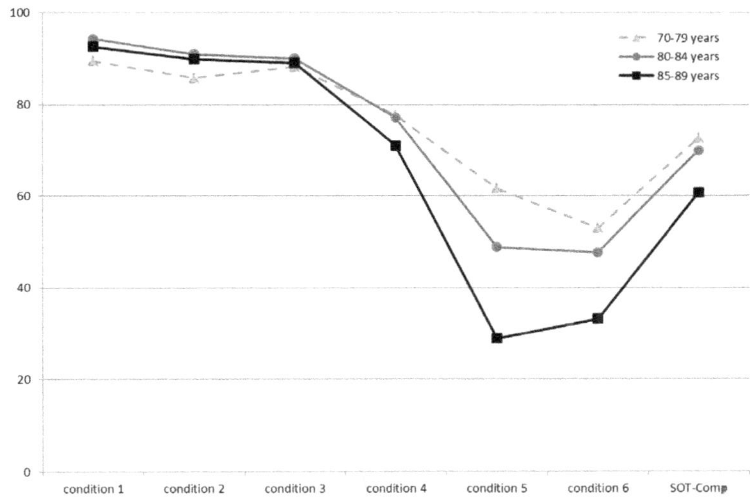

FIGURE 2 | Mean values for the three age groups in the six conditions and for the composite Sensory Organization Test data. The lowest values in condition 5 describe an age-related worsening of vestibular function. Data for the 70–79 age group are provided by NeuroCom® International Inc. (2003).

TABLE 3 | Descriptive, variance analysis, and normative data for each condition and composite SOT for three age groups: 70–79 years (data provided by NeuroCom® International Inc., 2003), very old (VO, 80–84 years), and oldest old (OO, 85–89 years).

Age group	70–79 years	VO 80–84 years	OO 85–89 years	VO vs. OO	70–79 years	VO	OO
	Mean ± SD	Mean ± SD (Median)	Mean ± SD (Median)	Variance analysis	SOT normative data		
Condition 1	89.4 ± 11.4	94.3 ± 1.3 (94.3)	92.6 ± 1.7 (92.6)	$p < 0.000$	70	92	90
Condition 2	85.8 ± 13.5	91.1 ± 3 (91.6)	89.9 ± 2.7 (89.8)	$p < 0.048$	63	86	85
Condition 3	88.2 ± 3.8	90 ± 7.6 (91.3)	89.1 ± 3.4 (89.6)	$p < 0.098$	82	77	83
Condition 4	77.6 ± 5.5	77.2 ± 8.3 (79.0)	71.2 ± 10.4 (74.3)	$p < 0.018$	69	63	54
Condition 5	61.6 ± 10.2	48.8 ± 17.5 (48.0)	28.9 ± 24.6 (21.8)	$p < 0.005$	45	20	0
Condition 6	53.0 ± 15.5	47.7 ± 20.5 (53.6)	33.2 ± 27.3 (34.6)	$p < 0.064$	27	13	0
Composite SOT	72.8 ± 5.4	69.9 ± 8.4 (73.0)	60.7 ± 10.3 (58.5)	$p < 0.003$	64	56	43

SOT, Sensory Organization Test.

(Peters, 2006), and physiological changes in postural control and balance (Kaye et al., 1994; Camicioli et al., 1997; Nardone et al., 2000), related to sensory deficits (Judge et al., 1995), CNS integration abnormalities (Morris and McManus, 1991), and musculoskeletal aging (Judge et al., 1996). From this point of view, a reduction in neurological performance can be defined as a sequela of neuroanatomical and neurofunctional changes (Morris and McManus, 1991; Papegaaij et al., 2014). The risk of falling increases in older adults, and balance impairment is one of the main targets of rehabilitation treatment (Chang et al., 2004).

As expected, mean values decreased in both VO and OO groups from Condition 1 (i.e., all sensory information available) to Condition 5 (i.e., visual information absent and proprioception not reliable). In the variance analysis, we observed that the scores for all conditions and for the composite SOT were statistically different between the VO and OO, with the exception of condition 6 and, broadly, of condition 3. A similar observation for condition 3 has already been provided in a previous study (Pletcher et al., 2017). In that paper statistical differences were seen between military groups with different tactical demands in all SOT conditions with the exception of condition 3; the authors hypothesized that the similar distribution of the SOT scores for condition 3 and somatosensory scores among groups might reflect the disadvantage to the visual system due to the sway-referenced surround. In our sample this result may suggest that aging can affect the use of proprioceptive information less than vestibular information with respect to balance control. However, this aspect requires further investigation.

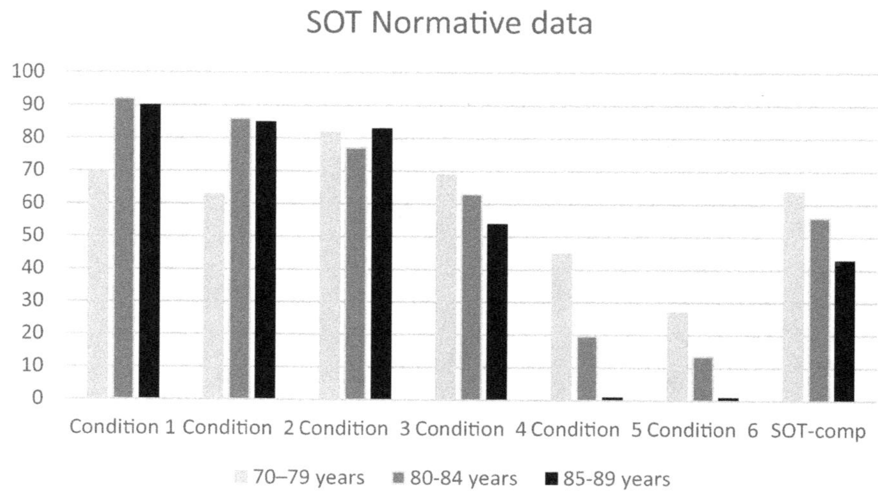

FIGURE 3 | Normative data for the six conditions and for the composite Sensory Organization Test data in the three age groups considered in this study. The striking reduction in norm values in conditions 5 and 6 is due to the wide standard deviation in those conditions. Data for the 70–79 age group are provided by NeuroCom® International Inc. (2003).

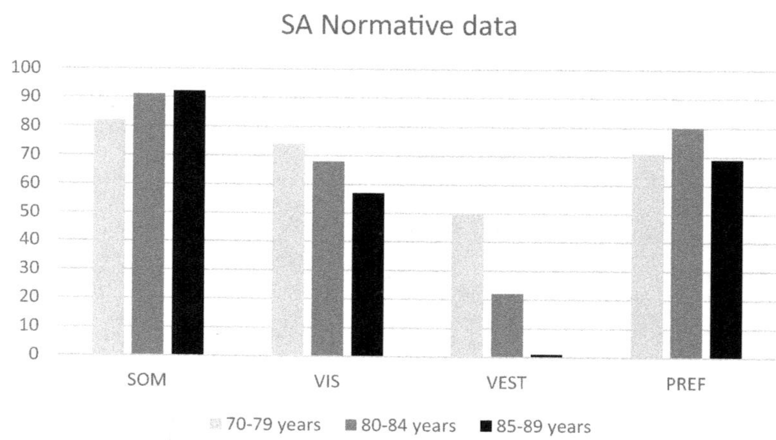

FIGURE 4 | Normative data for sensory analysis (SA) for the three age groups considered in this study. Data for the 70–79 age group are provided by NeuroCom® International Inc. (2003).

The normative data for conditions 1 and 2 are similar between VO and OO. In the OO group the norms for conditions 5 and 6 are equal to zero, and this evidence may imply that vestibular information are not sufficient for OO for maintaining balance control, and that a low vestibular score at the SOT could be considered as "normal" (whereas it would still be considered as pathological in the VO population).

Moreover, the comparison of normative data for the six SOT conditions, composite SOT and SA for VO and OO with those of the previous decade (**Tables 3, 4**) suggests some thoughts:

- The normative data for conditions 1 and 2 for the two groups in our sample were higher than those stated by NeuroCom for the 70–79 years age group. The reason for this discrepancy could have various origins. First, the sample adopted by NeuroCom for the 70–79 age group was smaller (n = 29, 14 female) than ours. Although declared asymptomatic, their sample was not previously evaluated for functional performance and medication intake. Second, aging for our subjects occurred 20 years later than the NeuroCom original study, so that health care conditions might have improved. Third, subjects who survived for a long time without health concerns could have had a functional advantage during aging. Fourth, the mediterranean environmental context might have fostered a healthier aging.
- The greatest differences with the NeuroCom 70–79 years group can be found for Conditions 5 and 6 norms: both VO and OO display lower values than the 70–79 group. This evidence may suggest that a reduction in the efficiency of

TABLE 4 | Sensory analysis (SA) descriptive (mean ± SD, median) and normative data for three age groups: 70–79 years (data provided by NeuroCom® International Inc., 2003), very old (VO, 80–84 years), and oldest old (OO, 85–89 years).

	70–79 years	VO		OO		SA normative data		
	Mean ± SD	Mean ± SD	Median	Mean ± SD	Median	70–79 years	VO	OO
SOM	95.1 ± 7.9	96.5 ± 3	97	97.1 ± 3.1	97	82	91	92
VIS	85 ± 0.066	81.8 ± 8	82	76.9 ± 11.7	80	74	68	57
VEST	67.3 ± 10.4	51.8 ± 18	52	31.4 ± 27	23	50	22	0
PREF	94.9 ± 14.4	98.5 ± 11	100	105.1 ± 21.8	101	71	80	69

SOM, somatosensory; VIS, visual; VEST, vestibular; PREF, visual preference.

TABLE 5 | Interclass correlation coefficients (ICC) for each condition and for composite SOT in the whole sample between T0 and T1.

	ICC
Condition 1	0.52
Condition 2	0.79
Condition 3	0.55
Condition 4	0.73
Condition 5	0.71
Condition 6	0.67
composite SOT	0.76

SOT, Sensory Organization Test.

the vestibular system can be involved in the increasing rate of falling in the elderly.

The reliability of the measures of SOT scores and of the composite SOT were found to be moderate to good. The reliability of SOT scores for Conditions 1-6 were comparable to those reported in previously published papers for individuals aged 20–80 + (19) and above 65 years of age (Ford-Smith et al., 1995). As already pointed out by Forth et al. (2007), there is a considerable variability in the ICCs of the different SOT conditions, ranging from 0.52 to 0.79 in our sample.

The normative data provided by this work may lead clinicians and researchers in defining the degree of balance impairment in individuals aged 80–89 years old. Moreover, the identification of the impaired sensory systems can guide the development of rehabilitation programs tailored on the patient and the measurement of rehabilitation outcomes. This information, together with other validated tool, will help in assessing the risk of falls in elderly people.

CONCLUSION

This study provided normative data for SOT and SA assessed by the EquiTest® System in healthy older subjects. Poor postural stability is a risk factor for falls and subsequent injury. To our knowledge, this study is the first to present SOT and SA norms for subjects aged 80+ years. Moreover, we investigated subjects in the oldest old category (85–89 years). Data from our research can assist both clinicians and researchers who deal with balance in older subjects.

LIMITS OF THE STUDY

The recorded data for the sample were not normally distributed. The variance analysis revealed how the vestibular performance decreased suddenly over a 5-year horizon (80–84 years vs. 85–89 years) and suggested an opportunity for studies with an older and wider span of older healthy subjects. However, it is not easy to find a large number of healthy subjects aged 85 + years. More studies focused on subjects aged 85 + or 90 + years will be possible and easier in the future, considering the global phenomenon of aging.

ETHICS STATEMENT

The studies involving human participants were reviewed and approved by Comitato Etico—Istituto Auxologico Italiano IRCCS. The patients/participants provided their written informed consent to participate in this study.

AUTHOR CONTRIBUTIONS

LP designed the study. LP and SF collected the data. LP, AR, and SS analyzed and interpreted the data. AR wrote the manuscript. LP and SS reviewed the manuscript. All authors contributed to the article and approved the submitted version.

FUNDING

This trial has been funded by the Italian Ministry of Health.

ACKNOWLEDGMENTS

We thank Anna Simone for the statistical support. We would like to thank Editage (www.editage.com) for English language editing.

REFERENCES

Alahmari, K. A., Marchetti, G. F., Sparto, P. J., Furman, J. M., and Whitney, S. L. (2014). Estimating postural control with the balance rehabilitation unit: measurement consistency, accuracy, validity, and comparison with dynamic posturography. *Arch. Phys. Med. Rehabil.* 95, 65–73.

Anacker, S. L., and Di Fabio, R. P. (1992). Influence of sensory inputs on standing balance in community-dwelling elders with a recent history of falling. *Phys. Ther.* 72, 574–575. doi: 10.1093/ptj/72.8.575

Brandstater, M. E., de Bruin, H., Gowland, C., and Clark, B. M. (1983). Hemiplegic gait: analysis of temporal variables. *Arch. Phys. Med. Rehabil.* 64, 583–587.

Buatois, S., Gauchard, G. C., Aubry, C., Benetos, A., and Perrin, P. (2007). Current physical activity improves balance control during sensory conflicting conditions in older adults. *Int. J. Sports Med.* 28, 53–58. doi: 10.1055/s-2006-924054

Camicioli, R., Panzer, V. P., and Kaye, J. (1997). Balance in the healthy elderly: posturography and clinical assessment. *Arch. Neurol.* 54, 976–981. doi: 10.1001/archneur.1997.00550200040008

Chang, J. T., Morton, S. C., Rubenstein, L. Z., Mojica, W. A., Maglione, M., and Suttorp, M. J. (2004). Interventions for the prevention of falls in older adults: systematic review and meta-analysis of randomised clinical trials. *BMJ* 328:680. doi: 10.1136/bmj.328.7441.680

Christensen, K., Doblhammer, G., Rau, R., and Vaupel, J. W. (2009). Ageing populations: the challenges ahead. *Lancet* 374, 1196–1208. doi: 10.1016/S0140-6736(09)61460-4

Ferber-Viart, C., Ionescu, E., Morlet, T., Froehlich, P., and Dubreuil, C. (2007). Balance in healthy individuals assessed with Equitest: maturation and normative data for children and young adults. *Int. J. Pediatr. Otorhinolaryngol.* 71, 1041–1046. doi: 10.1016/j.ijporl.2007.03.012

Ferrer, A., Formiga, F., Plana-Ripoll, O., Tobella, M. A., Gil, A., and Pujol, R. (2012). Risk of falls in 85-year-olds is associated with functional and cognitive status: the Octabaix Study. *Arch. Gerontol. Geriatr.* 54, 352–356. doi: 10.1016/j.archger.2011.06.004

Folstein, M. F., Folstein, S. E., and Mchugh, P. R. (1975). "Mini-Mental State". A practical method for grading the cognitive state of patients for the clinician. *J. Psychiat. Res.* 12, 189–198. doi: 10.1016/0022-3956(75)90026-6

Ford-Smith, C. D., Wyman, J. F., Elswick, R. K., Fernandez, T., and Newton, R. A. (1995). Test-retest reliability of the sensory organization test in noninstitutionalized older adults. *Arch. Phys. Med. Rehabil.* 76, 77–81. doi: 10.1016/S0003-9993(95)80047-6

Forman, D. E., Berman, A. D., McCabe, C. H., Baim, D. S., and Wei, J. Y. (1992). PTCA in the elderly: the "young-old" versus the "old-old". *J. Am. Geriatr. Soc.* 40, 19–22. doi: 10.1111/j.1532-5415.1992.tb01823.x

Forth, K. E., Metter, E. J., and Paloski, W. H. (2007). Age associated differences in postural equilibrium control: A comparison between EQscore and minimum time to contact (TTCmin). *Gait Posture* 25, 56–62. doi: 10.1016/j.gaitpost.2005.12.008

Garfein, A. J., and Herzog, A. R. (1995). Robust aging among the young-old, old-old, and oldest-old. *J. Gerontol. B Psychol. Sci. Soc. Sci.* 50, S77–S87. doi: 10.1093/geronb/50b.2.s77

Guskiewicz, K. M., Riemann, B. L., Perrin, D. H., and Nashner, L. M. (1997). Alternative approaches to the assessment of mild head injury in athletes. *Med. Sci. Sports Exerc.* 29, S213–S221. doi: 10.1097/00005768-199707001-00003

Judge, J. O., King, M. B., Whipple, R., Clive, J., and Wolfson, L. I. (1995). Dynamic balance in older persons: effects of reduced visual and proprioceptive input. *J. Gerontol. A Biol. Sci. Med. Sci.* 50, M263–M270. doi: 10.1093/gerona/50a.5.m263

Judge, J., Ounpuu, S., and Davis, R. I. (1996). Effects of age on the biomechanics and physiology of gait.pdf. *Clin. Geratr. Med.* 12, 659–678.

Kaye, J. A., Oken, B. S., Howieson, D. B., Howieson, J., Holm, L. A., and Dennison, K. (1994). Neurologic Evaluation of the Optimally Healthy Oldest Old. *Arch. Neurol.* 51, 1205–1211. doi: 10.1001/archneur.1994.00540240049015

Koo, T. K., and Li, M. Y. A. (2016). Guideline of Selecting and Reporting Intraclass Correlation Coefficients for Reliability Research. *J. Chiropr. Med.* 15, 155–163. doi: 10.1016/j.jcm.2016.02.012

Linacre, J. M., Heinemann, A. W., Wright, B. D., Granger, C. V., and Hamilton, B. B. (1994). The structure and stability of the Functional Independence Measure. *Arch. Phys. Med. Rehabil.* 75, 127–132.

Magni, E., Binetti, G., Bianchetti, A., Rozzini, R., and Trabucchi, M. (1996). Mini-Mental State Examination: a normative study in Italian elderly population. *Eur. J. Neurol.* 3, 198–202. doi: 10.1111/j.1468-1331.1996.tb00423.x

Morris, J. C., and McManus, D. Q. (1991). The neurology of aging: normal versus pathologic change. *Geriatrics* 46, 51–54.

Murray, M. P., Seireg, A. A., and Sepic, S. B. (1975). Normal postural stability and steadiness: quantitative assessment. *J. Bone Jt. Surg. Ser. A* 57, 510–516. doi: 10.2106/00004623-197557040-00012

Nardone, A., Galante, M., Corna, S., Grasso, M., Tarantola, J., and Schieppati, M. (2000). "The effects of aging on static and dynamic equilibrium" in *The Ageing Motor System and its Adaptations to Training.* eds P. Capodaglio and M. Narici (Pavia: PI-ME Press). 101–108.

Nashner, L. M., and Peters, J. F. (1990). Dynamic posturography in the diagnosis and management of dizziness and balance disorders. *Neurol. Clin.* 8, 331–349. doi: 10.1016/s0733-8619(18)30359-1

NeuroCom® International Inc. (2003). *Instructions for Use: EQUITEST® SYSTEM OPERATOR'S MANUAL. Version 8.* Clackamas: NeuroCom® International Inc.

Papegaaij, S., Taube, W., Baudry, S., Otten, E., and Hortobágyi, T. (2014). Aging causes a reorganization of cortical and spinal control of posture. *Front. Aging Neurosci.* 6:28. doi: 10.3389/fnagi.2014.00028

Pedalini, M. E. B., Cruz, O. L. M., Bittar, R. S. M., Lorenzi, M. C., and Grasel, S. S. (2009). Sensory organization test in elderly patients with and without vestibular dysfunction. *Acta Otolaryngol.* 129, 962–965. doi: 10.1080/00016480802468930

Peterka, R. J., and Black, F. O. (1990). Age-related changes in human posture control: Sensory organization tests. *J. Vestib. Res.* 1, 73–85. doi: 10.3233/ves-1990-1108

Peters, R. (2006). Ageing and the brain. *Postgrad. Med. J.* 82, 84–88. doi: 10.1136/pgmj.2005.036665

Pierchała, K., Lachowska, M., Morawski, K., and Niemczyk, K. (2012). [Sensory Organization Test outcomes in young, older and elderly healthy individuals–preliminary results]. *Otolaryngol. Pol.* 66, 274–9.

Pletcher, E. R., Williams, V. J., Abt, J. P., Morgan, P. M., Parr, J. J., Wohleber, M. F., et al. (2017). Normative Data for the NeuroCom Sensory Organization Test in US Military Special Operations Forces. *J. Athl. Train.* 52, 129–136. doi: 10.4085/1062-6050-52.1.05

Rogers, M. W., and Mille, M.-L. (2003). Lateral stability and falls in older people. *Exerc. Sport Sci. Rev.* 31, 182–187. doi: 10.1097/00003677-200310000-00005

Tesio, L., Alpini, D., Cesarani, A., and Perucca, L. (1999). Short form of the Dizziness Handicap Inventory: construction and validation through Rasch analysis. *Am. J. Phys. Med. Rehabil.* 78, 233–241.

Tesio, L., Perucca, L., Franchignoni, F. P., and Battaglia, M. A. (1997). A short measure of balance in multiple sclerosis: validation through Rasch analysis. *Funct. Neurol.* 12, 255–265.

United Nations Department of Economic and Social Affairs [UNDESA] (2020). *World Population Ageing 2019 (ST/ESA/SER.A/444).* United States: United Nations Department of Economic and Social Affairs.

Voorhees, R. L. (1990). Dynamic posturography findings in central nervous system disorders. *Otolaryngol. Head Neck Surg.* 103, 96–101. doi: 10.1177/019459989010300114

World Health Organization [WHO] (2013). *Definition of an Older or Elderly Person. Proposed Working Definition of an Older Person in Africa for the MDS Project.* Switzerland: World Health Organization.

Zizza, C. A., Ellison, K. J., and Wernette, C. M. (2009). Total water intakes of community-living middle-old and oldest-old adults. *J. Gerontol. A Biol. Sci. Med. Sci.* 64, 481–486. doi: 10.1093/gerona/gln045

Permissions

All chapters in this book were first published by Frontiers; hereby published with permission under the Creative Commons Attribution License or equivalent. Every chapter published in this book has been scrutinized by our experts. Their significance has been extensively debated. The topics covered herein carry significant findings which will fuel the growth of the discipline. They may even be implemented as practical applications or may be referred to as a beginning point for another development.

The contributors of this book come from diverse backgrounds, making this book a truly international effort. This book will bring forth new frontiers with its revolutionizing research information and detailed analysis of the nascent developments around the world.

We would like to thank all the contributing authors for lending their expertise to make the book truly unique. They have played a crucial role in the development of this book. Without their invaluable contributions this book wouldn't have been possible. They have made vital efforts to compile up to date information on the varied aspects of this subject to make this book a valuable addition to the collection of many professionals and students.

This book was conceptualized with the vision of imparting up-to-date information and advanced data in this field. To ensure the same, a matchless editorial board was set up. Every individual on the board went through rigorous rounds of assessment to prove their worth. After which they invested a large part of their time researching and compiling the most relevant data for our readers.

The editorial board has been involved in producing this book since its inception. They have spent rigorous hours researching and exploring the diverse topics which have resulted in the successful publishing of this book. They have passed on their knowledge of decades through this book. To expedite this challenging task, the publisher supported the team at every step. A small team of assistant editors was also appointed to further simplify the editing procedure and attain best results for the readers.

Apart from the editorial board, the designing team has also invested a significant amount of their time in understanding the subject and creating the most relevant covers. They scrutinized every image to scout for the most suitable representation of the subject and create an appropriate cover for the book.

The publishing team has been an ardent support to the editorial, designing and production team. Their endless efforts to recruit the best for this project, has resulted in the accomplishment of this book. They are a veteran in the field of academics and their pool of knowledge is as vast as their experience in printing. Their expertise and guidance has proved useful at every step. Their uncompromising quality standards have made this book an exceptional effort. Their encouragement from time to time has been an inspiration for everyone.

The publisher and the editorial board hope that this book will prove to be a valuable piece of knowledge for researchers, students, practitioners and scholars across the globe.

List of Contributors

Fabio V. dos Anjos, Talita P. Pinto, Marco Gazzoni and Taian M. Vieira
Laboratorio di Ingegneria del Sistema Neuromuscolare, Dipartimento di Elettronica e Telecomunicazioni, Politecnico di Torino, Torino, Italy

Jean-Louis Honeine and Oscar Crisafulli
Department of Public Health, Experimental and Forensic Medicine, University of Pavia, Pavia, Italy

Marco Schieppati
Department of Public Health, Experimental and Forensic Medicine, University of Pavia, Pavia, Italy
Centro Studi Attività Motorie (CSAM), Fondazione Salvatore Maugeri (IRCSS), Scientific Institute of Pavia, Pavia, Italy

Manh-Cuong Do
Faculty of Sport Science, Complexité, Innovations, Activités Motrices et Sportives (CIAMS), Université Paris-Saclay, Orsay, France

Paolo Cavallari, Francesco Bolzoni, Carlo Bruttini and Roberto Esposti
Human Motor Control and Posture Lab, Section Human Physiology of the Department of Pathophysiology and Transplantation, Università degli Studi di Milano, Milan, Italy

Clint Hansen
Research Department, Aspetar Qatar Orthopaedic and Sports Medicine, Doha, Qatar

Qin Wei
School of Information Engineering, Wuhan University of Technology, Wuhan, China

Jiann-Shing Shieh
Department of Mechanical Engineering, Yuan Ze University, Chung-Li, Taiwan

Paul Fourcade
URCIAMS – Motor Control and Perception Team, University Paris-Sud, Orsay, France

Brice Isableu
PSYCLE, Aix Marseille University, Aix-en-Provence, France

Lina Majed
Sport Science Program, College of Arts and Science, Qatar University, Doha, Qatar

Alain Hamaoui
Laboratoire de Physiologie de la Posture et du Mouvement, Centre universitaire de formation et de recherche Jean-François Champollion, Albi, France
Laboratoire Mouvement, Equilibre, Performance, Santé (EA 4445), Université de Pau et des Pays de l'Adour, Tarbes, France

Caroline Alamini-Rodrigues
Laboratoire Mouvement, Equilibre, Performance, Santé (EA 4445), Université de Pau et des Pays de l'Adour, Tarbes, France
Laboratoire de Physiologie de la Posture et du Mouvement, Institut National Universitaire Champollion, Albi, France

Jacques Abboud
Département D'anatomie, Université du Québec à Trois-Rivières, Trois-Rivières, QC, Canada

Arnaud Lardon
Pôle Recherche Clinique Chiropratique, Institut Franco-Européen de Chiropraxie, Ivry-Sur-Seine, France
Département des Sciences de L'activité Physique, Université du Québec à Trois-Rivières, Trois-Rivières, QC, Canada

Frédéric Boivin and Claude Dugas
Département des Sciences de L'activité Physique, Université du Québec à Trois-Rivières, Trois-Rivières, QC, Canada

Stefania Sozzi
Centro Studi Attività Motorie (CSAM), Fondazione Salvatore Maugeri (IRCCS), Pavia, Italy

Antonio Nardone
Posture and Movement Laboratory, Physical Medicine and Rehabilitation, Fondazione Salvatore Maugeri (IRCCS), Veruno, Italy
Department of Translational Medicine, University of Eastern Piedmont, Novara, Italy

Matthew J. Bancroft and Brian L. Day
Sobell Department of Motor Neuroscience and Movement Disorders, UCL Institute of Neurology, University College London, London, UK

Trieu Phat Luu, Yongtian He, Sho Nakagome, Kevin Nathan, Samuel Brown, Jeffrey Gorges and Jose L. Contreras-Vidal
Noninvasive Brain-Machine Interface System Laboratory, Department of Electrical and Computer Engineering, University of Houston, Houston, TX, United States

Rajal G. Cohen
Department of Psychology and Communication Studies, University of Idaho, Moscow, ID, USA

John G. Nutt
Department of Neurology, Oregon Health and Science University, Portland, OR, USA

Fay B. Horak
Department of Neurology, Oregon Health and Science University, Portland, OR, USA
Research Department, Veterans Affairs Portland Health Care System, Portland, OR, USA

Tony J. Szturm
Mobility and Cognition Lab, College of Rehabilitation Sciences, University of Manitoba, Winnipeg, MB, Canada
Department of Physical Therapy, University of Manitoba, Winnipeg, MB, Canada

Vedant S. Sakhalkar
Mobility and Cognition Lab, College of Rehabilitation Sciences, University of Manitoba, Winnipeg, MB, Canada
School of Medical Rehabilitation, University of Manitoba, Winnipeg, MB, Canada

Anuprita Kanitkar
Mobility and Cognition Lab, College of Rehabilitation Sciences, University of Manitoba, Winnipeg, MB, Canada
Applied Health Sciences, University of Manitoba, Winnipeg, MB, Canada

Mayur Nankar
Mobility and Cognition Lab, College of Rehabilitation Sciences, University of Manitoba, Winnipeg, MB, Canada

Teddy Caderby, Nicolas Peyrot, Xavier de Viviés, Bruno Bonazzi and Georges Dalleau
Laboratoire IRISSE, UFR des Sciences de l'Homme et de l'Environnement, Université de la Réunion, Ile de la Réunion, France

Eric Yiou
Laboratoire CIAMS, Université Paris Sud, Université Paris-Saclay, Orsay, France
Laboratoire CIAMS, Université d'Orléans, Orléans, France

Elisabeth Kaminski, Maike Hoff, Viola Rjosk and Bernhard Sehm
Department of Neurology, Max Planck Institute for Human Cognitive and Brain Sciences, Leipzig, Germany

Christopher J. Steele
Department of Neurology, Max Planck Institute for Human Cognitive and Brain Sciences, Leipzig, Germany
Department of Psychiatry, Cerebral Imaging Centre, Douglas Mental Health Institute, McGill University, Montreal, QC, Canada

Christopher Gundlach
Department of Neurology, Max Planck Institute for Human Cognitive and Brain Sciences, Leipzig, Germany
Faculty of Psychology, Department of Experimental Psychology and Methods, University of Leipzig, Leipzig, Germany

Arno Villringer
Department of Neurology, Max Planck Institute for Human Cognitive and Brain Sciences, Leipzig, Germany
Mind and Brain Institute, Charité and Humboldt University, Berlin, Germany

Patrick Ragert
Department of Neurology, Max Planck Institute for Human Cognitive and Brain Sciences, Leipzig, Germany
Faculty of Sport Science, Institute for General Kinesiology and Exercise Science, University of Leipzig, Leipzig, Germany

Normand Teasdale
Département de Kinésiologie, Faculté de Médecine, Université Laval, Quebec City, QC, Canada
Centre de Recherche sur les Soins et les Services de Première Ligne de l'Université Laval (CERSSPL-UL), Quebec City, QC, Canada

Mariusz P. Furmanek
Human Motor Behavior Laboratory, Department of Human Motor Behavior, The J. Kukuczka Academy of Physical Education, Katowice, Poland

Mathieu Germain Robitaille, Fabio Carlos Lucas de Oliveira and Martin Simoneau
Département de Kinésiologie, Faculté de Médecine, Université Laval, Quebec City, QC, Canada

Mariève Houle
Department of Anatomy, Université du Québec à Trois-Rivières, Trois-Rivières, QC, Canada

Jean-Daniel Bonneau and Andrée-Anne Marchand
Department of Chiropractic, Université du Québec à Trois-Rivières, Trois-Rivières, QC, Canada

Martin Descarreaux
Department of Human Kinetics, Université du Québec à Trois-Rivières, Trois-Rivières, QC, Canada
Département des Sciences de L'activité Physique, Université du Québec à Trois-Rivières, Trois-Rivières, QC, Canada

Fausto G. Baldissera
Retired, Milan, Italy

Luigi Tesio
Department of Biomedical Sciences for Health, Università degli Studi di Milano, Milan, Italy
Department of Neuro-Rehabilitation Sciences, Istituto Auxologico Italiano-IRCCS, Milan, Italy

Sanghee Moon
Department of Physical Therapy, Ithaca College, Ithaca, NY, United States
Laboratory for Advanced Rehabilitation Research in Simulation, Department of Physical Therapy, Rehabilitation Science, and Athletic Training, University of Kansas Medical Center, Kansas City, KS, United States

Chun-Kai Huang, Maryam Sadeghi and Hannes Devos
Laboratory for Advanced Rehabilitation Research in Simulation, Department of Physical Therapy, Rehabilitation Science, and Athletic Training, University of Kansas Medical Center, Kansas City, KS, United States

Abiodun E. Akinwuntan
Laboratory for Advanced Rehabilitation Research in Simulation, Department of Physical Therapy, Rehabilitation Science, and Athletic Training, University of Kansas Medical Center, Kansas City, KS, United States
Office of the Dean, School of Health Professions, University of Kansas Medical Center, Kansas City, KS, United States

Laura Perucca and Stefano Scarano
Department of Neurorehabilitation Sciences, IRCCS Istituto Auxologico Italiano, Milan, Italy
Department of Biomedical Sciences for Health, University of Milan, Milan, Italy

Antonio Robecchi Majnardi
Department of Neurorehabilitation Sciences, IRCCS Istituto Auxologico Italiano, Milan, Italy

Silvia Frau
Department of Biomedical Sciences for Health, University of Milan, Milan, Italy

Index

www.ingramcontent.com/pod-product-compliance
Lightning Source LLC
LaVergne TN
LVHW081033210926
848485LV00004B/1015
* 9 7 8 1 6 3 9 2 7 9 3 1 9 *